Editor

JOHN MARQUIS CONVERSE, M.D.

Lawrence D. Bell Professor of Plastic Surgery,
New York University School of Medicine

Assistant Editor

JOSEPH G. McCARTHY, M.D.

Associate Professor of Surgery (Plastic Surgery),
New York University School of Medicine

Editor, section on The Hand

J. WILLIAM LITTLER, M.D.

Chief of Plastic and Reconstructive Surgery,
The Roosevelt Hospital, New York City

SECOND EDITION

RECONSTRUCTIVE PLASTIC SURGERY

Principles and Procedures
in Correction, Reconstruction
and Transplantation

VOLUME THREE
THE JAWS
THE LIPS AND CHEEKS
FACIAL BURNS
THE CERVICAL REGION
THE EARS
FACIAL PALSY
THE AGING FACE

W. B. SAUNDERS COMPANY
Philadelphia   London   Toronto   Mexico City   Rio de Janeiro   Sydney   Tokyo

W. B. Saunders Company: West Washington Square
Philadelphia, PA   19105

1 St. Anne's Road
Eastbourne, East Sussex BN21 3UN, England

1 Goldthorne Avenue
Toronto, Ontario M8Z 5T9, Canada

Apartado 26370 — Cedro 512
Mexico 4, D.F., Mexico

Rua Coronel Cabrita, 8
Sao Cristovao Caixa Postal 21176
Rio de Janeiro, Brazil

9 Waltham Street
Artarmon, N.S.W. 2064, Australia

Ichibancho, Central Bldg., 22-1 Ichibancho
Chiyoda-Ku, Tokyo 102, Japan

Complete Set   0-7216-2691-2
Volume 1   0-7216-2680-7
Volume 2   0-7216-2681-5
Volume 3   0-7216-2682-3
Volume 4   0-7216-2683-1
Volume 5   0-7216-2684-X
Volume 6   0-7216-2685-8
Volume 7   0-7216-2686-6

Reconstructive Plastic Surgery

Last digit is the print number: 9   8   7

CONTRIBUTORS

TO VOLUME THREE

HANS ANDERL, M.D.

Surgeon in Chief, University Hospital for Plastic and Reconstructive Surgery, Innsbruck, Austria.

RICHARD J. BELLUCCI, M.D.

Professor and Chairman, Department of Otolaryngology, New York Medical College. Surgeon Director and Chairman, Department of Otolaryngology, Manhattan Eye, Ear and Throat Hospital; Attending Otolaryngologist, Flower Fifth Avenue Hospital, Metropolitan Hospital, St. Luke's Hospital, and New York Hospital, New York.

BURT BRENT, M.D.

Assistant Clinical Professor and Research Advisor in Plastic Surgery, Stanford University School of Medicine. Surgeon, Stanford University Medical Center and Affiliated Hospitals, Stanford, California.

PETER J. COCCARO, D.D.S.

Research Professor of Clinical Surgery (Orthodontics), New York University Medical Center. Associate Professor of Clinical Orthodontics, New York University College of Dentistry. Director of Craniofacial Research, Center for Craniofacial Anomalies, Institute of Reconstructive Plastic Surgery, New York University Medical Center, New York.

JOHN MARQUIS CONVERSE, M.D.

Lawrence D. Bell Professor of Plastic Surgery, New York University School of Medicine; Director, Institute of Reconstructive Plastic Surgery, New York University Medical Center; Director of Plastic Surgery Service, Bellevue Hospital; Consultant in Plastic Surgery, Manhattan Eye, Ear and Throat Hospital and Veterans Administration Hospital, New York.

THOMAS D. CRONIN, M.D.

Clinical Professor of Plastic Surgery, Baylor University College of Medicine. Director, Plastic Surgery Residency Program, St. Joseph's Hospital; Chief, Plastic Surgery, St. Luke's Episcopal Hospital and Texas Children's Hospital; Chief Emeritus, Plastic Surgery, Hermann Hospital; Emeritus Staff, Methodist Hospital; Active Staff, Twelve Oaks and Park Plaza Hospitals, Houston, Texas.

NICHOLAS G. GEORGIADE, M.D., D.D.S.

Professor and Chairman, Division of Plastic, Maxillofacial and Oral Surgery, Duke University Medical Center. Attending Plastic Surgeon, Duke University Medical Center, Watts Hospital, and Lincoln Hospital; Consultant in Plastic, Maxillofacial and Oral Surgery, Veterans Administration Hospital, Durham, North Carolina.

CARY L. GUY, M.D.

Clinical Associate Professor of Surgery (Plastic Surgery), New York University School of Medicine. Associate Attending Surgeon, Institute of Reconstructive Plastic Surgery, New York University Medical Center; Assistant Visiting Surgeon, Bellevue Hospital; Attending Plastic Surgeon, Manhattan Eye, Ear and Throat Hospital, New York.

HENRY K. KAWAMOTO, JR., M.D., D.D.S.

Assistant Clinical Professor, Division of Plastic Surgery, UCLA Center for the Health Sciences, Los Angeles. Attending Plastic Surgeon, Saint John's Hospital and Health Center and Santa Monica Hospital Medical Center, Santa Monica, California.

DUANE L. LARSON, M.D.

Professor of Surgery and Director of the University Burn Unit, The University of Texas Medical Branch. Chief of Staff and Chief Surgeon, Shriners Burns Institute, Galveston, Texas.

JOSEPH G. McCARTHY, M.D.

Associate Professor of Surgery (Plastic Surgery), New York University School of Medicine. Associate Director, Institute of Reconstructive Plastic Surgery, New York University Medical Center. Attending Surgeon, University Hospital, Bellevue Hospital, Manhattan Eye, Ear and Throat Hospital, and Veterans Administration Hospital, New York.

DANIEL C. MORELLO, M.D.

Clinical Instructor in Surgery (Plastic Surgery), New York University School of Medicine. Associate Attending Surgeon, United Hospital, Port Chester; Assistant Attending Surgeon, Manhattan Eye, Ear and Throat Hospital, Northern Westchester Hospital, St. Agnes Hospital, and White Plains Hospital, New York.

RADFORD C. TANZER, M.D.

Clinical Professor of Plastic Surgery Emeritus, Dartmouth Medical School, Hanover, New Hampshire; Consultant in Plastic Surgery, Veterans Administration Hospital, White River Junction, Vermont.

NOEL THOMPSON, M.S., F.R.C.S.

Clinical Tutor and Specialist Examiner in Plastic Surgery, University of London. Consultant Plastic Surgeon, The Middlesex Hospital, London, and the Plastic Surgery Centre, Mount Vernon Hospital, Northwood, Middlesex, England.

DONALD WOOD-SMITH, M.B., F.R.C.S.E.

Associate Professor of Surgery (Plastic Surgery), New York University School of Medicine. Surgeon Director, Department of Plastic Surgery, Manhattan Eye, Ear and Throat Hospital; Attending Surgeon, Institute of Reconstructive Plastic Surgery, New York University Medical Center; Visiting Surgeon in Plastic Surgery, Bellevue Hospital; Attending Surgeon, Veterans Administration Hospital; Consultant, New York Eye and Ear Infirmary, New York.

CONTENTS

RECONSTRUCTIVE PLASTIC SURGERY

CHAPTER 30

DEFORMITIES OF THE JAWS

John Marquis Converse, M.D.,
Henry K. Kawamoto, Jr., M.D., D.D.S.,
Donald Wood-Smith, F.R.C.S.E.,
Peter J. Coccaro, D.D.S.,
and Joseph G. McCarthy, M.D.

The mandible and the maxilla constitute a major portion of the facial skeleton. Because of this and the intimate interrelationship of the facial bones, small alterations can produce a wide range of facial deformities. These deformities can be classified into three main groups.

Congenital Malformations. Congenital malformations of the jaws may be unilateral or bilateral. They are often associated with such conditions as mandibulofacial dysostosis (Treacher Collins syndrome), craniofacial microsomia, craniofacial dysostosis, and other types of anomalous development of the first and second branchial arches (see Chapters 54, 55 and 56).

Developmental Malformations. Developmental malformations can be caused by several factors. These include:

1. *Congenital anomalies of adjacent structures.* Jaw malformations associated with congenital facial paralysis, hemangioma, or torticollis are examples of this type.

2. *Trauma.* Faulty development due to injury in early life results in varying degrees of deformity. These injuries can assume diverse forms: a fall on the chin producing an unnoticed condylar fracture and injury to a growth center (see Chapter 26), a facial burn with tight, deficient, and contracted soft tissues compressing and deforming the underlying skeleton.

3. *Abnormal neuromuscular patterns.* Asymmetrical maxillary and mandibular growth following facial nerve paralysis sustained during the period of early mandibular development is an example of this type of malformation. Another example is an open-bite produced by faulty tongue habits.

4. *Infection.* Osteomyelitis or adjacent soft tissue infection, particularly if it occurs early in life, may result in severe deformity.

5. *Endocrine imbalance.* The classic example of this type of deformity is mandibular prognathism associated with acromegaly.

6. *Nutritional deficiencies.* These are rare in developed countries. Vitamin D deficiency represents an appropriate example.

Acquired Deformities. Loss of bone as the result of partial or total resection of the mandible or maxilla in the treatment of malignant tumors produces severe deformities when the bone loss is extensive. The deformities and their repair are also discussed in Chapters 60, 61, and 62.

Traumatic deformities of the mandible are the result of: (1) loss of mandibular bone, which is not replaced at or soon after the time of injury; (2) malunion of fractures of the mandible; or (3) temporomandibular joint derangement, with or without ankylosis.

These deformities may affect any portion of the jaw—the dentoalveolar process, the denser bone of the body, the ramus, or the mandibular condyle. Similarly, deformities of the maxilla can involve the central nasomaxillary complex, the dentoalveolar process, or the entire maxilla.

Malocclusion of the teeth is a frequent accompaniment of the deformity. Correction of the malocclusion often provides a guide for planning the reconstructive procedure.

Developmental Malformations of the Jaws

General Considerations. Most of the problems discussed in this chapter relate to the harmony and balance of facial proportions. It must be emphasized at the outset that facial beauty is an emotion experienced by the viewer rather than an intrinsic physical property possessed by a particular human countenance. Thus, despite the work of countless investigators from the time of Leonardo da Vinci to the present, no valid norm for beauty has been established (see Chapter 1). The individual's concept of pleasing facial proportions and symmetry merely reflects his personal, ethnic, cultural, and esthetic background and experiences and constitutes a subjective and personal opinion rather than a universal criterion.

The problems of facial malformation require that decisions be made concerning the restoration of harmony and balance; the successful attainment of these objectives is the surgeon's goal. The patient and clinician must agree on the basic source of distress before correction is attempted. Exceptionally, overemphasis on minor facial blemishes occurs because of emotional difficulties; conversely, a patient with a quite obvious malformation may prefer to accept the deformity rather than undergo rehabilitative procedures. In most instances, however, an agreement must be reached on the nature of the facial malformation before it is possible to plan the corrective procedure. In the consideration of jaw malformations, the term "malformation" may be interpreted variously: to the anatomist and physiologist, it represents the effects of morphologic and functional deviation; the geneticist and anthropologist are concerned with hereditary and evolutionary components; the orthodontist is concerned with malocclusion of the teeth and facial harmony; to the plastic surgeon, the esthetic balance and the appearance of the integumental contour are the principal interests. These views are complementary, and some appreciation of each aspect is of great assistance in the diagnosis and treatment of these malformations.

Component Concept of Jaw Malformations. Establishing a diagnosis and a plan of treatment is simplified by analyzing a jaw deformity in terms of its components: (1) facial hard and soft tissues, (2) dentoalveolar complex, and (3) skeletal relations of the maxilla and mandible to each other and to the cranium (cephalometry). Each part should be analyzed separately. This will help clarify and define the problem.

HARD AND SOFT TISSUES OF THE FACE. Anatomic landmarks are displaced or absent in malformations of the jaws. From a reconstructive standpoint, it is convenient to use simple morphologic descriptions, supplemented, when indicated, by pertinent information regarding neuromuscular dysfunction.

Anthropometric points of the face are used in categorizing facial malformations (Figs. 30–1 and 30–2). Commonly used landmarks are *trichion*, the midpoint at the hairline of the forehead; *nasion*, the most anterior point of the midline of the frontonasal suture; *subnasale*, the point beneath the nose where the columella merges with the upper lip in the midsagittal plane; and *menton*, the lowest median point of the mandible. *Gnathion* is a bony chin point defined by the bisection of the angle formed by the mandibular and facial planes. *Tragion* is the notch immediately above the tragus of the ear; *orbitale* is the lowest point on the infraorbital margin; the Frankfort horizontal passes through these points.

The width of the face is divided in half by a vertical mid-sagittal line passing through trichion, nasion, subnasale, and gnathion (Fig. 30–2). The height of the face is divided in approximately equal thirds by horizontal lines drawn through nasion and subnasale. The

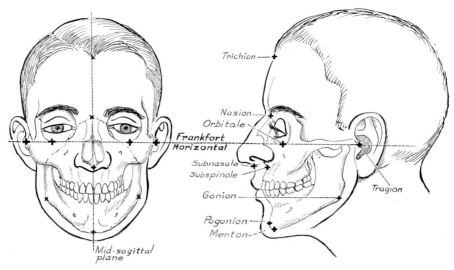

FIGURE 30–1. Anthropometric landmarks. These points of reference are essential in orienting the face.

lower third of the face, subnasale to gnathion, can be further subdivided into three equal parts. The lips should meet near the junction of the upper and middle thirds. These subdivisions can be used as a general guide in classifying and assessing the degree of existing facial deformity.

An acceptable facial profile is one in which the chin is situated between two vertical lines which cross the Frankfort horizontal at right angles: the anterior line tangential to the supraorbital ridge, and the posterior line drawn downward through orbitale (see Fig. 30–2, *A*). Gonzalez-Ulloa and Stevens (1968) placed the

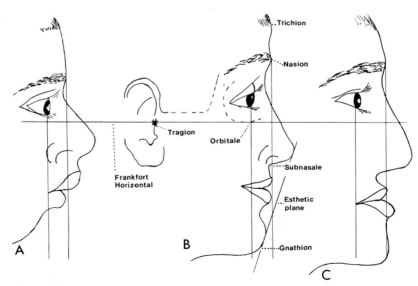

FIGURE 30–2. Determining the correct anteroposterior chin position. The anterior plane is tangential to the forehead and descends at a 90-degree angle with the Frankfort horizontal. The posterior plane also descends at right angles to the Frankfort horizontal from orbitale. *A*, In mandibular micrognathia, the chin and lower lip are posterior to the anterior plane. *B*, In the average profile, the chin is situated between the anterior and posterior planes. The lips are contained within the "esthetic plane," which is drawn tangentially from the tip of the nose to the chin. The upper lip is slightly more posterior to the plane than is the lower lip. *C*, In mandibular prognathism, the chin and lower lip protrude beyond the anterior plane.

anterior silhouette of the chin on a vertical line beginning at nasion and drawn at right angles to the Frankfort horizontal.

Lip posture and position are prominent features of the lower facial profile. In an acceptable profile, the lips are situated near the anterior line that is tangential to the supraorbital ridge. The upper lip is anterior to the lower. Ricketts (1957) correlated the lip, nose, and chin profile to a line drawn tangential to the nose and the chin, which he called the esthetic plane (see Fig. 30–2). The lips are contained within this line, with the upper lip slightly posterior to the lower lip when it is related to the line.

Lip posture is closely related to the position and forward inclination of the maxillary incisor teeth (Jackson, 1962). Changes in vertical intermaxillary distance will also influence lip posture. The anteroposterior skeletal jaw relationship can alter the lip profile; a change in lip posture following correction of a prognathic mandible is a good example.

Competent lip posture implies adequate lip seal: the lips are able to contact one another naturally without strain of the orofacial musculature when the mandible is in a position of physiologic rest. *Incompetent lip posture* occurs when the lips are unable to form a seal under similar unstrained conditions; this is a characteristic of certain malocclusions as well as of more serious facial deformities (Fig. 30–3).

Incompetent lip posture is functionally re-

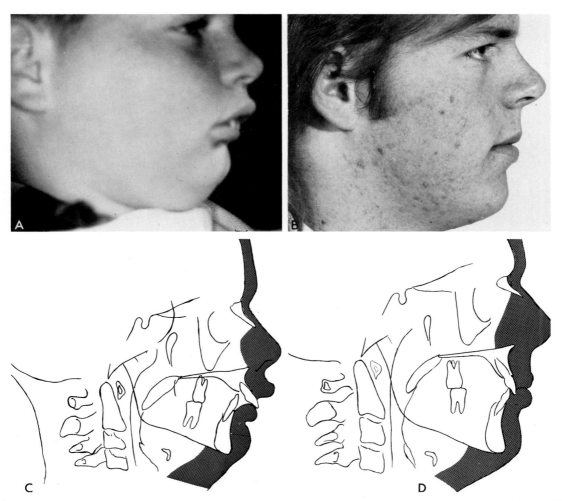

FIGURE 30–3. Malocclusion as a cause of incompetent lip posture. *A,* Photograph of child showing incompetent lip posture and malocclusion. *B,* Improved lip posture after orthodontic treatment. *C,* Tracing of cephalogram showing malocclusion (Class II, Division 1) prior to orthodontic treatment. Note the incompetent lip posture caused by maxillary dentoalveolar protrusion. *D,* Tracing showing improved lip posture following orthodontic therapy.

lated to the soft tissue contour of the chin. In an attempt to achieve lip seal, particularly in deglutition, the patient with incompetent lips contracts the mentalis muscle. Habitual contraction of the mentalis muscle eliminates the concavity of the labiomental fold and imparts a chinless appearance. The bony chin is often also affected.

The bony chin becomes more prominent throughout childhood and adolescence (Meredith, 1957), but a disturbance in the orofacial muscular balance may interfere with this pattern.

This basic discussion of lip incompetence illustrates the complex interplay between soft tissue form, skeletal support, and neuromuscular patterns.

THE DENTOALVEOLAR COMPLEX. Poor dentoalveolar relationship is a major cause of facial imbalance. The parts of the lower face most frequently affected by the position of the dentoalveolar structures are the upper and lower lips and the lower portion of the nose; these areas are bounded laterally by the nasolabial folds and below by the chin (Case, 1921).

The interdigitation of the cusps of the upper and lower teeth establishes what is known as the occlusal relationship, often referred to as the dental occlusion. Normally the mandibular dental arch is posterior to and smaller than the maxillary arch. The buccal or lateral cusps of the upper teeth project laterally from the buccal cusps of the lower teeth. The upper incisor teeth and canines (cuspids) overlap the corresponding lower teeth anteriorly. The mid-sagittal line passes between the central incisors. The mesiobuccal cusp of the maxillary first molar is aligned axially with the mesiobuccal groove of the mandibular first molar. When these relationships are disturbed, a malocclusion is produced.

Classification of malocclusion. Angle's (1899) classification of malocclusion is widely accepted in the United States. It is based on the mesiodistal (anteroposterior) relationship of the maxillary and mandibular first permanent molars (Fig. 30–4).

Class I (neutroclusion). The first molars are in adequate relationship. Irregularities of the anterior teeth may be present because discrepancy between tooth size and arch length causes a crowding and malocclusion of the anterior teeth.

Class II (distoclusion). The buccal groove of the lower first molar is distal (posterior) to the mesiobuccal cusp of the upper first molar.

> *Division 1.* In addition to the distoclusion of the posterior teeth, the upper arch is narrow and the incisors protrude.

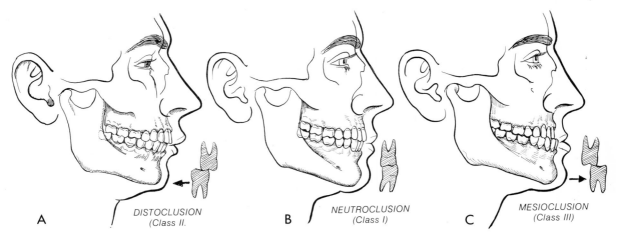

A   DISTOCLUSION (Class II.)   B   NEUTROCLUSION (Class I)   C   MESIOCLUSION (Class III)

FIGURE 30–4. Angle's classification of malocclusion. The classification is based on the mesiodistal (anteroposterior) relationships of the maxillary and mandibular first permanent molar teeth. The relationship between the position of the jaws and the facial profile is also illustrated.

A, Class II (distoclusion). The mandible is retrognathic, and the lower face appears to be recessed. The mandibular first molar occupies a more posterior (distal) position than normal. *B*, Class I (neutroclusion). The facial profile falls within the normal range. The maxillary and mandibular first molar teeth are in an ideal anteroposterior relation. The mesiobuccal cusp of the maxillary first molar is aligned correctly with the mesiobuccal groove of the mandibular first molar tooth. *C*, Class III (mesioclusion). Dental occlusion found in mandibular prognathism. The mesiobuccal groove of the mandibular first molar is mesial (anterior) to the mesiobuccal cusp of the maxillary first molar.

Division 2. The posterior teeth are in distoclusion. The upper incisors are inclined in a lingual direction and are crowded.

Class III (mesioclusion). The buccal groove of the lower first molar is mesial (anterior) to the mesiobuccal cusp of the upper first molar. The mandibular teeth are in an anterior relationship to the corresponding maxillary teeth.

The original Angle classification describes dental malocclusion between the mandibular and maxillary teeth. These anteroposterior *dentoalveolar* malocclusions are often reflected in the facial profile (Fig. 30–4). A patient with a Class I malocclusion generally has a normal facial profile; the patient with a Class II, division 1 malocclusion may have the typical "bird-face" profile; and the patient with a Class III malocclusion appears to have a protruding lower jaw. However, these correlations do not always exist, and not all types of malocclusion affect the facial profile. For this reason, the Angle classification is inadequate to appraise dentofacial balance; it is also misapplied to describe malocclusion caused by *skeletal* jaw deformities.

SKELETAL RELATIONS OF MAXILLA AND MANDIBLE (CEPHALOMETRY). The dentoalveolar structures are supported by the skeletal portion of the jaws. Changes in skeletal relationships have direct bearing on the dentoalveolar complex. Skeletal relationships are best studied with the aid of the cephalometric roentgenogram.

By means of cephalometric roentgenography, a simultaneous record of the dental, skeletal, and soft tissue components of the face is obtained, as well as a proper evaluation of the relationship of these elements. With this technique, the patient, the film, and the X-ray tube are positioned accurately in a fixed relationship within the cephalometric apparatus. Numerous efforts have been made to correlate certain dental and skeletal relationships seen on the cephalometric roentgenogram with the characteristics of a well-balanced face (Tweed, 1946; Downs, 1948; Steiner, 1953). Considerable variability is apparent even among individuals specifically selected for study because of satisfactory facial balance (Riedel, 1957; Burstone, 1958; Peck and Peck, 1970).

The use of cephalometric roentgenography was first proposed as an aid in the diagnosis and planning of surgical-orthodontic treatment of facial malformation in 1954 by Converse and Shapiro. At present it is widely used for

this purpose; in addition, it provides a valuable record for studying postoperative changes.

Anthropologists and orthodontists have established cephalometric landmarks which can be used to follow facial growth patterns and to study skeletal jaw relationships. The common landmarks (Figs. 30–5 and 30–6) include:

S (sella): the center of sella turcica.

N (nasion): the frontonasal suture.

ANS: anterior nasal spine.

Point A (subspinale): the most posterior point between the anterior nasal spine and the crest of the maxillary alveolar process.

Point B (supramentale): the most posterior point between pogonion and the crest of the mandibular alveolar process.

Po (pogonion): the most anterior point of the symphysis of the mandible.

Gn (gnathion): the point on the chin determined by bisecting the angle formed by the facial and mandibular planes.

G (gonion): the most posterior and inferior point at the angle of the mandible.

P (porion): the superior edge of the bony auditory meatus.

O (orbitale): the most inferior point on the infraorbital rim.

FH (Frankfort horizontal): a line drawn from porion to orbitale.

MP (mandibular plane): a line at the lower border of the mandible tangential to the most inferior point of the gonial angle and the profile image of the symphysis.

UI (upper incisor): a line drawn through the long axis of the upper cental incisor.

LI (lower incisor): a line drawn through the long axis of the lower central incisor.

The angles formed by the intersection of the lines drawn through various points are used to analyze the skeletal and dentoalveolar deformities.

The angles used to measure skeletal deformities relate the mandible and the maxilla to each other and to the cranial base (SN). These angles are illustrated in Figure 30–6. The angles used to measure dentoalveolar deformities relate the maxillary and mandibular teeth to each other and to their respective jaws. These angles are illustrated in Figure 30–6.

A summary of the cephalometric angles, what they represent, and their interpretation is shown in Table 30–1. Angular values used in the table apply to Caucasian patients. The range of angles will differ in the Oriental face and the Negro face (Cotton, Takano and Wong, 1951).

The component by component analysis of jaw malformations helps to minimize errors and provides maximum insight and understanding of the problem. Analysis of each com-

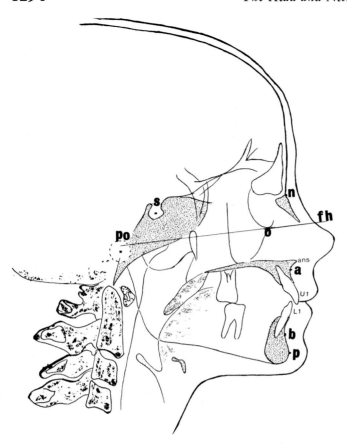

FIGURE 30–5. Cephalometric landmarks. Basic points used in cephalometric analysis.

ponent cannot stand alone. The skill with which the clinician interprets and integrates the individual parts will go a long way in determining the success of the treatment.

It must be emphasized that measurements are useful in evaluating the deformity; the final planning of the corrective surgery requires careful study of hard and soft tissue cephalometric tracings. The projected changes in facial contour are made first by modifying the tracings.

Classification of Jaw Malformations. Jaw malformations can be classified in various ways. The Angle classification is commonly used to describe both the dentoalveolar and skeletal malocclusions (Salzmann, 1966). Sassouni (1969) devised a classification to differentiate between skeletal and dentoalveolar malocclusions and to determine the various effects they have on facial soft tissue contours.

The nomenclature and classification employed in this chapter are shown in Table 30–2.

When mandibular development is impaired, as in cases of injury to the condylar area in childhood, hypoplasia of the mandible results in a typical birdlike appearance of the face, and the condition is referred to as *mandibular micrognathia* (small jaw). *Mandibular retrognathism* (backward jaw) describes a condition in which the jaw, normal in size, is retruded. *Microgenia* designates a small chin; the chin may be abnormal in an otherwise well-developed jaw. Displacement of the chin to one side, due either to unilateral underdevelopment or infrequently to overdevelopment of the jaw owing to condylar hyperplasia, results in a deviation from the mid-sagittal plane and a posterior crossbite; such a condition is designated by the term *laterognathism* (deviated jaw).

Prognathism (forward jaw), which may af-

FIGURE 30–6. Cephalometric lines and angles. Basic cephalometric lines and angles used to analyze dentoalveolar and skeletal relationships of the jaws to the anterior cranial base (SN). The esthetic plane is drawn from the tip of the nose to the chin, as reviewed on profile.

U1-SN (upper central incisor–sella nasion): represents the inclination of the maxillary central incisors; indicates the degree of protrusion or retrusion of the maxillary dentoalveolar arch.

L1-MP (lower central incisor–mandibular plane): measures the inclination of the mandibular central incisors; indicates the degree of mandibular dentoalveolar arch protrusion or retrusion.

U1-L1 (upper central incisor–lower central incisor): relates axial inclination of the central incisor teeth of both jaws; shows tendencies of bimaxillary protrusion.

SNA (sella–nasion–point A): shows the anteroposterior relation of the maxilla to the cranial base; used to determine the degree of maxillary prognathism or retrognathism.

SNB (sella–nasion–point B): represents the anteroposterior relation of the mandible to the cranial base; used to determine the degree of mandibular prognathism or retrognathism.

ANB (point A–nasion–point B): relates the mandible to the maxilla in an anteroposterior direction; used to determine discrepancy between the two jaws.

MP-SN (mandibular plane–sella nasion): denotes the total facial height; indicates tendency toward open and closed bite.

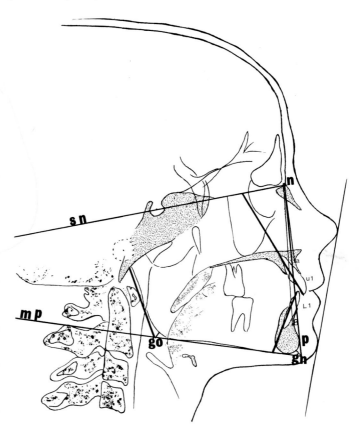

fect the mandible or the maxilla, is characterized by an anterior displacement of the jaw, the teeth of the affected jaw being anterior to the teeth of the opposing jaw. This can be due to either an enlargement of the jaw or an alteration in its relationships. The term "progenie" (forward chin) is used in the German literature for mandibular prognathism.

When the maxilla is underdeveloped, the term *maxillary hypoplasia* is employed; *maxillary micrognathia* describes a small jaw retarded in its growth. The term *maxillary retrognathism* suggests that the maxilla is normal in size and retroposed. An example would be the posterior position of the maxilla in malunited fractures. This condition may give an illusion of mandibular prognathism; however, the deformity is often a *pseudomandibular prognathism,* the mandible being within the norm in size and position and the maxilla being retruded.

When both the maxillary and mandibular anterior teeth protrude, the condition is called *bimaxillary protrusion.* This is normally seen in the Oriental and the Negro. *Apertognathism* (open bite) is present when the vertical intermaxillary distance is increased to a point where the teeth fail to occlude. When this occurs between the incisor teeth, it is termed an anterior open bite. When the premolars and molars fail to contact, the term posterior open bite is used. Normally the mandibular teeth are lingual to their corresponding teeth in the maxillary arch. When the reverse is present, a *crossbite* is produced (Fig. 30–7). Crossbites occur in the anterior as well as the posterior arches. Overbite refers to the vertical overlap of the teeth when the jaws are in normal full closure; the horizontal overlap is termed *overjet* (Fig. 30–8).

Diagnosis

FACIAL DIAGNOSIS. In addition to the clinical examination, full-face and profile photographs are taken, the face positioned in accord with the Frankfort horizontal and the

TABLE 30–1. *Cephalometric Analysis Summary*

COMPONENT	MEASURE-MENT	RELATIONSHIP	NORMAL VALUES		INTERPRETATION	
			Range (Degrees)	Mean (Degrees)	Increase	Decrease
Skeletal	SNA	Maxilla to cranial base	79–85	82	Maxillary prognathism	Maxillary retrognathism (micrognathism)
	SNB	Mandible to cranial base	76–84	80	Mandibular prognathism	Mandibular retrognathism (micrognathism)
	ANB	Maxilla to mandible	0–4	2	Varies according to facial divergence	
	SN-MP	Vertical facial height	–	–	Tendency toward Class II malocclusion	Tendency toward Class III malocclusion
Dentoalveolar	UI-SN	Upper central incisor to cranial base	100–110	104	Maxillary protrusion	Maxillary retrusion
	LI-MP	Lower central incisor to mandibular plane	87–99	93	Mandibular protrusion	Mandibular retrusion
	UI-LI	Upper central to lower central incisor	120–140	130	Bimaxillary retrusion	Bimaxillary protrusion

TABLE 30–2. *Classification of Jaw Malformations*

Skeletal
    Prognathism... maxillary
                                                           mandibular

    Retrognathism... maxillary
                                                           mandibular

    Micrognathism (micrognathia) (hypoplasia) .... maxillary
                                                            mandibular

    Laterognathism .... unilateral mandibular hyperplasia
                                                            unilateral mandibular hypoplasia

    Microgenia .... small or retruded chin

    Macrogenia .... large or protruding chin

    Nasomaxillary hypoplasia or retrusion .... with mandibular prognathism
                                                                (pseudomandibular prognathism)
                                                            without mandibular prognathism

    Midface hypoplasia or retrusion .... involves the entire midface skeleton

Dentoalveolar
    Protrusion .... anterior maxillary
                                                            anterior mandibular
                                                            bimaxillary

    Retrusion .... anterior maxillary
                                                           anterior mandibular
                                                            bimaxillary

Skeletal or dentoalveolar or both
    Apertognathism (open bite) .... anterior
                                                           posterior
                                                            anterior and posterior

    Crossbite .... anterior
                                                           posterior

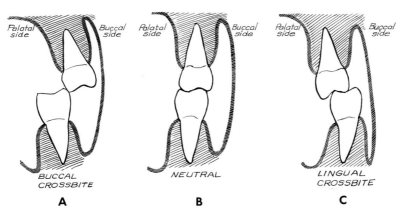

FIGURE 30–7. Buccolingual relationships of the teeth. *A,* Buccal version. Malocclusion is due to the tilting of the maxillary tooth toward the cheek. *B,* Neutral (centric) occlusion. Ideal relationship in which the buccal cusp of the upper tooth overlaps that of the lower tooth. *C,* Crossbite malocclusion caused by the lingual displacement of the upper teeth in relation to the lower teeth. Note that the buccal cusp of the upper tooth no longer overlaps that of the lower tooth.

mid-sagittal planes (see Fig. 30–1). Accurately oriented photographs are of great help in analyzing the facial soft tissue deformity (see Chapter 1). Horizontal lines, passing through trichion, nasion, and subnasale, on the full-face photograph divide the face into approximately three equal parts. The mid-sagittal plane of the face is useful in determining facial asymmetry and in defining deviation from the midline.

The study of the profile is helpful in establishing relationships between the lower and middle portions of the face. The relative position of the nose, lips, and chin can be judged by using the vertical lines described earlier in this chapter.

ORAL AND DENTOALVEOLAR DIAGNOSIS. Clinical and roentgenographic (intraoral and panoramic) examinations are necessary to evaluate the condition of the teeth and their supporting structures. Intraoral photographs are also useful. Dental caries and other intraoral disease require preoperative treatment. Unsalvageable teeth should be extracted. Since the teeth are utilized for postoperative fixation appliances and intermaxillary fixation, it is imperative that the teeth and supporting structures be in optimal condition.

Clinical examination and study of dental casts (generally referred to as "models" by the dentist) aid in determining the type of dentoalveolar malocclusion and in planning the corrective treatment. The dental casts serve as a record of the original condition and also as "working" models; two sets of dental casts are therefore made for each case. Study models

made in plaster are physically easier to section; those made of dental stone are harder and more durable.

When the surgical correction of malocclusion is being planned, the working casts are articulated and then cut to simulate the separation of the bone following the osteotomies (Fig. 30–9). The extent of the displacement of the fragments is evaluated preoperatively in this manner, thus facilitating the plan of osteotomy and the design of the appliance for fixation.

CEPHALOMETRIC AND SKELETAL DIAGNOSIS. The skeletal aspect of the malformation is best studied by cephalometric analysis. The development of standardized cephalometric roentgenograms has emphasized the importance of relating the teeth and their supporting structures to the face and skull. These techniques offer a dynamic approach to the study of facial growth.

Cephalometric tracings made on transparent acetate paper aid in planning facial profile changes. They are used to predict the overall changes in facial contour brought about by a corrective rhinoplasty or a change in chin shape or position (Fig. 30–10). Cut-outs of the outline of the deformed jaw are made. Repositioning these patterns aids in the choice of the type of osteotomy and provides an estimate of the amount of bone which must be advanced, recessed, or grafted (see Fig. 30–63).

In addition, cephalometric records are valuable in assessing the postoperative changes and in obtaining longitudinal studies. Relapse can be accurately measured. Changes in the relationship between the underlying bone and the soft tissue profile can also be followed serially.

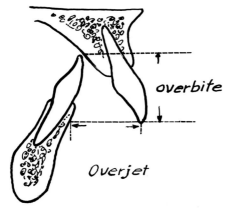

FIGURE 30–8. Relationship of the incisal edges. Overbite is the vertical overlap of the biting edges. Overjet refers to the labiolingual relationship of the incisal edges.

Preoperative Planning. The establishment of stable occlusal relationships between the teeth of the maxilla and the mandible is essential. The dental occlusion serves as a guide in the surgical correction of jaw deformities. Frequently, the establishment of adequate occlusal relationships also corrects the facial deformity. In many cases, however, a satisfactory facial contour demands a more than acceptable dentoalveolar position, because the deformity affects other portions of the jaws and additional corrective procedures are required. Other features of the face, principally the nose, may also require modification to improve the patient's facial profile.

Study of cephalometric roentgenograms showing both soft and hard tissue contour (see

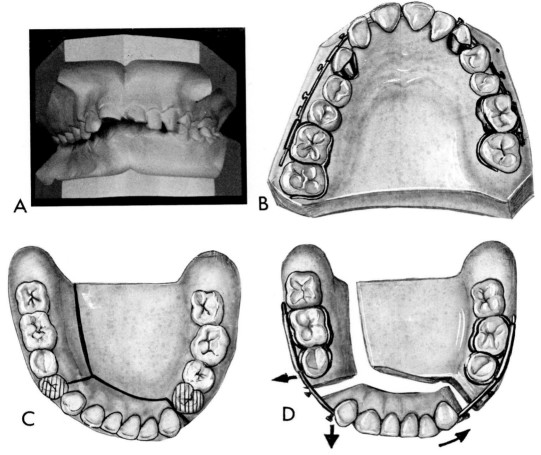

FIGURE 30–9. Planning of the osteotomies using dental casts. *A*, The plaster study casts show the malocclusion caused by a deformity of the mandible. *B*, Cast of the upper teeth showing the design of the appliance for intermaxillary fixation. *C*, Cast of lower dentition showing the lines of the proposed osteotomy to correct the deformity. The shaded teeth are to be extracted because of their poor condition. If the teeth are in good health, an interdental osteotomy is performed, preserving the adjacent teeth. *D*, Sectioned casts showing the extent of the planned displacement and rotation and advancement of the mandibular fragments. Fixation appliance is also illustrated. (From Kazanjian and Converse.)

Fig. 30–10) and of photographs taken with the patient's face placed in accordance with the Frankfort horizontal and the mid-sagittal plane provides valuable information. The cephalometric facial profile tracing is modified; contour changes are determined; and measurements and the necessary advancement or recession are planned. For example, let us consider a patient with an elongated lower third of the face resulting from an anterior open bite. Cephalometric analysis may show that, in addition to the closure of the open bite, a diminution in the vertical dimension of the symphysis and an increase in the projection of the chin are required.

Reconstructive surgery of jaw malformations is now highly developed and has been proved safe. Analysis of the facial soft tissue contour, the dentoalveolar complex, and the skeletal base provides a clear picture of the malformation. Once defined, the skeletal deformity can be corrected. In the past, most patients who appeared to have mandibular prognathism underwent a recession of the lower jaw, since this type of surgery is relatively simple. The actual deformity may have been maxillary hypoplasia, giving an illusion of mandibular prognathism (pseudoprognathism). This type of deformity is commonly seen in patients with cleft lip and palate. Presently, the preferred treatment is advancement of the maxilla to correct the deformity.

Each case is planned to satisfy the demands of the various individual problems. Because

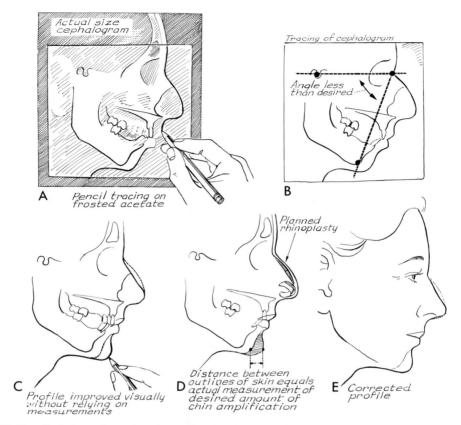

FIGURE 30–10. Cephalometric tracings for profile planning. *A,* Tracing of soft tissue and bone contour is made on transparent acetate. *B,* Sella turcica–nason–pogonion (SNPo) angle should be approximately 82 degrees. Angular measurements are of assistance but are not indispensable, as illustrated in *C* and *D. C,* Establishing the modified profile line. *D,* Shaded areas indicate the amount of nasal reduction and chin augmentation that is desired. *E,* Tracing of profile after rhinoplasty and chin augmentation.

treatment often involves surgical separation of the dentoalveolar and skeletal portions of the jaws, the planning must include a means of fixation of the repositioned parts. The action of the muscles of the jaws upon each fragment (see Chapter 24, Figs. 24–81 and 24–82) must also be considered.

FIXATION APPLIANCES. Fixation appliances are essential to achieve immobilization of separated fragments in their proper relationships following surgery. Such appliances should be kept simple and should minimize the problems of maintaining oral hygiene during the period of fixation. A degree of flexibility should be designed into the appliance. Adjustment may be required on the operating table because the amount of excised bone or the lines of osteotomy are often at slight variance with the preoperative plan; even the most careful preoperative planning is not always infallibly precise.

Orthodontic appliances appear to be most satisfactory. They are sufficiently flexible to permit adjustment at the time of operation or even during the immediate postoperative period. The appliances are placed preoperatively over the maxillary and mandibular teeth. Intermaxillary fixation in the planned occlusal relationship is maintained by either wires or orthodontic elastic bands. After completion of the operative procedure, a continuous thin coating of quick-curing acrylic covers the appliance, protects the mucosa of the lips, and provides additional stabilization. If minor adjustments are required postoperatively, it is preferable to dispense with the acrylic coating.

Arch bars similar to those used in treating jaw fractures are used if orthodontic support is not available (Fig. 30–11). The arch bars are preferably applied preoperatively to reduce operating time.

The disadvantage of cast dental cap splints

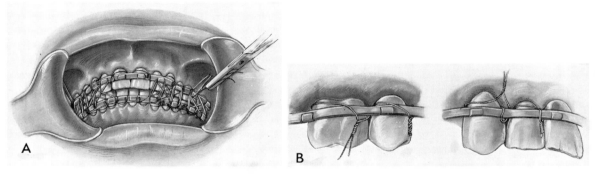

FIGURE 30–11. Application of arch bars. *A,* Prefabricated malleable arch bars are contoured to adapt to the curvature of the teeth, and fixation to the teeth is established by wires passed around the necks of the individual teeth. The wire is twisted to secure the arch bar to the teeth. Elastic bands can be used to provide intermaxillary traction to bring the teeth into occlusion. *B,* Note the technique used on the anterior teeth to avoid downward slippage of the arch bar.

and other mechanical appliances rigidly conceived and constructed on the anatomical articulators is that complete accuracy cannot always be relied upon. The appliance must often be adjusted in the operating room, as surgery cannot always reproduce the exact position which was preplanned on the articulator. Minor adjustments of the appliance must be possible.

Acrylic splints of various design are also used. In edentulous patients and in patients in whom the teeth are not serviceable, prosthodontic appliances ensure fixation of the separated fragments of the jaws. Acrylic splints, often of the segmental type, are joined after positioning of the fragments by the addition of quick-curing acrylic in the operating room (Fig. 30–12). The appliances are usually maintained by internal craniofacial suspension wiring or by circumferential wiring in edentulous patients; they can also be anchored with wires to the remaining teeth in the partially edentulous patient. Dentures (Fig. 30–13), bite-blocks with bite-guides (Fig. 30–14), and flanges are also necessary accessories in some patients. The type of splint illustrated in Figure 30–15 is of particular value in a partially edentulous mandible.

FIGURE 30–12. When teeth are present but are not serviceable because of their poor condition, this type of appliance can be employed. *A, B,* Excessive protrusion of the maxillary dentoalveolar process (Class II). Acrylic splint is made in two parts (*C* and *D*). *C,* After the maxillary set-back has been accomplished and the bone is removed to allow recession of the anterior maxillary segment. *D,* The anterior and posterior portions of the acrylic splint are joined in the operating room by quick-curing acrylic. The acrylic splint is anchored by transalveolar wire fixation to the pyriform aperture. This type of appliance requires the services of an expert maxillofacial prosthodontist (appliance made by Augustus J. Valauri, D.D.S.).

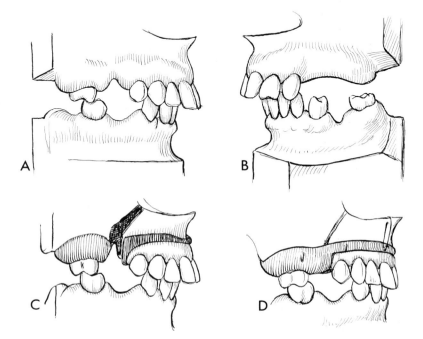

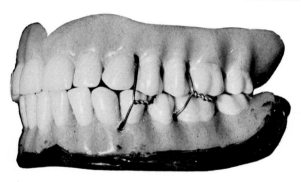

FIGURE 30–13. Intermaxillary fixation using dentures. If necessary the denture is relined for better adaptation to the alveolar arch. The upper denture is fixed by internal craniofacial suspension wires. The lower denture is held in place by circumferential wiring around the mandible.

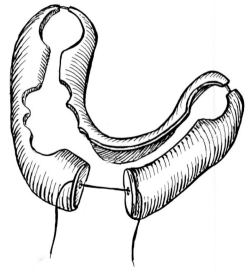

FIGURE 30–15. Acrylic splint to show how the splint is expanded to permit its placement over the dentoalveolar arch. The splint is tightened in position with an anterior stainless steel wire. Note the wire in the posterior end of the splint which permits the splint to open.

Orthodontics and Surgery. *The orthodontist is an indispensable member of the team.* He provides valuable aid during all phases of treatment. The best results are attained when close cooperation exists between the orthodontist and the surgeon.

Two different types of occlusal disharmony relate directly to facial appearance (Converse and Horowitz, 1969). The first type includes patients with maxillary, mandibular, or bimaxillary dentoalveolar protrusion. In this group of patients, the orthodontist is usually able to correct the malocclusion, and following dentoalveolar realignment, the soft tissue contour of the face is usually also improved. When favorable growth and development of the face occurs concurrently, the improvement in facial balance and harmony is dramatic and pleasing.

The second type, in contrast, includes dentoalveolar disharmony that is the result (rather than the cause) of facial malformation. Most skeletal deformities involving the lower third of the face are reflected to some extent in the dentition. This type of malocclusion, arising either from congenital facial anomalies or from trauma in early life, is characterized by deviant growth patterns. The resultant malocclusion is generally too severe to be corrected solely by traditional orthodontic procedures. Treatment requires the joint efforts of the reconstructive surgeon, the orthodontist, and, on occasion, other dental specialists.

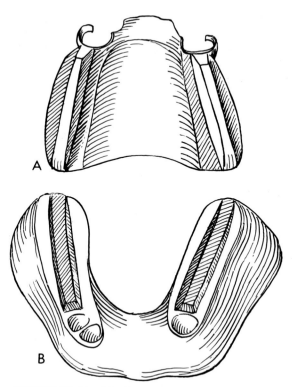

FIGURE 30–14. Maxillary and mandibular bite-blocks for edentulous and partially edentulous patients. Cranial fixation is established by internal suspension wiring.

When a skeletal facial malformation is the basic underlying problem, concurrent occlusal disharmony may develop (1) in anteroposterior jaw relationships (for example, mandibular prognathism); (2) in vertical balance (severe skeletal open bite); and (3) in the horizontal plane (left/right symmetry). If the congenital malformation is complex, as is often the case, the dentition frequently shows complex deviations from the normal relationships.

PREOPERATIVE AND POSTOPERATIVE ORTHODONTIC THERAPY. The timing of the orthodontic therapy and the surgical procedures varies according to the needs of the patient and the philosophy of the team. The necessary realignment of the dentition, the expansion of the dentoalveolar arch, and the achievement of optimal arch form should usually be obtained by the orthodontist prior to surgery. Thus maxillary-mandibular disparity is minimized, and the surgical results are also improved by the favorable interdigitation of the cusps of the teeth. In favorable cases the orthodontist and the surgeon can cooperate in achieving "instant" restoration of occlusion by dentoalveolar osteotomy (see p. 1304).

In many cases, the cooperation of the orthodontist in the operating room is desirable. Postoperative orthodontic therapy and surveillance are also necessary for minor occlusal adjustments, maintenance of the new relationships, and cephalometric follow-up.

Prosthodontics and Surgery. Appliances for fixation are required in edentulous patients and in patients whose dentition cannot withstand the forces exerted against them by other types of appliances. Occlusal bite planes may be required to maintain vertical space, to provide for overcorrection, or to compensate for gross occlusal discrepancies that cannot be corrected preoperatively. A prosthesis is always necessary in restoring a sulcus or a retentive alveolar ridge and in providing a serviceable denture for the reconstructed jaw. The prosthodontist is an essential member of the team (see Figs. 30–12 to 30–15).

Types of Osteotomies for Surgical-Orthodontic Correction in Jaw Deformities. In the surgical-orthodontic (surgical-orthognathic) correction of jaw malformations, osteotomies are performed in three different ways.

1. SKELETAL OSTEOTOMY. The osteotomy is performed through the entire thickness of the body of the bone (Fig. 30–16). It can be either a simple transection with resection of a segment or a transection with addition of bone

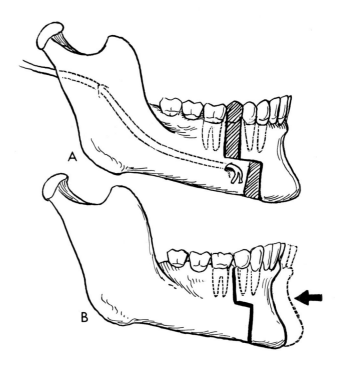

FIGURE 30–16. Skeletal osteotomy through the body of the mandible. *A*, The shaded areas represent the amount of bone to be resected to allow shortening of the mandibular body. The step osteotomy is placed above and anterior to the mental foramen to avoid injury to the inferior alveolar neurovascular bundle and mental nerve. (From Converse, J. M., and Horowitz, S. L.: The surgical-orthodontic approach to the treatment of dentofacial deformities. Am. J. Orthod., 55:214, 1969.)

by grafting. The segments are repositioned
and held securely by fixation in an improved
dentoalveolar and skeletal relationship.
Osteotomies through the ramus are also
employed to correct the gross malocclusions of
prognathism and micrognathia (see p. 1319).

2. DENTOALVEOLAR OSTEOTOMY. In contrast, the osteotomy can be confined to the
tooth-bearing portion of the jaw. The bone is
sectioned at the base of the dentoalveolar segment, leaving sufficient bone to protect the
apices and vascular supply of the teeth. The
dentoalveolar block containing several teeth
and their supporting structures is then moved

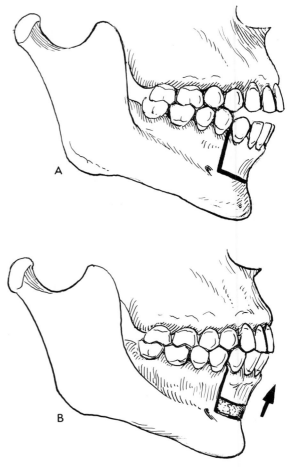

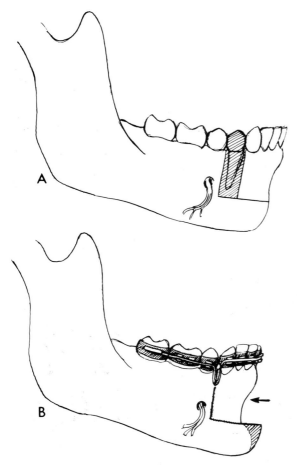

FIGURE 30–18. Dentoalveolar osteotomy for the correction of anterior open bite. *A,* Anterior dentoalveolar
segment outlined. *B,* The segment is mobilized vertically,
the open bite is closed, and bone grafts are placed in the
resulting bony defect. This technique is employed when
the lower third of the face has an acceptable contour. A
similar procedure can be used in the upper dentoalveolar
process.

FIGURE 30–17. Dentoalveolar osteotomy. *A,* When
the dentoalveolar segment is to be recessed, it may be
necessary to remove a tooth as well as the alveolar bone.
The line of the osteotomy extends vertically through the
alveolus and horizontally below the apices of the teeth.
B, The anterior dentoalveolar segment is repositioned and
immobilized by a monomaxillary fixation appliance. The
chin contour is improved by resecting the area represented
by the shading. (From Converse, J. M., and Horowitz,
S. L.: The surgical-orthodontic approach to the treatment
of dentofacial deformities. Am. J. Orthod., 55:214, 1969.)

to the planned new position (Fig. 30–17).
Movement is directed vertically, anteriorly
or posteriorly, or laterally. A combination of
directions can be used to suit the needs dictated by the deformity (Fig. 30–18). In these
procedures, blood supply is maintained by
the mucoperiosteal attachments.

3. CORTICAL OSTEOTOMY. The cortical osteotomy extends only through the cortical
bone of the alveolar process. The osteotomy
weakens the resistance of the bone to orthodontic forces. The procedure permits rapid displacement of the dentoalveolar segment, which
cannot be achieved by usual orthodontic therapy. It is particularly of value in the maxillary

arch and has its major application in the correction of the hypoplastic maxilla of the cleft palate patient (Fig. 30–19). The technique includes placement of an orthodontic appliance or a palatal acrylic split-plate expanded by a jackscrew that incorporates strong expansion forces following the surgical weakening of the alveolar bone support by the cortical osteotomy (Fig. 30–20). This procedure produces rapid expansion by lateral slippage of the entire alveolar bone support, without tipping of the teeth (see Fig. 30–19, *E, F*).

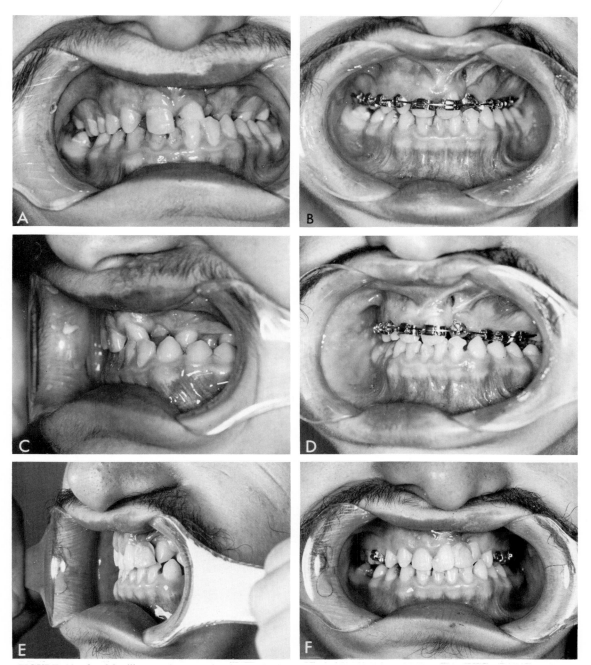

FIGURE 30–19. Maxillary arch expansion by cortical osteotomy. *A,* Malocclusion with crossbite prior to orthodontic therapy. *B,* After completion of orthodontic therapy. *C,* Oblique view prior to orthodontic therapy. *D,* Oblique view after orthodontic therapy. Note the inadequate result. Occlusal relationships have not been reestablished between the left maxillary and mandibular teeth because of the lingual displacement of the left maxillary arch. *E, F,* After cortical osteotomy and expansion by the appliance shown in Figure 30–20.

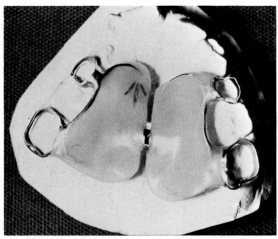

FIGURE 30–20. Palatal split-plate appliance expanded by a jackscrew is used to expand the alveolar arch which was weakened by a cortical osteotomy.

TREATMENT OF MANDIBULAR MALFORMATIONS

Surgical Approach

Various types of osteotomies combined with the displacement of bone, the resection of bone, or the addition of bone by grafting are performed either upon the body of the mandible or upon the ramus; in some cases, both the body and the ramus will require osteotomies.

Every mandibular operation requires adequate exposure; for this purpose various types of incisions and approaches are available. Dissection is facilitated and blood loss minimized if the area is infiltrated with a local anesthetic solution with epinephrine before the incision is made.

Extraoral and Intraoral Approaches to the Body of the Mandible

EXTRAORAL APPROACH. A submandibular incision placed in a strategic position for exposure of a portion of the mandible has been used and is still applied in some present-day techniques. Extraoral incisions have been largely supplanted by intraoral incisions. The body of the mandible is approached through a cutaneous incision, and the dissection is con-

tinued down to the bone. Precautions must be taken to avoid injury to the marginal mandibular branch of the facial nerve. The landmarks described by Dingman and Grabb (1962) should be observed.

The mental symphysis can be exposed through an incision in the submental fold or immediately below the chin along the posterior edge of the inferior border of the symphysis. The latter incision usually leaves a less conspicuous scar than the incision in the submental fold.

Cutaneous incisions should be avoided in patients who tend to form hypertrophic scars or keloids.

The extraoral approach was routine in the preantibiotic era. If a bone grafting procedure was in process to restore the continuity of the mandible and the oral mucosa was inadvertently torn and the oral cavity penetrated, the operation was interrupted and the bone grafting was postponed until the area of communication was healed. Contamination by saliva and the bacterial flora of the oral cavity was considered, probably justifiably so, a contraindication to completion of the operation. Clinical observation of the consolidation of loose jaw fragments exposed to the oral cavity, however, encouraged the development of the intraoral approach.

INTRAORAL APPROACH. The intraoral approach provides a wide exposure of the mandible without the disadvantage of an external scar. It affords an unrivaled exposure of the body of the mandible, which can only be achieved in the extraoral approach by an extensive submandibular incision. The risk of facial nerve damage is avoided.

Converse (1950) was the first to use the intraoral approach to transplant contour-restoring bone grafts. Success depends upon satisfactory soft tissue coverage of the osteotomy and bone graft site. Necrosis of bone, infection, sequestration, and nonconsolidation of the fragments are complications which occur when the soft tissue is poor in quality or lacking in quantity. Healing is compromised by a deficient blood supply and the absence of a protective seal. When the body of the mandible is elongated, the soft tissue is placed under tension and may not be adequate to provide coverage. It is important, therefore, to employ a technique of exposure that will provide as much intraoral tissue as possible for the coverage of the site of osteotomy.

The intraoral approach has been employed

not only for contour bone grafting of the skeletal framework of the face but also for osteotomies performed on both the ramus and the body of the mandible (Converse and Shapiro, 1952; Converse, 1954; Kazanjian and Converse, 1959, 1974b). Many jaw malformations can be corrected by the intraoral approach; it permits osteotomy for bending or elongation of the bone, resection of the bone to shorten or modify the shape of the jaw, or bone grafting for contour restoration.

The labiobuccal vestibular incision. This incision is made on the buccal aspect of the

vestibule, at least 1 cm above the frenulum (Fig. 30–21). The frenulum should not be sectioned; it is difficult to restore, and it heals poorly. The length of the incision depends upon the extent of the procedure. The mucosa is raised from the musculature of the cheek or lip, and sharp dissection is continued until the mandible is reached. At this point the periosteum is incised, and exposure is obtained by mucoperiosteal elevation.

When the symphysis area is to be exposed, the incision extends through the mucosa above the level of the frenulum. The mucosa is dissected from the orbicularis oris muscle. The periosteum is then incised, and the symphysis is exposed by subperiosteal elevation. Care must be taken to avoid injuring the mental nerve at its exit from the mental foramen.

The gingival incision. An incision made at the level of the mucogingival junction (Fig. 30–22) provides rapid and excellent exposure of the mandible. Tension produced by lengthening procedures, however, results in tearing of the gingival tissues and loss of soft tissue cover over the healing bone at the site of the osteotomy. Reinforcement of the gingival suture line can be obtained by placing the sutures through the gingiva between the teeth and looping them around the teeth.

The labiobuccal vestibular incision is preferred over the gingival incision when the jaw is to be lengthened, because ample coverage of

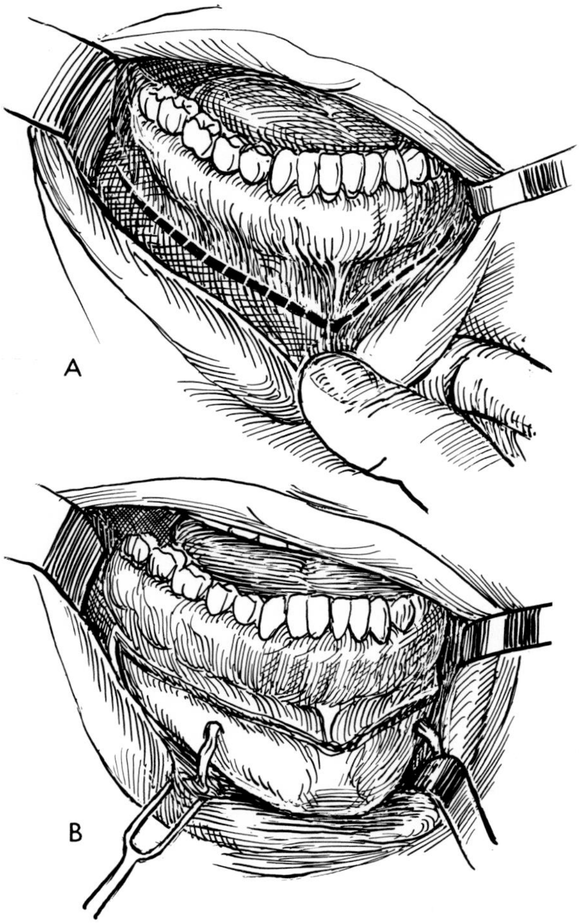

FIGURE 30–21. Labiobuccal vestibular incision and the "degloving" technique. *A,* The buccal vestibular incision is made on the buccal aspect of the vestibule above the origin of the frenulum. *B,* Degloving of the entire anteroinferior portion of the mandible can be achieved by subperiosteal dissection. (From Converse, J. M.: *In* Kazanjian, V. H., and Converse, J. M.: The Surgical Treatment of Facial Injuries. Copyright 1959. The Williams & Wilkins Company, Baltimore.)

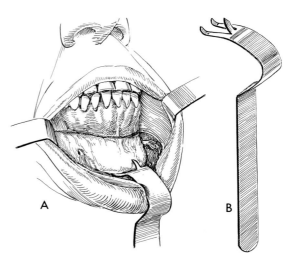

FIGURE 30–22. Gingival incision for the degloving technique. *A,* An incision is made through the gingiva above the level of the mental foramina, and the tissues are retracted. *B,* Obwegeser's three-pronged retractor for exposure of the mental symphysis.

the bone can be obtained from the adjacent tissue; a flap of mucous membrane which extends laterally onto the lip or cheek provides the needed extra tissue.

The degloving procedure. The degloving procedure described by Converse (1959, 1964b) provides excellent exposure of the anterior portion of the mandible. Either the labiobuccal vestibular incision or the gingival incision is extended from the premolar region across the midline to the contralateral premolar area; the major portion of the body and symphysis can be exposed (see Figs. 30–21 and 30–22). The labiobuccal incision is preferred if an advancement procedure is planned, as excessive soft tissue tension and disruption of the wound are avoided.

The risk of tearing the mental nerve during the operative procedure is a major one. To diminish this risk, when wide exposure is being obtained, the three branches of the mental nerve are carefully dissected free from the soft tissues (Fig. 30–23). Thus freed, the mental nerve and its branches are retracted with less danger of tearing or sectioning as the subperiosteal exposure is continued posterior to the mental foramen.

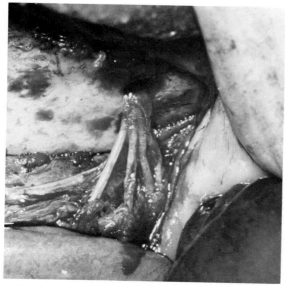

FIGURE 30–23. Dissection of the left mental nerve. To avoid avulsion of the mental nerve when the degloving technique is used, the three branches of the nerve are dissected free of the soft tissues. This precaution will permit the surgeon to work around and below the mental foramen and the inferior alveolar canal without endangering the nerve.

Extraoral and Intraoral Approaches to the Mandibular Ramus

EXTRAORAL APPROACH. The technique most frequently used is an incision below the angle of the mandible, occasionally referred to in the United States and Canada as the Risdon approach. The incision is placed in or parallel to a skin fold of the neck, thus minimizing the appearance of the subsequent scar. The angle of the mandible is reached by blunt dissection under the platysma muscle in order to avoid injury to the marginal mandibular branch of the facial nerve. The systematic exposure of the mandibular marginal branch of the facial nerve to protect the nerve from injury has been abandoned by the authors because a number of patients developed unnecessary temporary paresis following this maneuver.

The preauricular incision which curves into the supratragal notch provides another route to the upper ramus and condyle; it is extended upward into the scalp for additional exposure. The preauricular incision combined with a submandibular incision is particularly useful when both the upper and lower portions of the ramus require exposure; the parotid gland, facial nerve, and masseter muscle are raised between the two incisions.

The preauricular incision can also be extended around the lobe of the ear and backward in the retroauricular fold, over the mastoid process into the hairline; this extended incision is similar to that used in face lift operations. The incision provides wide exposure of the parotid, masseter, and submandibular areas.

INTRAORAL APPROACH. The intraoral approach to the mandibular ramus is through a vertical incision placed along the anterior border of the ramus. The incision extends downward and outward following the oblique line, a bony ridge which extends from the anterior border of the ramus to the mental tubercle. The entire ramus can be exposed through this incision.

COMBINED EXTRAORAL AND INTRAORAL APPROACH. In certain complex deformities of the jaws, it may be advisable to obtain exposure of both the body and the ramus of the mandible. This can be done by a dual intraoral and extraoral approach. The body of the mandible is exposed through the usual intraoral approach; the ramus is exposed through a submandibular incision. The two incisions are joined after the periosteum of the bone has been raised.

Mandibular Prognathism

John Hunter in 1778 defined mandibular prognathism as follows: "the lower jaw projecting too far forwards, so that the fore teeth pass before those of the upper jaw, when the mouth is shut; which is attended with inconvenience, and disfigures the face" (Fig. 30–24).

The lower jaw is oversized (macrognathia) and protruded. The dentoalveolar relationships in mandibular prognathism are characteristic of Class III (Angle) malocclusion. Dentoalveolar relationships, however, cannot be used as the sole criterion in the diagnosis of mandibular prognathism. It is possible to have a Class III dentoalveolar malocclusion without mandibular prognathism. A skeletal reference must also be included. Skeletal analysis using cephalometric tracings will show that the mandible is relatively anterior to the cranial base: the SNB angle is greater than normal.

Incipient mandibular prognathism can often be recognized in the primary dentition stage of dental development. More frequently, clear evidence of the condition is not apparent until the second decade of life. Mandibular prognathism tends to increase in severity throughout adolescence, and facial imbalance occurs because of the skeletal development of the mandible; it is the continued development of the mandible throughout this period that causes the malocclusion (Class III). The occlusion of the teeth and the form of the face are interdependent characteristics which rely on many factors to bring them into harmonious relationship (Hellman, 1932).

ETIOLOGY

Mandibular prognathism can be due to hereditary causes, trauma, or disease. The prevalence of prognathism in members of the same family in certain ethnic groups is cited in support of the hereditary factor in prognathism. The Habsburg family of Europe is a well-known historical example (the "Habsburg jaw") (Grabb, 1968). Many patients, however, have no family history of the deformity.

The role of trauma in mandibular prognathism is poorly defined and probably minor. Injury to the condyle appears to be a major cause of condylar and mandibular hyperplasia, which are also usually unilateral conditions. Mandibular prognathism can be caused by early childhood injury to the condyles, which can in-

duce growth rather than inhibit growth, as in the cases of micrognathia. This is probably a rare occurrence. Malunion following fractures of the jaw can lead to a prognathic deformity, abnormal occlusion of the teeth, and an open bite. Severe burn contractures of the neck in children cause protrusion of the anterior portion of the mandible. The first surgical correction of mandibular prognathism described in the American literature (Hullihen, 1849) was performed to correct such a deformity (see Fig. 30–140).

Patients with extensive hemangiomas which involve half of the face and tongue often have prognathism; this is due to the abnormally abundant blood supply, to the excessive size of the tongue, or to both of these factors. Acromegaly is a well-known cause of prognathism due to endocrine imbalance; acromegalic patients, however, are rarely candidates for reconstructive surgery. More esoteric examples are patients with Klinefelter's syndrome or Paget's disease.

Underdevelopment of the maxilla, which varies in degree but appears to be present in most cases of mandibular prognathism, accentuates the mandibular deformity.

CLASSIFICATION

Because of numerous variations in mandibular body and ramus size and shape, many studies have been made measuring the size and shape

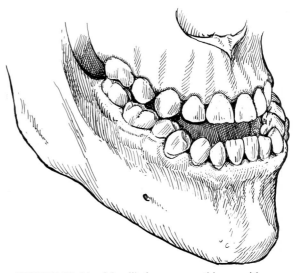

FIGURE 30–24. Mandibular prognathism with an anterior open bite. (After Hunter, 1835–1837.)

of the cranial base and craniofacial patterns using cephalometric techniques.

Theoretically, prognathism can result from variations in either the morphologic relationships of various craniofacial segments or their dimensions. Jaw length, for example, seems to be a less significant factor than the shape and size of the cranial base (Björk, 1947). Horowitz, Gerstman and Converse (1969), in reviewing 52 cases of mandibular prognathism, concluded that mandibular prognathism is not primarily a problem of size discrepancy but the result of a complex disturbance of the craniofacial relationships. Relative changes in the position and the form of the mandible contribute to the deformity. Sanborn (1955) was of the opinion that the basic fault lies in the area of the gonial (mandibular) angle, as the angle is more obtuse than normal. In the typical case, the length of the body and the height of the ramus are not significantly greater than normal. He concluded that the Class III malocclusion is not mainly one of overgrowth but one of abnormal angulation between the ramus and the body. This conclusion may apply to the most common cases, but a review of the various types of mandibular prognathism suggests that the deformity can be produced by overgrowth; prognathism associated with acromegaly is such an example.

At least four distinct craniofacial patterns can be differeniated (Fig. 30–25):

1. A maxilla developed within the normal range with a well-developed dental arch; an abnormally large mandible that results in a prominence of the lower third of the face.

2. Underdevelopment of the maxilla combined with an overdevelopment of the mandible. This is a frequent occurrence in most cases of mandibular prognathism. Studies have shown that the maxilla is frequently below the normal range of development. An accentuated "underbite" is present, the lower incisor teeth overlapping the upper teeth in a Class III occlusal relationship.

3. Anterior open bite combined with mandibular prognathism. The clinical and cephalometric examination in most of these cases shows an abnormally wide (obtuse) gonial angle and a downward inclination of the body of the mandible (steep mandibular plane). The prognathic deformity is compounded by the inability to occlude the anterior teeth.

4. Bimaxillary prognathism (or protrusion) in which both the maxilla and the mandible are prognathic.

Sanborn (1955) (Fig. 30–26) classified mandibular prognathism according to anteroposterior jaw position: (1) maxilla within the normal range, mandible anterior to the normal range; (2) maxilla posterior to the normal range; (3) both maxilla and mandible within the normal range of prognathism; and (4) maxilla posterior to the normal range and mandible anterior to the normal range.

Pseudoprognathism of the Mandible. This is a condition in which the mandible is within the normal range of development but appears prognathic because of hypoplasia of the maxilla. The deformity usually shows considerable irregularity and crowding of the maxillary teeth and a high palatal vault. The prognathic appearance is alleviated by expanding and advancing the recessed maxilla (see p. 1440).

TREATMENT OF MANDIBULAR PROGNATHISM

Proper timing of the operation is essential. Correction of the mandibular prognathism should be delayed until the adolescent mandibular growth spurt is passed. In the male patient, the growth spurt is usually completed around the age of 17 or 18; females generally complete this phase a few years earlier. Additional growth occurs during the late adolescent years, but the amount of growth is usually not sufficient to cause postponement of surgery. In extreme cases, earlier operation may be recommended with the understanding that a second procedure may be required.

There is no unequivocal dividing line between a Class III dentoalveolar malocclusion (an orthodontic problem) and a mandibular skeletal prognathism (a developmental deformity). For practical purposes, the severity of facial imbalance provides an acceptable guide to treatment. A lesser degree of facial change is to be expected from orthodontic treatment alone than after mandibular surgical recession. The decision is thus based on the degree of esthetic improvement considered to be desirable in a given case, the attainment of a balanced dental occlusion being taken into consideration.

Orthodontic Versus Surgical Treatment. Orthodontic therapy is often attempted in a child developing mandibular prognathism after the eruption of the permanent dentition. Angle, as early as 1898, in discussing severe prognathism of the mandible, condemned orthodontic

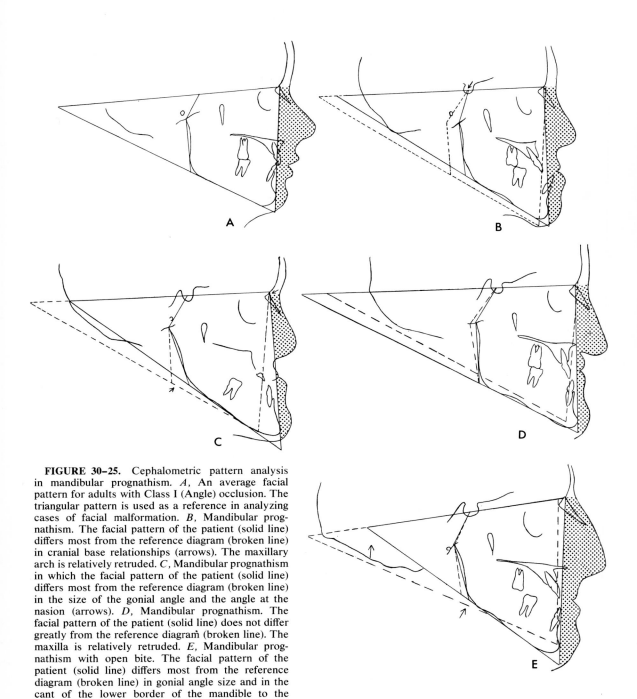

FIGURE 30–25. Cephalometric pattern analysis in mandibular prognathism. *A*, An average facial pattern for adults with Class I (Angle) occlusion. The triangular pattern is used as a reference in analyzing cases of facial malformation. *B*, Mandibular prognathism. The facial pattern of the patient (solid line) differs most from the reference diagram (broken line) in cranial base relationships (arrows). The maxillary arch is relatively retruded. *C*, Mandibular prognathism in which the facial pattern of the patient (solid line) differs most from the reference diagram (broken line) in the size of the gonial angle and the angle at the nasion (arrows). *D*, Mandibular prognathism. The facial pattern of the patient (solid line) does not differ greatly from the reference diagram (broken line). The maxilla is relatively retruded. *E*, Mandibular prognathism with open bite. The facial pattern of the patient (solid line) differs most from the reference diagram (broken line) in gonial angle size and in the cant of the lower border of the mandible to the cranial base line (arrows). (After Horowitz, Gerstman and Converse, 1969.)

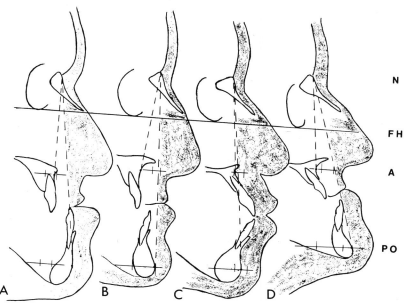

N

FH

A

PO

A   B   C   D

FIGURE 30–26. Cephalometric tracings representing the four main groups of Class III facial skeletal and soft tissue profiles. The short vertical lines at point A and PO designate the normal range or standard deviation of maxillary and mandibular prognathism. *A*, Those Class III patients presenting a maxilla within the normal range of prognathism but a mandible beyond the normal range of prognathism. *B*, Those with a maxilla below the normal range of prognathism and a mandible within the normal range of prognathism. *C*, Those with both maxilla and mandible within the normal range of prognathism. *D*, Those with a maxilla below the normal range of prognathism and a mandible beyond the normal range of prognathism. (After Sanborn, 1955.)

interference. He stated that these cases should be avoided by the orthodontist and that the limitations of orthodontic therapy should be recognized.

Orthodontic treatment produces changes in the position and form of the dentoalveolar segment of the jaw, but it does not significantly influence the position and the shape of the skeletal structures, the body and ramus of the mandible.

Orthodontic therapy, however, while incapable of completely correcting the skeletal deformity, is essential in the preparation for surgery and in the postoperative period to ensure a balanced, stable occlusion of the teeth.

Preoperative Planning. Preliminary planning is required to estimate the amount of recession of the mandible either by an operation on the ramus or by the resection of a measured section from the mandibular body. The differential diagnosis of prognathism is of practical significance in planning the surgery, since one technique may be more appropriately applied to a particular problem than another.

Study of the dental models is essential in planning the improved postoperative dentoalveolar relationships and in evaluating the degree of required mandibular recession. Casts of the upper and lower teeth are placed in occlusal relationship (Fig. 30–27, *A*). A vertical line is traced through the mesiobuccal cusp of the first maxillary molar tooth and extended to the underlying mandibular tooth. The casts are then placed into a more suitable dental occlusal relationship, and the vertical line on the upper molar is again extended downward to cross the lower tooth (Fig. 30–27, *B*). The distance between the lines on the lower cast indicate the extent of posterior displacement of the mandible which is required. The measurements should be made bilaterally; it is often necessary to recess one side more than the other when asymmetry is present.

Another method of estimating how much recession of the mandible is required is illustrated in Figure 30–28. When the casts are placed in the optimal dental occlusal relationships, wax or plaster is added to the posterior aspect of the maxillary cast until the casts maintain the corrected dentoalveolar position.

If an anterior open bite deformity is present and requires closure by section of the man-

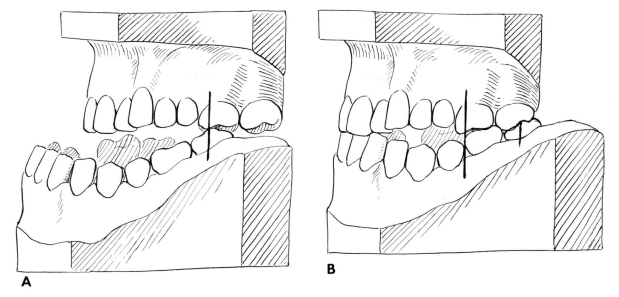

FIGURE 30–27. Dental casts in planning the correction of prognathism. *A,* Casts of upper and lower teeth are placed in the existing occlusal relationships. A vertical line is traced through the mesiobuccal cusp of the first maxillary molar and continued on the lower one. *B,* The casts are repositioned into the planned occlusal relationships. The vertical line on the maxillary molar is again extended downward on the mandibular cast. The distance between the anterior and posterior lines drawn on the lower cast represents the extent of posterior mandibular displacement required. (From Kazanjian, V. H.: The surgical treatment of prognathism. An analysis of sixty-five cases. Am. J. Surg., *87*:691, 1954.)

dibular body, the mandibular cast is cut at the appropriate level to allow for the correction. In a favorable case, the open bite is closed by recessing the mandibular cast and tilting the anterior part upwards, suggesting that an operation in the ramus may correct both deformities. In other instances, the open bite is the result of the malposition of the maxillary anterior segment; an anterior maxillary segmental osteotomy may be more suitable in this case (see p. 1428).

The interdigitation of the cusps of the teeth is studied. Spot grinding of the interfering cusps may be required; this can be done either preoperatively or during the operation to obtain a more favorable occlusion. Preoperative or postoperative orthodontic therapy needs must also be determined. An acrylic occlusal bite-plane (wafer) is used if overcorrection is desired or if extreme occlusal interference is present.

The skeletal deformity is assessed on the cephalometric roentgenogram. Cut-outs of the tracings are useful in the planning. Although, in the last analysis, the patient is more concerned about his facial contour, the planning of the postoperative dental occlusion is the most important step in achieving a satisfactory postoperative result.

Many variations in the deformity influence the decision as to the choice of procedure. Precise definition of the deformity permits the selection of the most desirable restorative procedure.

Evolution of Techniques for the Correction of Mandibular Prognathism. It is rewarding to look back and review the techniques that have been used in the past and to observe their gradual evolution toward present-day techniques.

Three approaches for the correction of mandibular prognathism have been followed throughout the years. The first operative procedure on the mandible to correct an anterior open bite in the United States was performed on the body of the mandible by Hullihen in 1849 (see Fig. 30–140). The second approach was directed to the condylar area almost a half century later by Jaboulay (1895). The ramus was the last region to be explored; Babcock sectioned the ramus horizontally in 1910 to correct mandibular prognathism.

EVOLUTION OF OPERATIONS ON THE MANDIBULAR BODY. Hullihen's patient was a young woman with a mandibular dentoalveolar deformity caused by a lower facial and neck scar contracture resulting from a childhood

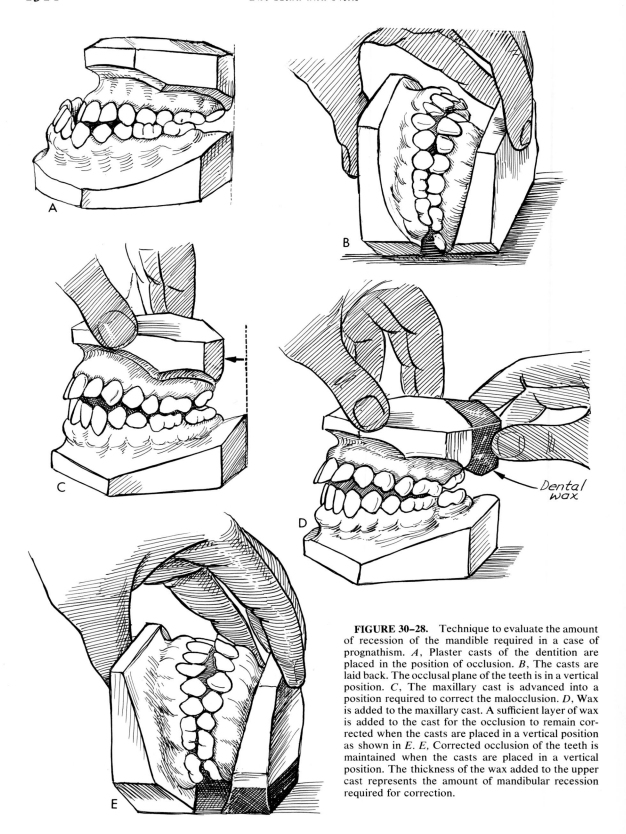

FIGURE 30–28.   Technique to evaluate the amount of recession of the mandible required in a case of prognathism. *A*, Plaster casts of the dentition are placed in the position of occlusion. *B*, The casts are laid back. The occlusal plane of the teeth is in a vertical position. *C*, The maxillary cast is advanced into a position required to correct the malocclusion. *D*, Wax is added to the maxillary cast. A sufficient layer of wax is added to the cast for the occlusion to remain corrected when the casts are placed in a vertical position as shown in *E. E*, Corrected occlusion of the teeth is maintained when the casts are placed in a vertical position. The thickness of the wax added to the upper cast represents the amount of mandibular recession required for correction.

burn. Hullihen, using a saw, sectioned the mandible transversely below the anterior teeth and removed a V-section from the premolar region. The V-section extended only through the upper two-thirds of the body of the mandible. Tilting the anterior mandibular fragment backward and upward corrected the protrusion of the teeth and the open-bite deformity. Blair did a similar operation successfully in 1887; his second operation was not as successful. The two operations were reported by Angle (1898). In the second case, total loss of the mandibular fragment occurred through necrosis. This disaster was attributed to failure of fixation; fixation was limited to the use of a Barton bandage and direct interosseous wiring between the bone fragments. Angle emphasized the importance of postoperative stabilization of the fragments, advice well heeded even to this day.

In 1906 von Eiselsberg described a step osteotomy of the body of the mandible to increase the surface contact. Lane (1905), Pickrell (1912), and Pichler (1918) used vertical straight-line ostectomies. Cryer (1913) removed a curvilinear section from the mandibular angle. Aller (1917) recommended the resection of a wedge of bone extending through the entire height of the mandibular body.

Little regard was given to the protection of the inferior alveolar neurovascular bundle until Harsha in 1912 performed a vertical section of the body posterior to the molar teeth, removing a segment of bone and preserving the neurovascular bundle. New and Erich (1941) removed a segment of bone from the tooth-bearing portion of the mandible in a one-stage procedure. Dingman (1944) advocated a two-stage straight-line ostectomy with preservation of the inferior alveolar neurovascular bundle. In the first stage, the teeth in the line of the resected bone were removed. Through an intraoral approach, the dentoalveolar portion of the bone was removed to the level of the inferior alveolar canal. The second stage was done four weeks later through an extraoral submandibular approach. The bone below the inferior alveolar canal was resected, thus completing the correction of the prognathism. Thoma (1948) suggested a similar procedure performed entirely through the intraoral approach in a single stage. Converse and Shapiro (1952) developed a technique which combined the advantages of the step ostectomy, the intraoral approach, and a one-stage operation. The intraoral step ostectomy is

made anterior to the mental foramen, when possible, thus preserving the inferior alveolar nerve, the mental nerve, and the sensory innervation of the lower lip. When a resection behind the mental foramen is indicated, the inferior alveolar neurovascular bundle is exposed by removing the outer cortical plate over the canal. The bone is then resected, keeping the nerve protected under direct observation. The step ostectomy offers a wide bony surface of contact and thus decreases the chance of delayed union or nonunion, complications which occur more frequently with the straight-line resection.

A C-shape variation of the step ostectomy of the mandibular body was described in 1966 by Toman. To provide additional contact between the fragments, Mayer (1971) reported a technique based on the sagittal splitting principle to shorten the body. Both these techniques have limited application since they require the removal of more than one tooth.

Evolution of Operations on the Mandibular Condyle. Bilateral condylectomy was advocated by Jaboulay (1895) for the correction of prognathism. Dufourmentel (1921) was a proponent of this method and resected a measured section of the condyle. González-Ulloa (1951) and Merville (1970), using a similar technique, evaluated the amount of resection in the condylar area by cephalometric measurements. The predetermined amount of the head of the condyle was then removed to permit correction of the prognathism. Because of the partial destruction of the temporomandibular joint and the associated secondary deformities and complications, condylectomy has generally been discontinued.

Section of the condylar neck using the Gigli saw technique (see Fig. 30–33) was popularized by Kostecka (1928). Kostecka later employed a similar technique to perform a horizontal osteotomy of the ramus. The blind operation, using a Gigli saw, has numerous disadvantages: soft tissue laceration, facial nerve injury, limited recession of the mandible, and frequent nonunion at the site of the osteotomy, establishing a pseudoarthrosis and eliminating condylar function.

In 1945, Moose described an intraoral technique for subcondylar osteotomy which he performed with a long-shank dental handpiece and a round burr. Smith and Robinson in 1954 reported a procedure for correction of mandibular prognathism by removal of bone below the sigmoid notch and a section of the base of the condylar process. Satisfactory bony contact is obtained by this operation, and the lateral pterygoid muscle, by its forward pull, assists in maintaining the bony contact.

Shortening the neck of the condyle is another technique, applicable to the unusual deformity characterized by elongation of this structure (see Figs. 30–103 and 30–104).

EVOLUTION OF OPERATIONS ON THE MANDIBULAR RAMUS. Lane (1905) used a horizontal osteotomy of the ramus for correction of retrognathism. Babcock (1909) applied this technique to the correction of mandibular prognathism. A Gigli saw was looped around the ramus. The saw was introduced through an intraoral puncture and passed through the skin posterior to the ramus. The other end of the saw was brought out through the skin anterior to the ramus. Ragnell (1938) and Hogeman (1951) made an opening through a postauricular incision to expose the posterior border of the ramus and sectioned the ramus with a saw placed above the mandibular foramen. Kazanjian (1954) advocated direct exposure of the ramus through a submandibular incision and a beveled cut made with an osteotome above the inferior alveolar foramen (Fig. 30–29). This

method increased the surface of contact between the bony fragments and decreased the tendency for separation of the fragments by the contraction of the lateral pterygoid muscle. Schuchardt (1954a) through an intraoral approach, used a step osteotomy which further increased the surface of contact.

Pichler and Trauner (1948) recommended an "inverted L" ramisection. The horizontal part of the "L" was made above the mandibular foramen, and the vertical limb was dropped down behind the foramen, parallel to the posterior border of the ramus.

A major contribution to the surgery of prognathism was made by Caldwell and Letterman in 1954. They described an operation for prognathism in which the ramus is split vertically from the sigmoid notch downward to a point just anterior to the mandibular angle (Fig. 30–30). The posterior fragment overlaps the anterior fragment laterally when the mandibular body is recessed to correct the prognathic deformity. Robinson (1956) made the osteotomy from the sigmoid notch to a point posterior to the mandibular angle: the oblique osteotomy of the ramus.

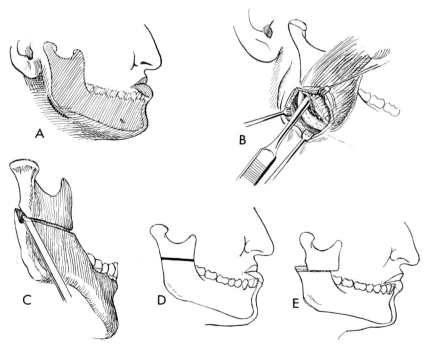

FIGURE 30–29. Technique of horizontal osteotomy of the ramus through the extraoral approach. *A*, The incision is made below the angle of the jaw. *B*, The periosteum and the masseter muscle are raised from the lateral aspect of the ramus. *C*, The osteotome cuts obliquely through the ramus of the mandible, above the level of entry of the inferior alveolar nerve. *D, E*, Backward displacement of the mandible after osteotomy. (After Kazanjian, 1954.)

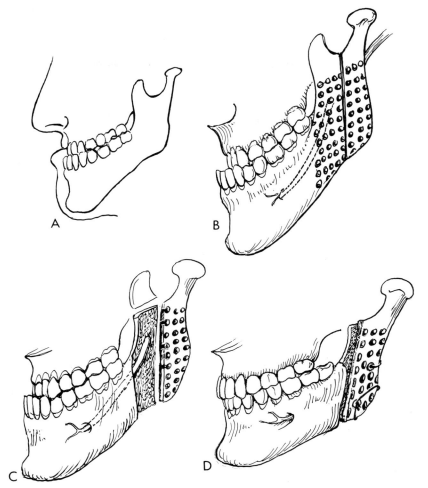

FIGURE 30–30. Caldwell and Letterman's operation for the correction of prognathism. *A,* Outline of a prognathic mandible. *B,* The ramus is exposed, and a series of drill holes are made through the cortex of the bone. The ramus is split by a vertical osteotomy. *C,* The outer table of the anterior fragment is removed, exposing the inferior alveolar neurovascular bundle. The coronoid process is amputated. *D,* The mandible is recessed; the fragments overlap. Care is taken to avoid compression of the inferior alveolar nerve. (After Caldwell and Letterman, 1954.)

In 1957 Obwegeser, enlarging upon the step osteotomy of Schuchardt, introduced an intraoral splitting of the ramus in a sagittal plane, thus increasing the contact between the bony surfaces of the fragments; Dal Pont (1961) suggested an anterior extension of the osteotomy to include the lateral cortical plate over the posterior aspect of the body of the mandible, thus further increasing the surface of contact between the fragments and aiding in the stability of the fragments (see Fig. 30–40). Dautrey (1975) modified the technique of sagittal splitting of the ramus, performing a subcortical section, thus remaining lateral to the inferior alveolar canal (see Fig. 30–44).

At present, the most commonly employed techniques to recess the mandible are the sec-

tion of the ramus along a frontal plane (the vertical or oblique osteotomy) and the section along a sagittal plane (the sagittal split osteotomy). Both of these techniques provide adequate bony contact between the fragments and rapid consolidation.

Surgical Correction of Mandibular Prognathism

OSTEOTOMIES OF THE BODY OF THE MANDIBLE

Indications. The principal indications for shortening the body of the mandible by removal of a measured segment of bone from each side are (1) a wide disparity in the arch shape between the maxilla and mandible; (2) the presence of an open bite, necessitating an upward tilting of the anterior portion of the mandible; and (3) the presence of edentulous gaps in the dental arch resulting from prior removal of teeth.

It is difficult to obtain satisfactory occlusal relationships when a well-developed maxillary arch is opposed by an abnormally shaped mandibular arch and when there is a posterior crossbite. It must be kept in mind that an osteotomy of the mandibular ramus permits anteroposterior and rotational displacements but does not modify the shape of the arch. When the prognathic mandibular arch is excessively wide and shows considerable disparity in shape when compared with the maxillary arch, reduction of the width of the mandibular arch is necessary, in addition to an anteroposterior recession (Fig. 30–31).

Resection of bone from the mandibular body

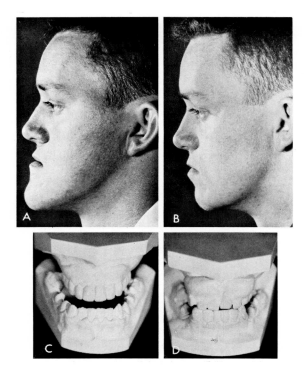

FIGURE 30–31. Mandibular prognathism treated by resection of a segment of the body of the mandible. *A*, Preoperative profile of the patient. *B*, Postoperative profile. *C*, Dental casts showing the gross disparity between the maxillary and mandibular arches. *D*, Postoperative dental occlusion.

is also indicated to correct prognathism with severe anterior open bite deformities. The best results have been obtained by a bilateral resection of bone from the mandibular body, combined with an upward displacement or tilt of the anterior fragment to close the open bite. Alternatively, a two-stage procedure is employed; first, a vertical or sagittal osteotomy of the ramus is performed; second, an osteotomy of the body for correction of the open bite deformity is accomplished (see later section on prognathism with open bite).

Technique of Ostectomy of the Mandibular Body. Patients with prognathism often have poor dentition. When mandibular teeth are absent in the premolar or first molar area, sacrifice of the remaining dental units is usually not necessary. Exposure of the body of the mandible is obtained by the intraoral approach; a cutaneous scar is thus avoided. In most operations on the body of the mandible, the bone and the mental nerves can be exposed by the degloving technique. Excellent exposure is obtained, facilitating the ostectomy.

A step osteotomy is preferable to a linear osteotomy because it affords increased bony contact between the fragments; the danger of delayed union or nonunion is thus diminished.

When possible, it is advantageous to place the osteotomy anterior to the mental foramen (see Fig. 30–16). This procedure is particularly indicated when an open bite deformity is present. The inferior alveolar canal and nerve are avoided, and the mental nerve is preserved. Sectioning the anterior extension of the inferior alveolar nerve, which provides sensory innervation to the anterior teeth, is of minor clinical importance.

The position of the area of section is often dictated by gaps in the dentition. When the osteotomy is made posterior to the mental foramen, crushing or pinching of the inferior alveolar nerve is avoided by wide decompression of the canal (Fig. 30–32).

The osteotomy can also be performed in the retromolar area, thus avoiding the extraction of healthy teeth in the dental arch. There are two disadvantages of an osteotomy in this region: (1) an extraoral approach must be used to provide exposure, and (2) it is difficult to control the position of the edentulous posterior fragments and to prevent a recurrence of the deformity caused by the forward shifting of the posterior fragment.

Regardless of the choice of location, the osteotomy is begun by outlining the measured

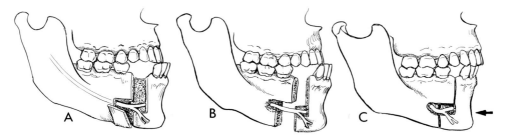

FIGURE 30–32. Mandibular body osteotomy through an edentulous portion of the mandible. *A,* The outer cortex has been removed by splitting the body with an osteotome. The inferior alveolar and mental nerves are exposed. *B,* The inner cortex and the remainder of the bone are resected. *C,* The anterior fragment is recessed. The technique is useful in unusual deformities when the molar teeth are in adequate occlusion and when the operative site is edentulous. The technique of exposing the inferior alveolar nerve is demonstrated.

area to be resected by means of a small fine fissure bur or a small round cutting bur activated by a high-speed drill. The outer cortical plate is cut through and removed using a bur or a sharp osteotome. If a tooth is present in the area of the osteotomy, it must be extracted. The inferior alveolar canal and nerve are exposed when the area of bone resection is posterior to the mental foramen. The nerve is kept under direct vision and protected as the lingual cortical plate is removed to complete the osteotomy.

The posterior fragment is placed in occlusion and maintained in position with intermaxillary fixation. The anterior fragment is displaced backward and placed in contact with the posterior fragment to close the gaps. Minor adjustments may be required. Excess bone requires additional resection; a bone gap between the fragments can be filled with bone chips from the resected bone. Removal of a small amount of bone from the horizontal branch of the step osteotomy aids in adjusting the occlusion of the anterior teeth. Once the anterior fragment is in correct occlusal relationship it is maintained by intermaxillary fixation.

The lower border of the posterior fragment, despite the intermaxillary fixation, tends to rotate lingually as a result of contraction of the medial pterygoid and the mylohyoid muscles. Interosseous fixation with 24-gauge stainless steel wire near the lower border of the fragments helps maintain the alignment and fixation. The intraoral incision is closed, and a compressive dressing is applied and held in place by a figure-of-eight Barton bandage. Intermaxillary fixation is continued for six to eight weeks. Dependent suction drainage prevents hematoma formation.

Edema following the operation may result in temporary loss of sensibility in the lower lip. When decompression and exposure of the inferior alveolar nerve is done, the loss is temporary; sensibility gradually returns, heralded by a feeling of "pins and needles" in the lower lip (for further details concerning operations on the body of the mandible, see Elongation Osteotomies, p. 1347).

OSTEOTOMIES IN THE CONDYLAR REGION

Condylectomy has generally been abandoned as a technique to correct mandibular prognathism. Destruction of a normal temporomandibular joint is a drastic procedure and need not be performed now that simpler, less disabling corrective methods are available.

Osteotomies of the condylar neck have also declined in popularity. Blind osteotomy (Kostečka, 1928) is needlessly dangerous in view of safer contemporary techniques (Fig. 30–33). In addition, the amount of mandibular recession is limited, and the small condylar fragment is difficult to control.

The sigmoid notch operation (Smith and Robinson, 1954) is now rarely used. It is a difficult operation which can be time-consuming; facial nerve injury is also a risk.

OSTEOTOMIES OF THE RAMUS

Horizontal Osteotomy of the Ramus. The horizontal osteotomy was the first osteotomy of the ramus to be used to correct mandibular prognathism (Babcock, 1909). A similar operation was used by Blair (1915). An intraoral or an extraoral approach can be used. The tech-

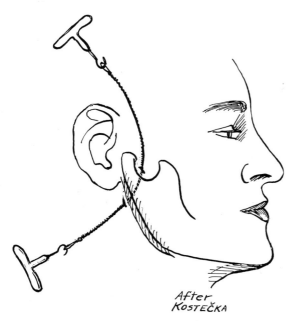

After
KOSTEČKA

FIGURE 30–33. Kostečka's technique of osteotomy through the neck of the condyle with a Gigli saw. Kostečka used a similar technique to perform a horizontal osteotomy of the ramus.

nique is simple, but the number of complications is high. The area of contact between the fragments is small. Contraction of the temporalis and lateral pterygoid muscles tends to distract the upper fragment an average of 15 degrees away from the lower tooth-bearing fragment (Hogeman, 1951; Björk, Eliasson and Sörensen, 1970). Muscle interposition into the gap leads to delayed union or nonunion. A long period (ten weeks) of intermaxillary fixation is necessary. Furthermore, Nordendram and Waller (1968) reported a relapse incidence of 52 per cent (between 1 and 15 mm), 55 per cent persistent paresthesia of the lower lip, and 31 per cent root resorption of the anterior incisors in patients followed at least one year postoperatively. Injury to the facial nerve was also reported.

Vertical Osteotomy of the Ramus. Caldwell and Letterman (1954) introduced the vertical osteotomy of the ramus for the correction of mandibular prognathism (see Fig. 30–30). The ramus was split vertically through an external approach from the sigmoid notch to a point anterior to the mandibular angle. The cortical surface of the anterior fragment was removed in the area of contact. The posterior fragment was wired in position lateral to the anterior

fragment. The coronoid process was detached at its base to neutralize the pull exerted by the temporalis muscle.

Robinson (1956) and Hinds (1957) proposed a variation when they placed the osteotomy posterior to the mandibular angle: the oblique osteotomy. A vertical osteotomy with additional modifications was described by Georgiade and Quinn (1961), Smith and Chambers (1962), Van Zile (1963), and Converse (1964a).

The techniques of vertical osteotomy and oblique osteotomy of the ramus are essentially the same. The oblique section places the line of osteotomy further posterior to the mandibular foramen but furnishes a smaller posterior fragment. The vertical section provides a wider bony surface of contact.

Technique of Vertical Osteotomy of the Ramus (External Approach). The cutaneous incision is made in one of the natural flexion lines of the neck below the angle of the mandible (Fig. 30–34, *A*). If the incision is properly placed, the resulting scar will be inconspicuous. Individuals predisposed to keloid formation, Black patients in particular, should be operated upon by an intraoral technique.

The patient should have his teeth in occlusion so that the mandibular angle can be located by palpation. An incision 3 to 5 cm in length usually provides sufficient exposure. The dissection is maintained beneath the platysma muscle until the angle of the mandible is reached. Blunt dissection with a hemostat under the platysma muscle exposes the angle of the mandible without endangering the marginal mandibular branch of the facial nerve.

Exposure of the Lateral Surface of the Ramus. Although the skin incision is short, careful retraction with the appropriate retractor will give sufficient exposure. The periosteum is incised along the lower border of the mandible, the angle, and the posterior border (Fig. 30–34, *B*). The masseter muscle is raised from the bone with the periosteum (Fig. 30–34, *C*). The subperiosteal elevation is continued superiorly to the sigmoid notch and the base of the condylar process, anteriorly as far as the base of the coronoid process. The stylomandibular ligament insertion on the posterior border of the ramus above the angle of the mandible is also detached. The subperiosteal disinsertion of the muscular ligamentous attachments exposes the posterior border of the ramus, which is an important

FIGURE 30–34. Vertical oste-otomy of the ramus by the external approach for the correction of mandibular prognathism. *A,* The principal anatomical structures and the outline of the skin incision are shown. The incision is placed in a skin fold of the neck below the angle of the mandible. *B,* After incision of the subcutaneous tissues and periosteum, the lateral surface of the ramus is exposed by subperiosteal dissection. *C,* The essential landmarks in this technique are identified by exposing the angle and the posterior border of the ramus. (From Converse, J. M., and Horowitz, S. L.: The surgical-orthodontic approach to the treatment of dentofacial deformities. Am. J. Orthod., 55:217, 1969.)

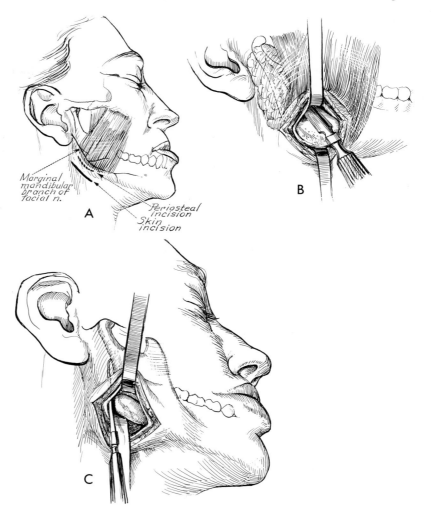

landmark as the vertical section is made parallel to it (Fig. 30–34, *C*).

Good illumination is essential, and a fiberoptic lighted retractor is particularly helpful. The angulated retractor should have a lip that fits into the sigmoid notch (Fig. 30–35, *A*). Thus the entire lateral surface of the ramus and the posterior border are exposed; the neck of the condyle and the sigmoid notch are readily identified.

The importance of careful subperiosteal detachment of the muscles and ligaments must be emphasized. Recurrence of the deformity is a complication which occurs when muscular disinsertion is not complete and when the sectioned fragments are repositioned without completely changing the direction of the pull and function of the muscles of mastication.

The pull of the powerful musculature of mastication cannot be counteracted unless the muscles are rendered temporarily impotent. The tendency to displace the fragments is minimized while bony consolidation occurs. The muscles find new points of insertion on the modified mandibular skeleton.

In cases of extreme prognathism, subperiosteal disinsertion of the temporalis tendon over the coronoid process is advisable. Caldwell (1964) stated that the coronoid process must be sectioned if the correction is greater than 10 mm to allow unrestricted posterior movement of the jaw. According to Hinds and Kent (1972), sectioning the base of the coronoid is rarely required; they have recessed the mandible up to 23 mm without coronoid process sectioning. In our own series of

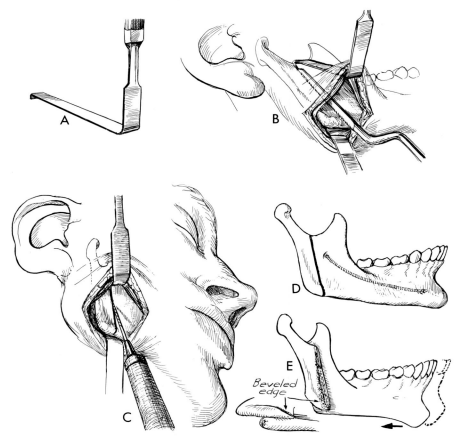

FIGURE 30–35. Vertical osteotomy of the ramus by the external approach. *A,* Retractor designed to engage the sigmoid notch. *B,* Subperiosteal reflection of the overlying masseter muscle and detachment of the fibers of the medial pterygoid muscle have been completed. A saw is used to score the bone along the proposed line of section. *C,* The Lindemann spiral bur completes the vertical osteotomy parallel to the posterior border of the ramus. *D,* Note that the line of section is posterior to the lingula and inferior alveolar neurovascular bundle. The linear osteotomy can also be performed by means of a reciprocating saw (Hall). *E,* The fragments overlap. (From Converse, J. M., and Horowitz, S. L.: The surgical-orthodontic approach to the treatment of dentofacial deformities. Am. J. Orthod., *55*:217, 1969.)

cases, the coronoid process has not been detached. When an associated anterior open bite is also closed, Hinds and Girotti (1967) have recommended resection of the coronoid process to overcome the pull of the temporalis muscle.

EXPOSURE OF THE MEDIAL SURFACE OF THE RAMUS. A curved periosteal elevator is used to detach the medial pterygoid muscle. This muscle is inserted by a strong tendinous lamina into the inferior and posterior portion of the medial aspect of the ramus, thus inferior and posterior to the inferior alveolar foramen. Digital palpation of the medial aspect of the ramus will locate the lingula. Care must be taken to limit the subperiosteal dissection to this level to avoid injuring the inferior alveolar nerve and artery. If the dissection is done along a subperiosteal plane, injury to the internal maxillary

artery and to the deeper situated pterygoid venous plexus is avoided.

THE OSTEOTOMY. In order to protect the structures deep to the ramus, a pliable retractor is placed between the medial surface of the ramus and the soft tissues. A specially designed retractor (Fig. 30–35, *A*) is hooked into the sigmoid notch and exposes the lateral surface of the ramus (Fig. 30–35, *B*). Overenergetic retraction can produce facial paralysis by placing traction upon the seventh cranial nerve branches.

The posterior border of the ramus serves as the landmark for the design of the osteotomy. It should be visible at all times. The posterior edge of the retractor should lie parallel to the posterior border of the ramus and extend downward to a point anterior to the angle, thus indicating the line of osteotomy. The line of section is directed to a point anterior to the angle of the mandible and parallel to the posterior border of the ramus. Injury to the inferior alveolar neurovascular bundle as it enters the inferior alveolar foramen is avoided. It is helpful to outline the osteotomy by scoring the cortical plate with a bur. The osteotomy (Fig. 30–35. *B, C*) is performed with an air-turbine-driven reciprocating saw with a vertical cutting blade, a bayonet saw, a Lindemann spiral bur, or any other instrument preferred by the surgeon. Beveling the osteotomy in a posterior direction increases the cancellous bony surface of contact. If required, a sharp osteotome is used to complete the line of section.

OVERLAP OF THE FRAGMENTS. The vertical osteotomy delimits a long posterior fragment which is easy to control. A side surface of contact occurs when the mandibular body is retropositioned as the posterior fragment overlaps the lateral aspect of the anterior fragment (Fig. 30–35, *D, E*). Bony consolidation is rapid because of the wide surface of contact, as compared to that of the oblique osteotomy (see later in text).

Similar steps are followed on the contralateral mandibular ramus. The body of the mandible can now be displaced backward to establish the preplanned occlusal relationships with the maxillary teeth. Prior to intermaxillary fixation, an essential precaution is to ensure that the posterior fragment overlaps the lateral aspect of the anterior fragment (Fig. 30–35, *D, E*) and that each condylar head is in the glenoid fossa and not riding forward on the articular eminence. The lower end of the posterior fragment should be beveled to avoid excessive protrusion under the masseter muscle (Fig. 30–35, *E*); this has not proved to be a problem in our series of patients and can be decreased further by removing the cortex over the surface of contact of the anterior fragment.

Interosseous fixation of the fragments is not necessary. Coaptation of the two bone surfaces is afforded by continuous traction of the lateral pterygoid muscle, which exerts a forward and medial pull and maintains firm contact between the bony fragments (Fig. 30–36). An advantage of not using interosseous wiring is that early postoperative occlusal changes can be made during intermaxillary fixation, if necessary; the posterior fragment is free to find a new position because it is not held by wire fixation. The wound is closed in layers, and a subcuticular running suture approximates the skin edges. A well-padded, firmly applied pressure dressing, maintained in position by a figure-of-eight Barton bandage, completes the procedure. Suction drainage, though not indispensable, is helpful in avoiding hematoma formation. Intermaxillary fixation is discontinued after approximately six weeks.

Technique of Oblique or Vertical Osteotomy of the Ramus (Internal Approach). The internal approach avoids the objections of the cutaneous scar and possible injury to the marginal mandibular branch of the facial nerve. Winstanley (1968) described an intraoral oblique subcondylar osteotomy approached from the lateral surface of the ramus. Herbert, Kent, and Hinds (1970) and Wilbanks (1971) brought the osteotomy further down, posterior to the

FIGURE 30–36. Direction of pull of the lateral pterygoid muscle. *A*, Note the insertion and the direction of the pull exerted by the lateral pterygoid muscle. *B*, The lateral pterygoid muscle tends to exert medial traction upon the condylar fragment, thus maintaining the fragments in close apposition after vertical section of the ramus. Direct interosseous wiring is not required.

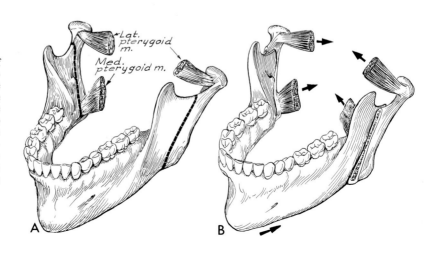

mandibular angle. A similar technique can be employed to achieve a vertical osteotomy with good results (Fig. 30–37).

The lateral surface of the ramus is exposed through an incision from the coronoid process to the buccal sulcus opposite the second molar tooth. This long incision is essential to provide the needed retraction and exposure. Muscular and ligamentous attachments are stripped from the angle and the posterior border of the ramus by use of a curved periosteal elevator. The sigmoid notch, neck of the condyle, and coronoid process are exposed by means of a retractor such as the one shown in Figure 30–38. The soft tissues around the area of section should be protected to avoid injuring the internal maxillary artery. The medial surface of the ramus is undisturbed to avert any danger to the inferior alveolar neurovascular bundle.

The osteotomy is performed with a Stryker right-angle oscillating saw with a short blade (6 mm) (see Fig. 30–38). An oblique line of section, as indicated by the broken lines on Figure 30–37, is easier to perform than the vertical section. Greater stability and a wider surface of contact between the overlapped posterior fragment and the ramus are achieved by the vertical osteotomy. A curved osteotome may be necessary to complete the osteotomy. The posterior fragment is now loose and is displaced laterally by retruding the mandible. As the posterior fragment is rotated laterally,

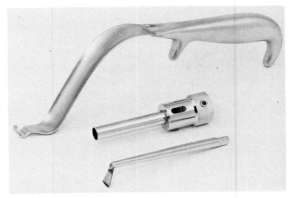

FIGURE 30–38 *Above,* L and M retractor for intraoral osteotomies of the ramus. *Below,* Side-cutting Stryker saw with attachment for use in the intraoral procedure. The blade of the saw is 6 mm long.

the periosteum is stripped from its medial surface, and the segment is allowed to find its position over the lateral aspect of the anterior fragment. After the contralateral osteotomy is completed in a similar manner, intermaxillary fixation is established. The position of the posterior fragments is confirmed. The intraoral wound is closed by catgut sutures, and a pressure dressing is applied.

Advantages and Disadvantages of the Vertical and Oblique Osteotomies of the Ramus (External and Internal Approaches). The main advantages of these techniques are the facility of execution and avoidance of injury to the inferior alveolar nerve. Teeth do not have to be sacrificed as is sometimes required in the body section techniques.

The disadvantage of the external approach is the cutaneous scar; however, if the incision is properly placed, the scar is difficult to detect. The intraoral approach should be used in patients with hypertrophic and keloid scar tendencies and in patients who object to having an external scar. The intraoral technique is more difficult to perform, and this must be carefully considered before the procedure is undertaken in patients with limited jaw opening and in patients with heavy masseteric musculature, as adequate exposure is difficult to obtain in these patients. In addition, the angle of mandibular divergence should be measured on a submental vertex roentgenogram (Massey, Chase, Shrmas, and Kohn, 1974). When the angle is less than 130 degrees, the intraoral technique is more difficult to perform.

THE SHAPE OF THE MANDIBLE FOLLOWING VERTICAL OR OBLIQUE OSTEOTOMY OF THE RAMUS. Patients with mandibular prognath-

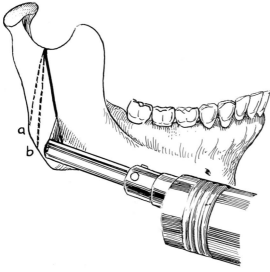

FIGURE 30–37. Ramus osteotomy through an intraoral approach. An angulated blade on an oscillating saw is used for the vertical or oblique (broken line) osteotomy of the ramus.

ism generally have a mandibular angle that is more obtuse than normal. This gives an unpleasant "straight-line" appearance to the lower jaw from the condyle to the chin. It is widely believed that the vertical and oblique sections of the ramus will improve this contour defect. This belief has not been confirmed by longitudinal data. During the immediate postoperative period, the gonial angle is less obtuse, and the mandibular contour appears more acceptable. However, cephalometric follow-up studies (Kelsey, 1968; Cunat and Gargiulo, 1973) made one to two years after the operation have shown that the angle remodels itself to its preoperative configuration.

POSTOPERATIVE CONDYLAR CHANGES. Temporomandibular joint dysfunction has not been a postoperative problem. When the posterior (condylar) fragment is overlapped laterally over the anterior fragment, a change in relation between the condyle and the glenoid fossa occurs. Ware and Taylor (1968) studied this problem with serial roentgenograms (Fig. 30–39). Three months after the operation, the condylar head was found to be displaced downward and forward out of the glenoid fossa. The displacement is probably due to the unopposed action of the lateral pterygoid muscle. The condyle, then, slowly moves in an upward and backward direction toward a normal position. At the end of one year, the condyle was found to be in its preoperative location. It was concluded that the postoperative condylar change was most likely due to remodeling.

RELAPSE. Postoperative cephalometric studies (Poulton, Taylor and Ware, 1963; Hinds and Kent, 1972; Bell and Creekmore, 1973) show an anterior movement of pogonion of 1 to 3 mm. The skeletal relapse becomes stabilized during the first year. The dentoalveolar intermaxillary relationship does not appear to be unfavorably changed; this is probably due to the improved cuspal interdigitation and accommodation of the pliable alveolar bone.

NERVE INJURY. Injury to the marginal mandibular branch of the facial nerve is always a possibility once the dissection is begun deep to the platysma muscle. The auriculotemporal (Frey) syndrome (Kopp, 1968) and parotid fistula formation (Goldberg, Marco and Googel, 1973) have also been reported as complications following the external approach. These complications, although rare when the technique is correctly performed, should not occur following the intraoral approach.

Technique of the Sagittal (Sagittal-split) Osteotomy of the Ramus. The technique of the vertical section of the ramus divides the ramus along a frontal plane. In contrast, the technique of sagittal section, as its name implies, divides the ramus along a sagittal plane.

As mentioned earlier in the chapter, Schuchardt (1954b) described a step osteotomy through the intraoral approach directed along the sagittal plane of the ramus, thus increasing the surface of contact between the fragments. Obwegeser (1957) refined this concept and further increased the surface of contact. The vertical distance between the medial and lateral horizontal cuts of the ramus was increased and the ramus was split with an osteotome between these two cuts along a sagittal plane. Dal Pont (1959, 1961) increased the surface of contact still further by including the retromolar lateral cortical plate of the body of the mandible (Fig. 30–40). The wide surface of contact and the avoidance of an external incision have made

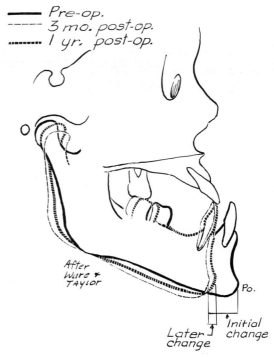

FIGURE 30–39. Cephalometric tracing showing changes of the mandible following vertical osteotomy of the ramus. Three months postoperatively, the condylar head is out of the glenoid fossa, and pogonion (Po) is in the most retruded position. One year postoperatively, the condylar head returns to a more normal relationship with the glenoid fossa. A small degree of relapse has occurred at pogonion. Note also that the mandibular angle contour remains essentially unchanged. (After Ware and Taylor, 1968.)

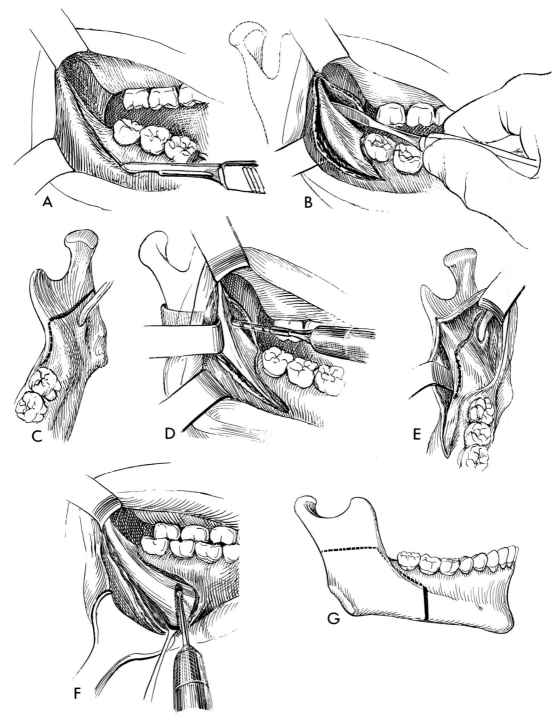

FIGURE 30–40. Technique of Obwegeser-Dal Pont sagittal osteotomy of the ramus. *A*, An incision is made along the anterior border of the ramus following the oblique line. *B*, Subperiosteal elevation of both the medial and lateral surfaces is begun. *C*, The medial cortical osteotomy is placed above the level of the mandibular foramen and is continued anteriorly along the oblique line. *D*, Bone can be removed from the medial aspect of the anterior border of the ramus to permit a better view of the lingula and the mandibular foramen region. The Lindemann spiral bur cuts the medial cortex above the foramen. *E*, The medial section of the cortex is completed. *F*, A vertical cut through the lateral cortex in the region of the second molar tooth is made with a small round bur. *G*, The cortical line of section is indicated by the broken line over the medial aspect of the ramus and along the anterior border. The solid line represents the vertical cut through the lateral cortex of the body of the mandible.

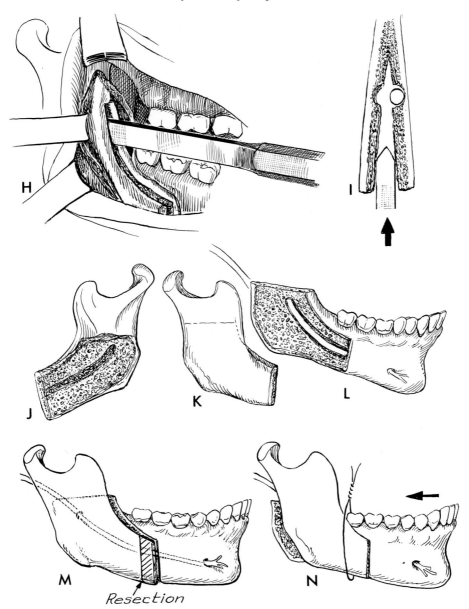

FIGURE 30–40. *Continued.* *H.* The sagittal splitting of the ramus is performed with a thick osteotome. *I,* The thick osteotome also acts as a wedge as it splits the ramus. *J,* View of the medial aspect of the lateral (condylar) fragment. *K,* The lateral aspect of the lateral (condylar) fragment. *L,* The medial (tooth-bearing) fragment. *M,* Excess bone (shaded area) must be resected from the anterior portion of the lateral fragment to allow for bony apposition after posterior displacement of the tooth-bearing fragment. *N,* Final position of the tooth-bearing portion of the mandible. A buried circumferential wire around the fragments or an interosseous wire is placed to approximate the fragments. (After Obwegeser, 1957.)

the Obwegeser–Dal Pont sagittal-split osteotomy popular in recent years.

The operation is performed through an incision made along the anterior border of the ramus and extended downward and laterally over the buccal surface of the body of the mandible (Fig. 30–40, *A*). The portion of the incision along the anterior border of the ramus should be kept lateral to the oblique line. Lateral placement of the incision facilitates wound closure after intermaxillary fixation is applied.

Subperiosteal dissection of the medial and lateral aspects of the ramus is begun (Fig. 30–40, *B*). The masseter muscle is disinserted from the lateral aspect of the ramus. When the periosteum is being elevated over the medial aspect of the ramus, care must be taken in the area of the lingula to avoid injuring the inferior alveolar neurovascular bundle as it enters the inferior alveolar foramen. The periosteum is carefully raised above the neurovascular bundle, which, with retraction and good illumination, can readily be seen. The subperiosteal dissection is extended around the posterior border of the ramus with a curved elevator. The stylomandibular ligament is detached. Specially designed retractors, of which there are various models (see Fig. 30–41), are then hooked onto the posterior border of the ramus to provide additional exposure. Obwegeser advocated using a bur to remove some bone from the medial aspect of the ramus, which is continuous with the oblique line. The lingula, the inferior alveolar neurovascular bundle, and the posterior border of the ramus then come into the operator's line of vision as a result of the removal of bone.

The ramus is now exposed and ready for the sagittal splitting procedure. The sigmoid notch is an essential landmark and should be located by palpation with a curved hemostat. A horizontal cut is made through the medial cortex approximately 1 cm above the lingula using a spiral drill or round bur (Fig. 30–40, *C, D*). Bleeding from the cancellous bone can be used as a guide to determine if the cortical bone has been penetrated. A series of drill holes placed along the anterior border of the ramus, medial to the oblique line, facilitates the sagittal osteotomy (Fig. 30–40, *E*). A second cut is made vertically through the lateral cortex of the body of the mandible in the area of the first or second molar (Fig. 30–40, *F*). Care should be

taken not to endanger the roots of the teeth. An outline of the proposed osteotomy is shown in Figure 30–40, *F* and *G*. Obwegeser recommended the use of a thick chisel or osteotome to split the ramus before the neurovascular bundle is reached (Fig. 30–40, *H, I*). The ramus is held by a retractor (Fig. 30–41) hooked around its posterior border during the splitting procedure. The retractor also acts to limit the backward trajectory of the chisel, thus preventing injury to the structures behind the ramus, notably the facial nerve.

It should be recalled that the inferior alveolar canal courses obliquely through the ramus as it continues into the body; thus, the inferior alveolar neurovascular bundle lies closer to the anterior border of the ramus as it descends through the ramus (Fig. 30–42). Care should therefore be taken as the osteotome courses the anterior one-third of the ramus to reduce the danger of direct injury to the neurovascular bundle. The medial toothbearing fragment contains the inferior alveolar neurovascular bundle and is continuous with the body of the mandible; the lateral fragment is continuous above with the condyle and the temporomandibular joint (see Fig. 30–40, *J* to *L*). The inferior alveolar nerve can be seen in its canal within the medial segment. Upon completion of the splitting, the body of the mandible is retruded into the predetermined occlusal relationship with the maxillary teeth (Fig. 30–40, *M*). Spot grinding of interfering cusps may be required before intermaxillary fixation is established.

When the tooth-bearing fragment is recessed, an overlap of bone occurs in the area of the line of osteotomy in the molar region (the Dal Pont extension) (Fig. 30–40, *M*). This excess of lateral cortical plate is resected, thus establishing a butt joint at the vertical osteotomy site. Obwegeser places a buried circumferential wire around the fragments in the retromolar area to maintain the respective position of the fragments and their close apposition (Fig. 30–40, *N*).

The condyle, under the influence of the lateral pyerygoid muscle pull, has a tendency to drift forward and downward from its position in the glenoid fossa. The condyle must be returned to its position in the glenoid fossa prior to the wiring of the fragments.

The intraoral incision is closed with interrupted sutures of plain 4–0 catgut. A pressure dressing is applied. Some surgeons prefer to omit the compressive dressing and allow the spontaneous resolution of the edema. Undue

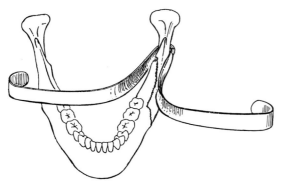

FIGURE 30–41. Obwegeser retractors facilitate exposure of the ramus in the sagittal splitting operation. Other types of retractors are also available (see Fig. 30–46).

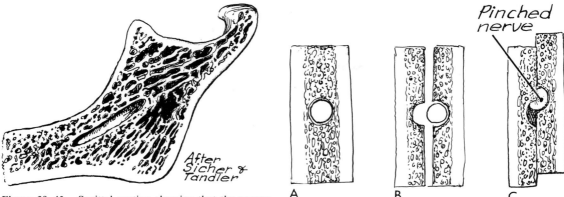

Figure 30-42. Sagittal section showing that the course of the inferior alveolar neurovascular bundle is closer to the anterior border of the ramus than is generally appreciated.

FIGURE 30-43. Diagram illustrating the mechanism by which the inferior alveolar nerve may be compressed by the split segments of the ramus, resulting in loss of the conductivity of the nerve.

swelling or hematoma is thus permitted to expand laterally away from the oropharyngeal space; the risk of possible embarrassment of the airway, although unusual, is decreased. Suction drainage is the best technique to avoid accumulation of blood and serum; the drain is brought out through the skin in the submandibular area.

ADVANTAGES AND DISADVANTAGES OF THE SAGITTAL SECTION OF THE RAMUS. The intraoral approach and the avoidance of an external scar are the distinct advantages of this technique. The wide surface of contact of cancellous bone between the split fragments ensures rapid bone consolidation, and the period of intermaxillary fixation can be reduced. Hunsuck (1968) advocated four weeks of intermaxillary fixation. However, the usual recommended period of fixation is five to six weeks. Delayed union and nonunion are rare.

The wide surface of contact also allows great latitude in the positional change between

FIGURE 30-44. The Dautrey modification of the sagittal split of the ramus. *A*, A conscious effort must be made to keep the cutting edge of the osteotome against the lateral cortical plate. Note the tendency of the posterior border of the ramus to flare laterally. *B*, By passing laterally or tangentially to the inferior alveolar canal, the possibility of directly injuring the nerve is lessened. *C*, The osteotome should not enter the inferior alveolar canal. *D*, By remaining immediately under the lateral cortex, injury to the nerve is avoided.

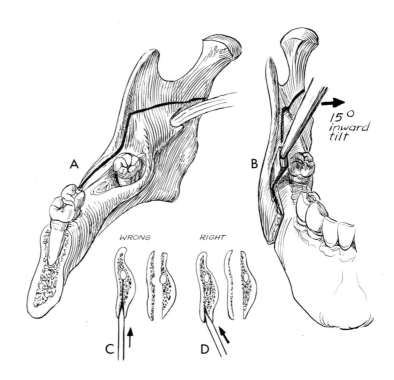

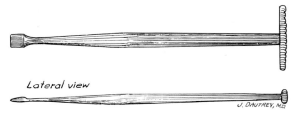

FIGURE 30-45. Dautrey's osteotome. The cutting edge is 1.5 mm thick.

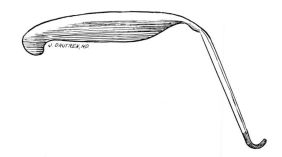

FIGURE 30-46. Dautrey's retractor with a handle providing a strong grip.

the fragments. This versatility has contributed to the popularity of the sagittal section procedure. The tooth-bearing fragment can be retruded, advanced in cases of mandibular retrusion, and rotated to close an anterior open bite.

Another advantage of the sagittal splitting technique is the improvement in the contour of the mandibular angle. In addition, lateral rotation of the condylar fragment is minimal. The condyle–glenoid fossa relationship remains essentially unchanged. The muscles of mastication quickly adapt to their new anatomical and biomechanical relationships. Rusconi, Brusati and Bottoli (1970) found no electromyographic changes of the masseter and temporalis muscles in their immediate and one-year postoperative studies.

The main disadvantage of the sagittal splitting procedure is the high incidence of loss of sensibility of the lower lip. Guernsey and De-Champlin (1971) reported an 80 per cent incidence of bilateral hypoesthesia immediately after the operation. With time, sensibility returns to all but 20 to 45 per cent of the patients (White and coworkers, 1969; Koblin and Reil, 1972; Pepersack and Chausse, 1974). All patients in the Pepersack and Chausse study were examined at least five years after the operation: 45 per cent of the patients had some degree of permanent decrease in sensibility of the lower lip. Both the teaching and the private cases of the University of Zurich were included in this report. A smaller incidence of diminished lip sensibility was present in the patients of the more experienced surgeons.

Niederdellmann and Dieckmann (1974) warned of the dangers involved in exposure of the medial aspect of the ramus: direct injury or stretching of the inferior alveolar nerve, or hematoma formation in the area. Another possible cause of diminished lip sensibility is compression of the inferior alveolar nerve between the two fragments of the ramus because of the change in the relationships between the sections (Converse, 1974b) (Fig. 30–43).

Other complications of the Obwegeser–Dal Pont procedure reported in a survey by Behrman (1972) are hemorrhage, airway obstruction, necrosis or sequestration, infection, and facial nerve disturbance, complications that have not occurred in our own series of cases.

THE DAUTREY MODIFICATION. The Dautrey modification (1975) of the Obwegeser–Dal Pont sagittal split of the ramus was devised to avoid the complications caused by injury or compression of the inferior alveolar nerve.

After exposure of the ramus by subperiosteal elevation as described earlier in the text, a small, round, perforating bur is used to make a line of section 3 mm deep in a horizontal plane through the cortex above the lingula on the medial aspect of the ramus (Fig. 30–44, *A*) and in a vertical direction along the external oblique line. The line of section with the bur is extended forward through the cortex of the lateral aspect of the mandibular body to a point situated between the first and second molars where it turns at a right angle downward

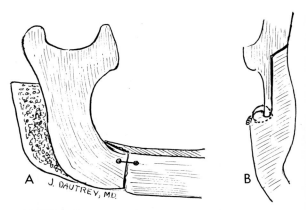

FIGURE 30-47. *A*, Final position of the fragments. An interosseous wire joins the two cortices. *B*, The antero-superior angle of the condylar fragment joins the tooth-bearing fragment in a mortise-like fashion, preventing a lateral displacement and vertical tilt postoperatively.

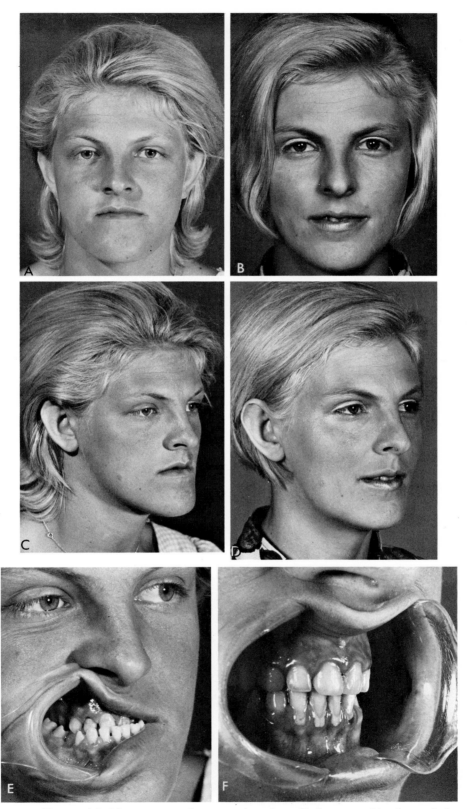

FIGURE 30–48. Change of facial appearance after correction of mandibular prognathism by vertical osteotomy of the ramus. *A, C,* Preoperative facial appearance. *B, D,* Postoperative appearance. *E,* Preoperative occlusal view. *F,* Postoperative occlusal view.

1331

to the lower border of the mandible. The key instrument for the operation is an osteotome which is extremely thin and 5 to 7 mm wide (Fig. 30–45). The sagittal splitting of the ramus is achieved by the osteotome progressing posteriorly at a gradually deeper level in order to follow a plane which is immediately deep to the lateral cortex of the ramus (Fig. 30–44, *D*). To avoid injury to the inferior alveolar neurovascular bundle (Fig. 30–44, *C*), the osteotome must be directed along a plane which is parallel to the lateral cortex (Fig. 30–44, *D*). The line of cleavage is facilitated by the groove already made by the bur. One should avoid any rotation of the osteotome for fear of provoking a fracture of the lateral cortex, which could occur at various levels. The osteotome gradually reaches the posterior and inferior borders of the ramus, where it comes into contact with the retractor which is displaced to follow the various positions of the osteotome. The retractor (Fig. 30–46) has a strong handle and narrow blade so that it can be readily hooked around the posterior border of the ramus. The splitting procedure requires striking the osteotome with a mallet with considerable force; the retractor stabilizes the jaw during the procedure. A suction tip with fiberoptic illumination provides satisfactory visibility during the operation.

Dautrey feels that the use of a circumferential wire to appose the fragments (see Fig. 30–40, *N*) is contraindicated, as it tends to compress the neurovascular bundle. After intermaxillary fixation and resection of the excess bone from the anterior portion of the Dal Pont extension, an interosseous wire joins the cortices of the two fragments. As the condylar fragment is thinner than the tooth-bearing fragment, it is joined to the latter in a mortise-like fashion (Fig. 30–47).

The technique splits the entire ramus anteroposteriorly. Thus the surface of contact between the fragments is maximal, and stability between the fragments is guaranteed; the anterior mortise also provides stabilization of the fragments, preventing any vertical tilt that might produce an anterior open bite postoperatively.

With the Dautrey modification in which the sagittal split occurs lateral to the inferior alveolar canal, the problem of lip paresthesia has been drastically reduced. The chance of direct nerve injury is reduced, since the canal is not grossly violated. The possibility of nerve compression between the two fragments is also eliminated. Over 300 operations have been performed by Dautrey utilizing the technique described. Transitory loss of sensibility or paresthesias for a period of two to three months were noted in 10 per cent of patients; no patient had permanent anesthesia of the lower lip.

Comminution of the condyle-bearing fragment can be a problem. When the ramus is thin and when the Dautrey modification is used, extreme care must be exercised during the osteotomy to avoid this complication. Guernsey and De Champlain (1971) recommend placing the medial horizontal osteotomy closer to the lingula instead of in the thinner subsigmoid region. Neuner (1976) has proposed an oblique sagittal osteotomy through an intraoral approach after subperiosteal exposure of the ramus and identification of the lingula and inferior alevolar neurovascular bundle, performed with a reciprocating saw placed immediately

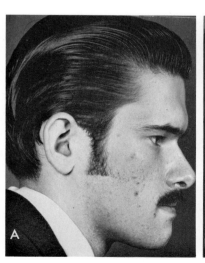
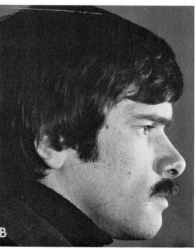

FIGURE 30–49. Mandibular prognathism corrected by vertical osteotomy of the ramus. *A*, Preoperative. *B*, Postoperative.

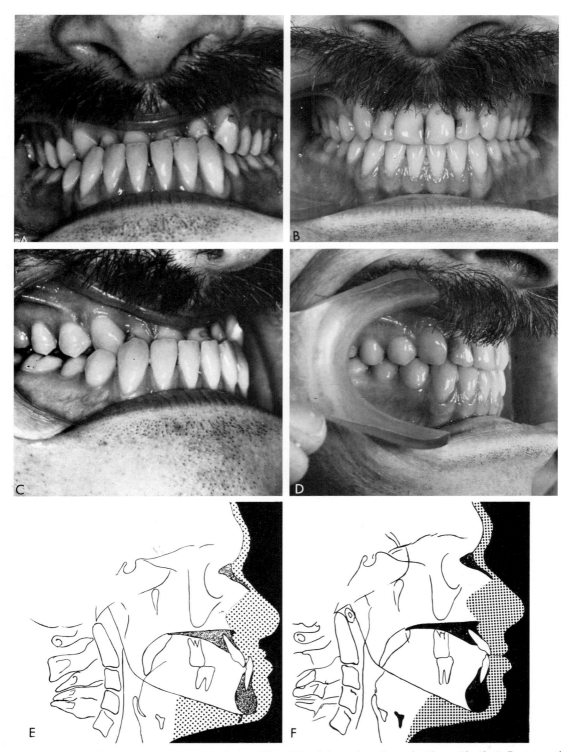

FIGURE 30–50. *A*, Preoperative dental occlusion (Class III) of the patient shown in Figure 30–49. *B*, Postoperative intraoral view. *C*, *D*, Additional views of the occlusion before and after surgical correction. *E*, Preoperative cephalometric tracing. *F*, Postoperative cephalometric tracing.

posterior to the inferior alveolar foramen and above the lingula.

Relapse. Relapse rate following the sagittal split technique is approximately the same as that observed following a vertical ramus section. A one-year cephalometric roentgenographic follow-up study by Egyedi (1965) showed an average relapse of 2 mm.

Results. Examples of patients with mandibular prognathism without anterior open bite whose deformity has been corrected by vertical or oblique osteotomy of the ramus are shown in Figures 30–48 through 30–53. The treatment of mandibular prognathism with anterior open bite is discussed on page 1418. When the maxilla is grossly hypoplastic in a prognathic patient, it must be advanced and the mandible recessed (see p. 1466).

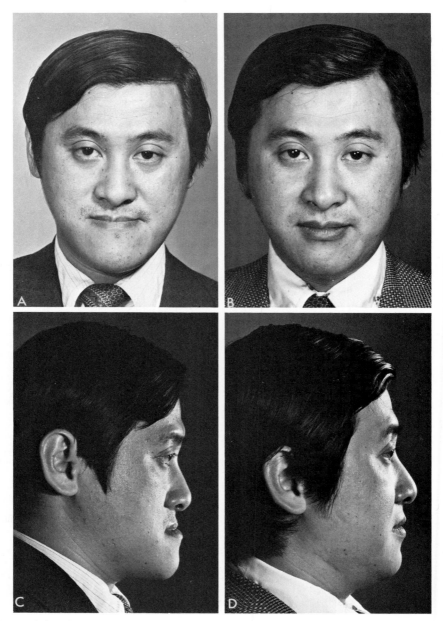

FIGURE 30–51. Oriental prognathic patient corrected by vertical osteotomy of the ramus. *A*, Preoperative full-face appearance. *B*, Postoperative. *C*, Preoperative profile view. *D*, Postoperative.

Treatment of the Edentulous Prognathic Patient. In the edentulous patient, various degrees of diminution of the vertical height of the alveolar process (Fig. 30–54) may complicate the problem of correcting mandibular prognathism. In certain cases the progressive resorption of bone results in exposure of the inferior alveolar nerve (Fig. 30–54, *C*). This condition makes it impossible for the patient to wear a denture and requires reconstruction of

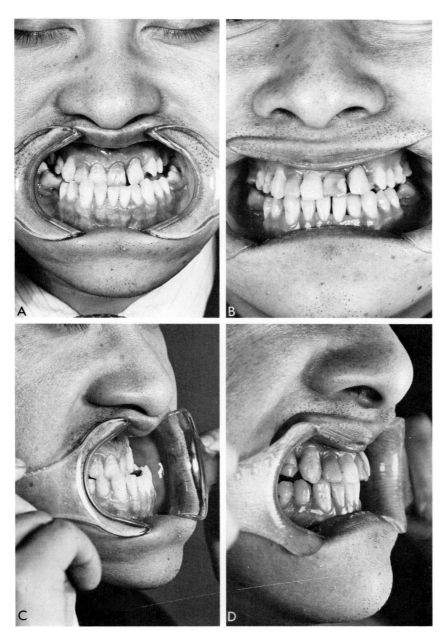

FIGURE 30–52. *A*, Preoperative intraoral view of the patient shown in Figure 30–51. *B*, Postoperative frontal view. *C*, Preoperative lateral view of the occlusion. *D*, Postoperative. *E*, Preoperative cephalometric tracing. *F*, Postoperative cephalometric tracing.

Illustration continued on the following page

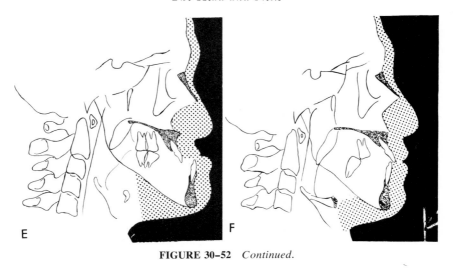

FIGURE 30–52 *Continued.*

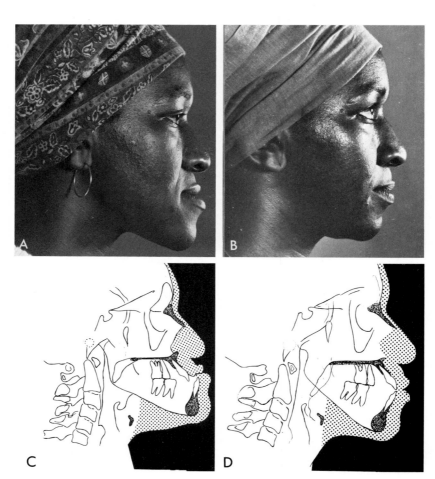

FIGURE 30–53. African prognathic patient corrected by vertical osteotomy of the ramus. *A*, Preoperative appearance. *B*, Postoperative. *C*, Preoperative cephalometric tracing. *D*, Postoperative cephalometric tracing.

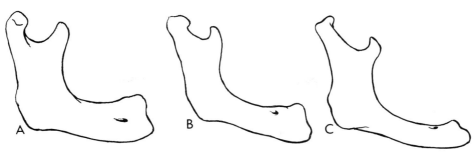

FIGURE 30–54. Progressive loss of height of the body of the mandible in the edentulous jaw. (After Grant, 1951.)

the alveolar process to cover the nerve and provide a retentive alveolar process for the denture (see Fig. 30–254, p. 1508).

In the moderately prognathic edentulous patient, the prosthodontist can usually provide efficient dentures to compensate for the faulty relationship of the alveolar processes. Surgical correction is required, however, when mandibular prognathism is more severe (Figs. 30–55 and 30–56). According to the deformity, the

techniques of mandibular body or ramus osteotomy are indicated. While the ramus approach is preferable, mandibular body osteotomy has its indications.

The mental foramen and the lateral surface of the body of the mandible are exposed. When the inferior alveolar nerve in an edentulous mandible is being exposed prior to the osteotomy, a practical consideration to bear in mind is the superficial position of the mental fora-

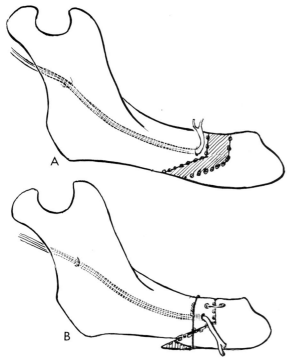

FIGURE 30–55. Technique for the correction of mandibular prognathism in the edentulous patient. *A,* Resection of bone after reverse L-shaped osteotomy of the body of the mandible. *B,* Circumferential wiring is used to immobilize the fragments after the excess bone is resected. (After Kazanjian.)

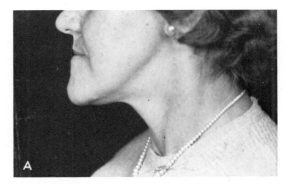

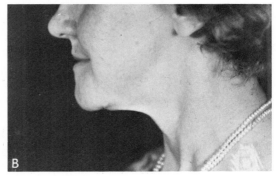

FIGURE 30–56. Mandibular prognathism in an edentulous patient treated by body section. *A,* Edentulous patient with mandibular prognathism. *B,* Result obtained after resection of bone from the body of the mandible, as illustrated in Figure 30–55.

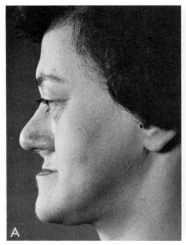
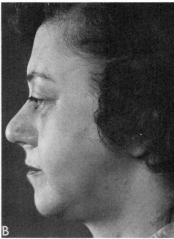

FIGURE 30–57. Mandibular prognathism in an edentulous patient treated by ramus section. *A*, Preoperative profile view. *B*, Result obtained after bilateral section of the ramus. The patient's upper denture was maintained in craniofacial fixation by internal suspension wires. The lower denture was maintained in intermaxillary fixation with the upper denture and circumferential wiring was used to fix it to the mandible.

men and inferior alveolar nerve due to resorption of the alveolar process.

A square section of alveolar bone of predetermined size is removed. The anterior segment is then recessed into its new position. Interosseous wires are used to secure the fragments.

Figure 30–57, *A* shows an edentulous patient with mandibular prognathism in whom the deformity was corrected by bilateral osteotomies of the ramus. The patient had worn dentures over a number of years. Preliminary studies had shown that satisfactory jaw relationships could be obtained by bilateral vertical section of the ramus. The patient's dentures were used as fixation splints. The upper denture was maintained in fixation by internal perizygomatic suspension wiring and the lower denture by circumferential wiring. A satisfactory correction was obtained (Fig. 30–57, *B*).

Children and Adolescents with Prognathism. Adolescent patients with prognathic tendencies show a rapid accentuation of mandibular prominence soon after the eruption of the permanent teeth. The deformity becomes more striking as the facial bones, particularly the mandible, attain full development. Immediate improvement results if the deformity is corrected by early surgery. The growth of the mandible, however, is not arrested. Thus recurrence of the prognathism can be anticipated with further growth, although to a lesser degree than before the operation (Fig. 30–58).

Children with extreme prognathism and an inadequate masticatory mechanism should not be neglected. A corrective procedure should be recommended with the understanding that additional corrective surgery will be required after completion of mandibular growth. A ramus operation is followed by a second definitive surgical intervention after the completion of growth. A body section cannot be performed in children because of the presence of unerupted teeth.

Mandibular Prognathism with Open Bite. This type of mandibular deformity presents special problems of treatment. These will be discussed after the section of this chapter concerned with the treatment of open bite (see p. 1418).

Mandibular Prognathism with Microgenia. It seems paradoxical that the large protruding jaw of the prognathic patient can be microgenic. The large size of the jaw does not preclude an inadequate development of the mental symphysis—hence the anomalous clinical situation of a patient whose prognathism has been corrected and who requires one of the procedures for increase in chin projection described on page 1385.

Choice of Procedure in the Correction of Prognathism. The advantages of sectioning the ramus are that (1) it is usually a relatively simple operative procedure; (2) when it is correctly performed, there is no interference with the conduction of the inferior alveolar nerve; and (3) greater efficiency in mastication is obtained, since the teeth are not sacrificed. The latter is the most important factor in favor of the ramus approach.

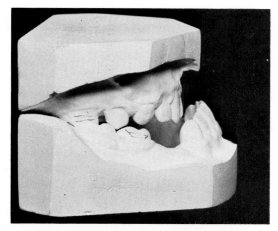

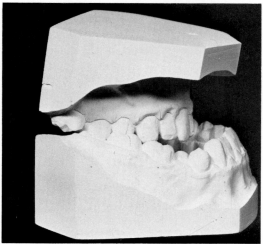

FIGURE 30–58. The upper set of casts shows the dentoalveolar relationships in a 12 year old boy with mandibular prognathism. The lower dental models are of the same patient at the age of 16 years; the distance between the upper and lower incisors has increased by 5 mm. (From Kazanjian, V. H.: The surgical treatment of prognathism. An analysis of sixty-five cases. Am. J. Surg., *87*:691, 1954.)

The body section techniques are indicated in cases of mandibular prognathism with severe disparity between the mandibular and maxillary arch forms and in some cases of anterior open bite deformity. Body section techniques allow changes to be made in (1) a selective segmental vertical direction, (2) arch length, and (3) arch width. A better mandibular arch can be obtained in the severely prognathic and hypertrophied jaw as a result of reducing jaw size and modifying the curve of the dental arch.

Disadvantages of the osteotomies through the body of the mandible include a more laborious surgical procedure, the possibility of nonunion, danger of injury to the inferior alveolar nerve, the sacrifice of teeth, and possible postoperative wound infection, a rare complication with contemporary surgical techniques and antibiotic coverage. If the resection of bone is carefully planned, the chances of inadequate bony contact and nonconsolidation are slight. After a period of approximately eight to ten weeks, in the rare case in which there is no evidence of consolidation, the area can be reinforced by bone chips and a thin onlay graft of iliac bone. If during the operation the area of contact between the fragments appears to be insufficiently intimate to ensure consolidation, chips of bone from the resected segments of the mandible can also be inserted into the defect at the ostectomy site.

Injury to the inferior alveolar nerve can be avoided if the resection is done anterior to the mental foramen and the inferior alveolar canal is not penetrated. In body osteotomies posterior to the mental foramen, adequate exposure will reduce the risk of nerve injury.

Body osteotomy procedures can be used advantageously in selected patients with missing teeth. As previously stated, many prognathic patients are partially edentulous. The gaps in the dental arch are convenient sites for osteotomies and bone resection; after reduction of the length of the body, the gaps are closed and the continuity of the dentition is restored.

One of the objections to the ramus osteotomy has been that the normal line of action of the powerful muscles of mastication is disrupted. It is not possible to push the mandible back to any great degree without completely changing the line of pull and function of these muscles. This problem has been resolved by subperiosteal elevation of the muscles from their insertions on the medial and lateral aspects of the ramus and, on rare occasions, section of the base of the coronoid process to release the traction of the temporalis muscle.

In certain cases of extreme prognathism, the posterior displacement can result in excessive retrusion of the posterior border of the ramus with impingement on the facial nerve. The hazard is eliminated by resecting the retruding posterior border of the ramus or removing a wedge of bone at the osteotomy site (Van Zile, 1963).

Because the sagittal split of the ramus (Obwegesser–Dal Pont procedure) is frequently complicated by loss of sensibility in the lower lip, the Dautrey modification is promising, since it minimizes the chance of producing permanent lip paresthesia. It can also be employed for advancement procedures and in favorable cases of anterior open bite (see prognathism with open bite in the section of this chapter concerning open bite deformities, p. 1418).

The sagittal split procedure is advantageous in that it causes only a minimal disturbance of the position of the condyle; the vertical section results in an outward rotation of the condyle in the glenoid fossa. Nevertheless, clinical observation of any dysfunction of the temporomandibular joint as a result of this rotation is rare. This finding is attributed to the ability of the condyle to adapt and remodel itself (Ware and Taylor, 1968).

The choice between an extraoral and an intraoral approach is determined by the possible contraindication of an external scar. In the patient who is predisposed to hypertrophic scars or keloids, the external incision is contraindicated. Female patients may object to an external scar; an intraoral approach is favored in such cases. In the muscular male patient with hypertrophied masseter muscles or in patients with limited opening of the mouth, an intraoral procedure on the ramus is technically difficult. Retraction of the soft tissue and muscles is difficult, and the exposure of the bone is poor. In this group of patients, the vertical osteotomy through an external approach is the technique of choice.

An additional advantage of the external approach is that antibiotic coverage can be dispensed with. Zallen and Strader (1971) are of the opinion that prophylactic antibiotics are not warranted when the extraoral approach is employed.

Regardless of the technique employed, gratifying restoration of facial balance and harmony is obtained. The stigma of aggressiveness and belligerence associated with the face having a prominent lower jaw is eliminated. Natural fullness of both lips is obtained, and the upper lip assumes a more adequate length and anteroposterior position (Knowles, 1965; Aaronson, 1967). For psychologic reasons, prognathic patients tend to hold their heads in a forwardly inclined position to minimize the chin prominence (Fromm and Lungberg, 1970). Postoperatively, the head is carried in a more normal upright position. Even with the change in the suprahyoid muscle posture, the hyoid bone position remains the same (Takagi, Gamble, Proffit and Christensen, 1967), and disturbances in respiration, swallowing, and speech do not occur.

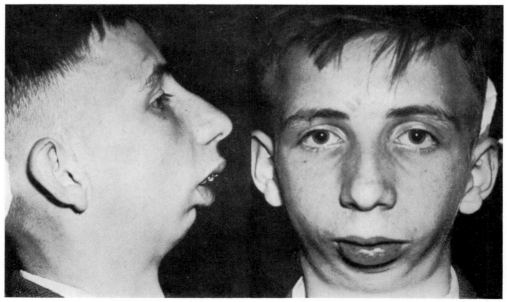

FIGURE 30–59. Typical appearance of mandibular micrognathia with temporomandibular ankylosis. Patient had fallen on his chin at the age of 2 years. (From Kazanjian and Converse.)

Mandibular Micrognathia and Retrognathism

From its Greek derivation, the term *micrognathia* signifies a small jaw. The micrognathic mandible is usually in retrusion in relation to the upper jaw. *Mandibular hypoplasia* results in a small mandible due to failure of growth and development (micrognathia). *Retrognathism* is used to describe a jaw that is posteriorly displaced. The use of the term *mandibular atresia* should be discouraged; atresia, derived from the Greek, means "no perforation." Because of the characteristic appearance of the face, the Germans have used the term *Vogelgesicht* (bird-face) to describe micrognathia. In the United States, the deformity is familiarly referred to as the "Andy Gump" facies because of its identification with the well-known car-

toon personality. The prominence of the lower third of the face is absent; the anteroposterior dimension is decreased, and the height of the lower face is shortened. Excessive forward and downward displacement of the anterior maxillary teeth and the nose and, in some cases, an accumulation of soft tissue under the micrognathic mandible complete the bird-like profile (Figs. 30–59 and 30–60).

ETIOLOGY

Micrognathia can be classified according to its etiology as congenital, developmental, or acquired.

One of the most frequent causes of *congenital* micrognathia is maldevelopment of the first and second branchial arches. Involvement can be unilateral, affecting only one ramus or the

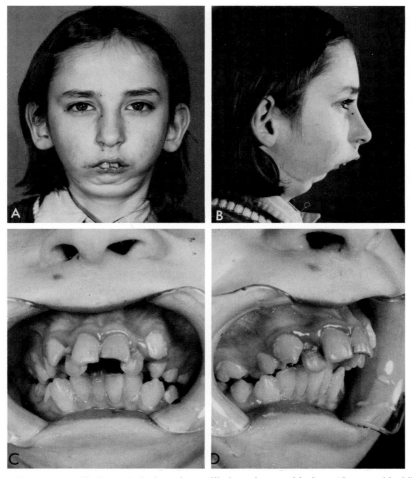

FIGURE 30–60.   Temporomandibular ankylosis and mandibular micrognathia in a 10 year old child. *A, B,* Typical micrognathic appearance. *C, D,* Intraoral views.

body of the mandible, or bilateral, the entire mandible being symmetrically underdeveloped. A relatively frequent deformity of the congenital type is observed in bilateral craniofacial microsomia (Chapter 54) and in mandibulofacial dysostosis (Chapter 55). In association with auricular malformation, underdevelopment of one or both sides of the skull is characteristic; the mastoid process and the petrous bone are poorly developed, and the middle ear bones are malformed. The condyle, ramus, and body are small; the condyle is situated in a medial position in relation to the infratemporal surface (see Chapter 54). Micrognathia of the Robin anomalad type may be the result of intrauterine compression; it is the only type of micrognathia which is usually self-correcting during the postnatal period (see Chapter 50). Fetal maldevelopment of the condylar region can result in temporomandibular ankylosis in the newborn. Agenesis of the temporomandibular joint, a rare condition with congenital absence of the ramus, has been observed in severe forms of craniofacial microsomia.

The *developmental* type of mandibular micrognathia is probably more frequent than is usually assumed. Injury by the application of forceps at birth can result in compression of the temporomandibular region and subsequent ankylosis. A fall in infancy can cause damage to the condyle and impair mandibular growth. Temporomandibular ankylosis adds a functional disability to the deformity. Causes other than trauma also interfere with condylar growth—for example, rheumatoid arthritis or suppurative disease originating in the mastoid process, and extending into the temporomandibular joint, a complication less frequent since the advent of antibiotics. The injudicious use of radiation therapy is another source of condylar growth arrest.

Acquired mandibular micrognathia is produced by bone resection for tumor or by the loss of bone due to a gunshot injury, when the fragments are allowed to collapse and the anterior portion of the mandibular arch is displaced posteriorly; on occasion, the arch is actually resected or destroyed.

VARIATIONS OF MANDIBULAR MICROGNATHIA AND THE ASSOCIATED FUNCTIONAL DISTURBANCES

Deficiencies in the length as well as the width of the ramus and the body characterize man-

dibular micrognathia. The degree of involvement of the ramus or body or both varies; unilateral and bilateral deformities occur.

When the deformity is *bilateral*, generalized micrognathia is observed (see Figs. 30–59 and 30–60). The mandibular body is short and often thick and shows a characteristic accentuated antegonial notch. The height of the ramus is decreased, and the condyles are deformed. In a number of patients in whom the condyles had been eliminated as sequestra during a septic episode in infancy or in whom there was agenesis of the ramus, the mandible articulates with the skull by means of the coronoid processes.

The chin of a patient with bilateral micrognathia is usually in retrusion in the midsagittal plane. The chin eminence is small and indistinct. The lower lip is retracted downward and is often unable to form a seal with the upper lip. Lip posture can be improved by orthodontic treatment and, occasionally, by surgical retraction of the anterior maxillary dentoalveolar arch. The anterior teeth of the retruded mandible are more posterior and lingual to their maxillary counterparts; the anterior mandibular teeth are usually inclined labially.

Interference with the growth of one side of the mandible, the consequence of *unilateral* injury, occurs more frequently than bilateral impairment of growth and hypoplasia. Although the initial site of disturbance is confined to one side, the entire mandible is eventually affected. The affected side of the mandible is shorter, and the chin is deviated toward the shortened side. The unaffected side of the mandible is flat and appears to be the deformed portion to an uninitiated observer (Fig. 30–61). The disparity in length of the two halves of the body of the mandible is evident when measurements from the midpoint of the chin to the mandibular angle are made.

The degree of deformity in mandibular micrognathia depends upon the age at which the injury to the growth centers has occurred: the earlier the injury, the greater the ensuing deformity. The asymmetry is clinically insignificant in early childhood, but it becomes more apparent as growth progresses. When the jaw is severely retruded, the patient suffers a serious disfigurement.

External facial asymmetry, due to the disproportionate growth of the two halves of the mandible, is accompanied by disturbed dental occlusion. The malocclusion is generally of the Angle Class II, division 1 type. Laterognathism and posterior cross bite are usually present.

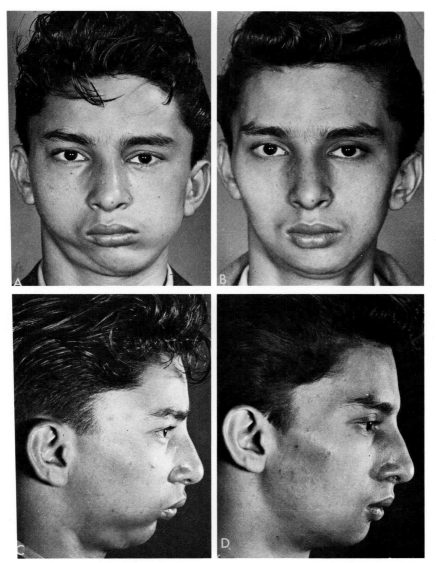

FIGURE 30–61. Developmental malformation of the mandible due to arrested growth on the left side as a result of a fall in childhood. *A*, The unaffected right side is flat and can be mistaken for the deformed side. *B*, Appearance following corrective mandibular surgery. *C*, Preoperative profile. *D*, Postoperative profile. See Figure 30–62 for the type of surgical osteotomy employed. (From Converse, J. M., and Shapiro, H. H.: Treatment of developmental malformations of the jaws. Plast. Reconstr. Surg., *10*:473, 1952. Copyright 1952, The Williams & Wilkins Company, Baltimore.)

Disparity of ramus height is also a feature of unilateral underdevelopment of the mandible, the ramus on the affected side being shorter than the ramus on the unaffected side. The shortness of the ramus is obvious; the mandibular angle on the affected side is situated at a higher level and in some cases is poorly defined. The commissure of the mouth is elevated in repose. Intraoral examination shows that the occlusal plane is inclined to-ward the maxilla on the affected side, assuming an oblique cant. The body of the mandible curves upward to meet the short ramus.

When temporomandibular ankylosis complicates the deformity, a serious functional disability is added to the micrognathia. Restoration of temporomandibular function is a necessary preliminary operative procedure before reconstruction of the micrognathic jaw is undertaken. The ankylosis is relieved as early as possible in the child. However, relief of the ankylosis, although it does restore motion, does not solve all the patient's functional problems. Effective mastication does not result if the mandibular teeth are in a position excessively posterior to the maxillary teeth, nor can the problem of mastication be effectively solved by dentures in edentulous patients. The mandible must be elongated surgically to reestablish satisfactory relationships between the maxillary and mandibular arches and efficient masticatory function.

Restoration of chin contour by a skin graft inlay and a downward extension of the denture is a compromise method of treatment, but one that is justifiable in patients of the older age group (see Chapter 67). Contour restoration by bone grafts or other types of transplants is another compromise procedure, since the occlusal problem remains. In unilateral micrognathia, contour-restoring grafts recapture symmetry of the face in repose. Asymmetry reappears, however, when the mouth is opened. The chin swings over to the short side of the mandible, not only because the mandible is shorter on that side but also because of the loss of the propulsive function of the lateral pterygoid muscle.

TREATMENT OF MANDIBULAR MICROGNATHIA

Surgical elongation of the body of the mandible restores jaw relationships, corrects the asymmetry in unilateral cases, and improves the appearance of the patient. When a normal complement of teeth is present, dental occlusion is improved, and masticatory efficiency is increased.

Early Surgical-Orthodontic Planning. Early consultation with the orthodontist eliminates later misunderstandings. One should particularly avoid and advise against untimely orthodontic therapy which modifies the position of the dentition to conform to the malformed mandible and greatly complicates subsequent surgical treatment. Little is gained by the achievement of a satisfactory occlusion between the teeth if the body of the jaw remains malformed. Later surgical procedures to elongate the mandible will, of necessity, produce malocclusion. Such ill-advised presurgical orthodontic treatment could be avoided by early coordinated observation and planning by both orthodontist and the surgeon. Only the in-

dicated orthodontic therapy should be done prior to the surgery.

Preoperative Planning. Diagnosis and planning of surgical correction begins with the clinical examination of the patient. A number of laboratory records are required to plan the surgical strategy. These include photographs, cephalometric roentgenograms, and dental study models.

The clinical examination and the photographs are helpful in studying the soft tissue contour deficiency and the condition of the intraoral structures. The following must be particularly noted: (1) the vertical and horizontal facial balance and the patient's customary head posture; (2) the lateral shifting of the chin point when the mandible is depressed or elevated, movements indicative of temporomandibular joint dysfunction or neuromotor disability; (3) the orofacial musculature in repose and while functioning; (4) the condition of the soft tissues of the mouth, especially with respect to soft

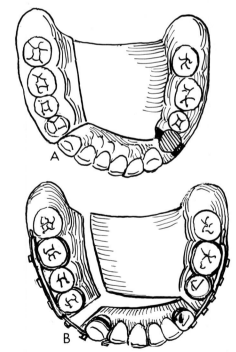

FIGURE 30–62. Planning the osteotomies on the dental casts of the patient shown in Figure 30–61. *A*, Casts are sectioned, advanced, and rotated to correct the jaw and occlusal relationships. Wax is used to join the fragments and represents the amount of advancement required. *B*, Note the larger amount of advancement that is necessary on the right side and the lesser amount required on the left side.

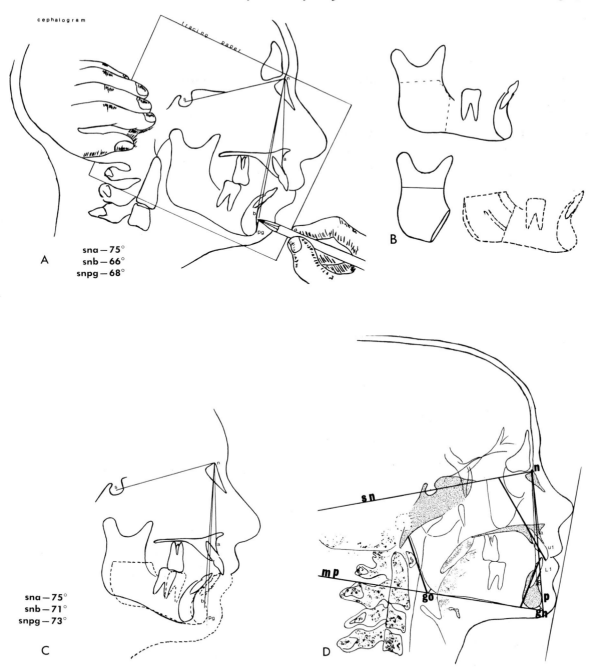

FIGURE 30–63. Cephalometric planning for mandibular advancement by a sagittal-split osteotomy of the ramus for the correction of mandibular micrognathia with retrusion and anterior open bite. *A*, Tracing of the cephalogram. Note the anterior open bite. Angles SNA and SNB confirm the mandibular retrusion. Note the preoperative angular measurements. *B*, Projected sagittal-split osteotomy of the ramus (*above*); the separated segments are shown (*below*). *C*, The medial tooth-bearing segment indicated by the broken-line tracing has been advanced and rotated to achieve the planned occlusal and skeletal relationships. Note the postoperative angular measurements. *D*, Final contour and occlusal relationships.

tissue lesions and periodontal disease. Retouched matte-finished photographs provide an opportunity to project the desired alteration in integumental contour.

The dentoalveolar relationships observed on the clinical examination are analyzed in detail using dental casts. The casts provide a record of arch length, width, and form, as well as of individual tooth position and occlusal relation-ships. Duplicate working casts are cut to sim-ulate the lines of osteotomy.

In mandibular micrognathia, as in mandibu-lar prognathism, an essential guide in preopera-tive planning is the condition of the dentition. A decision must be made as to whether ade-quate dental occlusal relationships between the mandible and the maxilla can be rees-tablished by osteotomies through the mandibu-lar ramus, the body, or both. The anterior portion of the sectioned dental working cast is

relocated to the desired position. The sections are then joined with dental wax (Fig. 30–62). The wax represents with reasonable accuracy the amount of elongation required. The sec-tioned cast can be mounted on a dental articu-lator; in most cases, however, comparison be-tween the permanent study cast and the work-ing cast provides sufficiently accurate in-formation.

In asymmetrical deformities, a greater amount of elongation is required on one side, and in some cases of mandibular asymmetry,

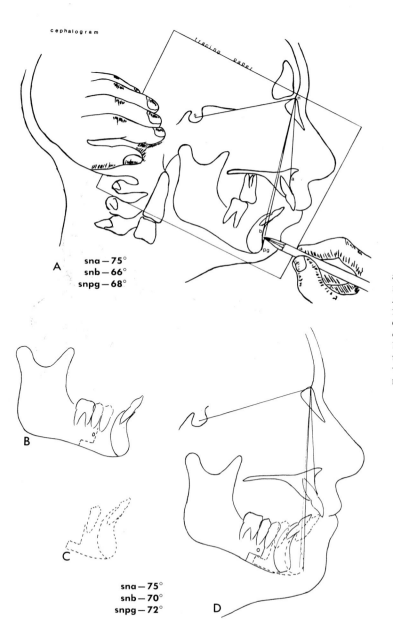

FIGURE 30–64. Cephalometric tracing and cut-out for surgical planning in micrognathia using a body osteotomy. *A,* Tracing of the osseous outline made from the cephalogram. *B,* The pattern is cut at the site of the proposed elongation osteotomy. *C,* Cut out of the portion to be advanced. *D,* The anterior portion of the cut pattern is shifted and rotated for-ward into a position improving the dental relationships and the facial contour.

the contralateral side must be shortened to achieve symmetry. Realignment to the mid-sagittal plane is used as a guide in positioning the anterior segment. In addition, a postero-anterior cephalometric roentgenogram can be used to determine the change required in the position of the chin point.

Cephalograms allow study of the skeletal deformity, as well as of the relationship of the overlying soft tissues to the osseous structures. The degree of mandibular retrusion is measured by the SNB angle; SNB values will be less than normal. The plane extending through the axis of the upper central incisor tooth is designated as UI; the plane extending through the axis of the lower central incisor tooth is labeled LI. The maxillary and mandibular anterior teeth are usually protruded. This is reflected by the increased angles of UI-SN and LI-MP, respectively. The cephalometric technique is illustrated in Figure 30–63.

The cephalometric roentgenogram is also of considerable assistance in determining the final position of the fragments following the osteotomy. The new facial contour can be estimated by tracing both the soft and hard tissue outlines (Fig. 30–63, *D*).

When the correction of mandibular micrognathia with retrusion and anterior open bite (Fig. 30–63, *A*) is being planned, cephalometric analysis will assist in confirming the correction that can be achieved by a sagittal split osteotomy of the ramus (Fig. 30–63, *B*). The tracing is cut, and the anterior portion is rotated into a forward position to simulate the amount of advancement and rotation required to correct the deformity.

If the cephalometric analysis and the clinical findings indicate that an elongation osteotomy of the body of the mandible is indicated, the tracing is sectioned and the anterior portion of the body of the mandible is advanced to restore harmonious occlusal relationships with the maxillary teeth (Fig. 30–64).

Further contour restoration may be required—a horizontal advancement osteotomy of the inferior portion of the mandible combined with bone grafting, for example (see p. 1387).

When a nasal plastic operation or chin recontouring procedure is indicated to improve the patient's profile, a tracing of the correction should be made to assess its influence on the projected facial profile (see Fig. 30–10).

A panoramic roentgenogram is a valuable document, especially in patients who have an associated temporomandibular ankylosis.

Throughout the preoperative planning period, the orthodontist and the prosthodontist should be consulted. The cephalometric analysis, the timing of orthodontic movement of the teeth, the spot grinding of interfering cusps, and the type of fixation appliances indicated require discussion.

An important part of the treatment planning is the choice of the site of osteotomy, as well as the choice of the type of osteotomy and the surgical approach to the mandible. The anterior maxillary alveolar process and teeth, unopposed by the retruded mandibular teeth, tend to drift forward and downward. A segmental maxillary set-back (see p. 1428) may be indicated as a procedure either preliminary or subsequent to the mandibular surgery.

Elongation Osteotomies of the Body of the Mandible: General Considerations. The line of osteotomy ˙and its location in the body of the mandible vary according to the deformity and the status of the dentition. Various types of osteotomy are available (Fig. 30–65), but the basic associated problems common to all body lengthening osteotomies require further consideration.

The surgical problems involved in the mandibular body osteotomies include (1) maintenance of contact between the bony fragments to ensure consolidation; (2) preservation of the continuity of the inferior alveolar neurovascular bundle; and (3) provision of soft tissue coverage over the area of the elongation osteotomy.

MAINTENANCE OF CONTACT OF THE BONY FRAGMENTS. The L-osteotomy (Fig. 30–65, *A* to *D*), the step osteotomy (Fig. 30–65, *E* to *H*), or sagittal splitting of the mandibular body (Fig. 30–66) are preferable to the vertical line osteotomy because they provide an increased area of contact between the fragments. Maintenance of contact between the fragments is ensured by the fixation appliance and direct interosseous or circumferential wiring. If the surface of contact between the bone fragments is inadequate, bone grafts are placed in the line of osteotomy to facilitate consolidation.

PRESERVATION OF THE INFERIOR ALVEOLAR NEUROVASCULAR BUNDLE. The inferior alveolar nerve divides into two terminal branches, the mental and incisive nerves. The mental nerve exits from the mental foramen and divides into three branches which provide the sensory innervation to the skin of the chin and the mucous membrane and skin of the lower lip. The other terminal branch, the incisive nerve, is an anterior extension of the nerve within the mandible. It supplies the sen-

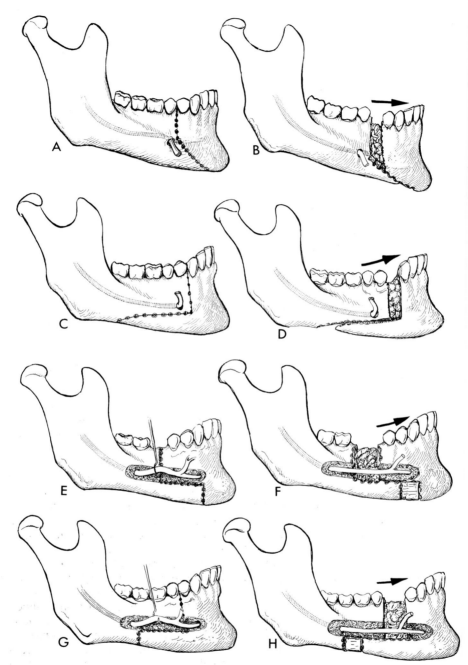

FIGURE 30–65. Four variations of osteotomy lines to lengthen the body of the mandible. *A*, L-osteotomy placed anterior to the mental foramen. *B*, Elongation obtained by the L-osteotomy. Iliac bone chips fill the resulting gap. *C*, The reverse L-osteotomy is a preferred technique for elongation of the body of the mandible. It is designed in the shape of an L resting on its back. *D*, Elongation obtained by the reverse L-osteotomy. *E*, Step osteotomy placed posterior to the mental foramen with exposure of the inferior alveolar neurovascular bundle. *F*, Elongation obtained by the step osteotomy. A bone graft is wedged into the gap along the lower border of the mandible, and bone chips are placed in the upper gap. *G*, Reverse step osteotomy with exposure and preservation of the main trunk and also the incisive branch of the inferior alveolar nerve. *H*, Elongation obtained by the reverse step osteotomy.

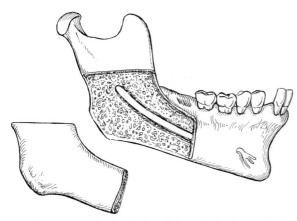

FIGURE 30-66. Sagittal splitting of the body of the mandible and ramus prior to the osteotomies required in a complex deformity. The outer table of the bone is removed, exposing the inferior alveolar neurovascular bundle which is protected as the mandible is divided. (After Obwegeser.)

sory innervation to the canine and incisor teeth. Whereas tearing or sectioning the mental nerve at the mental foramen results in permanent loss of sensibility of half of the lower lip, section of the incisive nerve abolishes the sensibility of the anterior teeth, a complication of little clinical significance.

The mental foramen is the landmark used to determine the position of the osteotomy. Osteotomy of the body of the mandible is preferably made anterior and inferior to the mental foramen, and the step osteotomy is completed by a horizontal or oblique osteotomy below the level of the inferior alveolar nerve and canal (see Fig. 30-65, *C*, *D*). The incisive nerve is sectioned, but the mental nerve is preserved. However, when an osteotomy through the body must be done posterior to the mental foramen, the inferior alveolar neurovascular bundle must be exposed to avoid severing it.

Gaps in the dental arch due to missing teeth offer a convenient site for the line of osteotomy, as possible injury to the adjacent teeth is avoided. When the osteotomy line is located posterior to the mental foramen (see Fig. 30-65, *E*, *F*), continuity of the nerve is preserved by the following technique. The outer cortical plate, posterior to the mental foramen, is removed by a motor-driven large round bur or by an osteotome. The nerve is thus decompressed. When a wide area must be exposed, the sagittal splitting technique affords the greatest exposure (see Fig. 30-66). The resected outer cortex is replaced over the inferior alveolar canal after the procedure is completed. Care should be taken to avoid compression of

the nerve. When the osteotomy is performed anterior to the mental foramen, the conduction of the inferior alveolar nerve and of the mental nerve is generally preserved. Loss of sensibility in the anterior teeth has not been a cause of complaint on the part of the patients. When the osteotomy is performed posterior to the mental foramen, decompression of the nerve may suffice to preserve conduction when the lengthening of the mandibular body is moderate. If, however, tension on the nerve becomes evident when considerable advancement is required, two techniques can be employed to decrease tension and prevent the loss of nerve conduction. The first is complete decompression of the neurovascular bundle from the mental foramen to the area of osteotomy; the second method, indicated in cases requiring greater lengthening, is nerve grafting. The inferior alveolar nerve is separated from the vessels using visual magnification with binocular loupes or the operating microscope (Hausamen, Samii

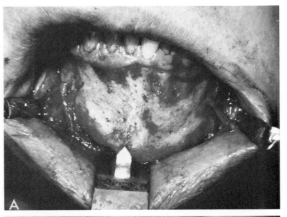

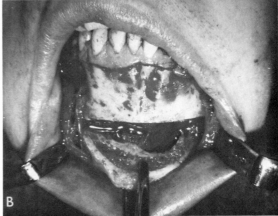

FIGURE 30-67. The degloving procedure. *A*, Exposure obtained by the degloving technique. Note that the mental nerves have been liberated from the soft tissues. *B*, The lower portion of the mandible has been sectioned by a horizontal osteotomy and is being advanced.

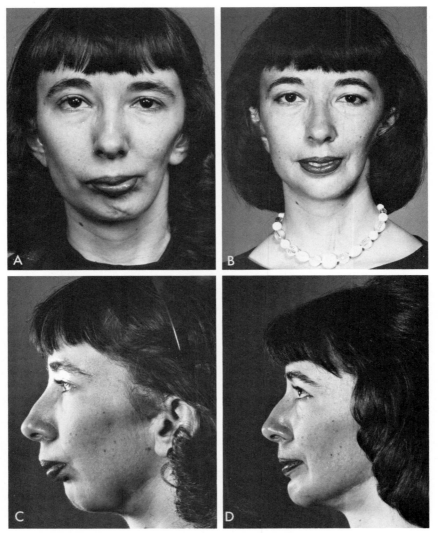

FIGURE 30–68.   Micrognathia resulting from irradiation of the left side of the mandible in childhood. *A*, Appearance of the patient with micrognathia and considerable shortening of the left half of the mandible. *B*, Postoperative appearance following bilateral osteotomy and bone grafting of the body of the mandible through the intraoral approach. *C*, Preoperative profile. *D*, Postoperative profile showing elongation of the body of the mandible. (From Converse, J. M.: Micrognathia. Br. J. Plast. Surg., *16*:197, 1963.)

and Schmidsetter, 1973). The nerve is sectioned and allowed to retract, and a nerve graft is sutured to the sectioned ends of the nerve, applying Millesi's tension-free principle (see Chapter 76).

PRESERVATION OF SOFT TISSUE COVERAGE. The best technique of exposure is the degloving procedure (Fig. 30–67). The major portion of the body is exposed, and preservation of the mental nerves is facilitated. Detachment of the suprahyoid musculature, which resists the mandibular advancement, is advisable. An ex-

cellent surgical access to the bone for the osteotomy is provided.

The labiobuccal vestibular incision, made well above the cul-de-sac of the sulcus and continued backward over the inner aspect of the cheek, provides ample tissue to ensure coverage in the average elongation osteotomy and is preferable to the gingival incision. The rigid gingival tissue is more difficult to suture under tension and is apt to tear.

When an unusual amount of elongation is required (Figs. 30–68 and 30–69), adjacent

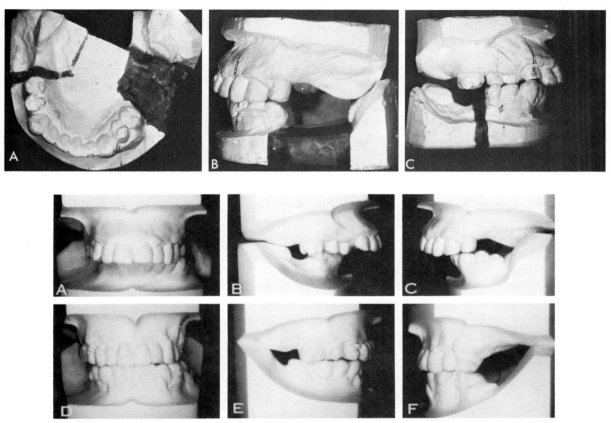

FIGURE 30–69. *Above,* Planning the osteotomies on the dental casts of the patient shown in Figure 30–68. The casts are sectioned, advanced, and rotated to correct the jaw and occlusal relationships. Wax is used to join the fragments and represents the amount of advancement required. Note the larger amount of advancement that is necessary on the left side and the lesser amount required on the right side.

Below, Dental casts showing the occlusal relationships. *A, B, C,* Preoperative occlusal relationships of the patient shown in Figure 30–68. *D, E, F,* Postoperative relationships.

soft tissue must be used to cover the area of the osteotomy or the bone graft interposed between the fragments. Usually, as in the patient shown in Figure 30–68, the portion of the body to be elongated is edentulous. If the resulting bony defect is extensive, sufficient bony contact cannot be expected between the fragments if an L-shaped or step osteotomy is used; a bone graft must be interposed (see also the planning of the mandibular lengthening in Fig. 30–62).

Prior to the osteotomy of the mandibular body (Fig. 30–70, *A*), a wide, rectangular, cheek-based flap is outlined which will overlap the grafted area (Fig. 30–70, *B*). The distal portion of the flap extends from the floor of the mouth and includes the mucoperiosteum over the bone and the mucosa of the sulcus and cheek. The base of the flap is on the cheek wall below the parotid duct orifice. The flap is raised, exposing the mandible. The mandible is sectioned and elongated; the fragments are placed in their new position, and the resulting gap is filled with an iliac bone graft (Fig. 30–70, *C, D*). The flap is drawn lingually and sutured in position (Fig. 30–70, *E, F*). To avoid tension, the buccal sulcus is bridged and thus temporarily obliterated (Fig. 30–70, *E* to *H*). The fragments are immobilized by intermaxillary fixation. Primary healing is expected if the flap has been designed wide enough to ensure coverage and if tension is avoided. After the bone graft has healed, a new buccal sulcus is established by the skin or mucosa inlay technique, which restores an alveolar ridge for the support of a denture (see Fig. 30–251).

A transposition flap of mucoperiosteum and vestibular mucous membrane is another technique for providing coverage of the exposed

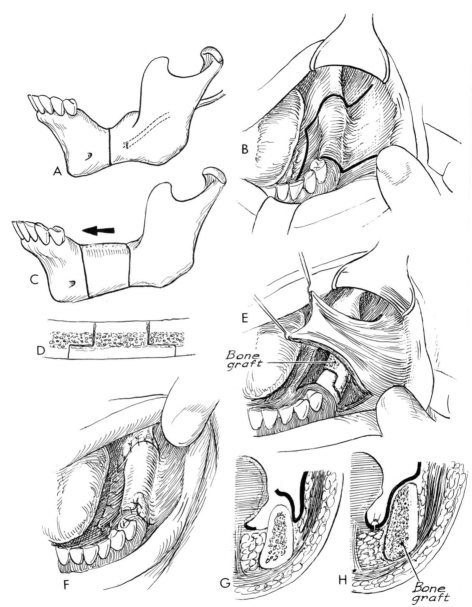

FIGURE 30–70.   Covering a bone graft when an unusual amount of elongation is required. *A*, The line of osteotomy of the body of the mandible is indicated. *B*, Outlining of the cheek-based flap which is raised prior to the osteotomy. *C*, The bone graft in position after the mandible has been lengthened. *D*, Cross section illustrating the greater surface of contact with the host bone achieved by the overlapping flanges of the bone grafts. *E*, Mucosal flap is advanced over the grafted area. *F*, Suturing is completed. *G*, Frontal section illustrating the flap being raised prior to the osteotomy. *H*, Flap sutured in position to cover the bone graft. The buccal sulcus is obliterated and will be restored at a later date by the skin graft inlay technique.

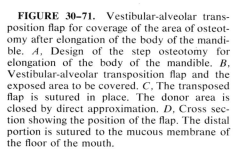

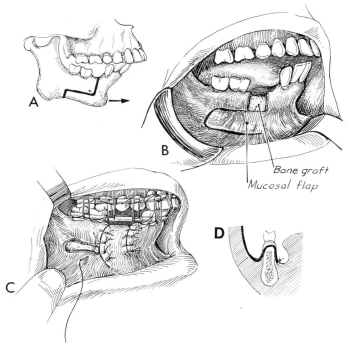

Bone graft
Mucosal flap

FIGURE 30–71. Vestibular-alveolar transposition flap for coverage of the area of osteotomy after elongation of the body of the mandible. *A,* Design of the step osteotomy for elongation of the body of the mandible. *B,* Vestibular-alveolar transposition flap and the exposed area to be covered. *C,* The transposed flap is sutured in place. The donor area is closed by direct approximation. *D,* Cross section showing the position of the flap. The distal portion is sutured to the mucous membrane of the floor of the mouth.

bone graft (Fig. 30–71). The flap will only cover narrow gaps but has the advantage of eliminating the need for a second operation to restore the buccal sulcus.

Techniques for Lengthening the Mandibular Body. The step osteotomy is frequently used to lengthen the shortened body of the mandible (see Fig. 30–65). Bony contact is maintained between the fragments by the horizontal portion of the step. This method was employed by von Eiselsberg (1906) to lengthen the body of the mandible and by Blair (1907) to correct an open bite.

The simplest technique of elongation step osteotomy is that of the reverse L-osteotomy (see Fig. 30–65, *C, D*). The osteotomy is made in the shape of an L which is resting on its back. The vertical branch extends anteriorly to the mental foramen, and the horizontal branch lies below and parallel to the inferior alveolar canal. The horizontal limb must be placed close to the lower border of the mandible, because the inferior alveolar canal often descends toward the lower border before ascending to reach the mental foramen. If the horizontal branch is made too close to the mental foramen, there is a risk of penetrating the

canal and sectioning the inferior alveolar nerve. Roentgenograms taken prior to surgery are helpful in locating the canal.

The reestablishment of conduction through a partially divided inferior alveolar nerve can occur. Furthermore, considerable overlay of the sensory innervation occurs in the denervated lower lip from the adjacent sensory nerves, but the lower lip rarely recovers full sensibility through this process. For this reason, preservation of the continuity of the inferior alveolar bundle should be a routine procedure.

The osteotomy is made by a small, oscillating, end-on Stryker saw blade or by a series of bur holes joined by a fissure bur or an osteotome. The angle between the two branches of the L is increased when an anterior open bite is to be closed. The increased angle allows the anterior segment to rise as it is advanced, closing the open bite deformity.

After completion of the osteotomy, the anterior segment is drawn forward and placed in its new position. The orthodontic arch wire is then applied, and it supports the anterior fragment; intermaxillary fixation completes the immobilization of the anterior and posterior fragments. The inferior border of the posterior fragment tends to tilt lingually from the con-

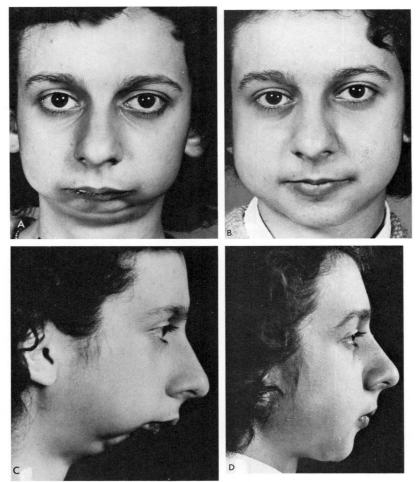

FIGURE 30–72. Bilateral temporomandibular ankylosis and mandibular micrognathia. *A, C,* Preoperative views. *B, D,* Postoperative appearance following (1) temporomandibular arthroplasty, (2) elongation osteotomy of the body of the mandible, and (3) restoration of mandibular contour by iliac bone grafting through the intraoral approach. (From Converse, J. M.: Micrognathia. Br. J. Plast. Surg., *16*:197, 1963.)

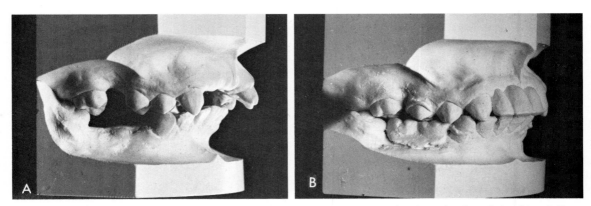

FIGURE 30–73. Dental casts of patient shown in Figure 30–72. *A,* Preoperative dentoalveolar relationships. *B,* Postoperative casts with improved occlusal relationships and prosthodontic restorations.

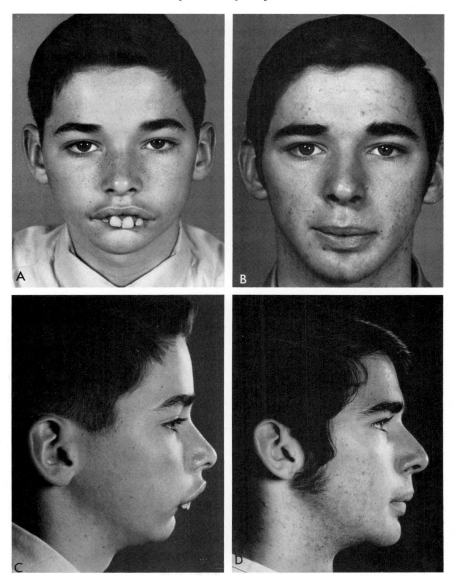

FIGURE 30–74. Mandibular micrognathia and maxillary protrusion treated by maxillary segmental premolar (set-back) osteotomy in a first stage, elongation osteotomy of the mandibular body in a second stage, and horizontal oste-otomy of the mandible with forward traction exerted by the stick-and-carrot appliance in a third stage (see Fig. 30–77). *A*, Appearance prior to surgery. Note the downward and forward protrusion of the maxillary dentoalveolar segment. A premolar set-back maxillary osteotomy was required to correct this deformity (see Fig. 30–163). *B*, Four years later after completion of three operative stages. *C*, Preoperative profile. *D*, Postoperative profile. Note adequate projection of chin and satisfactory lip seal.

traction of the medial pterygoid and mylohyoid muscles. Direct interosseous wire fixation is required (1) to stabilize the posterior frag-ments, (2) to assist in maintaining the forward position of the anterior fragment, and (3) to prevent a postoperative backward and down-ward tilt of the mental symphysis caused by the contraction of the suprahyoid muscles if these muscles are not detached.

Measured blocks of iliac bone are wedged into the gaps left by the steps. Any remaining interstices are filled with cancellous bone chips. The intraoral soft tissues are closed with catgut sutures. Six to eight weeks of postopera-tive fixation are usually required.

A patient with micrognathia who underwent an elongation osteotomy of the body of the mandible is shown in Figure 30–72. Iliac bone grafting for additional contour restoration followed. The occlusal relationship of the teeth before and after surgical and prosthodontic treatment is shown in Figure 30–73 (see also Fig. 30–74).

INTERDENTAL OSTEOTOMY. The vertical branch of the step osteotomy can be made through the alveolar bone between two adjacent teeth without injuring the dental roots. The extraction of a tooth is thus avoided. Interdental and panoramic roentgenograms give a clear picture of the position of the roots of the teeth and the amount of intervening alveolar bone. The buccal and lingual cortical bone along the proposed line of osteotomy between the adjacent teeth is removed with a small bur activated by an electrotorque. After the remain-

der of the step osteotomy has been completed, a narrow, tapered, shape osteotome severs the spongy bone remaining between the teeth.

VARIATIONS. When gaps in the posterior teeth are present, a step osteotomy posterior to the mental foramen can be used (see Fig. 30–65, *E*, *F*). An iliac bone graft is required to fill in the void left by the elongation. The inferior alveolar nerve is decompressed and lengthened. Moderate elongation of the inferior alveolar bundle is not a problem, and lengthening has been done without causing excessive tension on the nerve if the nerve is widely decompressed. The inferior alveolar canal should be decompressed to the mental foramen.

An osteotomy in the shape of an L with a wide angle between its branches and with a

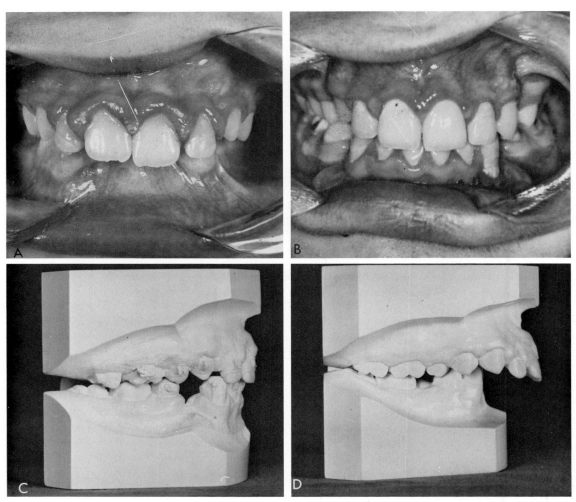

FIGURE 30–75. Intraoral views and dental casts (models) of the patient shown in Figure 30–74. *A*, Prior to surgical-orthodontic treatment. *B*, After completion of treatment. *C*, Before. *D*, After.

horizontal branch of the L extending forward and downward can be applied when lengthening of the mandible must be combined with a correction of an anterior closed bite and a short vertical lower facial height (Fig. 30–65, *A, B*).

MANDIBULAR MICROGNATHIA ASSOCIATED WITH MAXILLARY PROTRUSION. The problem of correction is well illustrated by the patient shown in Figure 30–74. The patient was first examined at the age of 12 years. The mandibular micrognathia was severe, and the soft tissues over the mental symphysis were tight and unyielding. The anterior maxillary dentoalveolar process had drifted forward and downward, resulting in an accentuated overjet and overbite (Fig. 30–75, *A*).

Treatment planning was achieved using cephalometric tracings and casts of the dentition. The first phase consisted of a premolar segmental maxillary dentoalveolar (set-back) osteotomy performed according to the technique shown in Figure 30–163.

After extraction of a premolar tooth on each side of the dental arch and removal of bone from the alveolar arch, from the hard palate, and above the apices of the teeth, the anterior maxillary dentoalveolar segment was displaced backward and upward into the predetermined position (Fig. 30–75, *B, D*). An edgewise orthodontic appliance maintained the fixation without intermaxillary fixation (Fig. 30–76).

After exposure of the mandible by the degloving technique, the body of the mandible was lengthened in a second stage by a step osteotomy (see Fig. 30–65, *E, F*). The step osteotomy was combined with a horizontal advancement osteotomy of the lower portion of the mandible (see p. 1387).

The tight soft tissues over the mental symphysis prevented adequate projection of the chin; however, the step osteotomy of the mandibular body achieved sufficient lengthening and improved the occlusal relationships (Fig. 30–75, *B, D*). Three months later, the mandible was again exposed by the degloving technique and a second horizontal advancement osteotomy was performed. To counteract the resistance of the soft tissues, the stick-and-carrot appliance was employed (Fig. 30–77). A cast vitallium splint with an outrigger extension made it possible to apply continuous forward traction on the mobilized segment by a stainless steel wire looped through a hole in the bone. The resistance of the soft tissues, intraoral as well as extraoral, was overcome (see Fig. 30–74, *B, D*). The cephalograms taken prior to the onset of treatment and 5 years after completion of treatment (Fig. 30–78, *A, B*) and the cephalometric tracings (Fig. 30–78, *C, D*) illustrate the skeletal and soft tissue contour changes.

COMBINED STEP OSTEOTOMY AND HORIZONTAL OSTEOTOMY OF THE BODY OF THE MANDIBLE. It is usually preferable to perform a horizontal or oblique advancement osteotomy of the anteroinferior portion of the mandible (see p. 1387) following the consolidation of the osteotomy used to elongate the mandibular body. However, when preoperative planning indicates the need for an increase in the projection of the symphysis portion of the mandible, occasionally a horizontal osteotomy and forward projection of the lower mandibular segment can be combined in the same stage with an elongation osteotomy of the mandibular body (see Fig. 30–125).

The mandibular symphysis and body are exposed using the degloving technique (see Fig. 30–67). A horizontal section of the mandible is extended backward, below, and posterior to the mental foramen. The osteotomy must remain

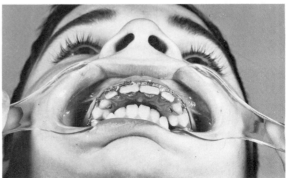

FIGURE 30–76. Edge-wise orthodontic appliance for fixation following premolar set-back osteotomy.

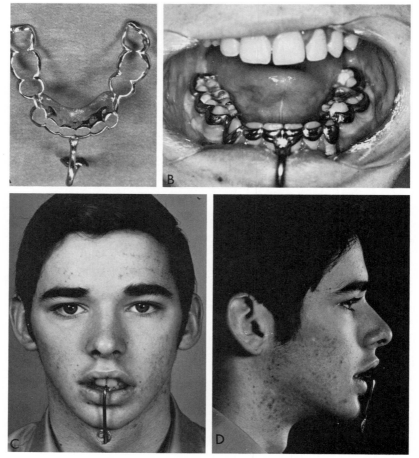

FIGURE 30–77.   The "stick-and-carrot" appliance. *A*, Vitallium splint with outrigger extension. *B*, Appliance fitted to the dental arch. *C*, Patient with appliance in position. *D*, Profile view with appliance. See also Figure 30–126.

well below the inferior alveolar canal. A vertical section is then made through the body of the mandible anterior to the mental foramen. The tooth-bearing anterior segment of the mandible is advanced and secured in position by intermaxillary fixation. The anteroinferior portion of the mandible, which has been separated from the body by the horizontal osteotomy, is advanced further, protruding beyond the anterior tooth-bearing segment of the mandible. Bone grafts will be needed to fill the space in the mandibular body and the defect along the lower border produced by the advancement of the bone. Flat pieces of cancellous bone are placed over the areas of junction between the various bony segments. This technique provides improved contour of the chin in addition to elongation of the micrognathic mandible in one stage. A second chin advancement may be necessary at a later stage if the covering soft tissues are tight.

ELONGATION BY SAGITTAL SPLITTING OF THE BODY OF THE MANDIBLE.   Dividing the body of the mandible along a sagittal plane is another technique that is employed in some unusual jaw deformities in which the shape of the mandible must be modified as well as elongated (see Fig. 30–66). The medial fragment carries the teeth and the inferior alveolar canal. The lateral segment includes the condyle and the remainder of the ramus. If the mandible is edentulous in the portion of the jaw that is to be operated upon, the procedure is easier to perform, since the only part that needs to be considered is the inferior alveolar neurovascular bundle. In the posterior portion of the mandibular body, the inferior alveolar canal is situated lingually (Fig. 30–79); thus,

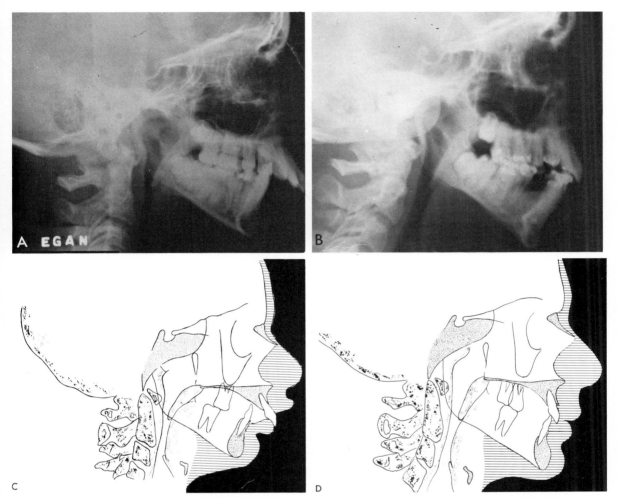

FIGURE 30–78. Preoperative (*A*) and postoperative (*B*) cephalograms of the patient shown in Figure 30–74. Preoperative (*C*) and postoperative (*D*) cephalometric tracings.

FIGURE 30–79. Trajectory of the inferior alveolar canal from the inferior alveolar foramen to the mental foramen. Note the oblique course of the canal. The inferior alveolar canal is situated on the lingual aspect of the mandible posteriorly and reaches the buccal surface of the mandible anteriorly.

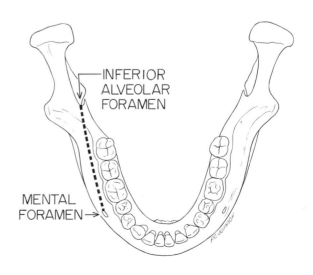

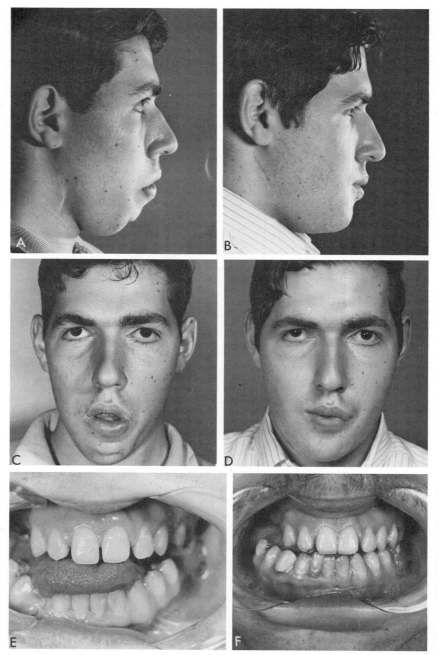

FIGURE 30–80. Complex mandibular deformity associated with an open bite. *A,* Preoperative profile view showing the downward and backward sloping of the chin and the steep mandibular plane. *B,* Postoperative appearance following multiple osteotomies to recontour the mandible: (1) sagittal section (see Fig. 30–66) of the right mandibular body; (2) osteotomy of the left mandibular body at the premolar region; and (3) transplantation of the lower border of the mandible over the mental symphysis (see Figs. 30–113 and 30–114). *C,* Preoperative appearance. Note the increase in the vertical dimension of the lower third of the face. *D,* Postoperative appearance. *E,* Preoperative intraoral view showing the open bite and the disparity between the upper and lower dental arches. *F,* Early result prior to orthodontic therapy and prosthodontic restoration.

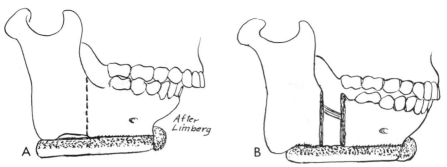

FIGURE 30–81. Limberg's technique using a retromolar lengthening osteotomy. A bone graft was initially placed along the lower border of the mandible to maintain bony continuity. (From Converse, J. M.: Micrognathia. Br. J. Plast. Surg., *16*:197, 1963.)

after sagittal section, a substantial amount of bone is present on the lateral segment.

Lengthening is obtained by sectioning and sliding forward the anterior tooth-bearing segment. Bony contact is maintained between the condylar and tooth-bearing fragments through the lateral segment. Bone grafts may be required for additional support over the buccal aspect of the lateral segment, particularly in the edentulous jaw. The lingual surface of the lateral fragment should be excavated to accommodate the inferior alveolar nerve and to avoid nerve compression when the fragments are approximated by a wire suture.

The patient shown in Figure 30–80 had a complicated mandibular deformity resulting from a neuromuscular deficiency associated with poliomyelitis in childhood. The mandibular deformity was characterized by prognathism with an anterior open bite (Fig. 30–80, *E*). The molar teeth had been extracted in a futile attempt to improve the open bite deformity. Partial facial paralysis was present on the left side. Remodeling the mandible required four

successive osteotomies placed in strategic positions along the length of the body from the angle to the incisive area; only sagittal splitting of the body of the mandible made possible the necessary corrective procedures while preserving the continuity of the inferior alveolar nerve and permitting the closure of the open bite and the correction of the prognathism (Fig. 30–80, *F*). The fragments were approximated by circumferential wires, and an acrylic splint (see Fig. 30–15) was maintained by circumferential wires.

THE RETROMOLAR STEP OSTEOTOMY. The retromolar osteotomy to lengthen the body of the mandible was employed by Limberg (1928). A bone graft was placed along the lower border of the mandible in a preliminary stage (Fig. 30–81, *A*). In a second stage, a vertical retromolar osteotomy was performed, the mandibular body was advanced, and the previously transplanted bone graft was used to maintain bony continuity (Fig. 30–81, *B*).

The retromolar step osteotomy, similar to that described for the correction of mandibular

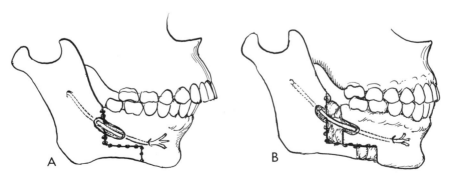

FIGURE 30–82. Retromolar elongation osteotomy. *A*, Outline of the step osteotomy and exposure of the inferior alveolar nerve. *B*, Position of the fragments after the anterior segment of the mandible has been advanced. Bone grafts were placed in the bony gap.

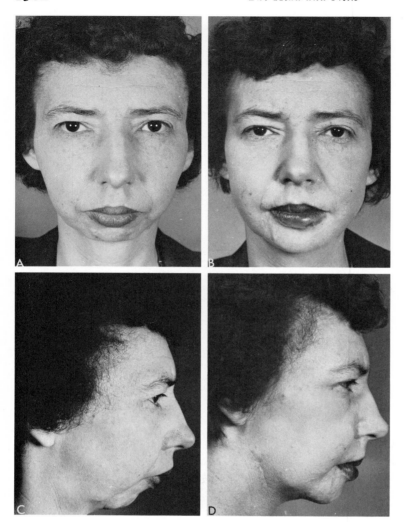

FIGURE 30–83. Mandibular micrognathia corrected by a retromolar elongation osteotomy. *A, C,* Preoperative appearance of the patient. *B, D,* Postoperative result following the elongation osteotomy.

prognathism, has the advantage of not producing a gap in the dental arch when the body of the mandible is elongated, but it is more difficult to perform (Fig. 30–82). The vertical cut of the step osteotomy is placed behind the last molar. Intraoral decompression of the inferior alveolar nerve is difficult in this area because of the lingual position of the nerve; an external approach is preferable. The sagittal splitting technique, illustrated in Figure 30–66, facilitates the procedure. Figure 30–83 shows a micrognathic patient who underwent a retromolar elongation osteotomy.

BONE GRAFTING ASSOCIATED WITH ELONGATION OSTEOTOMY. Iliac bone grafts, consisting mostly of cancellous bone, are used as flat pieces that cover the lines of osteotomy and as blocks of bone and small chips that fill

the gaps caused by the advancement. Resected segments of mandibular bone can also be employed when they are available. The bone grafts assure bony continuity, increase the chances of successful consolidation at the osteotomy sites, and improve the size and contour of the mandible. They will be successful only if they are covered with well-vascularized soft tissues.

OTHER ELONGATION OSTEOTOMIES OF THE BODY OF THE MANDIBLE. The oblique osteotomy through the body of the mandible was described by Blair (1907) and Kazanjian (1939). It is another technique which can be utilized in the edentulous mandible when the inferior alveolar nerve has been destroyed by trauma, disease, or ablative surgery of the mandibular body (Fig. 30–84).

EXTERNAL TRACTION APPARATUS. After

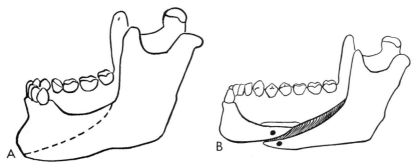

FIGURE 30–84. *A*, Oblique osteotomy of the mandible. The mandible is cut through diagonally after its lateral surface has been exposed intraorally. *B*, A hole is drilled at each end of the bone segments, which are sutured together with stainless steel wire following advancement. This type of osteotomy is indicated only when the inferior alveolar nerve has been destroyed.

lengthening procedures have been performed on the mandibular body, an external traction apparatus may be required to counteract muscular forces. These appliances are described later in the text (see p. 1371).

ADVANTAGES AND DISADVANTAGES OF BODY ELONGATION OSTEOTOMIES. The main indication for a body elongation osteotomy is the need for correction of mandibular arch form as well as length. A mandible of unequal body length and a distorted dental arch contour is best managed by these techniques.

The disadvantages of mandibular body osteotomies are (1) possible injury to the inferior alveolar nerve when the osteotomy must be placed behind the mental foramen; (2) gaps in the dental arch, which require later dental restoration; (3) technical difficulties in performing the osteotomy; (4) the need to provide additional soft tissue to cover the osteotomy sites; and (5) the need for bone grafts to ensure against delayed union and nonunion.

Operations on the Mandibular Ramus to Increase the Projection of the Mandible. Operations consisting of a horizontal osteotomy through the ramus above the inferior alveolar foramen to lengthen the mandible were practiced by Lane (1905) and Blair (1907). Such operations are subject to the three major complications previously enumerated in the section of this chapter concerning mandibular prognathism: (1) distraction of the fragments by the pull of the temporalis and lateral pterygoid muscles on the upper fragment, which allows interposition of soft tissue between the fragments and delayed union or nonunion; (2) occasional loss of the vertical dimension of the ramus through overlapping of the fragments, caused by the pull exerted by the masseter and the medial pterygoid muscles on the lower

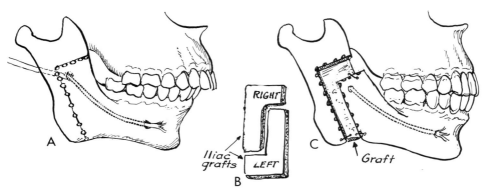

FIGURE 30–85. Wassmund's reversed L-shaped osteotomy of the ramus. *A*, Outline of the osteotomy. *B*, Iliac bone grafts (right and left). *C*, Operation completed. Bone graft in position.

fragment; and (3) relapse. These complications often result in an anterior open bite deformity. Because of these problems, the horizontal osteotomy has been abandoned.

Wassmund (1927) described a vertical section of the ramus in the shape of an upside-down L; the vertical osteotomy, instead of reaching the sigmoid notch, took a sharp forward angle above the lingula through the base of the coronoid process. Pichler and Trauner (1948) and Schuchardt (1958) also used this type of osteotomy to treat micrognathia. In this technique bone grafts are placed in the resulting defect to promote bony consolidation (Fig. 30–85).

The Babcock (1937) operation was revived by Trauner (1957); this consists of the insertion of cartilage in the temporomandibular joint

posterior to the condyle. The entire mandible is forced forward to improve the mandibular position and the occlusal relationship of the teeth. It is doubtful that surgical interference with the temporomandibular joint is justified in correcting micrognathia, since other techniques are available.

The evolution of surgical techniques for the treatment of mandibular micrognathia parallels that of the techniques used for the correction of mandibular prognathism. The surgical principles employed for the management of prognathism were also adapted to the elongation osteotomy through the ramus.

Caldwell and Amaral (1960) combined an iliac bone graft with a vertical section of the ramus. The coronoid process was resected to neutralize the pull of the temporalis muscle

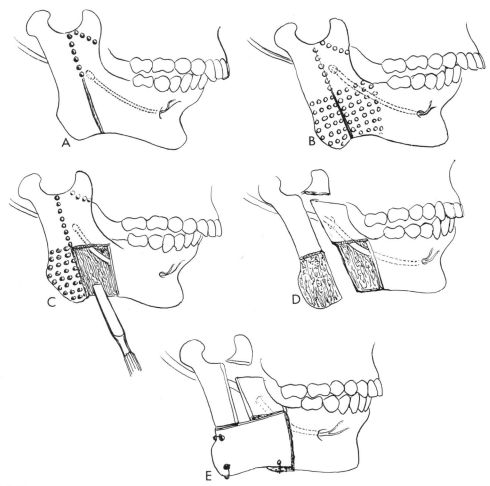

FIGURE 30–86. Vertical osteotomy of the ramus of the mandible combined with a bone graft for advancement of the body of the mandible. *A*, Lines of osteotomy. *B*, The outer cortex in the region of the angle is perforated by multiple drill holes. *C*, The outer cortex of the mandible is removed with an osteotome. *D*, The body of the mandible is advanced after completion of the osteotomy; the coronoid process is also detached. *E*, An iliac bone graft is wired in position to maintain bony contact between the separated mandibular fragments. (After Caldwell and Amaral, 1960.)

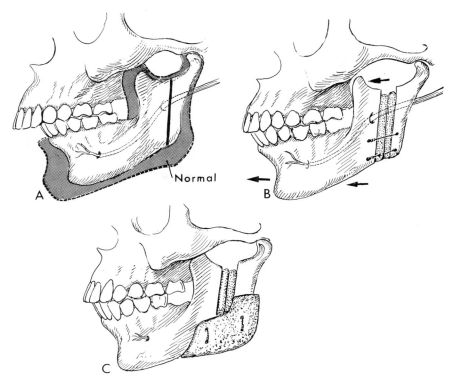

FIGURE 30–87. Elongation of the mandible by vertical section of the ramus and bone grafting. *A*, Micrognathic mandible is contrasted to the normally developed mandible (shaded). *B*, After vertical section of the ramus, bone grafts are interposed between the fragments and maintained by interosseous wiring. *C*, An onlay bone graft is added to reinforce the interposed bone grafts and augment the contour of the mandibular angle. (From Converse, J. M., Horowitz, S. L., Coccaro, P. J., and Wood-Smith, D.: The corrective treatment of the skeletal asymmetry in hemifacial microsomia. Plast. Reconstr. Surg., *52*:221, 1973. Copyright 1973, The Williams & Wilkins Company, Baltimore.)

and to eliminate the danger of impingement of the coronoid process on the posterior surface of the zygoma after the anterior fragment is advanced. An onlay iliac bone graft was placed over the lateral surface of the lower portion of the ramus after the cortical bone was removed. A bone graft was also placed to bridge the gap in the divided ramus (Fig. 30–86).

Robinson and Lytle (1962) reported a series of cases in which they omitted the section of the coronoid process and the addition of bone grafts. A V-shaped defect in the ramus was allowed to fill with bone formed by the investing periosteum. However, a 12-week period of intermaxillary fixation was required. Bone grafts would have accelerated the consolidation. Robinson (1957) performed an oblique osteotomy of the ramus and bone-grafted the gap.

In the vertical osteotomy technique, a vertical section of the ramus is performed bilaterally, the body of the mandible is advanced, and intermaxillary fixation is established. The surgical approach for elongation of the mandible by vertical section of the ramus is similar to that described previously for the correction of mandibular prognathism. The osteotomy is done with an air-turbine–activated bur anterior and parallel to the posterior border of the ramus. The space between the fragments, after advancement of the mandible and establishment of intermaxillary fixation, is filled with an iliac or a costal bone graft. In children, Longacre (1957) recommended wedging split rib grafts between the fragments. Crockford and Converse (1972) have shown that iliac bone grafts can be removed from children without injuring the growth centers of the ilium (see Chapter 13). Bone grafts are interposed between and over the fragments without removing the outer cortex. Onlay bone grafts are also added to increase the bulk of the ramus and to improve the overlying soft tissue contour (Fig. 30–87).

ADVANTAGES AND DISADVANTAGES OF THE VERTICAL OSTEOTOMY OF THE RAMUS. The principal advantage of the vertical section procedure of the ramus is its simplicity. Exposure is good, the osteotomy is easy to perform, and adequate advancement can be obtained. In contrast to body elongation techniques, the vertical osteotomy of the ramus avoids injury to the inferior alveolar nerve; edentulous areas are not produced in the dental arch; and soft tissue coverage of the osteotomy is not a problem. A small ramus can be increased in size, and contour restoration with bone grafts is possible at the same time.

When the ramus is hypoplastic, a vertical osteotomy combined with bone grafting will increase its anteroposterior dimension, thus advancing the body of the mandible. The degree of advancement is limited, however, by the presence of the zygoma, which checks the anteroposterior increase in the size of the ramus. The Wassmund technique (see Fig. 30–85) or the Hayes C-osteotomy (see Fig. 30–92) offers the advantage that the coronoid process does not participate in the advancement and does not abut against the zygoma.

INCREASING THE VERTICAL DIMENSION OF THE RAMUS. The hypoplastic mandible is usually deficient in both horizontal and vertical dimensions.

The vertical dimension of the ramus of the mandible may be elongated by a horizontal section of the ramus and the interposition of a bone graft between the segments. The ramus is exposed by wide subperiosteal elevation of the masseter and medial pterygoid muscles. If separation of the fragments is to be successfully achieved, the muscles must be completely disinserted. A block of iliac bone is wedged into the interval between the upper and lower fragments. It is essential to maintain the downward position of the lower fragment by means of an intraoral bite-block placed in the molar region. Converse did an operation of this type in collaboration with Rushton in 1941; follow-up of this patient was reported by Rushton (1942, 1944) and by Gillies and Millard (1957). A similar technique was employed by Osborne (1964). This technique has been employed in craniofacial microsomia (see Chapter 54).

A preferable technique is to combine the vertical osteotomy illustrated in Figure 30–87 with additional onlay bone grafts to lengthen the ramus and form a new mandibular angle.

Osteotomies of the ramus cannot be used to correct dental arch length discrepancies and severe posterior crossbite problems. A cutaneous scar may be objectionable to some patients and contraindicated in patients who are prone to form keloids. Injury to the marginal mandibular nerve is always a possibility. Another disadvantage is the need to place bone grafts. Although Robinson and Lytle (1962) have shown that bone grafts can be omitted, the 12 weeks of postoperative intermaxillary fixation is an excessive inconvenience for the patient. The bone graft interposed between the ramus fragments also prevents the forward displacement of the posterior fragment.

ELONGATION OF THE MANDIBLE BY SAGITTAL SECTION OF THE RAMUS. The ramus sagittal splitting technique provides a wide surface of contact between the fragments and has been employed to increase the anteroposterior dimension of the ramus (Fig. 30–88), thus advancing the mandibular body in patients with a retruded mandible (Fig. 30–89). The technique has been discussed previously (see Fig. 30–40). Similar steps are followed as described in the management of mandibular prognathism. The Dautrey modification (see Fig. 30–44) can be employed in order to avoid compression of the inferior alveolar nerve. The tooth-bearing portion is moved forward to elongate the mandible and is held in intermaxillary fixation.

Bone grafts are usually not required because of the wide surface of bony contact. Interosseous or circumferential wires are placed to complete the stabilization of the fragments (see Fig. 30–88). In the patient shown in Figure 30–89, adequate dental occlusal relationships have been attained (Fig. 30–90). The cephalometric tracings show the degree of advancement (Fig. 30–91). A horizontal advancement osteotomy of the anteroinferior portion of the mandible (see p. 1387) is indicated to improve the contour further.

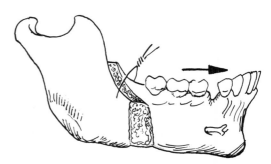

FIGURE 30–88. Advancement of the mandible by sagittal osteotomy of the ramus. The technical details of the sagittal osteotomy of the ramus are described in Figure 30–40. After the condyle is repositioned in the glenoid fossa, the tooth-bearing segment is advanced; intermaxillary fixation is established, and an interosseous wire retains the respective positions of the fragments. A bone graft has been wedged into the gap remaining in the cortex after advancement of the tooth-bearing segment of the mandible.

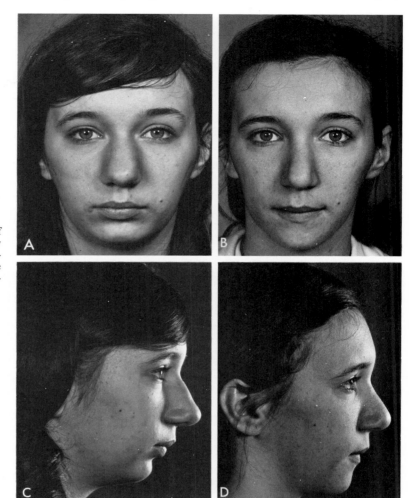

FIGURE 30–89. Advancement of the mandible by sagittal osteotomy of the ramus. *A*, Preoperative full-face appearance. *B*, Postoperative appearance. *C*, Profile view, preoperative. *D*, Postoperative.

Advantages and disadvantages of the sagittal section of the ramus. The advantage of the technique is the wide surface of bony contact afforded following advancement of the segments. Bone grafts are not needed to maintain bony contact. Consolidation of the fragments is rapid, and nonunion is rare. The anterior segment can also be rotated upward to close an anterior open bite (see p. 1418). The intraoral approach eliminates the external scar. Gaps are not produced in the dental arch.

A disadvantage is that the sagittal splitting technique is not feasible when hypoplasia of the ramus is severe. The chance of comminution of the condylar fragment and the risk of injuring the inferior alveolar nerve are greater in a hypoplastic ramus. In such cases the vertical section technique accompanied by an in-

terposition bone graft through an external approach is preferable.

OSTEOTOMY OF THE RAMUS AND BODY OF THE MANDIBLE FOR ELONGATION OF THE MANDIBLE. A C-shaped osteotomy of the mandibular ramus was described by Caldwell, Hayward and Lister (1968). It was originally referred to as an L-osteotomy, although the outline of the osteotomy is in the shape of a C. The vertical branch of the C spares the mandibular angle and extends forward below the inferior alveolar canal toward the body of the mandible; it is then angulated through the inferior border. A combined intraoral and extraoral approach was recommended in the original description of the technique. The insertions of the masseter and medial pterygoid muscles are reflected by subperiosteal dissec-

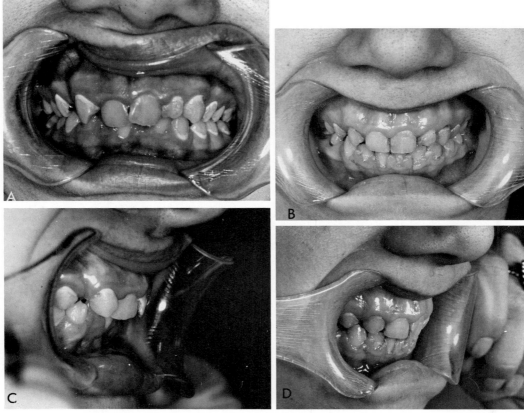

FIGURE 30–90. Intraoral views of the patient shown in Figure 30–89. *A*, Preoperative. *B*, Postoperative and after orthodontic therapy. *C*, Lateral view, preoperative. *D*, After completion of treatment.

tion. The upper horizontal branch of the C-osteotomy is made with a bur using an intraoral approach. The remainder of the osteotomy is done through the extraoral incision. The horizontal sections should be kept parallel to the plane of advancement. After the osteotomy is completed, the tooth-bearing fragment is advanced to the desired location, and intermaxillary fixation is applied. The condyle on the proximal fragment is returned to the glenoid fossa, and the fragments are joined by an interosseous wire. There may be sufficient bony contact to dispense with bone grafts unless they are needed to add bulk and form and to aid in the consolidation.

Hayes (1973) applied the principle of the sagittal osteotomy to increase the surface of contact along the inferior portion of the body of the mandible (Fig. 30–92). The operation is performed through an extraoral approach. An oscillating Stryker saw is used to cut the bone, in preference to burs, which remove an excessive amount of bone. Once the lower horizontal branch of the osteotomy reaches the body, the bone cut is made through the lateral cortical plate only (Fig. 30–92, *A*), thus achieving a sagittal split (Fig. 30–92, *B*, *C*, *D*). The medial portion of the lower horizontal osteotomy is dropped vertically to the inferior border, where the mandibular body begins. The distance between the medial and the lateral vertical sections of the lower horizontal extension should be approximately double the distance of the advancement to ensure adequate bony contact. The fragments are separated, and the tooth-bearing anterior fragment is held in its corrected relationship to the maxilla by intermaxillary fixation. A single interosseous wire is placed at the inferior border (Fig. 30–92, *B*).

Advantages and disadvantages of the C-osteotomy. The advantage of the C-osteotomy is that it provides sufficient bony contact so that a bone graft is not needed. The body sagittal split modification further increases the sur-

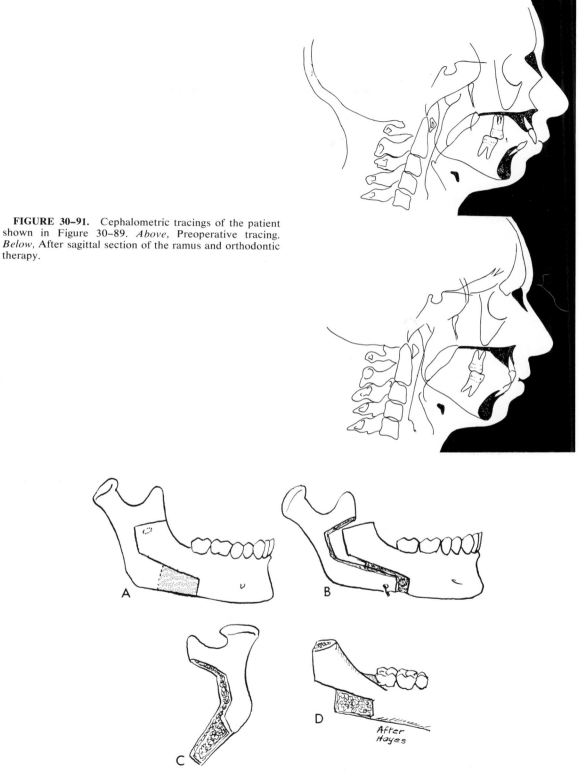

FIGURE 30–91. Cephalometric tracings of the patient shown in Figure 30–89. *Above,* Preoperative tracing. *Below,* After sagittal section of the ramus and orthodontic therapy.

FIGURE 30–92. The C-shaped ramus osteotomy with an anterior extension. *A,* Design of the osteotomy. Shaded area indicates where the sagittal splitting of the body is made. *B,* After completion of the advancement, a single interosseous wire is placed at the inferior border. *C,* Lingual view of the condylar segment showing the osteotomy and the sagittal split of the body. *D,* The tooth-bearing segment: the outer cortex of the sagittal split rests with the condylar fragment. (After Hayes.)

1369

face of contact. The C-osteotomy may be used when the ramus is small, whereas the sagittal splitting technique is not always possible in such cases. In addition, injury to the inferior alveolar nerve is less likely to occur, unless the lower horizontal section is unintentionally made too high through the inferior alveolar canal.

The external incision is a disadvantage, albeit minimal, of this technique. Care must also be taken when the sagittal splitting of the mandibular body is done. Excessive force can produce a fracture at the critical junction of the lower horizontal section with the vertical osteotomy of the ramus. Bone grafts are required in a small ramus.

INCREASE IN SIZE AND RESTORATION OF CONTOUR OF THE MANDIBLE IN MICROGNATHIA. The deformity produced by a small, retruded mandible is one of the most challenging jaw malformations to correct. An anatomical approach to the individual problem must be considered. If the ramus is small, short, or lacking in sufficient anteroposterior dimensions, it should be enlarged and lengthened and its anteroposterior dimension increased. An osteotomy and bone grafts are required to achieve these goals. If the mandibular body is small, short, and lacking in its anteroposterior dimension, it should be increased in size and lengthened by osteotomy and bone grafts. When the mandibular body and the ramus are both hypoplastic, an increase in the size of both structures in consecutive operations may be indicated.

The arch form of either the maxilla or mandible may require expansion. This is usually achieved by expanding the palate through a paramedian osteotomy combined with bone grafting. The mandibular arch is expanded by osteotomies of various designs in the mental area or in other portions of the body of the mandible combined with bone grafting, if necessary.

In addition to the problem of micrognathia, the surgeon must overcome the problems of tight soft tissue shortage, and possible associated maxillary deformities. Multiple staged procedures are often required.

Many patients with mandibular micrognathia also have an underdeveloped chin (microgenia) and inadequate contour of the elongated mandibular body. An additional procedure, such as a horizontal advancement osteotomy of the inferior border of the anterior portion of the mandible, may be needed to obtain a satisfactory result. Onlay bone grafts are also helpful in restoring contour.

Patients with temporomandibular ankylosis need multiple procedures to restore function and form. Rehabilitation of the patient usually begins with a temporomandibular arthroplasty (see Chapter 31).

CHOICE OF A TECHNIQUE FOR ELONGATION AND ADVANCEMENT OF THE MANDIBLE. There are many techniques, and the order of procedure varies in the treatment of mandibular micrognathia. Each case has its unique features and problems. Careful preliminary study and planning will aid in the choice of the most suitable reconstructive procedures and ensure the best final results.

Elongation osteotomy of the body of the mandible is a procedure limited to those patients in whom the secondary dentition has erupted; the presence of tooth buds in the body of the mandible precludes the use of this technique. For this reason, body osteotomies are usually performed after adolesence. Bilateral osteotomies of the ramus can be used in children to advance the body of the mandible, since the ramus contains no tooth buds.

In micrognathia, the ramus, although short, is often thick and amenable to the sagittal splitting technique.

In some unilateral mandibular cases of micrognathia when the upper and lower dental arch forms are favorable but malaligned to one another, various ramus osteotomies may be indicated. On the affected side, a sagittal or C-shaped osteotomy can be used to allow advancement of the body of the mandible without loss of bony contact; thus the need for bone grafts is eliminated. On the unaffected contralateral side, a vertical osteotomy is done to facilitate rotation of the mandible without unduly disturbing the temporomandibular joint. The unaffected side behaves more like a pivoting center, and bony contact is maintained.

When gross disparity and malalignment exist between the upper and lower dental arch forms, a body elongation osteotomy is indicated. Osteotomies of the ramus change the relative position of the mandibular dental arch but not its form. Dentoalveolar discrepancies can be corrected by the orthodontist, but an arch disparity due to skeletal deformities is best managed by surgical modification of the shape of the mandibular body.

AGE AT OPERATION. A major problem which remains controversial is the age at which the corrective procedure should be done in the developmental type of micrognathia. Temporomandibular ankylosis should be relieved early. A growing trend is toward operation in early childhood. An osteotomy to increase the size and anteroposterior dimension of the ramus is feasible when sufficient permanent teeth have erupted to permit adequate intermaxillary fixation. Further longitudinal studies of these patients will undoubtedly provide the answer.

POSTOPERATIVE RELAPSE. Postoperative regression of the advanced segment of the mandible is a major problem. Recent postoperative cephalometric studies have provided valuable information. Poulton and Ware (1973) observed patients treated by the sagittal splitting (ramus) technique. The follow-up period extended over three years. Serial cephalograms documented 50 to 80 per cent relapse during the period of study. McNeill, Hooley, and Sundberg (1973) noted similar relapse in their postoperative cephalometric studies. The major portion of the relapse occurs during the intermaxillary fixation period. Of interest is the observation that the dentoalveolar relationships are maintained by the intermaxillary fixation appliance, but the relapse occurs in the skeletal portion of the mandible, indicated by the regression of pogonion (bony chin point). Inadequate repositioning of the condyle during the operation cannot be blamed for the relapse; the anatomical position of the condyle in the glenoid fossa was verified by roentgenograms during the immediate postoperative period. Several soft tissue factors contribute to regression of the advanced mandibular skeleton. These will now be considered.

The suprahyoid musculature. The anterior belly of the diagastric, the mylohyoid, and the geniohyoid muscles exert a strong downward and backward pull on the anterior fragment, causing it to rotate. The stretching of the muscles, as the advancement is made, contributes further to the muscle pull. Three methods of counteracting the effect of the muscular contraction are employed: (1) subperiosteal disinsertion of the suprahyoid musculature, (2) external traction devices, and (3) external mandibular supporting appliances.

1. Disinsertion of muscle attachments. Subperiosteal disinsertion of the anterior belly of the digastric and of the geniohyoid muscles from the lower mental spines is of assistance in combating the tendency toward downward and backward rotation after the osteotomy is performed (Converse, 1963). Steinhauser (1973) recommended this technique in cases involving a steep mandibular plane or an anterior open bite. Tongue dysfunction and airway obstruction were not observed postoperatively. Disinsertion of the mylohyoid muscle and the genioglossi muscles from the upper mental spines is not advised because it may interfere with swallowing and cause retroposition of the tongue and airway obstruction.

2. External traction devices. An external apparatus which exerts traction on the mandible can be used to neutralize the pull of the suprahyoid musculature. Forward traction is particularly indicated in the treatment of severe micrognathia. The correction requires advancement and upward rotation of the symphyseal portion of the mandible to counteract the backward and downward rotation and the labial inclination of the incisor teeth. Various

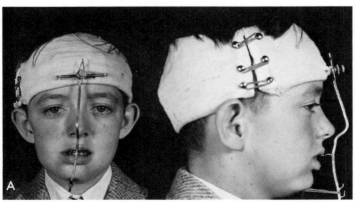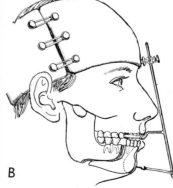

FIGURE 30–93. The Kazanjian extraoral traction appliance. *A,* The apparatus is embedded in a plaster head cap (at the present time mostly replaced by head frames). The vertical bar has a horizontal extension which acts as a fulcrum, resting on the labial aspect of the maxillary fixation appliance. Elastic traction is exerted on the lower border of the mandible. *B,* Details. Circumferential wire is shown around the symphysis; the ends are brought out through the skin near the lower border of the symphysis, are twisted in the shape of a hook, and are attached by an elastic band to the vertical bar. The bulky plaster headcap has been superseded by the head frame.

appliances have been devised to provide the necessary external traction.

The Kazanjian extraoral traction appliance (Fig. 30–93), which used a plaster head cap, has been replaced by head frames (see Fig. 30–94). A circumferential stainless steel wire is passed around the symphysis; the ends of the wire are brought out through the skin below the fat pad of the chin, and forward and upward traction is exerted. When the anterior portion of the mandible is exposed by the degloving technique, a hole is drilled through the lower border of the symphysis to accommodate the loop of wire. The Kazanjian appliance uses a rigid bar adjusted in front of the face between the forehead and the chin. A horizontal extension attached to this bar rests on the labial surfaces of the upper incisors, which serve as a fulcrum, and is fastened to the maxillary arch bar. The mandibular wire is secured to the lower end of the rigid bar. The inferior border of the symphysis of the mandible is thus retained in position, resisting the downward and backward displacement.

Various cranial fixation appliances have been developed. Georgiade's halo or "crown of thorns" appliance (Fig. 30–94) has been popular in the United States; the rear portion of the halo may be removed to allow the patient to rest his head on a pillow. Other head frames do not encircle the head.

Completion of the contour restoration often requires a horizontal advancement osteotomy of the lower portion of the body of the mandible (see Figs. 30–112 to 30–116). When the overlying soft tissues are tight and resist the

advancement, a stick-and-carrot appliance can be used (see Fig. 30–77). This appliance dispenses with the need for a cranial fixation device and is better tolerated by the patient.

3. External mandibular supporting appliances. Regression of the advanced mandibular segment can also be minimized by the use of external mandibular supporting devices. Poulton and Ware (1973) employed a Pitkin cervical collar to help neutralize the relapsing forces. The angle of force applied by the cervical collar, however, does not completely counteract the pull exerted by the suprahyoid muscles. The cervical collar is worn throughout the intermaxillary fixation period and at night for the next 6 to 12 months along with an acrylic occlusal splint. The amount of relapse was reduced from 50 to 80 per cent to 10 to 30 per cent. The cervical brace also helps to correct the forward movement of the hyoid bone and cervical vertebrae which occurs because of the tendency to drop the head during the postoperative period. Both the hyoid bone and the cervical vertebrae return to their original preoperative positions as the muscles readapt to their new positions.

Snyder, Levine, Swanson, and Browne (1973) have shown in animal studies that the mandible can be elongated by continuous external traction applied after the osteotomy. Abbott (1927) had previously used a similar method to lengthen the tibia and fibula. New bone formation occurs at the osteotomy site; bone grafts are not required.

Soft tissue deficiency. Tight soft tissues often cover the micrognathic mandible. Both the soft tissues and the underlying bone are hypoplastic. The patient has difficulty in occluding his lips, in achieving lip seal. The tight soft tissues resist the mandibular advancement. External traction appliances help to maintain the advanced position of the bone and to counteract the resistance of the soft tissues.

Wide elevation of the soft tissue around the osteotomy site may also be helpful. Vertical parallel incisions through the periosteum assist in overcoming the restrictive force of the periosteal capsule and in allowing for a moderate degree of expansion.

Resistance to advancement can also be caused by a deficiency of intraoral mucosal lining and musculature. A similar problem is encountered in providing adequate lining for the nose which is constricted because of loss or scarring of the nasal lining (see Chapter 29, p. 1199. Releasing the mucous membrane and

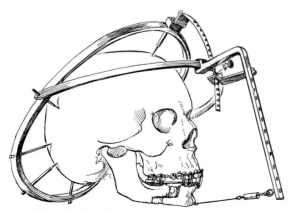

FIGURE 30–94. Georgiade's external traction apparatus. A number of such head frames have been designed.

the attached mental and suprahyoid muscles from the bone, as is done in the skin graft inlay technique for the reconstruction of the buccal sulcus (see p. 1503), permits a wide expansion of the overlying soft tissues. The buccal sulcus is incised, the mandible is advanced, and a skin graft inlay remedies the mucosal deficiency and expands the covering soft tissues.

When covering soft tissue deficiency is a problem, a chin implant of silicone expands the tissues preliminary to advancement of the bone. The implant must not be left in position for more than one or two months to avoid absorption of the underlying bone from the pressure exerted by the implant. The implant must be placed over the hard bone of the lower border of the symphysis and not be allowed to drift upward into the soft dentoalveolar bone and the roots of the teeth (see p. 1399).

The sphenomandibular ligament. The sphenomandibular ligament is a fibrous band extending from the angular spine of the sphenoid bone to the lingula of the mandibular ramus. In vertical and sagittal osteotomies of the ramus, the lingula remains on the advanced segment of the mandible. The inelastic ligament may hinder the anterior repositioning and play a role in the production of relapse (Hovell, 1970). The vertical position of the ligament, however, would appear to offer little resistance to the advancement.

Other techniques to prevent relapse. McNeill, Hooley, and Sundberg (1973) recommended prolonged maintenance of intermaxillary fixation combined with use of the Pitkin cervical collar until the relapse forces are expended. Serial cephalograms are used to judge the proper time to release the fixation and the collar.

Overcorrection of the micrognathic deformity may also be indicated. An acrylic occlusal bite guide is required to compensate for the dental intercuspal interferences. A posterior open bite should be incorporated in the design of the acrylic wafer (Poulton and Ware, 1973). The appliance helps to rotate the symphysis upward and anteriorly and provides more chin prominence. In addition, the posterior open bite will increase the posterior facial height, which is usually short in the mandibular micrognathic patient. The increase in the posterior vertical facial dimension is maintained as the posterior maxillary teeth extrude downward to close the artificial posterior open bite.

Secondary operations. If a relapse occurs, a secondary procedure usually achieves a satisfactory result. Additional procedures may be required, such as a horizontal advancement osteotomy of the lower portion of the anterior mandibular body, which may be combined with bone grafting (see Fig. 30–115).

Contour Restoration in Mandibular Micrognathia. After the mandible has been lengthened and advanced to correct the malocclusion and to improve the contour of the face, additional contour restoration is often needed.

Contour restoration of the ramus and the body of the mandible is best obtained by bone grafts. Augmentation by inorganic implants generally fares poorly in these regions; they are widely used with success, however, in the area of the mental symphysis. Costal and iliac bone grafts are also employed.

Wide subperiosteal contact between the bone grafts and the mandibular bone favors osteogenesis. Experimental data suggest that bone grafts with attached periosteum, applied as onlay bone grafts, survive more favorably (Thompson and Casson, 1970; Knize, 1974). The periosteum of the onlay bone graft may encourage more rapid revascularization. Failures in contour restoration by bone grafting will occur if the overlying soft tissues are under sufficient tension to cause pressure atrophy of the grafted bone. Bone grafts survive when they are subjected to functional stress, when they are rapidly revascularized (cancellous bone facilitates revascularization), and when bone is not transplanted in excessive amounts. Bone graft onlays on deformed mandibles are generally successful (Fig. 30–95), in contrast to bone grafts placed to correct the minor deformity of microgenia; the latter grafts often undergo a slow absorptive process. The success of onlay bone grafts is unpredictable. Partial absorption will require additional onlay bone grafting until the desired contour is obtained. Longacre and DeStefano (1957) showed that serial onlay bone overgrafting can be used to restore contour.

Many techniques are available for contour restoration of the chin. They will be discussed later in the section dealing with the management of microgenia.

LATEROGNATHISM: LATERAL DEVIATION OF THE MANDIBLE

A truly symmetrical face does not exist. When carefully studied, the right and left halves of the average face show some degree of asym-

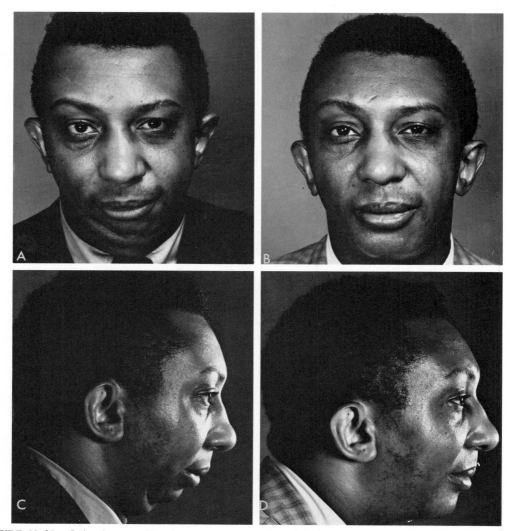

FIGURE 30–95. Onlay bone grafting for contour restoration of the mandible. *A*, Patient with temporomandibular ankylosis and micrognathia. The dental relationships were acceptable. *B*, Result four years after contour-restoring bone grafts were placed through the intraoral approach. *C*, Preoperative profile. *D*, Postoperative view.

metry. When the skeletal portion of the mandible deviates to one side beyond the average range, facial asymmetry becomes clinically pronounced, and mandibular laterognathism is produced: the mental symphysis is lateral to the mid-sagittal plane of the face. The midlines between the upper and lower central incisors do not coincide; posterior crossbite is usually present. In lesser deviations of the mandible, the dentoalveolar structures of the jaws achieve a compromised occlusal relationship to compensate for the skeletal deviation.

Etiology.   Trauma plays an important role in

producing lateral deviation of the mandible, facial skeletal asymmetry, and malocclusion (posterior crossbite). Unilateral micrognathia is often the result of injury to one condyle in early life. Laterognathism is also of congenital origin, i.e., the deformity characteristic of the maldevelopment of the first and second branchial arches (hemicraniofacial microsomia; see Chapter 54). Conversely, laterognathism can be caused by unilateral condylar hyperplasia or congenital hemifacial hyperplasia. The deformity may also be acquired; traumatic loss of a portion of the mandible results in lateral mandibular deviation, the mental symphysis being drawn toward the short side of the mandible. Loss of bone following the resection of tumors also produces laterognathism (see Fig. 30–68).

Preoperative Planning. Asymmetry of the face is usually readily detected on clinical examination. Determination of the defective side of the face may not be so easy; on casual examination, the unaffected side may appear to be the involved side. The position of the chin is used as a rough clinical guide. When the deformity is caused by an underdevelopment or loss of a portion of the mandible, the chin assumes a retruded position and deviates to the affected side. Conversely, when the deformity is caused by a unilateral hyperplasia of a portion of the mandible, the chin appears to be more prominent and is deviated to the contralateral side. The lateral movement of the chin when the jaw is opened, therefore, cannot be used as a reliable guide, since the chin will always deviate to the shorter side of the mandible. The side to which the chin has deviated may be shorter because of hypoplasia on that side or hyperplasia of the mandible on the opposite side.

Panoramic and cephalometric roentgenograms will confirm the clinical diagnosis. Dental casts should be trimmed to show any cant of the occlusal plane and anteroposterior mandibular asymmetry.

Condylar Hypoplasia

Injury to the condylar cartilage from delivery forceps at birth, a fall, other trauma, or sepsis in infancy or early childhood can lead to arrested growth. The degree of growth impairment is greater when the insult occurs in early postnatal life. Altered condylar growth is also seen in many congenital malformations.

Lund and Jacobsen (1971) reported the overgrowth of a hypoplastic mandibular ramus following the insertion of costal bone grafts after an osteotomy to lengthen the mandibular body. This 18-year longitudinal study began when the operation was done on a 9 year old patient who wore an orthodontic biteplane appliance until the age of 16. In another longitudinal study by the same authors, patients with less severe deformities resulting from condylar neck fractures were followed (Jacobsen and Lund, 1972). Immediately after the injury, the chin deviated to the affected side. After the adolescent skeletal growth spurt, the chin deviated to the contralateral

side. The condylar heads were re-formed (see also Chapter 24, p. 680).

Altered Muscular Activity and Condylar Injury. The condylar growth center is active until at least the twenty-first year and is generally regarded as one of the most active in the growing mandible. When it is traumatized, there is a definite deceleration in growth due to the inhibitory effect on the proliferation of cartilage and ossification, particularly during the preschool years. The progressive facial asymmetry which ensues is directly related to the injury's damaging effect upon the condylar growth center. There is radiographic evidence that the injury not only affects growth but also alters the anatomical relationships of the structures which give rise to the origin and insertion of the muscles of mastication. Thus, muscle length and direction are involved, contributing to abnormal mandibular movements during mastication and at rest. Soon afterward, facial asymmetry inevitably results.

Alteration of the balanced muscular relationships is a particularly serious condition. Stability and the functional movement of the mandible are disrupted. Hence, detrimental secondary skeletal changes occur to produce an asymmetry; symmetry can be restored by using the principles of myofunctional therapy.

Coccaro (1969) has shown that promoting muscular activity on the defective side helps the muscles achieve their maximal growth potential. The change in myofunction is directly reflected on the intimately related underlying bone. The patient, a 5 year old girl, had fallen on her chin at the age of 2 years. The examination showed a deviation of her chin to the right and a flattened appearance of the mandible on the left side (Fig. 30–96). When requested to move her jaw, the patient could move her mandible to the right with facility but had limited movement to the left. This finding suggested some disability of the lateral pterygoid muscle on the right side. The posteroanterior cephalogram (Fig. 30–97, *A*) showed a hypoplastic and medially displaced condyle and ramus on the right side.

At age 6 years, a sectional orthodontic appliance was constructed to fit over the left deciduous cuspid and molars. An occlusal registration was obtained, with the patient deviating the jaw laterally as far to the left as possible. With the appliance in position, the patient was compelled to move the mandible from the affected side to the unaffected side to achieve dental occlusion. The purpose of the appliance was to force the patient to use the muscles of mastication on the hypoplastic right side. The

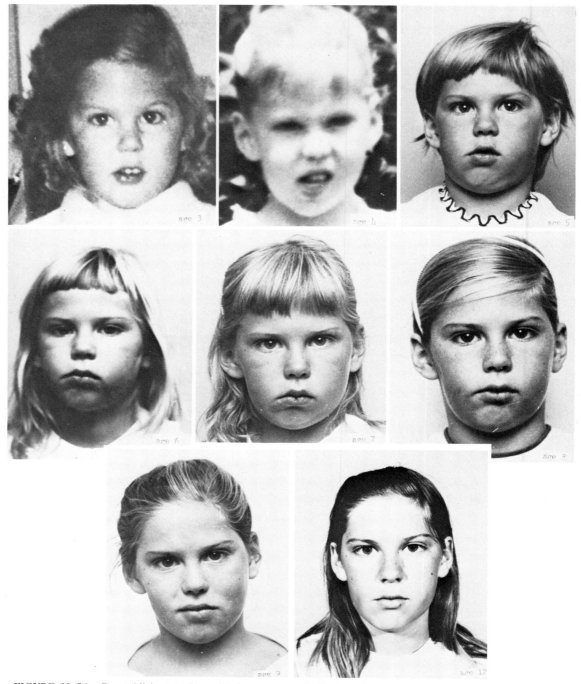

FIGURE 30–96. Reestablishment of mandibular symmetry by increased muscular activity. Asymmetry caused by a fall on the chin at the age of 2 years. The successive photographs show the improvement from the age of 5 years to the age of 12 years as a result of the treatment (see text). (From Coccaro, P. J.: Restitution of mandibular form after condylar injury in infancy (a 7-year study of a child). Am. J. Orthod., 55:32, 1969.)

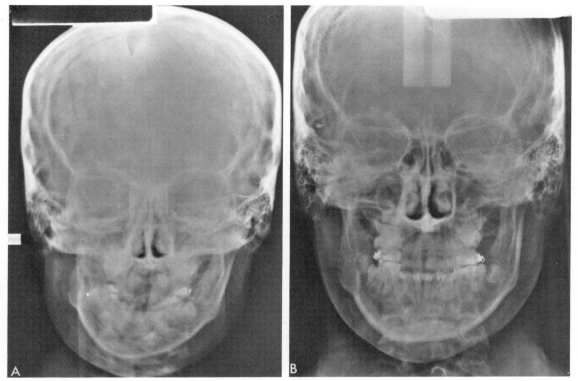

FIGURE 30–97. *A,* Posteroanterior cephalogram of the patient (Fig. 30–96) at the age of 5 years. *B,* Cephalogram at the age of 12 years. (From Coccaro, P. J.: Restitution of mandibular form after condylar injury in infancy (a 7-year study of a child). Am. J. Orthod., *55*:32, 1969.)

patient was instructed to wear the removable appliance at all times and to remove it only after meals for cleaning. Because of wear and changes in retention, second and third appliances were made at later dates. At age 8 years, growth of the affected side appeared to be progressing favorably.

When the use of the appliance was finally discontinued, the patient continued to move her jaw effectively to the unaffected side, even without the appliance. Restoration of symmetry continued as a result of the improved muscular function on the affected side. The discernible changes, with time, in ramus height and im-

FIGURE 30–98. Serial tracings of posteroanterior cephalograms superimposed in the midline and on the lesser wings of the sphenoid bone, showing growth changes contributing to the improvement in facial symmetry. Note the degree of serial reduction of the asymmetry. (From Coccaro, P. J.: Restitution of mandibular form after condylar injury in infancy (a 7-year study of a child). Am. J. Orthod., *55*:32, 1969.)

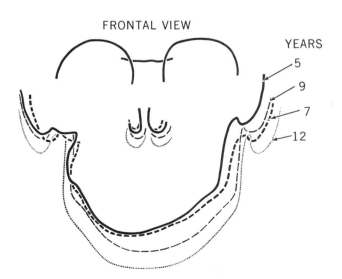

FRONTAL VIEW

YEARS

5

9

7

12

proved condyle-fossa relationships are documented in Figures 30–97, *B* and 30–98.

Attempts have been made to replace the deficient or defective condylar head with a bone graft having an epiphyseal growth center. Metatarsal grafts have been used by Stuteville and Lanfranchi (1955), Stuteville (1957), Entin (1958), Bromberg, Walden, and Rubin (1963), Dingman and Grabb (1964), and Glahn and Winther (1965). Costochondral grafts were also employed by Bromberg and his associates and by Ware and Taylor (1968), who also used the proximal head of the fibula. Longitudinal studies suggest that the epiphyseal growth center probably does not survive and that the growth observed is mainly appositional growth. The graft serves to restore anatomical relationships and function rather than to re-establish a growth center. This finding is in keeping with the functional matrix theory of Moss (1960).

In the adult, when the deformity is not too conspicuous and the deviation of the chin is the salient feature, a horizontal osteotomy and repositioning of the mental symphysis toward the midline will restore symmetry (see Fig. 30–118).

In some cases it is possible to restore symmetry by bilateral vertical osteotomy combined with orthodontic therapy. Overlap of the ramus fragments on the longer side will equalize mandibular length on both sides. More severe hypoplasia results in a unilateral micrognathic deformity discussed earlier in the chapter (see p. 1343).

CONDYLAR HYPERPLASIA AND UNILATERAL MANDIBULAR MACROGNATHIA

Condylar hyperplasia can result from injury during childhood. Gruca and Meiselles (1926), Ivy (1927), Rushton (1944), McNichol and Rogers (1945), Cernéa (1954), and others have reported on this condition. The condyle progressively enlarges and elongates, a characteristic finding in this type of hyperplasia.

The ramus and one-half of the body of the mandible enlarge in all dimensions. The occlusal relationships of the teeth are thus also affected. The patient shows a shift of the midpoint of the mandible toward the contralateral side. The posterior maxillary teeth on the involved side are usually in a buccal crossbite relationship. A posterior open bite is a frequent occurrence. Facial contour is prominent over the enlarged condyle, and roentgenograms confirm the increased size of the head of the condyle. No limitation of the temporomandibular joint motion is observed. The characteristic deformity is shown in Figure 30–99, *A*. There is often associated pain in the temporomandibular joint. The pain radiates in various

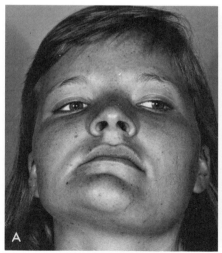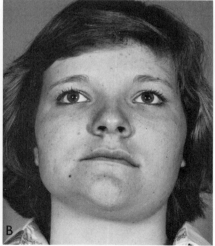

FIGURE 30–99. *A*, Patient with left-sided condylar hyperplasia. Note that the chin is deviated to the unaffected side. *B*, Appearance following staged condylectomy and recontouring of the inferior border of the mandibular body on the affected side.

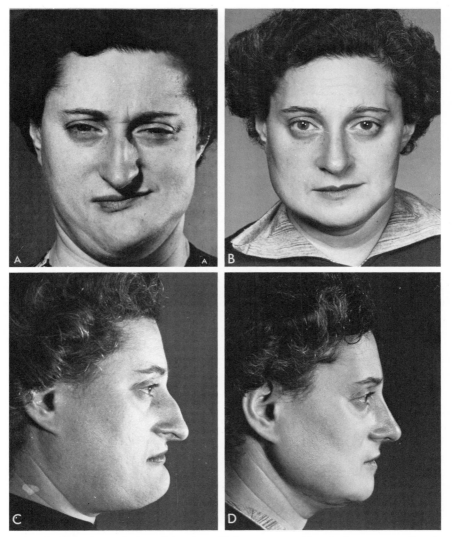

FIGURE 30–100. Condylar hyperplasia and hemimandibular macrognathia. *A*, Appearance of patient with lateral deviation, malocclusion, and macrognathia of the right hemimandible. *B*, After bilateral osteotomy of the body of the mandible to improve the dental occlusion (see Fig. 30–101), resection of the excess bone from the lower portion of the body of the mandible on the right (see Fig. 30–102), transplantation of the resected bone to improve the contour of the chin, and a corrective rhinoplasty. *C*, Preoperative profile. Note that the lower border of the mandible bows inferiorly. *D*, Postoperative appearance. (From Converse, J. M., and Shapiro, H. H.: Treatment of developmental malformations of the jaws. Plast. Reconstr. Surg., *10*:473, 1952. Copyright 1952, The Williams & Wilkins Company, Baltimore.)

directions and is more acute when the patient opens his mouth. Resection of the condylar head on the affected side interrupts progression of the asymmetry and relieves the symptoms (Fig. 30–99, *B*).

A patient with the characteristic deformity of unilateral macrognathia of the mandible is shown in Figure 30–100. In addition to the condyle, the entire half of the mandible is hyperplastic. The only relevant history was

that of an injury to the mandible following the removal of a molar tooth at the age of 12 years. Progressive enlargement of half of the mandible and elongation of the face on the same side continued until the patient was 28 years old. Figure 30–100 shows that the lower border of the mandible of the involved side bows inferiorly; the chin deviates to the left, and the angle of the mouth on the same side appears elevated. The overbite of the upper

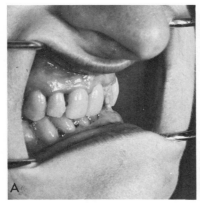
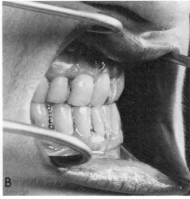

FIGURE 30–101. Preoperative (*A*) and postoperative (*B*) views of the dentition of the patient shown in Figure 30–100. The dental occlusion was improved by bilateral osteotomies through the body of the mandible.

anterior teeth is pronounced and is accompanied by a lingual version of the mandibular teeth and the alveolar process (Fig. 30–101, *A*). With the teeth in occlusion, the incisal edges of the upper anterior teeth contact the labial gingival tissues of the lower jaw. The mandibular anterior teeth are tilted toward the right.

Condylectomy is essential to arrest continued growth. The condyle is exposed through a preauricular incision. The root of the zygomatic arch is identified, and the capsule of the joint is incised transversely. The enlarged condylar head and a portion of the neck are removed.

Additional procedures are often required in patients with unilateral macrognathia. In the patient shown in Figure 30–100, a step osteotomy on each side anterior to the mental foramen was performed to correct the dental arch relationships (Fig. 30–101, *B*). Six weeks later the inferior border of the enlarged body of the mandible was resected. Care must be taken to identify the position of the inferior alveolar canal, since it may lie below the proposed line of the mandibular resection. The entire inferior alveolar canal was decompressed, and the neurovascular bundle was transposed to a higher level in a groove prepared in the mandible to permit resection of the necessary amount of bone to restore symmetry (Fig. 30–102). Final restoration of the contour of the symphysis was achieved at a later date by onlay bone grafts. A rhinoplastic operation completed the facial contour restoration (Fig. 30–100, *B*, *D*).

When the patient was first examined, hypertrophy of the right condyle was overlooked. Attention was focused on the facial deformity. Seven years after completion of the corrective surgery, the patient complained of increasing pain in the right condylar region which was referred to the area of distribution of the auriculotemporal nerve. Surgical resection of the hypertrophied condyle relieved the patient of her symptoms.

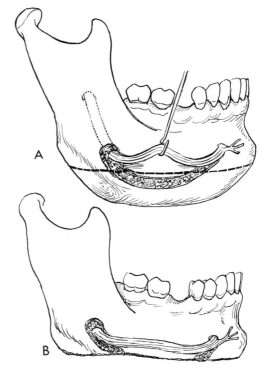

FIGURE 30–102. Transposition of the inferior alveolar neurovascular bundle. *A*, Resection of hypertrophied bone (shown by broken line). The neurovascular bundle has been lifted from the canal in order to preserve continuity. *B*, The mandible following resection of the hypertrophied bone.

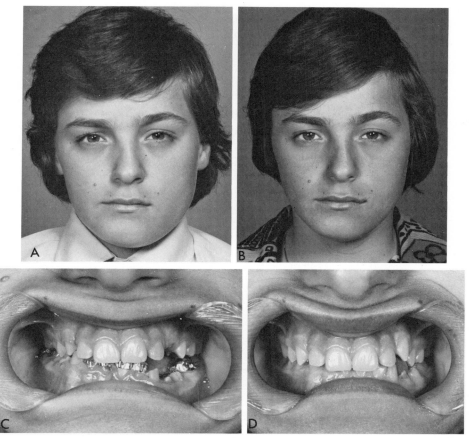

FIGURE 30–103. Lateral deviation of the mandible caused by elongation of the neck of the condyle. *A*, Patient with deviation of the chin to the right caused by an elongated condylar neck on the left side (see Fig. 30–104). *B*, After resection of a measured section of the neck of the left condyle. *C*, Occlusal relationships prior to the surgical correction. Note the deviation to the right. *D*, Dental occlusion after completion of the treatment.

FIGURE 30–104. *A*, Tracings of a panoramic roentgenogram showing the elongation of the neck of the condyle on the left side. *B*, After resection of a measured segment from the condylar neck.

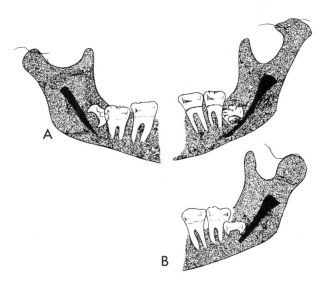

This case illustrates several points. First, it is necessary to resect the condyle to arrest the continued growth and eventual discomfort and pain resulting from the increased size of the condyle. Second, it shows the sequence of events that should be followed in treating a mandibular malformation with malocclusion. Initial treatment should be directed toward correction of the malocclusion. The next step is the restoration of contour of the mandible by removal of the excess bone and the addition of onlay bone grafts to areas of deficiency. Finally, the case emphasizes the need for longitudinal follow-up evaluation.

In the exceptional case in which the neck of the condyle is unusually elongated, causing laterognathism, resection of a measured segment of the condylar neck reestablishes symmetry and adequate dental occlusion (Figs. 30–103 and 30–104).

HEMIFACIAL HYPERPLASIA

Hemifacial hyperplasia is a rare congenital deformity that affects both the soft tissues and the bony tissues of the face. The terms facial hemihypertrophy, hemifacial hypertrophy, and hemifacial gigantism have also been used. Its etiology is unknown, and no heredity pattern is present. Rowe (1962), in reviewing the subject, found that the condition is more prevalent in males than in females and involves the right side of the face more frequently than the left. Histologic studies show an increase in the number of cells. The asymmetry is progressively accentuated through puberty. Abnormal enlargement generally ceases at the age of 17 to 18 years as skeletal maturation occurs.

Enlargement of the zygoma, maxilla, and mandible on the affected side is present. The inferior alveolar canal is also increased in size. The cranium may also be involved. Premature development and eruption of the teeth occur, as well as macrodontia of varying degrees. The overlying facial soft tissues are increased in bulk, and the auricle may be increased in size. Unilateral enlargement of the tongue and its papillae is also a feature. The entire ipsilateral side of the body, or in some cases the contralateral side, can be involved.

Treatment is difficult and consists of reducing the bulk of the facial soft tissues and repositioning the jaws to a more normal location. Surgical procedures similar to those used to correct unilateral mandibular macrognathia can be employed. Robinson, Shuken, and Dougherty (1969) recommended early con-

dylectomy on the affected side to reduce the ongoing asymmetrical growth.

LATERAL MANDIBULAR DEVIATION RESULTING FROM LOSS OF BONE

Acquired deformities due to bone loss usually require bone grafting and elongation osteotomy procedures similar to those described in the section concerning mandibular micrognathia (see p. 1348). Additional details concerning the correction of these deformities will be found later in this chapter (p. 1481).

FACIAL HYPERPLASIA

Pathologic states such as fibrous dysplasia, cherubism, and acromegaly result in increase of facial skeletal size. Facial hyperplasia of unknown origin is rare.

Acromegaly, an endocrine disorder characterized by enlargement of the bones of the head and gigantism due to dysfunction of the pituitary gland, is one of the best-known examples of facial hyperplasia. A patient with acromegalic features is shown in Figure 30–105. A thorough evaluation, while showing enlargement of the sella turcica, failed to demonstrate elevated growth hormone levels. A mandibular degloving procedure (see Fig. 30–21) was performed, and the mandibular angles were exposed through subangular incisions. A horseshoe segment of the lower portion of the body of the mandible, including the mandibular angles, was resected through a combined intraoral and extraoral exposure. The anterior portion of the resected horseshoe-shaped segment was transplanted over the remaining mandibular symphysis to restore adequate chin projection and the labiomental fold. An iliac bone graft was transplanted in a second operative session as part of a corrective rhinoplasty; in a later stage, a submental excision of redundant soft tissue was required (Fig. 30–105, *B, D*).

Deformities of the Chin

The position and contour of the chin are important components in facial harmony and balance. The chin deformity may be the only deformity, or it may coexist with malformations of the jaws or other facial structures.

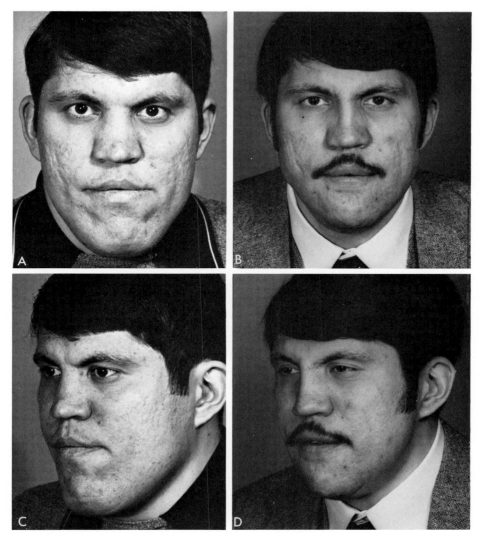

FIGURE 30–105. Patient with acromegalic features. *A, C,* Preoperative views. Note elongated face and flat nose. *B, D,* Appearance following removal of a horseshoe segment from the inferior border of the mandible and transposition to a position anterior to the symphysis. In a separate stage an iliac bone graft was placed over the nasal dorsum, and redundant submental soft tissue was resected.

Anatomical Considerations. The mandible fuses in the midline during prenatal life. At the junction of the two halves, there is a ridge, the mental symphysis, which divides below and encloses a triangular eminence, the mental protuberance. The base of the mental protuberance is depressed in its center. The raised portions on each side form the mental tubercles. On each side of the symphysis is a fossa, the incisive fossa, which gives origin to the mentalis and a small portion of the orbicularis oris muscle. A faint ridge, the oblique line, extends backward and upward from each mental tubercle and passes below the mental foramen; it is continuous with the ridge which forms the an-

terior border of the ramus. The mental foramen is an important surgical landmark, situated below and usually slightly anterior to the second premolar tooth. The quadratus labii inferioris and triangularis muscles are attached to the oblique line immediately lateral to the origin of the mentalis muscle. The platysma is attached to the lower portion of the lateral surface of the mandible below the oblique line.

On the lingual surface near the lower part of the symphysis are two pairs of small projections, the mental spines. The genioglossus muscles arise from the superior mental spines. The lower pair of spines serves as the origin of the geniohyoid muscles. An oval depression is present on each side below the level of the spines. The anterior bellies of the digastric muscles insert into the bony depressions. The mylohyoid muscle originates in the mylohyoid line, which extends posteriorly and upward from the lower part of the symphysis.

The function of the circumoral muscles is affected by the bony deformity of the chin. Alterations of the skeleton are accompanied by changes in soft tissue contour and function. For example, the patient with a small chin may experience difficulty in occluding the lips and achieving lip seal. This appears to be caused by the downward traction of the muscles of the lower lip. These muscles are placed under abnormal tension as a result of their attachment to the backward and downward inclined slope of the skeleton of the chin. An increase in the projection of the chin and the subperiosteal detachment of the musculature of the lower lip (mentalis, depressor labii inferioris, triangularis muscles) will improve this condition in many cases. The chin pad no longer rides upward obliterating the labiomental fold when the patient tries to occlude his lips. Relief of the abnormal tension thus improves the function of the muscles.

MICROGENIA

Microgenia, or "small chin," implies an underdevelopment of the region of the mental symphysis. The term should not be confused or interchanged with the term "micrognathia," in which the deformity involves the various components of the jaw.

Microgenia is often seen in patients with acceptable dentoalveolar relationships, as well as in patients with variable degrees of malocclusion. Frequently, the anterior maxillary dentoalveolar segment is protruded (Class II, division 1 malocclusion). Orthodontic therapy is helpful in de-emphasizing the deformity of the tooth-bearing structures and thus relatively accentuating the chin. Microgenia is also seen in patients with variable degrees of hypoplasia of the mandible (micrognathia) and, paradoxically, in mandibular prognathism.

Diagnosis and Preoperative Planning. Precisely oriented photographs and cephalometric roentgenograms help to confirm the clinical diagnosis. Various cephalometric measurements have been proposed to determine the ideal position of the chin (Ricketts, 1957;

Hambleton, 1964; Merrifield, 1966). These measurements are limited by their two dimensional nature and are useful only as guides; the final analysis depends more on the esthetic judgment of the surgeon.

The nose-chin relationship is an important aspect of vertical facial balance. The general appearance of the face is largely influenced by the size, shape, and position of the nose and chin. As stated earlier in the chapter, it has been proposed that a face divided into equal horizontal thirds represents the best artistic facial balance; however, many esthetically acceptable variations of the ideal ratio are found in nature. Analysis of the nose-chin variations is usually related clinically to the midline of the face, while anteroposterior abnormalities can best be assessed by means of cephalometric roentgenograms and photographs. The planning of the degree of increase in the projection of the chin can be determined, when necessary, by tracing the new position of the chin and measuring the distance between the new tracing and the tracing of the original contour (see Fig. 30–64). In the average case of microgenia, the surgeon is able to estimate the amount of chin augmentation by careful examination of a profile photograph of the patient's face.

Chin Augmentation. Nose-chin relationships to reestablish a balanced profile were emphasized by Aufricht (1934). Use of the dorsal hump of a large hump nose was one of the first means of increasing the projection of the chin. Stripped of mucoperiosteum and mucoperichondrium and shaped, the dorsal hump was introduced over the mental symphysis through a short submental incision. More recently, silicone rubber prostheses (Silastic) have become a popular means of achieving an improved contour of the chin.

Bone and cartilage grafts and a sliding advancement osteotomy of the lower border of the mental symphysis are other techniques which can be employed for remodeling the contour and increasing the projection of the chin.

SURGICAL APPROACH. Prior to draping of the face, a vertical ink line is traced on the skin in the proposed midline of the chin. This line serves as a landmark when the chin is being recontoured. An extraoral or an intraoral approach can be used for exposure.

Extraoral approach. When an extraoral approach is employed, the incision is made under the mental symphysis. In the submental area, a better quality scar is obtained when the incision is made along the inferior border of the mandible rather than in the submental fold. A subperiosteal pocket is made by incising and raising the periosteum. The pocket is only large enough to accommodate the implant or transplant, leaving no dead space (see Chapter 37, Fig. 37–27).

Intraoral approach. A horizontal intraoral incision (Converse, 1950) should be made above the vestibular sulcus, since an incision in this area is difficult to suture and may be placed under tension with eventual disruption; the vestibular cul-de-sac also permits the accumulation of saliva and food debris, which can interfere with the healing of the wound. Either the labiobuccal vestibular incision (see Fig. 30–106) or the gingival incision (see Fig. 30–22) provides adequate exposure. The labial incision is preferred in chin augmentation procedures, since it provides the extra tissue needed to accommodate the increased bulk of the chin. Augmentation procedures, particularly in the mental symphysis region, may place the soft tissues under tension, which can cause separation of the wound edges and exposure of the material used to project the chin. A single midline incision, or two vertical incisions placed laterally are optional techniques to introduce the transplant or implant.

The horizontal incision is made on the inner aspect of the lower lip above the origin of the frenulum. The mucosa alone is incised and raised from the orbicularis oris muscle downward to the bone (see Fig. 30–106, *A, B*). The periosteum is incised along a horizontal line. The extent of the subperiosteal dissection depends upon the size of the contour-restoring material.

If the elevation of the periosteum extends laterally, the mental nerve and vessels should be avoided at their exit from the mental foramen. Wide exposure downward to the inferior mandibular border is obtained, and the transplant or implant can thus be placed in the desired position over the lower portion of the mental symphysis.

Technique of Contour Restoration in Microgenia. Four techniques are available to correct microgenia of the mandible: (1) contour restoration by cartilage or bone grafts, (2) contour restoration by horizontal advancement osteotomy, (3) contour restoration by an inorganic implant, and (4) contour restoration by a skin graft inlay and prosthodontic support.

CONTOUR RESTORATION BY CARTILAGE OR

BONE GRAFTS. Two types of tissue are suitable for contour restoration of the symphysis: cartilage and bone. Allografts and xenografts of cartilage have been used but have their limitations—namely, progressive absorption. Autogenous cartilage grafts survive and maintain their contour but do not consolidate with the underlying bone. Although cartilage allografts have a tendency toward progressive absorption in patients with microgenia, the contour of the chin is preserved for a long period of time (Converse, 1964b).

Iliac bone grafts are generally preferred because they provide a greater proportion of cancellous bone as compared to costal bone grafts.

The amount of subperiosteal elevation is determined by the size of the graft. After intraoral exposure has been obtained (Fig. 30–106, *A, B*), the bone graft is contoured and placed over the mental symphysis (Fig. 30–106, *C*). When lengthening of the lower face is indicated, the graft is hooked under the mental symphysis (Fig. 30–106, *D*). The bone graft is removed from the medial aspect and/or the crest of the ilium and shaped as shown in Figure 30–106, *E*. A pressure dressing is also illustrated in Figure 30–106, *E*. Usually a smaller Elastoplast adhesive tape dressing suffices (see Fig. 30–108).

The surgeon has two alternatives in placing the bone graft over the mental symphysis: he can place it so that the cortex faces either the soft tissues or the host bone.

The cortical surface of the graft is placed against the host bone and the cancellous part toward the skin surface. This orientation of the cancellous surface of the graft has two advantages: (1) the cancellous surface of the graft can be carved and shaped more readily than the cortical surface; and (2) the contact of the cancellous surface with the overlying soft tissues ensures rapid revascularization of the graft. Additional bone chips can also be used to fill the space between the main graft and the host bone and the space lateral to the main graft.

If the surface of the mental symphysis is irregular and the mental tubercles are prominent, the recipient site is flattened with an osteotome or bur. Some of the cortex of the symphysis is removed to achieve a more intimate contact between graft and host.

If an osteoperiosteal graft is employed, the periosteal surface is placed toward the soft tissues. The periosteum plays an important role in minimizing the absorption of the onlay grafts

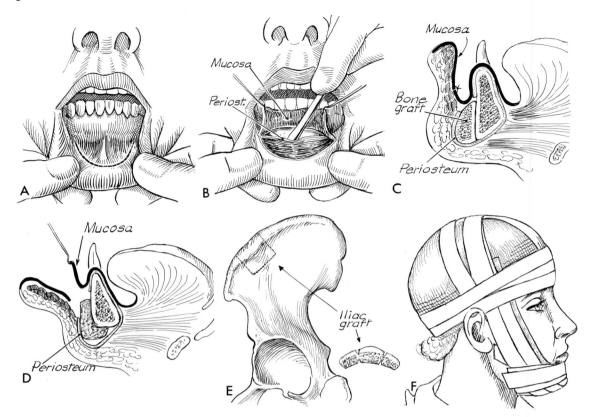

FIGURE 30–106. Iliac bone grafting through an intraoral approach for the correction of microgenia. *A,* Incision through the mucosa is made above the insertion of the frenulum. *B,* The periosteum is incised and raised after the mucosal flap is elevated. *C,* The bone graft is in position. *D,* When vertical increase as well as increased projection is indicated, the graft is hooked under the symphysis. *E,* Site of removal of the iliac bone graft from the medial aspect of the crest and inner aspect of the ilium. *F,* A "definitive" type of dressing as illustrated is usually not required (see Fig. 30–108).

(Thompson and Casson, 1970; Knize, 1974). Contour adaptation is obtained by bending the graft and making a concavity in the cancellous surface.

A guide-suture assists in the correct placement of the bone graft (Fig. 30–107). The guide-suture is removed after the intraoral incision is closed and the Elastoplast fixation dressing is completed. Catgut is used for the guide-suture, since it will be progressively dissolved should the suture break during its removal.

Elastoplast adhesive strapping helps immobilize the bone graft. A 2-cm wide strip of Elastoplast is initially placed in the labiomental fold to prevent upward displacement of the graft. A second strip is added along the lower border of the symphysis, supporting the graft from below. Additional strips are applied over the skin of the chin; the dressing is reinforced with plain adhesive tape for a period of one week (Fig. 30–108). The dressing need not

be continued beyond this time, for the autografts adhere to the underlying bone within a short period of time. Although the use of antibiotics makes bone grafting by the intraoral

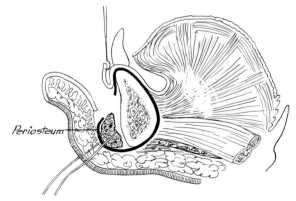

FIGURE 30–107. A guide suture is useful in placing the bone graft over the mental symphysis when the intraoral approach is used.

FIGURE 30–108. Pressure dressing for fixation of contour-restoring bone grafts. *A*, Strips of Elastoplast are placed in the labiomental fold and below the chin, thus limiting upward and downward displacement of the bone graft. *B*, Additional strips of Elastoplast are placed over the chin and are reinforced by strips of adhesive tape.

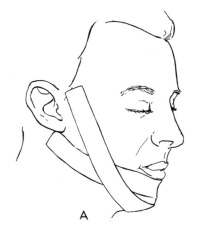
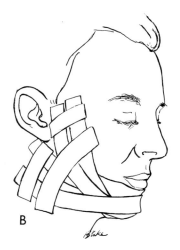

approach possible, it should be emphasized that the prevention of hematoma is essential to ensure the success of the operation. A noncollapsible, flat silicone tube is placed in a dependent position to drain any collection of blood; the tube pierces the skin under the chin and is connected to a continuous suction apparatus (Jackson-Pratt).

Intraoral bone grafting was used to correct the microgenia of the patient shown in Figure 30–109. Cephalometric tracings made preoperatively (Fig. 30–110, *A*) and four years postoperatively (Fig. 30–110, *B*) show maintenance of the size and shape of the graft.

The detachment of the musculature of the chin and the increase in chin projection facilitate lip closure (Fig. 30–109). Preoperatively forced muscular contraction was required to achieve a lip seal (Fig. 30–109).

Bone grafting through the extraoral ap-

proach, using an incision along the lower border of the mandible, is indicated in the more severe deformities (Fig. 30–111).

Onlay bone grafts are not uniformly successful, particularly when minor contour restoration is required. Progressive absorption has been observed in some of the grafts. The absorption appears to be caused by the absence of functional stress. It should be noted that the best results from onlay bone grafts are obtained in the more severe types of micrognathic deformities; serial onlay bone grafts, placed one over the other, have yielded excellent permanent restoration of contour in these cases.

CONTOUR RESTORATION BY HORIZONTAL ADVANCEMENT OSTEOTOMY. The techniques of horizontal osteotomy of the mandible (Hofer, 1942; Obwegeser, 1957; Converse and Wood-Smith, 1964) consist of detaching the

FIGURE 30–109. *A*, Microgenia with downward and backward slant of the lower lip. *B*, Improvement obtained by intraoral bone grafting over the mental symphysis and a corrective nasal plastic operation. (From Converse, J. M., and Campbell, R. M.: Bone grafts in surgery of the face. Surg. Clin. North Am., *34*:375, 1954.)

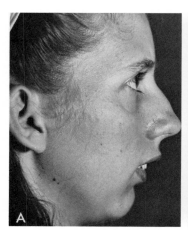
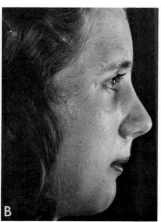

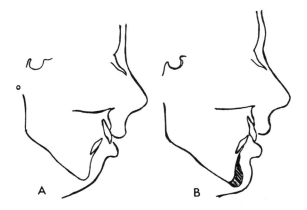

FIGURE 30–110. Cephalometric follow-up of a bone graft placed in the patient shown in Figure 30–109. *A*, Preoperative cephalometric tracing. *B*, Postoperative cephalometric tracing four years after bone grafting.

lower portion of the anterior mandibular body, usually moving it forward, occasionally laterally, and not infrequently transplanting it over the anterior aspect of the mandible. It is a highly versatile technique, and excellent results are obtained.

The horizontal osteotomy (Fig. 30–112) requires exposure of the body of the mandible by the degloving technique (see Fig. 30–21). A Stryker oscillating saw or a cutting bur and an osteotome are used to outline and complete the osteotomy. The level and the angle of the line of osteotomy can be varied to suit the deformity. However, the osteotomy must always be situated below the apices of the teeth. It extends posteriorly, according to the demands of the deformity, often reaching and continuing beyond the mental foramen below the level of the inferior alveolar canal. The position of the inferior alveolar canal is variable and should be identified on preoperative roentgenograms. The canal usually descends for a few millimeters

before reaching the mental foramen. Failure to verify the position of the canal can result in its penetration by the line of osteotomy and severance of the inferior alveolar nerve.

Vertical cuts through the reflected periosteum will allow for greater expansion of the pocket to accommodate the advanced segment of bone.

The surgeon at this point can choose among various alternatives to satisfy the needs of the particular deformity:

1. The inferior segment is advanced after partial or complete subperiosteal detachment of the suprahyoid musculature (Obwegeser, 1957).

2. The inferior segment is completely detached subperiosteally from the suprahyoid musculature and transplanted over the anterior mandibular cortex (Converse and Shapiro, 1952; Converse, 1959), either in two sections (Fig. 30–113) or in one section (Fig. 30–114). The technique is indicated when the vertical

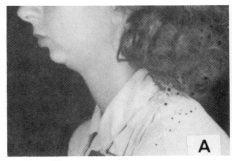
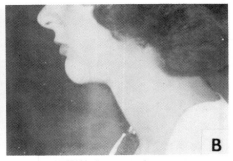

FIGURE 30–111. Mandibular micrognathia, the result of injury in childhood. A long period of orthodontic treatment maintained the teeth in satisfactory occlusion but had little effect on the development of the mandibular body. A previous operation in which preserved cartilage was used failed to correct the condition. *B*, Addition of iliac bone to the mental symphysis and resection of submental adipose tissue gave a satisfactory result. (From Kazanjian, V. H.: Bone transplanting to the mandible. Am. J. Surg., *83*:633, 1952.)

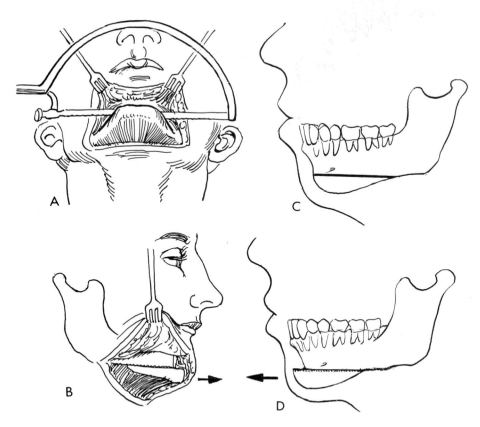

FIGURE 30–112. Horizontal osteotomy to advance the lower portion of the mandible. *A, B,* Hofer's technique (1942) of horizontal advancement osteotomy through an extraoral approach. *C,* Line of osteotomy passing below the mental foramen and inferior alveolar canal. *D,* Fragment is advanced to augment the contour of the chin.

FIGURE 30–113. Horizontal osteotomy and transplantation of bone from the lower portion of the body of the mandible. *A,* The osteotomy is performed with an oscillating saw. *B,* The lower fragment is split into halves and transplanted onto the anterior portion of the symphysis.

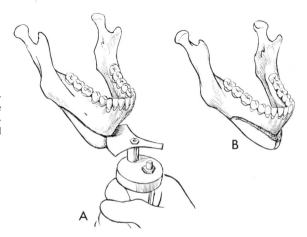

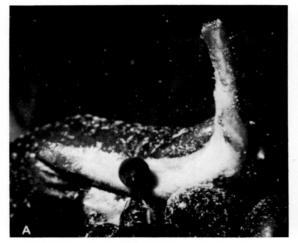
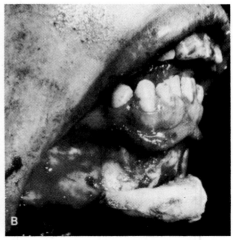

FIGURE 30–114. Horizontal osteotomy and transplantation of the lower fragment. *A*, A large round bur is used to contour the lingual aspect of the lower mandibular fragment to adapt it to the contour of the symphysis. *B*, The fragment is placed anteriorly over the symphysis. (From Kazanjian and Converse.)

FIGURE 30–115. The sandwich procedure. The horizontal osteotomy is combined with a bone graft for vertical elongation of the anterior portion of the mandible and for increasing the prominence of the chin. *A*, The line of osteotomy. *B*, The bone graft has been interposed, in a sandwich fashion, between the lower segment and the body of the mandible. Circumferential wiring immobilizes the bone graft and the detached lower segment. (Figs. 30–115 to 30–119 from Converse, J. M., and Wood-Smith, D.: Horizontal osteotomy of the mandible. Plast. Reconstr. Surg., *34*:464, 1964. Copyright 1964, The Williams & Wilkins Company, Baltimore.)

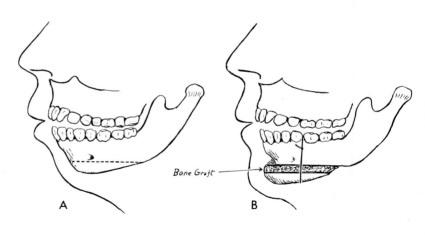

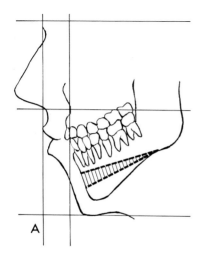
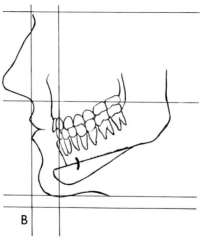

FIGURE 30–116. Horizontal osteotomy and resection of a segment of bone to shorten the vertical dimension of the anterior mandible. *A*, Outline of the segment to be resected. *B*, Advancement and upward repositioning of the lower segment after resection of bone.

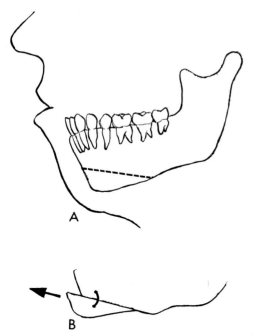

FIGURE 30–117. Oblique osteotomy for advancement and moderate shortening of the vertical dimension of the mandible. *A,* Design of the oblique osteotomy. *B,* Fragment is moved upward and forward and held in fixation by interosseous wiring.

dimension of the lower face is excessive and projection of the chin is desirable. An intimate contact between graft and host bone is obtained by adjusting the contour of the concave surface of the transplant with an air-turbine–driven large vulcanite cutting bur.

3. When increased vertical dimension is required, a bone graft is sandwiched between the mandibular body and the segment detached by the horizontal osteotomy (Fig. 30–115) (Converse and Wood-Smith, 1964).

4. In patients with an excessive vertical dimension of the symphyseal portion of the mandible, a horizontal section is removed between the fragment that is to be advanced and the bone below the apices of the teeth (Fig. 30–116). The resected bone should be limited posteriorly to the portion of the mandible situated below the inferior alveolar canal.

5. An oblique osteotomy (Fig. 30–117) will permit simultaneous advancement and shortening of the vertical dimension of the symphyseal area.

6. In lateral deviations of the mandible, when malocclusion of the teeth and shortening of the mandible on one side are relatively

minor (Fig. 30–118), a horizontal osteotomy permits replacement of the chin in the midsagittal plane (Fig. 30–119) (Converse and Wood-Smith, 1964). In more severe lateral deviations, after mandibular body or ramus lengthening, the midline repositioning of the chin can also be used as a final-stage procedure.

7. The double-step osteotomy (Neuner, 1965) consists of a two-tier osteotomy, two osteotomies made one above the other (Fig. 30–120). The upper segment is advanced first and wire fixation established; the lower segment is then advanced and wired to the upper segment. This is an excellent technique which can be used when the deformity requires considerable advancement (Fig. 30–121). Cancellous bone chips are molded between the fragments and over the interosseous wires to promote rapid consolidation of the fragments. Cephalometric tracings in Figure 30–122 illustrate the change in contour.

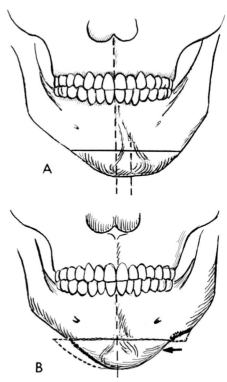

FIGURE 30–118. Correction of lateral deviation of the chin by horizontal osteotomy. *A,* Vertical dotted line shows the amount of deviation of the chin to the left. *B,* After the horizontal osteotomy. The lower mandibular segment is displaced toward the right. The broken line outlines the protruding bone that is resected to obtain a smooth contour.

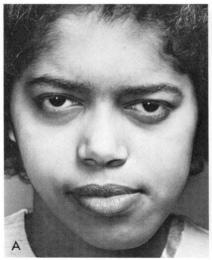
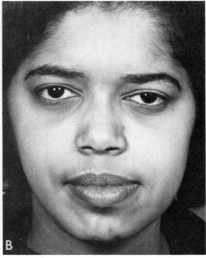

FIGURE 30–119. Patient with lateral deviation and retrusion of the chin corrected by the procedure shown in Fig. 30–118. *A*, Preoperative full-face view showing the lateral deviation of the chin to the left. *B*, Facial symmetry restored by the horizontal osteotomy and displacement of the lower mandibular segment forward and to the right.

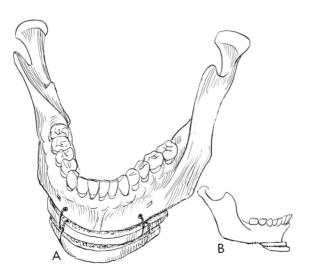

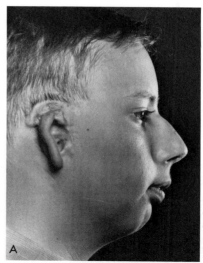

FIGURE 30–120. Double-step osteotomy. *A*, Advancement of the lower segment anterior to the upper segment by a two-tier osteotomy. Interosseous wire fixation is used to maintain the position of the fragments. *B*, Lateral view of the double-step osteotomy. Cancellous bone chips have been added to promote consolidation and to improve the contour. (After Neuner.)

FIGURE 30–121. Double-step osteotomy. *A*, Preoperative view showing microgenia. *B*, Postoperative appearance following a double-step osteotomy by the technique illustrated in Figure 30–120 and a corrective rhinoplasty in the same operative session. Ear reconstruction has also been performed.

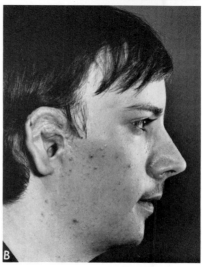

Fixation following horizontal advancement osteotomy. Fixation is efficiently maintained by interosseous wiring of the advanced fragment to the body of the mandible or by fixation of the two advanced segments to each other and to the body of the mandible. The twisted ends of the stainless steel wire are buried in one of the bur holes. The wires become incorporated into the bone and may remain permanently without causing local reaction, either in the soft tissue or in the bone. As with all well-tolerated, permanently buried, inert materials, the procedure is successful unless hematoma and local infection, fortunately rare complications, compel the surgeon to remove the wire.

One or more circumferential wires may be required to reinforce the fixation. The circumferential wires, looped around the jaw or an arch bar (Fig. 30–123), are well tolerated and can be left in position for several weeks without complications.

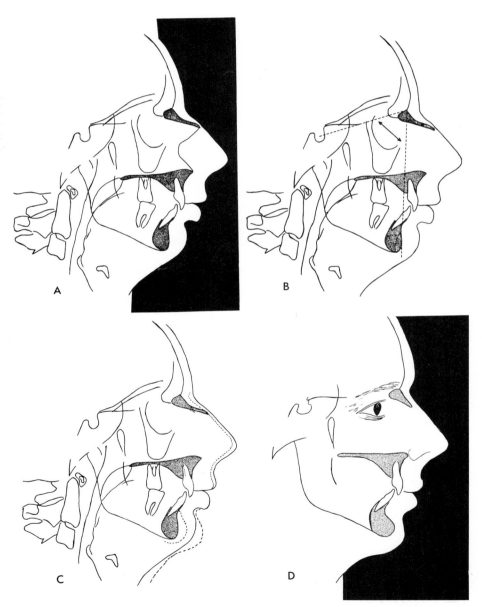

FIGURE 30–122. Cephalometric follow-up of patient shown in Figure 30–121. *A,* Preoperative tracing. *B,* Tracing showing the angle (SNB) denoting mandibular retrusion. *C,* Tracing with dotted lines to indicate anticipated corrections of the nose, chin, and soft tissue. *D,* Tracing with skeletal and soft tissue profile six months after corrective surgery.

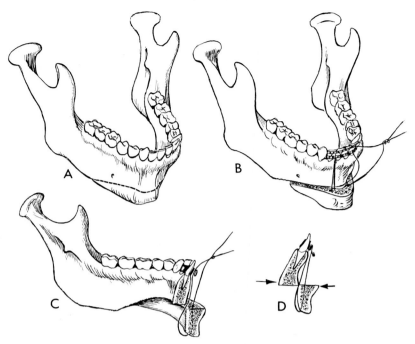

FIGURE 30–123. Circumferential wire fixation of the advanced mandibular segment to an orthodontic appliance after horizontal osteotomy. *A*, Design of the horizontal osteotomy. *B*, The lower fragment has been advanced. Wires are passed through drill holes placed through the posterior portion of the mobilized segment. *C*, Cross-sectional view showing the position of the fixation wire. *D*, Advancement of the mobilized inferior segment. Bony contact is maintained between the lateral portion of the fragment and the body of the mandible.

When the lower portion of the mandible is transplanted over the anterior aspect of the symphysis, wire fixation is not required. The pressure dressing (see Fig. 30–108) serves to anchor the graft.

Bone grafting in conjunction with horizontal advancement osteotomy of the lower portion of the mandible. Chips of cancellous bone assist in the consolidation of the segments and should be used whenever the fragments are mobilized for greater than average distances. When a single segment is advanced to a point where contact is lost between the posterior surface of the arch and the body of the mandible (Fig. 30–124), the intervening space must be filled with cancellous bone. In such cases, use of the double-step osteotomy technique with the addition of bone chips is preferable. Small chips of cancellous bone are placed in the interstices. A "buttonhole" incision over the iliac crest is used to remove the cancellous bone between the inner and outer cortices. In severe deformities, the horizontal advancement osteotomy can also be combined with onlay bone grafts placed over the lateral aspects of the body of the mandible.

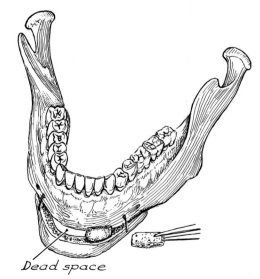

Dead space

FIGURE 30–124. When contact is lost between the advanced segment and the body of the mandible, bone grafts fill the void. The technique illustrated is recommended when such a degree of advancement is required.

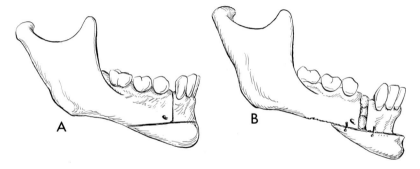

FIGURE 30–125. Combined step osteotomy to lengthen the body of the mandible and horizontal advancement osteotomy. *A*, Outline of osteotomies. *B*, Osteotomies completed. Bone grafts fill the gap in the mandible. It is usually preferable to perform the horizontal advancement osteotomy at a later stage.

The incision is closed with plain catgut sutures. The careful application of a pressure dressing, which relies on the compressive action of the Elastoplast strips, is an important final step. Elimination of the dead space diminishes the chance of hematoma formation and the development of infection in the hematoma. A fine-caliber, flat, noncollapsible, silicone suction drain brought out through the submental area is used to minimize this possibility; antibiotic therapy is routine.

The horizontal osteotomy following surgical lengthening of the jaw: The stick-and-carrot outrigger appliance. A horizontal advancement osteotomy is occasionally feasible in conjunction with a lengthening step osteotomy of the mandible (Fig. 30–125). Usually, however, a horizontal advancement osteotomy is performed as a secondary procedure to complete the restoration of contour.

Tight soft tissues over the mandibular symphysis resist the advancement of the lower portion of the mandibular body after the horizontal osteotomy. Posteriorly directed postoperative muscular forces and soft tissue pressure over the advanced segment of bone can result in gradual recession of the bone. The stick-and-carrot appliance (Fig. 30–126) counteracts this tendency. The appliance consists of a cast dental splint with a forward extraoral extension. The splint is anchored to the teeth of the mandible. A stainless steel wire is looped through a hole drilled near the lower border of the advanced bone segment. The ends of the wire are passed transcutaneously below the chin pad and are attached to the outrigger extension. Continuous forward traction is then exerted on the bone fragment. The soft tissue pressure is counteracted, and the downward and backward rotation of the advanced bone fragment is prevented. The forward traction is maintained until consolidation is well established and the soft tissues have become progressively distended. In one of our patients, the traction was maintained for 11 weeks.

Distension of the soft tissues with a silicone implant. The silicone implant is placed over the lower portion of the mental symphysis to distend the soft tissues. In the patient shown in Figure 30–127, the implant remained in position for four months. It was then removed, and the avascular capsule was carefully removed to restore the blood supply to the area. A horizontal osteotomy was then performed, and advancement of the bone encountered no soft tissue resistance. There was, however, some absorption of bone; it was concluded that the large implant should have been removed at two months.

Complications. After fixation is assured, there is little danger of a recession of the advanced fragment unless the soft tissues exert an unusually strong backward force. Possible means of relieving such pressure include (1) the addition of an adequate vestibular lining prior to osteotomy; (2) wide periosteal elevation; (3) vertical scoring of the periosteum; and (4) use of the stick-and-carrot traction appliance.

The main complication is formation of a hematoma, which provides a fertile medium for the growth of bacteria. Infection and abscess

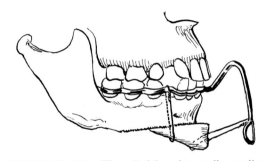

FIGURE 30–126. The "stick-and-carrot" appliance (see also Fig. 30–77).

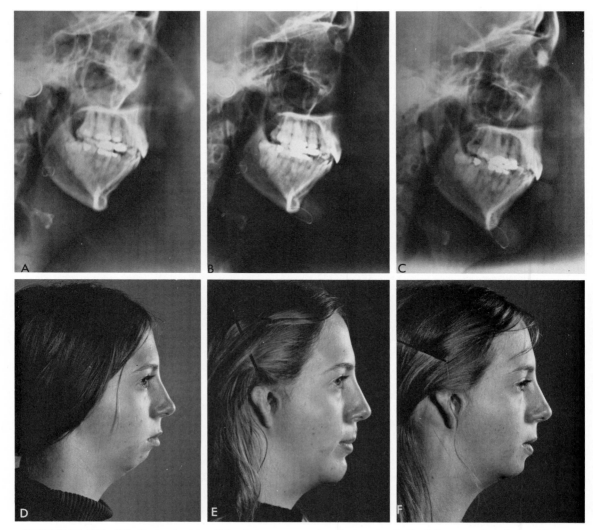

FIGURE 30–127. Silastic implant to distend the premental soft tissues. *A,* Cephalogram of patient with severe microgenia (craniofacial microsomia). *B,* Implant in position five days. The implant was wired to the lower border of the symphysis; however, the implant is being tilted upward. *C,* After four months, the implant has caused absorption of bone. *D,* Preoperative profile of the patient. Note the restrictive soft tissue. *E,* Appearance one month after implantation. *F,* Six months after removal of the implant and horizontal osteotomy. Because of the absorption of the bone by the implant, a lesser degree of advancement was obtained. The implant should not be left in position longer than two months to avoid erosion of bone caused by the pressure of the soft tissues over the implant.

formation require incision and dependent drainage and removal of buried wires.

Exposure of the bone grafts as a result of dehiscence of the intraoral mucosal incision should not occur if the incision is placed high above the sulcus. Although this complication is always worrisome when it occurs, healing by second intention usually closes the wound.

Results. The techniques of (1) horizontal advancement osteotomy and (2) horizontal osteotomy and transplantation of the segment as an onlay graft over the symphysis of the mandible have proved to be reliable and successful.

The procedures not only increase the projection of the mental symphysis but also widen the contour of the anterior portion of the mandible. The horizontally sectioned lower segment of the mandible is arch-shaped. As it is advanced, the lateral contour on each side of the mental symphysis increases. If the lateral protrusion is excessive, the excess bone should be reduced. If the lateral protrusion is unusually excessive, the advanced segment is sectioned in the midline, particularly when the bone is transplanted as an onlay graft.

A cephalometric survey of cases of horizon-

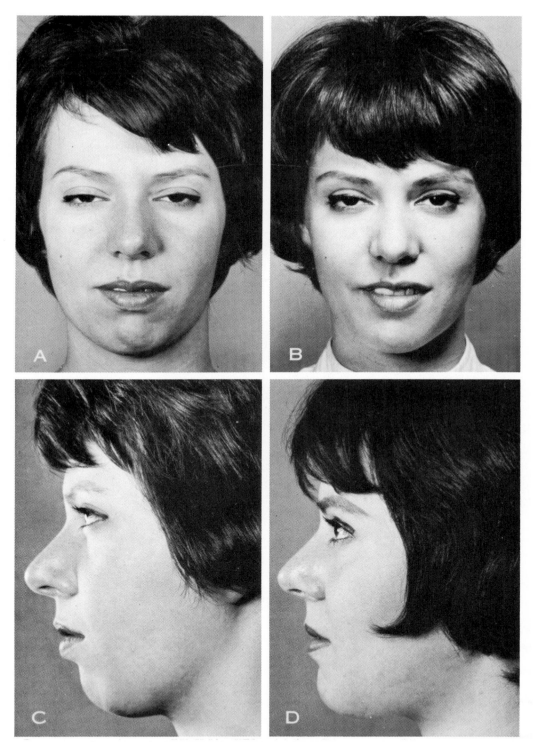

FIGURE 30–128. Correction of microgenia using a horizontal osteotomy. *A, C,* Preoperative views. *B, D,* Following horizontal osteotomy and advancement of the lower mandibular segment. (Figs. 30–128 and 30–129 from Converse, J. M., and Wood-Smith, D.: Horizontal osteotomy of the mandible. Plast. Reconstr. Surg., *34*:464, 1964. Copyright 1964, The Williams & Wilkins Company, Baltimore.)

tal osteotomy done over a period of 20 years has shown the procedure to be successful in a high proportion of cases. During the first year the edges of the advanced or transplanted bone become rounded, with minimal change in the degree of projection of the graft. In subsequent years a small loss of volume of the advanced or transplanted fragment occurs; this is not clinically significant, since the facial contour is maintained with relatively little change.

In the patient shown in Figure 30–128, the cephalometric roentgenograms taken prior to surgery (Figs. 30–129, *A* and 30–130), shortly after surgery (Figs. 30–129, *B* and 30–130), and seven years after surgery (Figs. 30–129, *C* and 30–130) show the remodeling process that has taken place. Loss of the projection of the advanced segment has not occurred.

The horizontal advancement osteotomy offers a distinct advantage over iliac bone graft onlays, since there is little absorption of the advanced bone. In mandibular micrognathia (as opposed to microgenia), it offers a particular advantage over inorganic implants, which are

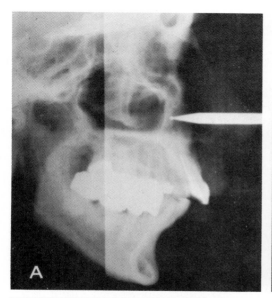

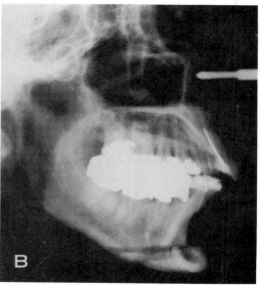

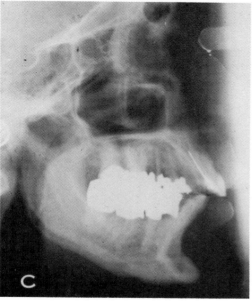

FIGURE 30–129. Cephalometric longitudinal study of the patient shown in Figure 30–128. *A*, Prior to surgery. *B*, During the postoperative period. *C*, Seven years after surgery. Note the rounding of the upper edge of the advanced bone as described in the text.

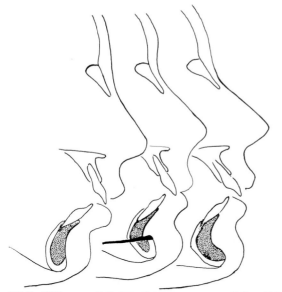

PRE-OP.   POST-OP. 7 YRS. POST-OP.

FIGURE 30–130. Tracings of the cephalometric longitudinal study of the patient shown in Figure 30–128.

best suited for less severe deformities (microgenia).

CONTOUR RESTORATION BY AN INORGANIC IMPLANT. Inorganic implants in the form of silicone rubber have their main application in microgenia. Prefabricated silicone implants are commercially available in various sizes and shapes. The solid silicone implant has been widely used. Recently a silicone implant filled with a gel (Snyder, 1975) and having a Teflon strip on its posterior to minimize slippage has become available; the implant is soft rather than hard. Clinical experience with this type of implant is limited.

The prefabricated solid implants can be used without modification of shape or can be trimmed to fit the individual deformity. The implants are placed in a supraperiosteal or subperiosteal pocket through either a submental incision or the intraoral approach. Because the operative procedure is simple, inorganic implants have become popular in the treatment of moderate degrees of microgenia and as adjuncts to a corrective rhinoplasty. The concomitant corrective procedures on the nose and the chin usually achieve a successfully balanced profile.

The body of the mandible is formed of hard, dense bone in its lower skeletal portion and of spongy bone with thin lingual and buccal cortices in its dentoalveolar portion. Robinson and Shuken (1969) reported bone absorption under inorganic implants and postulated pressure as the causative agent. As a result of misplacement of the implant or its upward displacement by the pressure of the overlying soft tissues, the implant may penetrate through the thin cortex into the softer cancellous bone and endanger the roots of the incisor teeth (Fig. 30–131). Figure 30–132 is a diagrammatic

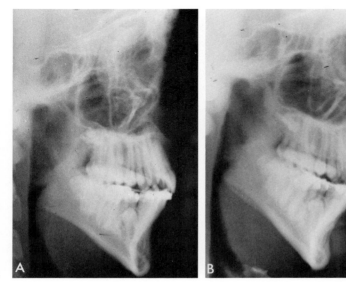
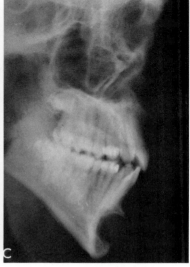

FIGURE 30–131. Penetrating silicone implant. *A,* Preoperative cephalogram. *B,* Four months after placement of the silicone implant. Note the erosion of the bone. *C,* Two years after surgery, the implant has penetrated the bone, endangering the roots of the teeth.

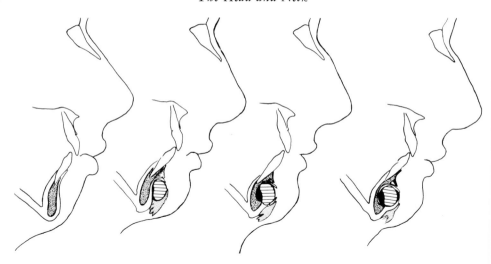

FIGURE 30–132. Cephalometric tracings illustrating the progressive penetration of the silicone implant over a two-year period. From left to right: preoperative; postoperative, 4 months; postoperative, 16 months; postoperative, 24 months. Although progressive incorporation of the silicone implant has occurred, note that the soft tissue profile improvement has been maintained.

illustration of the progressive incorporation of the implant into the bone. In this particular case, despite the sinking in of the implant, the roots of the teeth were spared. The implant was incorporated within the bone, and the surrounding capsule became calcified. Figure 30–133 shows a long-term follow-up of the patient, demonstrating maintenance of the restored contour.

Technique. The inorganic implant is usually introduced through an intraoral approach into a subperiosteal or supraperiosteal pocket. Implants placed over the periosteum tend to be less stable than implants positioned subperiosteally.

One may also elect to introduce the implant through a short submental (cutaneous) incision, although some female patients may object to this approach. The incision is made under the chin along the lower border of the mental symphysis. The periosteum is exposed and incised in a vertical fashion. Two subperiosteal pockets are prepared on each side of the incision through the periosteum. The pockets are sufficiently large to accommodate the implant, which is introduced into one lateral pocket, folded on itself, and placed into the contralateral pocket. Dead space should be avoided (see Chapter 37, Fig. 37–27, for technical details). The subcutaneous layer is

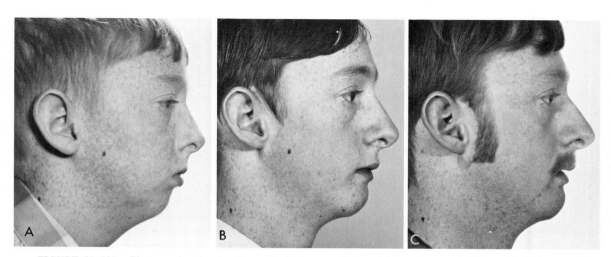

FIGURE 30–133. Photographs showing the patient whose cephalometric tracings are in Figure 30–132 at age 13 years, 16 years, and 20 years.

sutured; the operation is completed by suture of the skin. As the implant is fitted into a restricted space, it is maintained in position by the surrounding tissues, and the chance of hematoma formation is decreased.

Two precautions should be observed as the inorganic chin implant is inserted. The first is to place the implant over the hard and resistant bone of the mental symphysis, where it should be well adapted to avoid instability and dead space. The second is to prevent hematoma formation by making the pocket only large enough to accommodate the implant, by providing postoperative compression using an Elastoplast dressing, and, if deemed advisable, by providing submental continuous suction drainage.

Supraperiosteal placement of the implant has been advocated to prevent underlying bony absorption. While there is some suggestion that this technique causes less absorption of the subjacent bone, the important point is to position the implant over the hard bone of the lower portion of the symphysis.

A guide-suture (see Fig. 30–107) is an aid in positioning the implant. The following routine has been adopted: (1) a small notch is made with the scalpel in the midline of the upper border of the implant (if the solid silicone implant is used); (2) the midline of the chin is traced with ink; (3) the implant is inserted into its pocket with a double-armed (two straight needles) suture of catgut looped around the implant and through the midline notch; (4) the needles are passed through the skin; (5) traction is exerted upon the suture, and the implant is placed under direct vision in the midline of the lower portion of the symphysis and is maintained in the correct position while the intraoral wound is sutured with catgut suture; (6) Elastoplast strips placed into the labiomental fold exert pressure and immobilize the implant; and (7) the catgut suture is removed, and the dressing is completed.

Complications. The main complications are the upward displacement of the implant and erosion and penetration of the mandible. When the implant penetrates the mandible but does not endanger the apices of the teeth, as shown in the series of cephalometric tracings in Figure 30–132, it is encapsulated and incorporated into the bone. The capsule surrounding the implant becomes calcified.

When the implant penetrates the softer tooth-bearing portion of the mandible (see Fig. 30–131), the implant should be removed to save the teeth.

Figure 30–134, *A* to *C* shows a series of cephalometric tracings which illustrate a case in point. The bone absorption occurred

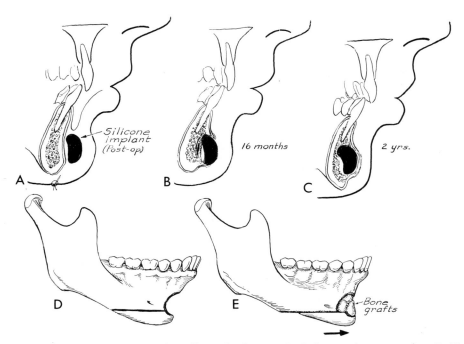

FIGURE 30–134. Treatment of a penetrating silicone implant. *A, B, C,* Progressive penetration. *D,* The implant is removed; a horizontal advancement osteotomy is outlined. *E,* After advancement and bone grafting of the defect.

rapidly over a two-month period. The degloving procedure was used to approach the symphysis and to remove the embedded implant. After the capsule which had formed around the implant was removed, a horizontal advancement osteotomy of the lower border of the mandible was performed, and chips of iliac bone were packed into the remaining cavity (Fig. 30–134, *D, E*). Because of the danger of bone absorption beneath an inorganic implant or its extrusion, the horizontal advancement osteotomy is a preferable method of treatment of the major types of microgenia.

Infection, usually resulting from a hematoma, requires removal of the implant. Extrusion as a result of excessive soft tissue pressure usually occurs through the newly healed oral wound. Occasionally, the implant can rotate in the soft tissues and produce an undesirable chin contour. Migration of the implant has also been observed.

Results. The clinical application of the in-

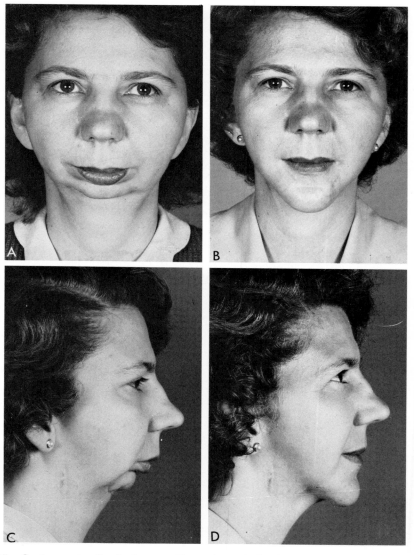

FIGURE 30–135. Contour restoration by bone grafting and prosthodontics in mandibular micrognathia. *A,* Preoperative chinless appearance. *B,* Restoration of contour obtained by bone grafting and a dental prosthesis. The labial sulcus was restored by the skin graft inlay technique to accommodate the overextended denture flange which helped to restore the chin contour. *C,* Preoperative birdlike facial profile. *D,* Postoperative profile view. (From Converse, J. M., and Shapiro, H. H.: Treatment of developmental malformations of the jaws. Plast. Reconstr. Surg., *10:*473, 1952. Copyright 1952, The Williams & Wilkins Company, Baltimore.)

organic implant should be limited to moderate cases of microgenia. When excessively large implants are placed, the pressure of the overlying tight tissues may cause bony erosion and absorption of the underlying mandible. Extrusion and migration of the implant are other problems which can follow injudicious use in such cases.

Erosion of the bone can be seen on the cephalometric roentgenogram within months. after implantation. When the overlying tissues are tight, soft tissue pressure appears to be the principal factor in this process. A small amount of erosion can actually be beneficial; it will allow the implant to "seat" itself and prevent displacement.

A cephalometric survey of 85 chin implants suggests that small and medium-sized implants are well tolerated in the absence of tight overlying soft tissues (Friedland, Coccaro and Converse, 1976). Although some degree of erosion was noted, it did not appear to progress for more than a few months after implantation. The survey also emphasized the advisability of placing the implant over the hard, resistant bone of the mental symphysis.

CONTOUR RESTORATION BY SKIN GRAFT INLAY AND DENTAL PROSTHESIS. The skin graft inlay technique, which is used for restoration of the buccal sulcus after reconstruction of the mandible, is discussed later in this chapter. It has been applied to achieve contour restoration in mandibular micrognathia when the mandible is edentulous. The labial flange of the denture is extended downward and has an anteriorly directed curvature in order to maintain the labiomental fold and adequate chin projection.

The technique (see Chapter 67) is not an entirely satisfactory method of restoring contour.

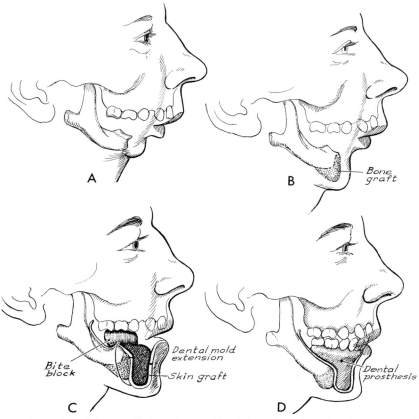

FIGURE 30–136. Correction of the mandibular micrognathia of the patient shown in Figure 30–135 by a combination of bone grafting, a skin graft inlay, and a dental prosthesis. *A,* Mandibular micrognathia with absence of the condyle. Note that the coronoid process of the mandible articulated with the infratemporal surface. *B,* An onlay bone graft is added to the anterior portion of the mandible in a preliminary operation. *C,* After healing of the bone graft, a skin graft inlay is done. The inlay is maintained by the downward extension of the bite-block into the newly formed sulcus. Circumferential wiring holds the prosthesis in position. *D,* Final denture with an enlarged labial flange which extends into the skin-grafted labial sulcus to restore the contour of the lower portion of the face.

It has its limitations, but it is a justifiable compromise in patients of the older age group.

A skin graft inlay procedure was done on the patient with mandibular micrognathia shown in Figure 30–135. Osteomyelitis had occurred following a fracture of the mandible resulting from the removal of a tooth early in childhood. The mandible had failed to develop beyond the childhood stage. The condyles were hypoplastic, and the mandible articulated with the base of the skull by way of the coronoid processes (Fig. 30–136, *A*). Because of the posterior position of the micrognathic mandible, a base for a lower denture capable of articulating with the teeth of the maxilla could not be provided. Sufficient bone was not available to permit an elongation osteotomy. It was decided that bone should be added to the mandible anteriorly to provide bony support for a denture (Fig. 30–136, *B*). The inferior labial sulcus, anterior to the bone graft, was deepened with a skin graft inlay (Fig. 30–136, *C*).

After the skin graft had healed, the compound mold was replaced by a denture constructed with a large labial flange which extended into the deepened sulcus. Denture retention was improved by the deepened sulcus, and the lower facial contour was also restored (Fig. 30–136, *D*).

MACROGENIA

Macrogenia describes specifically the overdevelopment of the chin area. This portion of the mandible develops independently from the rest of the mandible bone and is strongly influenced by hereditary factors. The chin protuberance, as are other facial dimensions, is larger in males. While a large chin is esthetically acceptable in the male, a similar mental protuberance in females produces an unpleasing prognathic appearance.

Macrogenia frequently occurs in conjunction with mandibular prognathism, but it is also seen as an independent malformation. The chief complaint of the patient usually centers on the lower facial imbalance and the prognathic appearance.

Surgical correction of macrogenia in the absence of true prognathism poses a difficult problem. Cephalometric tracings are used to determine the amount of reduction required to improve the facial contour. The degloving approach is used for subperiosteal exposure of the mental symphysis. Three procedures are available to correct macrogenia.

1. **Removal of the Excess Bone.** Removal of the bone from the symphyseal area usually does not result in appreciable improvement in the soft tissue contour of the chin. If the excess soft tissue drapes poorly over the newly contoured bone, a double chin appearance may result.

The thickness of the bone to be removed is indicated on the shank of a round cutting bur by an ink line. The bur is drilled into the bone until the ink line reaches the surface of the bone. This maneuver is repeated at a number of points over the symphysis. The drill holes are then filled with surgical ink. A large, pear-shaped cutting bur removes the excess bone until the depth of the guide bur holes is reached, as indicated by the presence of the ink stain. Care must be taken to avoid eliminating the labiomental fold by the excessive removal of bone.

2. **Horizontal Recession Osteotomy.** A horizontal section and retrusion of the symphyseal area inferior to the dentoalveolar segment can also be employed. The basic technique is the same as that described for the treatment of microgenia (see p. 1387). In patients with an excessive vertical dimension of the chin, a horizontal section of bone should be removed to restore facial balance. In some cases, improved soft tissue redistribution is achieved by leaving the soft tissue attached to the inferior border of the recessed segment.

3. **Osteotomies Similar to Those Used to Correct Mandibular Prognathism.** These procedures are rarely indicated in the treatment of macrogenia. Improved facial balance can be achieved, but at the expense of incurring a dental malocclusion.

Careful attention must be taken so that the soft tissue is repositioned by carefully applied strips of Elastoplast to minimize the danger of producing a postoperative double chin appearance.

Benign Masseteric Hypertrophy

Benign masseteric hypertrophy is characterized by an asymptomatic unilateral or bilateral increase in size of the masseter muscle. Bilateral involvement is more common. Legg (1880) first described the condition, and it has been subsequently reported by Boldt (1930) and

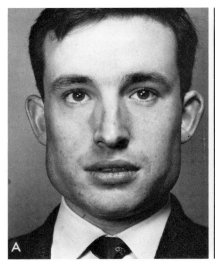 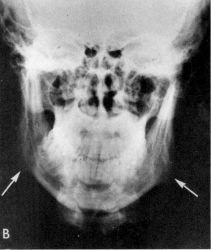

FIGURE 30–137. Bilateral masseteric muscle hypertrophy. *A,* Typical square jaw facial appearance. *B,* Roentgenogram showing hyperostosis in the region of the angle of the mandible.

Coffey (1942). The surgical treatment of the abnormality was described by Gurney (1947) and Adams (1949).

The deformity occurs with equal frequency in both sexes and has its highest incidence in the third decade of life (Wolhynski, 1936; Oppenheim and Wing, 1959). The patient is often emotionally unstable (Guggenheim and Cohen, 1959, 1960, 1961), and may have a "jaw-clenching" habit, lending substance to Gurney's "work hypertrophy" theory. The etiol-ogy is unknown in most cases (Waldhart and Lynch, 1971).

Diagnosis. The face has a square contour, with prominence of the preauricular and mandibular angle regions (Fig. 30–137, *A*). The diagnosis is confirmed by palpating the masseter muscles with the patient at rest and during biting. The condition has been mistaken for a parotid tumor or lymphangioma. Roentgeno-logic studies usually show hyperostosis with ac-

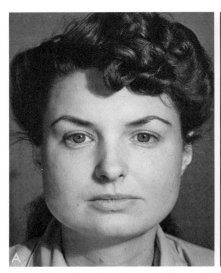 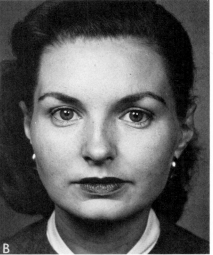

FIGURE 30–138. Bilateral masseteric muscle hypertrophy. *A,* Preoperative appearance. *B,* After resection of excess masseter muscle and removal of hyperostotic bone from the angle of the mandible by the intraoral approach.

centuation of the mandibular angle (Fig. 30–137, *B*). The neurologic examination and electromyographic studies are usually inconclusive. Biopsy studies have reported "normal striated muscle" (Coffey, 1942).

Treatment. Resection of the excess muscle is indicated to improve facial contour. The external inframandibular approach described by Adams (1949) exposes the inferior border of the mandible and the masseter muscle. The medial part of the muscle and the hyperostotic areas are removed under direction vision. Gurney (1947) excised only the lateral portion of the muscle. Converse (1951) used the intraoral approach for the resection of the hypertrophied muscles and the protruding hyperostotic bone at the angle of the mandible (Fig. 30–138). Ginestet, Frezière, and Merville (1959) also recommended the intraoral approach. This approach avoids an external scar and the danger of damage to the marginal mandibular branch of the facial nerve. The oral mucosa and the underlying buccinator muscle are incised over the anterior border of the masseter muscle, and the medial portion of the masseter muscle is resected.

Open Bite Deformities of the Jaws

The term open bite (apertognathism) is applied when the teeth fail to occlude when the jaws are brought together. An open bite occurs in the incisor segment (anterior open bite or apertura incisiva), in the premolar and molar segments (posterior open bite), or in both segments (lateral open bite) of the dentoalveolar arch. The deformity primarily affects the dentoalveolar complex but both the dentoalveolar segment and the body of the jaw can be involved. Dysfunction of the orofacial musculature almost always accompanies the malocclusion.

Anterior open bite, in particular, results in functional and esthetic disturbances. The functional disturbance is characterized by the absence of the concerted and coordinated action of the tongue and teeth in pronouncing certain consonants; in addition to the speech impairment, many patients with anterior open bite have difficulty in mastication. Anterior open bite is also frequently characterized by an elongation of the lower third of the face, a finding which may be sufficiently pronounced to constitute a conspicuous deformity.

Etiology. Numerous causes of open bite malformation have been proposed: vitamin deficiencies (for example, rickets), faulty mouth habits and neuromuscular patterns, temporomandibular joint arthritis, tumors, and trauma. The majority of open bite deformities are caused either by imbalance of the orofacial musculature or by trauma. Patients with open bite malocclusion frequently have a history of finger sucking or lip or tongue thrusting habits. Disturbance of neuromuscular patterns leads to tongue thrusting between the upper and lower teeth during the act of deglutition, and the subsequent development of an anterior open bite. The patients frequently have difficulty in obtaining lip seal, and hyperactivity of the mentalis muscle attempts to compensate for this deficit.

Traumatic Open Bite. Trauma is a common cause of the skeletal type of open bite. Kazanjian and Converse (1974a) listed the most frequent causes as follows:

1. Bilateral fractures of the ramus, especially at the level of the condylar neck. The backward and upward displacement of the tooth-bearing segment invariably causes a shortening of the vertical dimension of each ramus. Occlusal contact of the dentition occurs only in the region of the posterior molars.

2. Malunited fractures of the body of the mandible, which usually are not serious but often interfere with masticatory efficiency.

3. Fractures of the bones of the midface, with the maxilla being displaced backward, resulting in premature contact of the posterior teeth.

4. Untreated jaw fractures in children, with disturbance of the growth centers and the development of an increasing deformity with growth.

5. Distortion of the mandible by scar contractures following cervical burns.

It is essential to distinguish etiologic factors, if any, and the type of deformity present before beginning treatment.

PREOPERATIVE PLANNING. An appreciation of the vertical dimension of the face should be obtained during the clinical examination. The height of the lower third of the face will influence the surgical treatment. The orofacial musculature pattern must also be carefully observed. Failure to recognize faulty muscular activity invites relapse and a poor final result.

Dental casts are essential in studying the

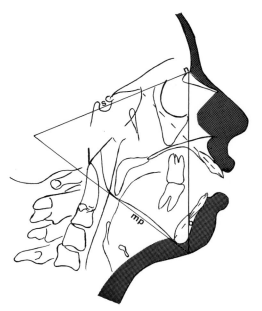

FIGURE 30–139. Cephalometric tracing of a patient with an anterior open bite. Note the increase in the facial height, the steep mandibular plane and the downward tilt of the anterior aspect of the mandibular body. The hard palate shows an unusual downward tilt.

dentoalveolar component of the deformity. Working dental casts are sectioned to determine the location of the osteotomies required to correct the deformity.

Cephalometric roentgenograms best define the skeletal component of the deformity. The anterior facial height is often elongated, and the mandibular plane (MP) is steep, as noted by the increased MP-SN angle (Fig. 30–139). Elongation of the lower third of the face is often caused by the downward tilt of the anterior portion of the body of the mandible, which increases the distance between the anterior nasal spine and menton. The vertical dimension of the ramus is often short, and mandibular prognathism (increased SNB) is a frequent concomitant deformity. The amount of eruption of the molar teeth and the inclination of the incisor teeth (Ll-MP and Ul-SN) should also be recorded, since they have a bearing on the type of treatment.

Occasionally, the lower third of the face is not elongated. Such a situation can be seen following a malunited fracture of the maxilla. Patients with craniofacial dysostosis also have an associated open bite without an increased vertical dimension of the lower third of the face. The maxillary hypoplasia compensates for any

tendency toward facial elongation (see Chapter 56).

An open bite malocclusion that affects primarily the dentoalveolar segment responds well to orthodontic treatment if concomitant improvement in the muscular forces acting on the dentoalveolar structures is also achieved. However, in patients with an open bite secondary to a developmental malformation of the jaw and craniofacial skeleton, the response to orthodontic therapy alone is often poor, and correction cannot be achieved without surgical-orthodontic treatment.

Open bite deformities can thus be associated with vertical displacement in all or part of the upper or lower dentoalveolar segments and with prognathism or retrognathism. In problems which are not amenable to orthodontic therapy alone, orthognathic surgery of the mandible or the maxilla or both can be of assistance. The choice of the corrective technique will depend on whether the open bite is primarily due to a malformation of the mandible or of the maxilla.

The differentiation between an anterior open bite of maxillary origin and a mandibular open bite is aided by study of the cephalogram. If the palatal plane reflects an upward deflection anteriorly and a downward deflection posteriorly, the diagnosis of maxillary anterior open bite is confirmed. In mandibular open bite, the palatal plane is level, and the anterior portion of the mandible shows a downward cant.

Treatment will also differ depending upon whether or not an elongation of the lower third of the face is present.

Thus, before surgery is attempted, the following questions must be answered: (1) Is the basic defect in the maxilla, in the mandible, or in both? (2) Is the deformity a dentoalveolar or a skeletal problem? (3) Is there a vertical increase of the lower third of the face?

Surgical-Orthodontic Treatment of Open Bite: Historical Background. As mentioned earlier, the first operation in the United States to correct an open bite deformity and a prognathism of the lower jaw was reported by Hullihen in 1849 (Fig. 30–140). The operation consisted of the resection of bilateral V-shaped segments of bone from the upper two-thirds of the mandible in the premolar region; a subapical horizontal osteotomy then connected the resected wedge-shaped areas. The anterior dentoalveolar segment was tilted backward and upward to close the open bite. Blair in 1897 (Angle, 1898) and von Eiselsberg (1906) per-

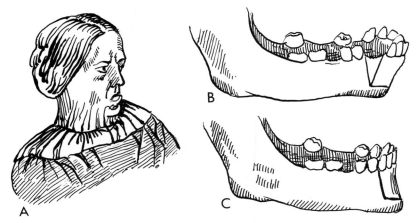

FIGURE 30–140.   Hullihen's operation for the correction of open bite. *A*, The open bite was caused by contractures due to a third degree burn. *B*, Outline of the V-shaped segment to be resected and the dentoalveolar osteotomy. *C*, Result of the operation.

formed similar operations. Lane (1905) and Pickrell (1912) corrected open bite deformities by the removal of a wedge-shaped segment of bone, which extended through the entire thickness of the mandible in the premolar area. Subsequently, osteotomies of the mandibular ramus and body to correct mandibular prognathism and micrognathism were adapted to close the open bite malocclusion. A reversed L vertical osteotomy of the ramus with resection of a V-shaped section of bone was described by Limberg (1925) for the treatment of micrognathia with an anterior open bite (Fig. 30–141). He later (1928) proposed the addition of a costal bone graft, a technique applied by Schuchardt (1958). Robinson (1957) used an iliac bone graft to fill the gap.

Selective movement of a segment of the dentoalveolar arch after osteotomy (segmental os-teotomies, see p. 1409) has also been used to correct an open bite. The principles for this type of operation were developed by Cohn-Stock (1921), Spanier (1932), Wassmund (1935), Schuchardt (1955), and Köle (1959a).

In general, most open bite deformities caused by dentoalveolar malrelationships can be corrected by selective *segmental alveolar osteotomies* of the jaws. *Skeletal open bite* caused by deformity of the main body of the jaw usually requires movement of a larger portion of the jaw.

Surgical-Orthodontic Correction of Dentoalveolar Open Bite.   Dentoalveolar open bite deformities are most frequently located in the anterior portion of the upper or lower jaws; the anterior maxillary or the anterior mandibular teeth, occasionally both, fail to attain a hori-

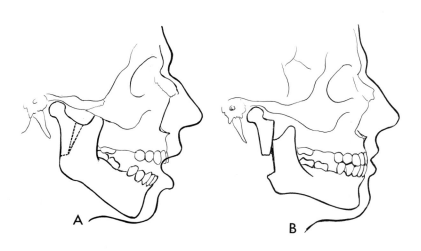

FIGURE 30–141.   Limberg's operation for correction of an anterior open bite. *A*, Outline of osteotomy with V-resection of bone from the ramus. *B*, After closure of the open bite.

zontal plane in relation to the occlusal plane. Often, the incisor teeth also protrude. Occasionally, overeruption of the posterior maxillary dentoalveolar segment causes the anterior open bite; premature contact of the molar teeth prevents the anterior teeth from occluding (see Fig. 30–142). The anterior as well as the posterior open bite deformity can be corrected by planned dentoalveolar osteotomies.

Segmental osteotomies require that the blood supply to the fragment be maintained through either a labial, buccal or lingual mucoperiosteal flap. Elimination of the blood supply from both flaps leads to the disastrous sequestration of the dentoalveolar segment. Parnes and Becker (1972) reported a case in which both the labial and palatal mucoperiosteum was elevated from the anterior maxillary segment. Necrosis of the entire segment occurred. Revascularization studies in animals by Bell (1969), Bell and Levy (1970), and Brusati and Bottoli (1970) confirmed the long-standing clinical observations that preservation of a single mucoperiosteal flap is essential.

POSTERIOR SEGMENTAL ALVEOLAR OSTEOTOMY FOR CORRECTION OF THE MAXILLARY ANTERIOR OR LATERAL DENTOALVEOLAR OPEN BITE. Schuchardt (1955) described a two-stage method applicable to the closure of a posterior open bite and also to the closure of an anterior open bite resulting from premature contact of overerupted upper posterior teeth (Fig. 30–142). In a first stage, after a palatal flap is raised, an anteroposterior osteotomy of the hard palate was performed along the base of the alveolar process on each side (Fig. 30–142, A). In a second stage six weeks later, a buccal mucoperiosteal flap was raised, and anterior and interdental osteotomies were performed in a vertical direction to a level above the apices of the teeth; the two vertical osteotomies were then joined by a horizontal osteotomy. Bone was resected above the apices of the teeth (Fig. 30–142, B), and the anterior open bite was closed (Fig. 30–142, C). When a posterior open bite was present, the mobilized fragment was lowered toward the occlusal plane to close the bite, and a bone graft was inserted in the resulting bony gap.

In the case of an anterior open bite, a segment of bone was resected superiorly, and the premolar-molar segment was elevated into the maxillary sinus to close the anterior open bite. Care must be taken when the hard palate osteotomy is being performed to direct the line of section into the maxillary sinus and not into the floor of the nose. If the osteotomy is misdirected into the floor of the nose, obstruction by the lateral wall of the nasal cavity will require that the lateral wall be comminuted, or partly resected, when the mobilized dentoalveolar segment is impacted into the maxillary sinus.

The operation is done in one stage if a mucoperiosteal flap is preserved for providing blood supply to the mobilized segment

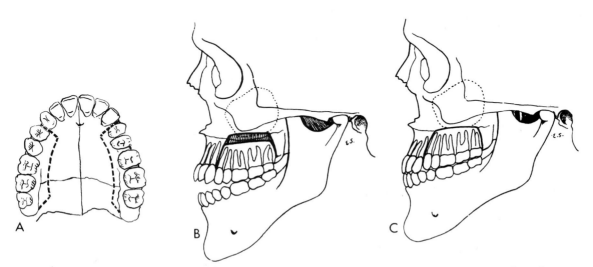

FIGURE 30–142. Schuchardt procedure for closure of an anterior open bite. *A*, In the first stage, bilateral osteotomies of the alveolar processes are performed as outlined. The palatal flap is reapplied, preserving the vascular supply. *B*, Six weeks later, a buccal mucoperiosteal flap is raised, and the lateral aspect of the maxilla is exposed. A segment of the maxilla above the apices of the teeth is resected as indicated by the shaded area. *C*, Correction achieved following vertical repositioning of the posterior maxillary segments; fixation is maintained by arch bars and intermaxillary wiring. (After Schuchardt.)

(Kufner, 1968). The buccal mucoperiosteal flap is raised, and after the buccal osteotomy is performed, a narrow, thin, tapered osteotome is introduced through the buccal osteotomy line, traversing the maxillary sinus to perform the osteotomy without injuring the palatal mucoperiosteal flap. Intermaxillary fixation is maintained for six to eight weeks.

West and Epker (1972) have applied a similar technique to correct unilateral or bilateral posterior maxillary crossbite and to reposition the posterior maxillary alveolus distally when there is insufficient space for an erupting canine or premolar tooth.

ANTERIOR SEGMENTAL ALVEOLAR OSTEOTOMY FOR THE CLOSURE OF MAXILLARY OPEN BITE.   An anterior premolar segmental osteotomy to close the open bite is done ac-

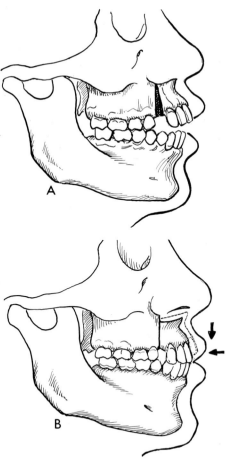

FIGURE 30–143.   Anterior segmental dentoalveolar osteotomy for the closure of a maxillary open bite. *A,* An anterior dentoalveolar segment is outlined. *B,* The segment is mobilized; the open bite is closed.

cording to a technique similar to that used in the procedure described in the correction of a mandibular open bite (Fig. 30–143). A mucoperiosteal palate flap maintains the vitality of the teeth on the mobilized segment (for details of the technique see Segmental Osteotomies, p. 1427).

ANTERIOR SEGMENTAL ALVEOLAR OSTEOTOMY FOR THE CLOSURE OF MANDIBULAR DENTOALVEOLAR OPEN BITE.   Since Hullihen's original operation (1849), the mandibular anterior segmental dentoalveolar osteotomies have been refined by Köle (1959b) and Schuchardt (1963). A labial mucoperiosteal flap is raised, and vertical osteotomies are made at the selected interdental spaces (see Fig. 30–18). A transverse osteotomy below the level of the apices of the teeth connects the lower limits of the vertical sections. A thin, tapered osteotome is used to complete the interdental vertical osteotomy. Blood supply is maintained by a lingual mucoperiosteal flap. The fragment is then elevated toward the occlusal plane to close the open bite deformity. Bone grafts are interposed into the resulting defect to support the transposed segment. Intermaxillary fixation is not required. The mobilized segment is secured by an orthodontic appliance or an arch bar which is reinforced by quick-curing acrylic. Fixation is maintained for a period of six weeks.

Advantages and disadvantages of segmental alveolar osteotomies.   Segmental osteotomy provides a means of selective surgical-orthodontic correction of a dentoalveolar malocclusion. Correction of only that part of the dental arch which is actually deformed is achieved. Body and ramus osteotomies can also be used, but they are more involved and may introduce a secondary malocclusion and an undesirable change in the facial contour. When the deformity is in the anterior portion of the dental arch, an additional advantage is that monomaxillary fixation is all that is required; intermaxillary fixation need be only temporary and can be released after the desired occlusion is ensured.

The disadvantages are minimized by careful attention to technique. The survival of the mobilized segment depends upon the preservation of either a lingual or a buccal mucoperiosteal flap. The flap should be protected throughout the operation. It should be designed to provide coverage of the lines of osteotomy and any bone grafts. These precautions and careful apposition of alveolar bone adjacent to the interdental osteotomy will decrease the risks of excessive alveolar bone loss and subsequent periodontal problems (Kent and Hinds, 1971; Bell, 1971). Thin, tapered osteotomes must be used to complete the interdental aspect of the osteotomy to prevent damage to the roots of the neighboring teeth. Injury to the apices of the teeth is always a possibility. Therefore, it is advisable to preserve at least 3 and preferably 5 mm of bone beyond the apices. The canine teeth have the longest roots and are the most apt to be injured. An estimate of their length can be obtained from intraoral dental roentgenograms. The teeth in the mobilized segment usually retain their vascularity and regain their sensibility if their apices are not directly damaged (Butcher and Taylor, 1951; Madritsch, 1968; Johnson and Hinds, 1969; Barton, 1973; Pepersack, 1973). In the study by Pepersack, 94.5 per cent of the maxillary teeth and 75 per cent of the mandibular teeth responded to stimuli one year postoperatively. The incidence of damage to the mandibular teeth was higher — 1.5 per cent as compared to 0.3 per cent involving the maxillary teeth. The increased number of cases involving nonresponse and injury to the lower teeth is explained by the greater difficulty of the surgical approach and the differences in the vascular and nerve supply. Teeth adjacent to the interdental osteotomy encounter the greatest risk. Poswillo (1972), in animal experiments, showed that progressive fibrosis and loss of odontoblasts occurs in the pulp of the mobilized teeth. Nerve fibers do not regenerate, but the teeth retain their viability and vascularity. Hutchinson and MacGregor (1969) postulated that the return of sensibility is due to the perivascular nerve supply.

Relapse is always a possibility, especially if orofacial musculature dysfunction is overlooked. Detrimental habits and neuromuscular patterns are difficult to correct, but their control is crucial to the success of the operation.

The posterior maxillary segmental osteotomy (Schuchardt procedure) has been abandoned by most surgeons because of the high incidence of relapse. However, Kufner (1968) and West and Epker (1972) have shown that this need not be the case if the mobilization is complete and the segment can be repositioned with ease. The transverse posterior palatal osteotomy (see Fig. 30–146), when indicated, is another technique which ensures complete mobilization and eliminates recurrence.

Since the maxillary sinus is entered during the operation, alterations in sinus function may theoretically occur. Such problems have not been reported (Young and Epker, 1972). It is important to evaluate preoperatively any history of sinus disease and to eliminate any pathology before the operation.

Surgical Correction of Skeletal Open Bite. Skeletal open bite deformities are also best managed by a combined orthodontic and surgical approach. The skeletal structures supporting the dentoalveolar structures must be altered to correct the open bite deformity. Osteotomies of the skeletal complex alone or in conjunction with a segmental dentoalveolar osteotomy may be required.

OPEN BITE WITH MAXILLARY MICROGNATHIA OR RETROGNATHISM. This type of open bite occurs as a result of the vertical displacement of the maxillary segment in whole or in part. The patient usually has an anterior open bite as a result of premature contact of the posterior teeth.

Maxillary micrognathia with an anterior open bite malocclusion is often seen in craniofacial malformations, such as cleft palate, Apert's syndrome, and Crouzon's disease (see Chapter 56). Early childhood injury can produce a hypoplastic and retruded maxilla with an open bite deformity. Retrognathism and an open bite malocclusion can be the result of a malunited fractured maxilla displaced posteriorly and superiorly. The choice of treatment depends upon the severity of the deformity. A low maxillary (LeFort I) osteotomy, a naso-orbitomaxillary osteotomy, a LeFort II osteotomy, or a craniofacial disjunction (LeFort III) osteotomy may be indicated to correct the deformity. These osteotomies are discussed later in the chapter.

OPEN BITE WITH INCREASE OF THE VERTICAL DIMENSION OF THE LOWER THIRD OF THE FACE. Anterior open bite of this type is associated with an abnormality of the ramus or the body. The mandibular plane is steep (increased MP-SN angle), and the anterior facial height is increased (see Fig. 30–139). Clinically, the chin appears excessively long. Close study of the cephalogram will show that the chin is of normal size; it appears to be elongated because of its inferior displacement. The basic problem is a short ramus, a downward slope of the mandibular body, and a wide gonial angle. In some cases, the gonial angle is so wide that the condyle and the chin are joined by a line that is nearly straight; there is no, or very little, mandibular angle.

When the vertical dimension of the ramus is short, an osteotomy of the ramus is indi-

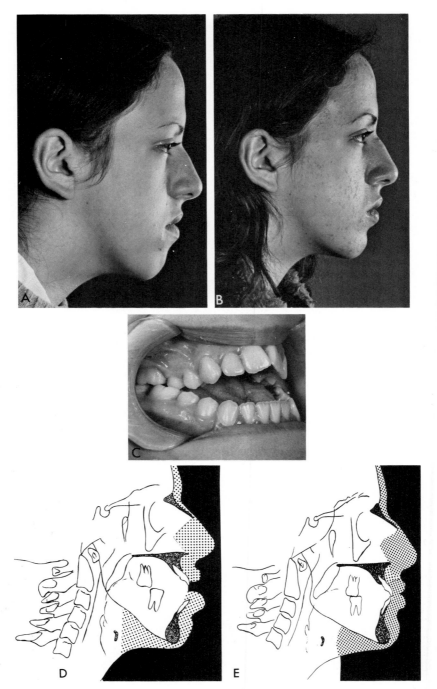

FIGURE 30–144.   Correction of an anterior open bite by bilateral sagittal osteotomies of the ramus. *A*, Preoperative appearance of the patient. Note the elongation of the lower third of the face and the downward cant of the jaw. *B*, After bilateral sagittal osteotomies of the ramus and rotation of the mandible to close the open bite (see *C* and *E*). *C*, The dental view showing the open bite. *D*, Preoperative cephalometric tracing. *E*, Postoperative cephalometric tracing. The open bite is closed.

cated. A sagittal splitting procedure (see p. 1326) and an L-osteotomy with bone grafts inserted into the resulting gap (see p. 1348) are the preferable techniques, since they leave the temporalis muscle undisturbed with the condylar fragment. The tooth-bearing segment of the mandible is rotated upward to close the open bite, and, as in the patient shown in Figure 30–144, the technique also corrects the mandibular prognathism.

Sagittal splitting or other types of osteotomies of the ramus will correct an open bite only in certain favorable cases. Our experience in using the sagittal osteotomy to close open-bite deformities is as follows. Closure of the open bite is achieved at the time of surgery. However, over a variable period of time, the bite progressively reopens to a degree much less than the original condition. A secondary osteotomy is required to treat the relapse. A dentoalveolar osteotomy is done if the vertical dimension of the lower face is satisfactory. An osteotomy through the body of the mandible is indicated if the vertical dimension of the lower face remains excessive. In some cases, additional reduction of the symphyseal height using a horizontal osteotomy procedure is necessary.

Open bite deformities caused by a downward slope of the mandibular body can be corrected by a bilateral body osteotomy through the portion of the dental arch where the open bite first appears. The anterior segment is raised to the desired occlusal level to correct the malocclusion. An interdental osteotomy avoids the extraction of a tooth unless such an extraction is indicated to obtain adequate occlusion. A vertical osteotomy through the body of the mandible can be used successfully (see ·Fig. 30–154); a reverse step osteotomy (Fig. 30–145), when feasible, is generally preferable, because it provides a wider surface of contact. A V-shaped wedge resection (after extraction of a premolar) may be required if the anterior teeth are inclined labially (Fig. 30–145). Small chips of bone from the resected mandibular bone are packed into the defect between the bone fragments to ensure consolidation; soft tissue coverage must also be provided.

After closure of an anterior open bite, the anterior facial height is reduced and facial balance is restored. The repositioned chin may appear adequate in size and shape.

TRANSVERSE POSTERIOR PALATAL OSTEOTOMY FOR CLOSURE OF AN ANTERIOR OPEN BITE. This procedure is occasionally indicated when the cephalogram shows an unusually downward cant of the hard palate (and the floor of the nose). This type of deformity has been observed in patients with an abnormal skeletal deformity due to a neuromuscular disease. The upward displacement of the floor of the nose in such patients does not interfere with the airway (Fig. 30–146).

For closure of an anterior open bite caused by premature contact of the molar teeth, the palatal mucoperiosteum is raised to preserve its blood supply by tunneling under it from one alveolar process to the other (Fig. 30–147). Through this tunnel, the hard palate and vomer are sectioned. A buccal anteroposterior horizontal supra-apical osteotomy is extended posteriorly to the pterygomaxillary junction. The pterygomaxillary junction is sectioned to free the entire posterior palatal-alveolar segment, which can then be displaced upward to

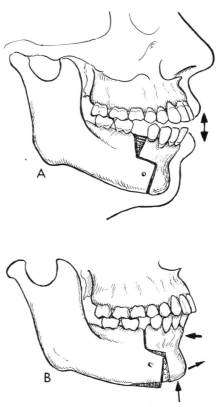

FIGURE 30–145. Reverse-step osteotomy for closure of an open bite. *A,* Reverse-step osteotomy. A V-shaped area of bone is resected from the alveolar process. *B,* Position of the mandibular segment after osteotomy. The gap between the fragments is filled with bone taken from the V-shaped segment resected from the alveolar process as shown in *A.* The lower border of the mandible is trimmed.

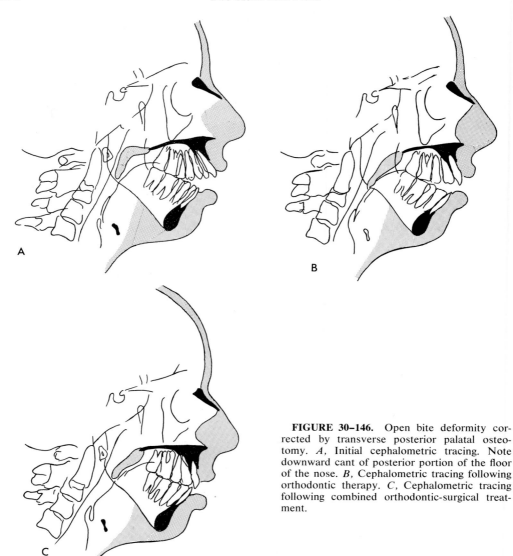

FIGURE 30–146. Open bite deformity corrected by transverse posterior palatal osteotomy. *A*, Initial cephalometric tracing. Note downward cant of posterior portion of the floor of the nose. *B*, Cephalometric tracing following orthodontic therapy. *C*, Cephalometric tracing following combined orthodontic-surgical treatment.

correct the anterior open bite after resection of an adequate segment of bone from the vomer and lateral wall.

No disturbance in velopharyngeal competence has been found following this type of operation.

The case of the patient shown in Figure 30–148 represents an excellent example of cooperation between surgeon and orthodontist. Presurgical orthodontic therapy was helpful in obtaining a satisfactory final dental occlusion after the operation. The patient's original position in repose is shown in Figure 30–148, *A*. The patient's molar teeth are in occlusion, but the anterior open bite prevents lip seal. The lips are occluded only under forced muscular contraction. The appearance after orthodontic therapy and the transpalatal osteotomy is shown in Figure 30–148, *B*. The occlusal views demonstrate the anterior open bite before (Fig. 30–148, *C, D*) and after (Fig. 30–148, *E*) surgical-orthodontic treatment.

TRANSVERSE POSTERIOR PALATAL OSTEOTOMY FOR CLOSURE OF A POSTERIOR OPEN BITE. A technique similar to that illustrated in Figure 30–147 is employed to close a posterior open bite. The posterior palatal segment is displaced downward, and bone grafts fill the gaps resulting from the downward displacement of the palate and alveolar processes.

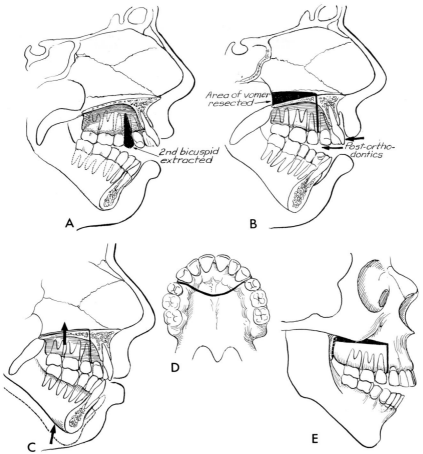

FIGURE 30–147. Technique of transverse posterior palatal osteotomy. *A*, Sagittal view showing cant of floor of nose. Second bicuspids were extracted. *B*, Lines of osteotomy and area of vomer resection. Note change in inclination of anterior teeth following orthodontic treatment. *C*, Following osteotomy and elevation of the posterior segment. *D*, Palatal view of line of osteotomy. *E*, Lateral view of line of osteotomy and maxillary resection.

FIGURE 30–147. *Continued. F, G,* The lines of osteotomy and the new position of the posterior portion of the palate. *H,* Postoperative intermaxillary fixation and craniofacial suspension. The interocclusal dental wafer is in place.

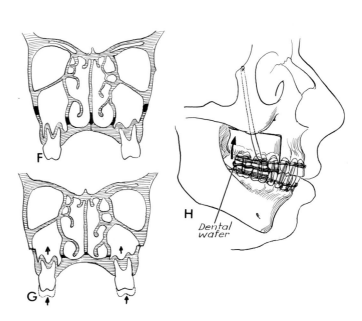

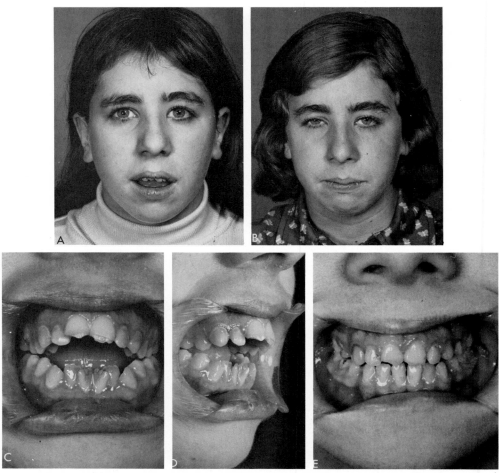

FIGURE 30–148. Closure of an anterior open bite by surgical-orthodontic treatment (see Fig. 30–147). *A,* Appearance of patient with open bite. Note the inability to occlude the lips in repose. *B,* After combined surgical (Fig. 30–147) and orthodontic therapy. *C, D,* Intraoral views showing the open bite. *E,* After completion of surgical orthodontic treatment.

ADDITIONAL PROCEDURES TO CLOSE THE ANTERIOR OPEN BITE AND DIMINISH THE VERTICAL DIMENSION OF THE FACE. When applicable, some of the procedures described in the previous pages are successful in closing an anterior open bite and diminishing the excessive height (vertical dimension) of the lower third of the face. Additional techniques may be required in lieu of those previously described.

Transplantation of the inferior mandibular segment after horizontal osteotomy (Converse, 1959). After the open bite has been closed by an osteotomy of the body of the mandible, the lower portion of the mandible is resected through a horizontal osteotomy to shorten the vertical dimension of the lower face. The resected bone is transplanted as a bone graft to increase the projection of the chin.

Transplantation of bone following dentoalveolar osteotomy (Köle, 1959b). Köle's technique consisted of a dentoalveolar osteotomy to correct the open bite malocclusion. The resected chin fragment is then inserted into the space between the elevated dentoalveolar process and the remaining mandibular body (Fig. 30–149). Fixation of the anterior segment is established by an orthodontic appliance or an arch bar reinforced with quick-curing acrylic. The fixation appliance is kept in place for six to eight weeks. The procedure can be used only when there is excessive vertical height of the mental symphysis; sufficient bone must be maintained in the remaining anterior portion of the mandible to preserve its strength and prevent accidental fracture. A greater incidence of dental injuries (6.5 per

FIGURE 30–149. The Köle procedure to close an anterior open bite and reduce the vertical height of the symphysis. *A*, Outline of the osteotomies. Sufficient bone must be preserved between the anterior segmental dentoalveolar osteotomy and the horizontal osteotomy of the lower border of the mandible. The transverse cut of the dentoalveolar segmental osteotomy is made at least 5 mm below the apices of the teeth. *B*, The anterior open bite has been closed, and the resulting gap is filled with bone taken from the horizontal osteotomy. Monomaxillary fixation stabilizes the fragment; intermaxillary fixation is not required.

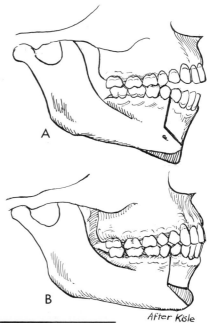

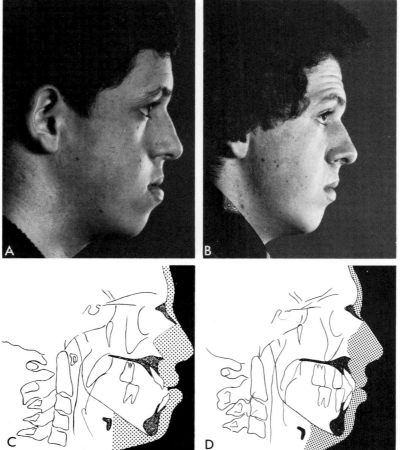

FIGURE 30–150. Mandibular prognathism with open bite. *A*, Patient with mandibular prognathism with open bite. Note the downward cant of the anterior portion of the mandible and the backward slope of the chin. *B*, After bilateral vertical osteotomy of the ramus and posterior and upward rotation of the tooth-bearing segment. The backward slope of the chin requires a horizontal advancement osteotomy to improve projection. *C*, Preoperative cephalometric tracing. *D*, Postoperative cephalometric tracing. The patient refused chin augmentation.

1417

cent) is associated with this technique (Pepersack, 1973). Because of the interposition of bone, the number of nonresponsive teeth is also increased (40 per cent).

MANDIBULAR PROGNATHISM WITH OPEN BITE. In mandibular prognathism with Class III malocclusion, correction of the deformity is usually relatively uncomplicated if the principles of treatment described in the earlier section of this chapter are followed (see p. 1310). When an open bite is also present, it is often caused by a downward cant of the anterior portion of the mandible, usually starting at the premolar level. When the anterior open bite is severe, considerable elongation of the lower portion of the face and a false impression of retrusion of the lower jaw are characteristics of the deformity (Fig. 30–150). Microgenia is also a feature in many of the patients with mandibular prognathism with open bite. As seen in the postoperative photograph of the patient in Figure 30–150, *B*, despite successful closure of the open bite and correction of the

Class III malocclusion, the chin remains deficient; a horizontal advancement of the lower portion of the mental symphysis is required to provide adequate projection of the chin.

The various operations for the correction of mandibular prognathism by an osteotomy of the ramus can be employed when preliminary studies show that closure of an anterior open bite and satisfactory dental occlusion can be achieved. In the patient in Figure 30–150, bilateral vertical osteotomies of the ramus with recession and upward rotation achieved satisfactory occlusal relationships (Fig. 30–151). Shortening of the vertical height of the lower face was also obtained (see Figs. 30–150, *D*, and 30–151). Bilateral vertical osteotomies of the ramus also achieved an equally good result in the patient shown in Figure 30–152.

Consecutive osteotomies of the ramus and body of the mandible in prognathism with open bite. In cases of prognathism with a wide anterior open bite (Figs. 30–153 to 30–156),

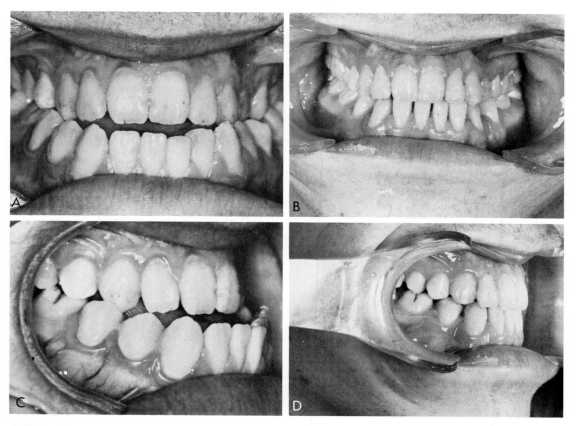

FIGURE 30–151. The dentition of the patient in Figure 30–150. *A, C,* Preoperative Class III malocclusion. *B, D,* Dental occlusion obtained following surgical-orthodontic treatment.

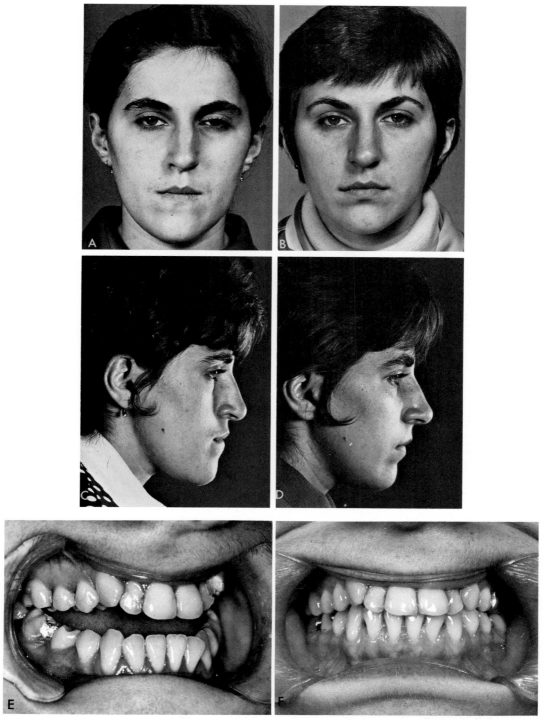

FIGURE 30–152. Closure of a mandibular anterior open bite by bilateral osteotomies of the ramus. *A*, Preoperative appearance of the patient. *B*, Postoperative view. *C*, Preoperative profile view. Note the increase in vertical height of the mental symphysis. *D*, Postoperative profile view. *E*, Intraoral view showing the open bite. *F*, Postoperative; the open bite is closed.

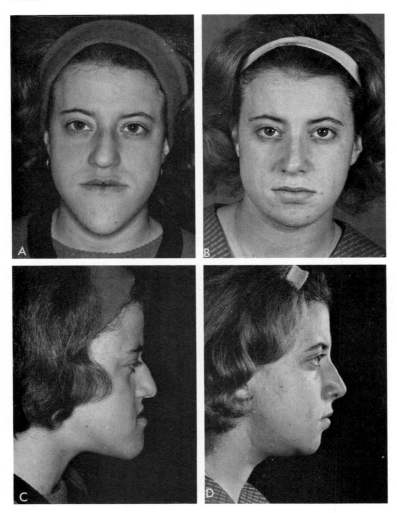

FIGURE 30–153. Mandibular prognathism corrected by consecutive osteotomies of the ramus and the body. *A, C,* Characteristic appearance of mandibular prognathism and anterior open bite. Note the elongation of the lower third of the face. *B, D,* After vertical section of the ramus to correct the anteroposterior relationships of the jaws and an osteotomy of the body to close the open bite. Patient also underwent a corrective rhinoplasty operation.

caused by the downward cant of the anterior portion of the mandible, it is often impossible to achieve the necessary upward rotation with a ramus or body section alone to close the open bite. A vertical osteotomy (see p. 1323) or a sagittal splitting osteotomy (see p. 1325) is done in a first stage to correct the anteroposterior skeletal discrepancy between the mandible and maxilla. In the patient shown in Figure 30–153, a bilateral vertical osteotomy was done in a first stage (Fig. 30–154, *A, B*). The molar teeth were brought into a corrected occlusal relationship. In a second stage, the open bite deformity was treated by a body osteotomy anterior to the mental foramen. To obtain the optimum occlusal relationships, a first premolar tooth was extracted (Figs. 30–154, *C, D* and 30–155).

A linear osteotomy was used instead of a step osteotomy because an upward and backward displacement of the fragment without a need for rotation corrected the open bite on the dental study models. The anterior segment of the mandible was moved upward to close the open bite. The preoperative and postoperative cephalometric tracings are shown in Figure 30–156.

Although the correction can be achieved in a single stage, a more precise orthodontic result is obtained by the two-stage procedure, which allows for the slight relapse which occurs following operations for prognathism (see p. 1317). In the second stage, permanent occlusal relationships are established to close the open bite and little or no postoperative orthodontic therapy is required.

Anterior open bite with mandibular prognathism and laterognathism. Bilateral sagittal

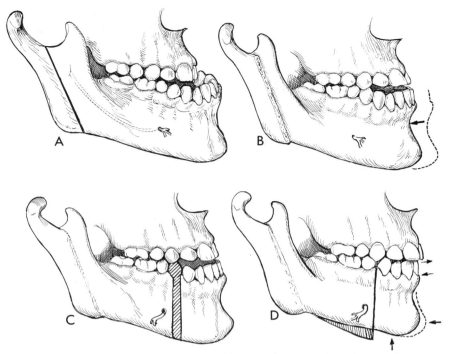

FIGURE 30–154. Consecutive osteotomies used on the patient in Figure 30–153. *A,* The line of vertical osteotomy in the ramus. *B,* Correction of the anteroposterior relationships by recessing the mandible. The anterior open bite remains. *C,* Final correction of the anterior open bite and prognathism. The shaded area represents the extracted tooth and the amount of bone resected from the body. *D,* The open bite is closed by moving the anterior segment upward. Protruding bone along the lower border of the mandible (shaded) is resected.

osteotomy of the ramus will correct moderate examples of the deformity. When treating a patient such as the one shown in Figure 30–157, *A,* an osteotomy of the body of the mandible is preferable. Prior to the operation, prosthodontic restorations were required in order to provide intermaxillary fixation.

A measured section of bone was removed from each side. The anterior portion of the jaw was repositioned posteriorly, rotated toward the midline, and raised until the dental relationships were reestablished by intermaxillary fixation. Adequate occlusal relationships were obtained (Fig. 30–157, *C, D*), and the patient's appearance was improved (Fig. 30–157, *B*).

Open bite with mandibular micrognathia. Where there is retrusion of the jaw in addition to the open bite, the operative procedure and postoperative care are more complicated. The mandible must be elongated and the anterior fragment retained in an advanced and superiorly rotated position to close the open bite. Elongation can be achieved by the various procedures discussed earlier in this chapter. It is usually advisable to employ a traction appliance to maintain the forward and upward posi-

tion of the anterior fragment (see Figs. 30–93 and 30–94).

DEFORMITIES OF THE MAXILLA AND MIDFACIAL SKELETON

Deformities of the maxilla are often more complex than those of the mandible. Although the actual defect may be confined to the maxilla, frequently other portions of the midfacial skeleton are involved because of the intimate relationships between the maxilla, the nasal skeleton, the orbit, and the zygoma. When the maxilla is hypoplastic, the nose is often affected and appears to be flat or depressed. The resulting nasomaxillary hypoplasia and recession produce a "dish-face" deformity. Deficiency of the zygoma may be reflected in a decrease in the prominence of the cheekbone. The inferior rim of the orbit may be depressed backward, not only in its medial maxillary portion but also in its lateral zygomatic portion. The lack of development of one bone, the maxilla in particular, can affect all of the other bones of the midface ("the domino effect").

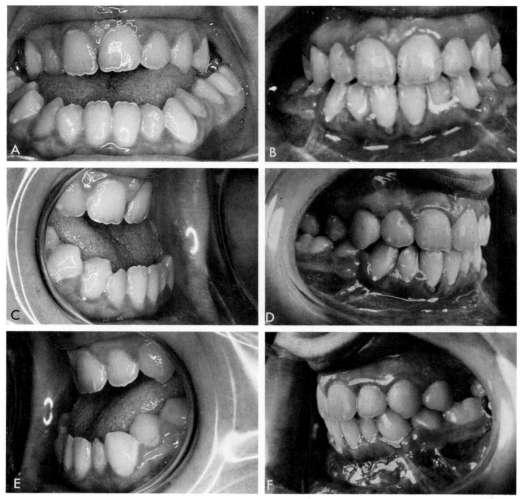

FIGURE 30–155.   Intraoral views of the patient shown in Figure 30–153. *A, C, E,* Appearance prior to treatment. *B, D, F,* Occlusion following the treatment outlined in Figure 30–154.

An understanding of the growth and development of the nasomaxillary complex is helpful when a nasomaxillary deformity is being assessed (see Chapters 26 and 42).

Classification of the Deformities

Because of the intimate interrelationship of the bones of the midfacial skeleton, maxillary deformities should be considered in terms of the *dentoalveolar* and *skeletal* components. Dentoalveolar malocclusions occur alone or in combination with a skeletal jaw deformity, which in turn can be associated with malformations of the adjacent bony structures. By dividing a complex deformity into its dentoalveolar

and skeletal parts, the analysis, diagnosis, and treatment are simplified.

Dentoalveolar Maxillary Deformities.   When the maxillary anterior teeth are projected more labially than normal, the term *maxillary protrusion* is used; when the teeth are inclined more lingually than normal, *maxillary retrusion* is present. A similar buccolingual malrelationship can be found between the posterior teeth. When the posterior maxillary arch width is excessive, a unilateral or a bilateral buccal crossbite is produced. Sagittal maxillary arch collapse, as seen in a cleft palate patient, leads to a lingual crossbite malocclusion of the posterior teeth (see Fig. 30–7, *C*).

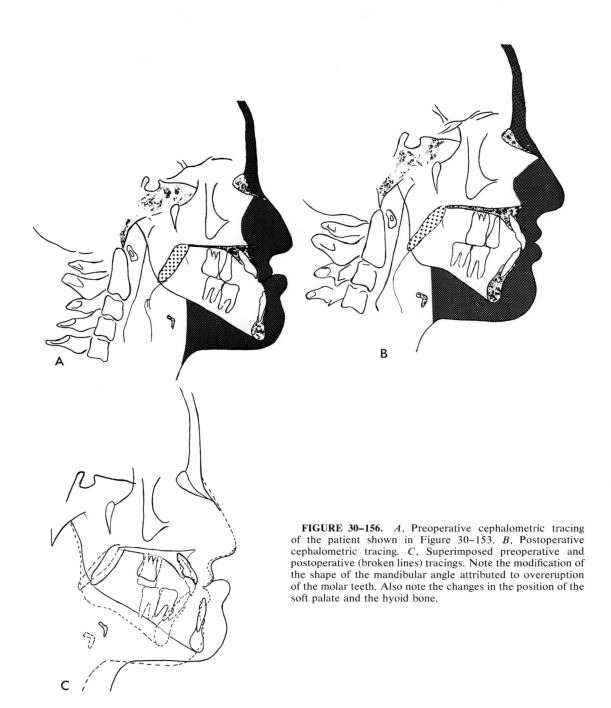

FIGURE 30–156. *A*, Preoperative cephalometric tracing of the patient shown in Figure 30–153. *B*, Postoperative cephalometric tracing. *C*, Superimposed preoperative and postoperative (broken lines) tracings. Note the modification of the shape of the mandibular angle attributed to overeruption of the molar teeth. Also note the changes in the position of the soft palate and the hyoid bone.

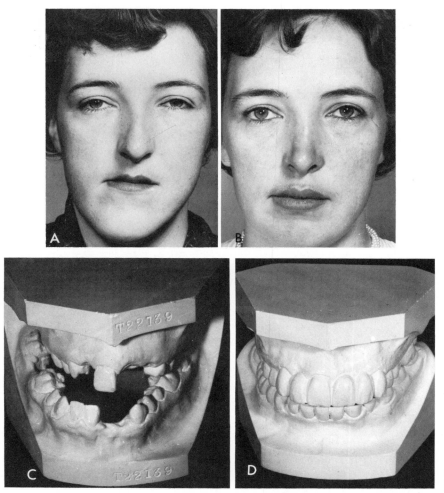

FIGURE 30–157. Correction of mandibular prognathism with lateral deviation and anterior open bite. *A*, Preoperative view showing deviation of the mandible to the right, prominence of the chin, and elongation of the lower face. *B*, After bilateral resection of measured sections of the body of the mandible with closure of the anterior open bite, dental restoration, and a corrective rhinoplasty. *C*, Preoperative dental casts illustrating the malocclusion. *D*, Postoperative dental casts showing the correction of the malocclusion and dental restoration.

Skeletal Maxillary Deformities. The condition characterized by a small, underdeveloped, retruded maxilla is termed *maxillary hypoplasia* or *micrognathia*. This type of malformation is often seen in the cleft palate patient or in the patient with craniofacial dysostosis (Crouzon's disease and Apert's syndrome). The maxilla is of normal size but in a retruded position in *maxillary retrognathia* (or *"retromaxillism"*). A common example is the retropositioned maxilla that is found following a malunited midfacial fracture. In all the above examples, the mandible, though normal in size, appears to be prognathic (mandibular pseudoprognathism).

Idiopathic maxillary prognathism, in which the entire maxilla is anteriorly positioned, is a rare condition. Usually the protrusion is localized in the anterior dentoalveolar segment, and the maxillary dentoalveolar segment drifts forward and downward. This type of maxillary deformity is seen in patients with mandibular micrognathia (see Fig. 30–74). With tumors such as fibrous dysplasia, either unilateral or bilateral (cherubism), the maxilla is often severely protruded.

The "dish-face" deformity is an example of a nasomaxillary skeletal deformity. The entire nasomaxillary complex is depressed and is displaced posteriorly. This type of deformity results from a malunited midfacial fracture. Congenital nasomaxillary hypoplasia (Fig. 30–204) or nasomaxillary deformity caused by trauma in early postnatal life usually affects the central portion of the maxilla and the nose (see Fig. 30–198).

Preoperative Planning and Diagnosis

The diagnosis made from the clinical examination of the patient is correlated with the analysis of the photographs, the dental study models, and the cephalometric roentgenogram.

Dental casts are invaluable aids in studying dentoalveolar malformations. A duplicate cast is sectioned and the fragments repositioned to simulate the maxillary osteotomies in a manner

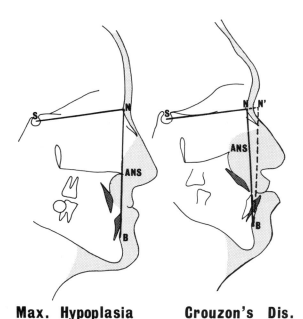

Max. Hypoplasia

SNB = 80

Crouzon's Dis.

SNB = 86

SN'B = 80

FIGURE 30–158. Relationship between sella-nasion (SN) and facial profile angles. Although the patient with maxillary hypoplasia and the patient with Crouzon's disease appear to have mandibular prognathism, neither of these patients has an abnormal lower jaw. The pseudoprognathic appearance is caused by hypoplasia of the maxilla. In the patient with maxillary hypoplasia, SNB = 80 degrees (which measures the projection of the mandible) is within the average range. In the patient with Crouzon's disease, SNB = 86 degrees; however, if SN were extended to a normal length (SN'), the SN'B angle would fall within the normal range. (From Firmin, F., Coccaro, P. J., and Converse, J. M.: Cephalometric analysis in diagnosis and treatment planning of craniofacial dysostoses. Plast. Reconstr. Surg., *54*:300, 1974. Copyright 1974, The Williams & Wilkins Company, Baltimore.)

similar to the planning employed in the correction of mandibular deformities (see Fig. 30–9).

Cephalometric measurements of primary concern are the SN length, SNA and SNB angles, midfacial height, and Ul-SN angles (Fig. 30–158). Cephalometric analysis provides a means of distinguishing the respective anatomical characteristics of nasomaxillary hypoplasia and craniofacial dysostosis (Firmin, Coccaro and Converse, 1974). When the midfacial advancement procedures are planned, it is helpful to record the SN length and the vertical midfacial dimension. The SNA and SNB angular measurements can be misinterpreted if the SN length is not taken into consideration. Smaller SN measurements contribute toward a larger SNB angle, indicating mandibular prognathism in the presence of an average size mandible (Fig. 30–158). SNA angles are similarly affected by the decreased SN length.

The hypoplastic nasomaxillary region may require an advancement as well as a downward rotation to provide the necessary forward projection and increase in vertical facial dimension. The amount of midfacial elongation needed is estimated from the vertical midfacial measurements. In addition to assessing the amount of displacement required, the cephalogram aids in indicating the size and volume of the bone grafts required to fill the voids in the skeletal framework.

The Ul-SN cephalometric measurement is used to assess the amount of protrusion or retrusion of the anterior maxillary dentoalveolar segment.

Henderson (1974) described a technique which combines the use of transparent cephalometric and photographic cut-outs to help predict the final facial profile. Photographs are enlarged to the dimensions of the cephalogram and are sectioned along the lines of the osteotomies. The parts of the photograph are recomposed to conform to the movement of the skeleton.

Surgical Approach to the Maxilla

The maxilla is exposed through an intraoral incision, an extraoral incision through the lower eyelid, a conjunctival approach, a coronal scalp flap, or through a combination of these incisions.

The Intraoral Approach. The oral cavity offers a direct approach to the bones of the face. Incisions in the oral vestibule, extended

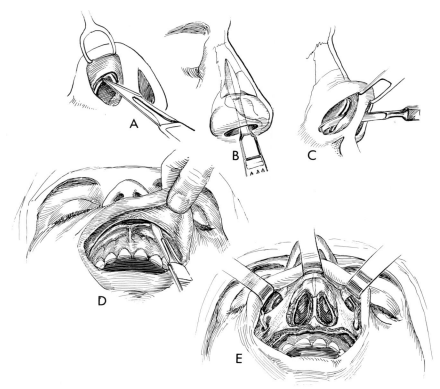

FIGURE 30–159. The midface degloving procedure. *A,* Bilateral intercartilaginous incisions are made as in a corrective rhinoplasty. *B,* The soft tissues are dissected over the lateral nasal cartilages bilaterally. *C,* The transfixion incision is illustrated. *D,* An incision is made through the mucosa on the labial aspect of the sulcus. *E,* The midfacial skeleton is exposed subperiosteally, respecting the infraorbital nerves. (From Casson, P. R., Bonanno, P. C., and Converse, J. M.: The midface degloving procedure. Plast. Reconstr. Surg., *53*:102, 1974. Copyright 1974, The Williams & Wilkins Company, Baltimore.)

through the periosteum, permit subperiosteal exposure of the bones. Through this approach the maxilla and zygoma are exposed up to the level of the infraorbital rims.

The two basic types of intraoral incisions described for the exposure of the mandible are also applicable to the maxilla. These are the labiobuccal vestibular incision and the mucogingival incision (see Figs. 30–21 and 30–22). The mucogingival incision has limitations, since it is more difficult to suture without tension if the maxillary skeleton is advanced or augmented with onlay bone grafts.

THE MIDFACE DEGLOVING PROCEDURE. Converse described the intraoral approach to the maxilla and the mandible in 1950 and the mandibular degloving procedure in 1959 (see Fig. 30–21). Casson, Bonnano, and Converse (1974) described a midfacial degloving procedure which is done in a similar fashion except that the nose is an obstacle to complete exposure; the nasal structures must be retracted. This is made possible by the following technique.

Bilateral intercartilaginous incisions are made between the alar and lateral cartilages (Fig. 30–159, *A*). The soft tissues over the lateral cartilages and the nasal bones are elevated (Fig. 30–159, *B*). A transfixion incision is extended down along the dorsal and caudal portions of the septal cartilage to the nasal spine (Fig. 30–159, *C*). An intraoral incision is made through the mucosa on the labial aspect of the upper vestibule (Fig. 30–159, *D*); the periosteum is raised, and the nasal spine and the pyriform aperture are exposed. The attachments of the nasal tissues to the pyriform aperture are exposed and severed. The premaxillary dissection is joined with the transfixion incision. Retractors are applied, and the subperiosteal elevation is continued upward to the inferior orbital rim, exposing and respecting the infraorbital nerve. Complete exposure of the midfacial skeleton can thus be obtained (Fig. 30–159, *E*). After the skeletal procedures are completed, the nasal tissues are carefully redraped, and the transfixion incision is sutured; the intranasal and labial incisions are also sutured. A nasal splint is applied for 48 hours to avoid hematoma formation. After occlusive sutures are placed through the eyelids, a moderately compressive dressing is applied over the entire midface.

The Lower Eyelid Approach. The lower eyelid incision is an excellent approach to the upper portion of the maxilla. The preferred incision is one made along the lower border of the tarsus; the septum orbitale is readily exposed, after a horizontal incision is made through the orbicularis oculi muscle, and is followed down to the orbital rim. This approach avoids penetration of the septum orbitale and the extrusion of orbital fat (see Chapter 25, Fig. 25–27).

Additional external incisions across the root of the nose and downward over the lateral nasal wall provide further exposure for osteotomies and bone grafting in this area.

The Conjunctival Approach. This approach through an incision in the conjunctiva of the lower eyelid is described in Chapter 25 (see Figs. 25–28 and 25–29). Because this approach may result in extrusion of the orbital fat and vertical shortening of the lower lid, the external incision below the tarsus is preferred. The lower eyelid incision combined with the midfacial degloving incisions and other supplementary incisions provides adequate exposure of the midface skeleton.

Exposure of the Midface Skeleton Through a Coronal Scalp Flap. The bifrontal scalp flap, which is often referred to as a "coronal" flap, extends behind the hairline from preauricular area to preauricular area. It is wise to place the incision sufficiently posterior to the hairline in male patients to allow for a receding hairline. The flap is raised through the areolar tissue between the galea aponeurotica and the pericranium. The pericranium is then incised 4 to 5 cm above the supraorbital rims and raised from the bone with a periosteal elevator.

The subperiosteal elevation is extended to the supraorbital rims and along the lateral orbital rims down to the zygomatic arch on each side. The elevator continues its subperiosteal trajectory over the zygomas. If additional exposure is required, the periorbita is raised from the roof, medial and lateral walls of the orbits, and along the bony dorsum of the nose. The scalp flap is thus loosened, providing exposure of a major portion of the midface skeleton (see also Chapter 56).

Segmental Osteotomies to Correct Maxillary Dentoalveolar Deformities

Segmental maxillary osteotomies correct a wide range of dentoalveolar deformities in any selected portion of the dental arch. These osteotomies have been discussed earlier in this chapter (see p. 1410).

Cohn-Stock (1921) described a surgical procedure for the correction of maxillary protrusion. Spanier (1932) performed a recession of the anterior portion of the maxilla for protrusion. The presently used one-stage set-back technique with its variations has been developed from Schuchardt's (1955) two-stage procedure for the preservation of the blood supply. Köle (1959a, b) and Wunderer (1962) advocated a one-stage set-back procedure, which was employed for maxillary advancement by Converse, Horowitz, Guy, and Wood-Smith (1964a). Variations of the premolar maxillary set-back have also been described by Kent and Hinds (1971).

Anatomical Considerations. Preservation of the blood supply to the mobilized segment is of paramount importance. The blood supply of the anterior maxillary teeth is derived from branches of the internal maxillary artery. The anterior-superior alveolar branches originate from the infraorbital artery within the infraorbital canal and descend through the anterior alveolar canals to supply the upper incisors and canine teeth and the mucous membrane. The posterior-superior alveolar artery originates from the internal maxillary artery in the pterygopalatine fossa. As it descends over the tuberosity of the maxilla, it divides into numerous branches to supply the molars and premolars. Other branches continue forward on the alveolar process to supply the gingiva. All of these vessels anastomose with various branches of the ophthalmic and external maxillary arteries which supply the face. The vascularity of the area permits the mucoperiosteal flap to maintain the blood supply of the detached anterior maxillary segment.

The descending palatine artery, a branch of the internal maxillary artery, descends through the pterygopalatine canal and emerges at the greater palatine foramen. It courses forward toward the incisive canal in a groove on the hard palate on the medial aspect of the alveolar border. The artery then anastomoses with branches of the posterior septal arteries, which pass through the canal.

The sphenopalatine artery, another branch of the internal maxillary artery, enters the

The Head and Neck

nasal cavity through the sphenopalatine foramen and terminates on the nasal septum in a number of posterior septal branches. These anastomose with branches of the descending palatine artery and the septal branch of the superior labial artery, among others.

The blood supply is sufficient if either the palatal or labial mucoperiosteal flap remains attached to the mobilized dentoalveolar maxillary segment.

Surgical-Orthodontic Correction of Maxillary Dentoalveolar Protrusion

Orthodontic therapy can often correct the inclined maxillary incisor teeth and result in competent lip posture and improved dentofacial balance. Orthodontic therapy is most commonly achieved during childhood or adolescence, and it has erroneously come to be regarded as a treatment available exclusively to the young. Age is not a limiting factor; treatment can be rendered at any time provided that the teeth and their supporting structures are in good physical condition.

Protrusion of the mandibular incisor teeth is often also associated with maxillary protrusion. This condition, "bimaxillary protrusion" (Case, 1921), imparts a displeasing convexity to the subnasal profile. Bimaxillary protrusion is a relative designation, as the dentoalveolar prominence results from overdevelopment of the maxillary and mandibular arches or from underdevelopment of the other skeletal components (Fig. 30–160). The soft tissue contour is an important diagnostic sign. Lip incompetency, "receding chin effect," and loss of the labiomental curve are frequently observed in these patients. Bimaxillary protrusion to a moderate degree is commonly seen in the Negroid and Oriental ethnic groups.

Satisfactory facial harmony and balance can be restored by surgical-orthodontic procedures when improvement in facial harmony cannot be achieved through orthodontic therapy alone or when an adult patient is unwilling to accept the required appliance therapy. Such procedures consist of osteotomies which modify the occlusion of the teeth and the contour of the face. Two types of osteotomies are employed: the *segmental osteotomy*, in which a segment of the dental arch only is displaced, and a *complete horizontal osteotomy*, in which the entire dental arch is displaced.

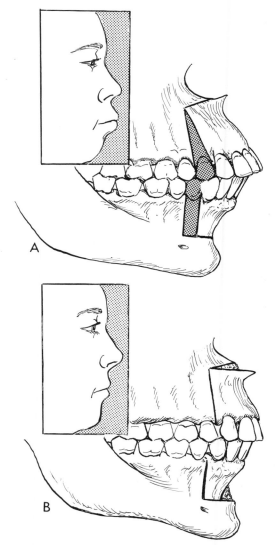

FIGURE 30–160. Correction of bimaxillary protrusion by dentoalveolar set-back osteotomy. *A*, The lines of osteotomy and the segments to be resected (shaded) are indicated. *B*, The position of the maxillary and mandibular segments after the set-back osteotomy.

The Premolar Recession (Set-back) Osteotomy. Wilhelm (1954), who described the surgical technique used by Schuchardt, favored a two-stage procedure for the correction of maxillary protrusion. In the first stage, the mucoperiosteum of the palate was raised, the second premolar teeth were extracted, and an osteotomy was performed through the palate and the alveolar arch. Three to four weeks later,

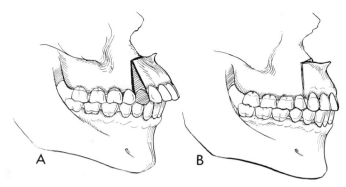

FIGURE 30–161. Premolar maxillary recession (set-back) osteotomy. *A*, Alveolar segment to be resected (shaded) after removal of the premolar tooth. *B*, Position of the anterior segment following surgical recession.

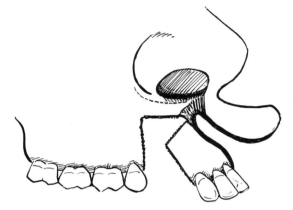

FIGURE 30–162. Labial mucoperiosteal flap. The blood supply to the mobilized maxillary segment is preserved by the anterior mucoperiosteal flap. (After Wunderer, 1962.)

the second stage completed the correction. Wilhelm considered the one-stage procedure dangerous. Wunderer (1962), however, disagreed and advocated a one-stage procedure (Fig. 30–161). He used an anterior mucoperiosteal flap (Fig. 30–162) to maintain the blood supply. The operation is performed without risk if either a labial or a palatal mucoperiosteal flap remains attached to the repositioned segment as previously mentioned (Fig.

30–162). The abundant blood supply of the area explains the success of these operations.

Extraction of a premolar tooth on each side of the arch is usually required. The palatal mucoperiosteum is reflected subperiosteally from the anterior portion of the hard palate. The incision should be made posterior to the incisive papilla to avoid injury to the vascular supply originating from the incisive canal. Direct exposure for the palatal osteotomy site

FIGURE 30–163. Premolar maxillary set-back osteotomy. *A*, Outline of the segment of bone to be resected when tilting of the dentoalveolar segment is not a problem and a straight set-back is desired. Resection of a triangular segment would be required to produce the tilting. *B*, The mucoperiosteal palatal flap has been elevated. The shaded area indicates the required resection of bone.

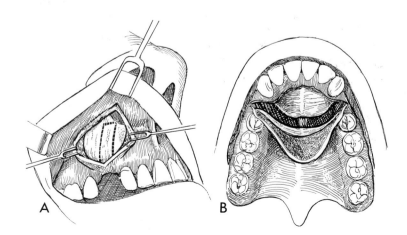

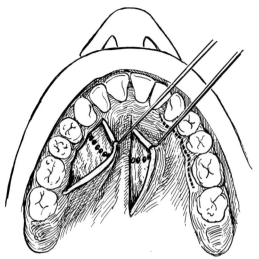

FIGURE 30–164. Tunneling technique to preserve the continuity of the blood supply of the palatal mucoperiosteal flap.

the area where bone consolidation must take place.

A more conservative technique is to raise a subperiosteal tunnel over the area of the proposed osteotomy for the resection of palatal bone and vomer. A short midline palatal mucosal incision aids in the exposure without jeopardizing the blood supply (Fig. 30–164). Figure 30–165 demonstrates that it is possible to incise the palatal mucoperiosteum at the site of the osteotomy without endangering the blood supply. The procedures illustrated in Figures 30–163 and 30–164 are obviously preferable.

A short period of venous congestion characterized by a bluish coloration of the mucosa may cause some anxiety; return to the color of healthy, well-vascularized tissue is, however, rapid.

The precaution should be taken to place the osteotomy in the recessed segment above the apices of the teeth so as to leave sufficient bone above the apices to ensure the blood supply to the teeth. Radiologic verification of the position of the teeth is essential.

The palatal and alveolar osteotomies with resection of bone are illustrated in Figure 30–163. A curved (Fig. 30–163, *B*) or V-shaped (Fig. 30–166, *A*) strip of bone from the hard palate and vomer is resected. The septal cartilage may also require a limited resection to accom-

is thus obtained. The required amount of bone is resected from the alveolar process (Fig. 30–163, *A*) and the hard palate (Fig. 30–163, *B*). The vertical buccal mucoperiosteal incisions in the premolar area should be placed posterior to the buccal osteotomy site. Designed in this manner, the incision will not lie directly over

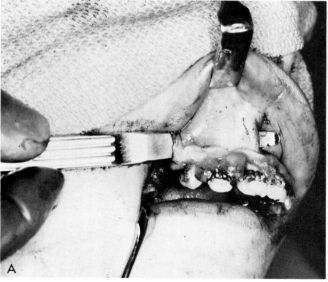
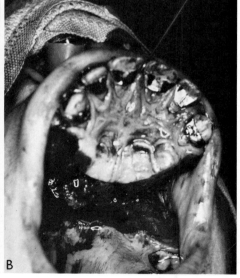

FIGURE 30–165. Operative view which demonstrates the rich blood supply of the anterior maxillary segment. The labial flap maintains the blood supply. *A*, The labial flap has been elevated subperiosteally. A short midline incision assists the procedure without jeopardizing the blood supply. *B*, To demonstrate the viability of the anterior maxillary segment attached only to an anterior mucoperiosteal flap, the mucoperiosteum and the hard palate were incised and sectioned. Raising the palatal flap in the usual fashion is preferable (see Figs. 30–163 and 30–164).

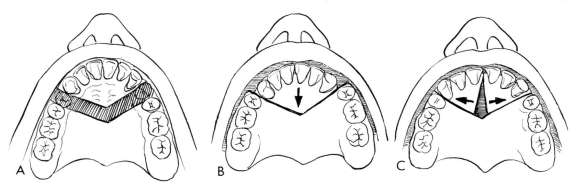

FIGURE 30–166. *A*, V-shaped osteotomy to prevent rotation of the recessed anterior maxillary segment. *B*, Loss of alignment of the dental arch after the set-back. *C*, A midline palatal osteotomy realigns the dental arch. A triangular bone graft fills the gap.

modate the maxillary recession and to permit repositioning of the anterior dentoalveolar segment. If a direct anteroposterior displacement is required, the V-shaped triangular resection of the palate prevents rotation of the anterior segment; if any degree of rotation is needed to achieve optimal occlusal relationships, a curved line of resection is imperative. The amount of maxillary recession is estimated by the double standard of reestablishment of correct occlusal relationships with the mandibular teeth and of attainment of an adequate facial contour.

Occasionally, a midline palatal splitting osteotomy is required to realign the dental arch (Fig. 30–166, *C*). The dental arch increases in width posteriorly. When the anterior segment is displaced backward, the discrepancy of the arch width results in a poor buccopalatal alignment of the teeth adjacent to the osteotomy (Fig. 30–166, *B*). A midline palatal splitting osteotomy corrects the alignment (Heiss, 1934; Dautrey and Pepersack, 1971; Steinhauser, 1972) (Fig. 30–166, *C*). Alignment of segments is necessary to decrease the chance of periodontal pocket formation and disease (Hinds and Kent, 1972). The palatal flap is then reapplied.

Fixation of the detached fragment is maintained by an orthodontic appliance or arch bars which provide monomaxillary fixation (see Fig. 30–172). The molar teeth provide anchorage for the appliance. A continuous labial coating of quick-setting tooth-colored acrylic assists in the stabilization during the six-week period of postoperative healing. Intermaxillary fixation is usually not necessary.

The maxillary set-back procedure is combined with a mandibular dentoalveolar set-back operation in patients with bimaxillary protrusion (see Figs. 30–160, 30–174 to 30–177 and also Fig. 30–74).

The Subnasal Dentoalveolar Segmental Osteotomy. In some cases, when it is not desirable to modify the position of the nasal spine and

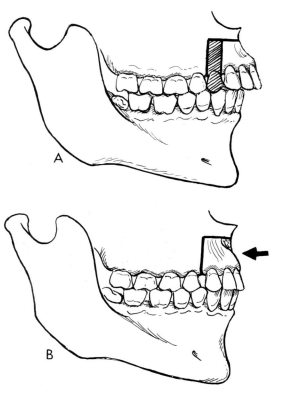

FIGURE 30–167. The subnasal premolar maxillary set-back osteotomy. *A*, The subnasal line of osteotomy. The bone to be resected is indicated by the shaded area. *B*, Relationships after completion of the procedure.

the anterior nasal floor, a more limited type of osteotomy may be indicated. In the subnasal premolar osteotomy technique, a dentoalveolar osteotomy, the edge of the pyriform aperture is exposed subperiosteally, and the line of section extends below the nasal spine and the floor of the nose. The procedure is otherwise similar to the premolar set-back osteotomy. The osteotomy is directed backward, transecting the bone above the apices of the teeth, then down-ward in the region of the premolars (Fig. 30–167).

The technique can be utilized to close an anterior open bite. The subnasal dentoalveolar segment is detached and displaced downward to close the open bite, and bone chips are packed into the resultant subnasal defect. Conversely, the subnasal osteotomy can be used to correct a deep overbite. Resection of a segment of bone above the apices of the teeth per-

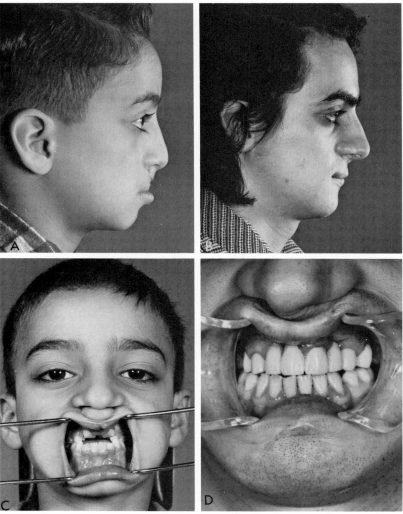

FIGURE 30–168.   Premolar segmental maxillary advancement osteotomy. *A,* A 10 year old patient with a repaired bilateral cleft lip and palate. The vermilion portion of the prolabial segment of the lip has been sacrificed, resulting in a tight upper lip. The premaxilla is loose and lingually inclined against the hard palate (see *C*). The occlusal relationships between the molar teeth are adequate. *B,* Thirteen years after the following procedures: (1) an Abbé flap reconstruction to relieve the tight upper lip and to lengthen the columella at the expense of the prolabial segment and a cantilever bone graft wired to the nasal bones to maintain the projection of the nasal tip; (2) orthodontic treatment to realign the premaxilla; (3) consolidation of the premaxilla to the adjacent dentoalveolar segments by bone grafting; (4) premolar segmental advancement osteotomy (see Fig. 30–169) to correct the anterior maxillary hypoplasia. *C,* The dentition prior to treatment. Note the premaxilla lingually inclined against the palate. *D,* Final appearance of the dentition. Dental restorations were required and were completed following surgical-orthodontic treatment. (From Converse, J. M., Horowitz, S. L., Guy, C. L., and Wood-Smith, D.: Surgical and orthodontic procedures in bilateral cleft lip and cleft palate. Cleft Palate J., *1*:153, 1964.)

mits the upward displacement of a maxillary anterior dentoalveolar segment which has drifted downward (see Fig. 30–74).

Surgical-Orthodontic Correction of Anterior Maxillary Dentoalveolar Retrusion

Occasionally, the anterior maxillary dentoalveolar complex is retruded but the molar occlusal relationships are satisfactory. A premolar segmental advancement osteotomy should be considered when this situation is seen (Converse, Horowitz, Guy and Wood-Smith, 1964a). This type of malocclusion is frequently associated with the cleft lip and palate deformity.

The Premolar Advancement Osteotomy. The outline of the premolar segmental osteotomy is similar to that of the premolar set-back osteotomy; the freed anterior maxillary segment is advanced to correct the anterior maxillary retrusion.

The degree of surgical advancement is planned preoperatively on the sectioned dental casts using the dental occlusion and the cephalometric roentgenograms as guides.

The patient shown in Figure 30–168 is a typical example of a complex case in which the premolar segmental advancement osteotomy is specifically indicated. The bilateral cleft lip and palate had been repaired. The vermilion portion of the prolabial segment had been sacrificed in the repair of the bilateral cleft lip. When the patient was first seen at the age of 10 years (Fig. 30–168, A), the upper lip was tight, the anterior portion of the maxilla was hypoplastic, and the premaxilla was loose, lying lingually on a plane nearly horizontal with the palate (Figs. 30–168, C and 30–169, A, B). In a first stage an Abbé flap from the lower lip was transposed to relieve the tight upper lip; the prolabial segment was used to lengthen the columella, and the tip of the nose was maintained in a forward projected position by a cantilever bone graft wired to the nasal bones. By orthodontic therapy, the premaxilla was realigned with the adjacent dentoalveolar segments. The premaxilla was then consolidated with the adjacent dentoalveolar segments by bone grafting. At this point the patient still had a retruded and hypoplastic maxilla. The occlusal relationships between the maxillary and the mandibular molar teeth were, however, adequate. Thus a premaxillary segmental osteotomy was indicated rather than a Le Fort I advancement osteotomy (see Fig. 30–182), which would have disturbed the

molar occlusal relationships. The planning of the premolar segmental osteotomy is shown in Figure 30–169, C, D, and the result of the premolar segmental osteotomy is shown in Figure 30–169, E, F.

To ensure mucoperiosteal coverage of the bone grafts and to allow for the advancement of the anterior maxillary segment, changes in the design of the incisors and flaps must be made (see Figs. 30–171 and 30–173).

The general outline of the osteotomy is similar to that of the set-back osteotomy (Fig. 30–170) except that the premolar teeth are retained, and bone is not removed from the hard palate. A labial mucoperiosteal tunnel is made over the proposed osteotomy site. With a small, round bur or an oscillating blade, the line of osteotomy is made from the edge of the pyriform aperture to a line extending upward from the interdental space between the premolar teeth (Fig. 30–170, A). A thin, tapered osteotome is used to make the interdental alveolar section, leaving sufficient bone on each side to protect the adjacent teeth. The palatal mucoperiosteum is raised (Fig. 30–171, A), and the osteotomy is continued across the hard palate, reaching the alveolar line of section of the contralateral side (Fig. 30–171, A). In the midline of the palate, the osteotomy must be extended upward across and through the vomer.

The nasal septal framework is exposed by careful elevation of the mucoperiosteum and mucoperichondrium. The nasal septal cartilage is divided at its line of insertion into the vomer groove to a point which reaches the osteotomy through the vomer.

The mobilized anterior segment of the maxilla is advanced and rotated downward, upward, or laterally as needed. The anterior fragment is maintained in monomaxillary fixation in the corrected position by an orthodontic appliance or arch bar, using the teeth in the posterior fixed portion of the maxilla for anchorage (Fig. 30–172). A continuous thin coating of quick-curing acrylic is used to provide additional stabilization; intermaxillary fixation is not necessary.

Small fragments of bone are wedged between the fragments to restore osseous continuity (Fig. 30–171, B, C). Interosseous wiring may be required for stabilization. Bone grafts may also be inserted around the edge of the pyriform aperture and over the anterior surface of the maxilla (Fig. 30–173) if additional reinforcement of the bony continuity or contour restoration is required. The mucoperiosteal incision is closed (Fig. 30–171, D, E).

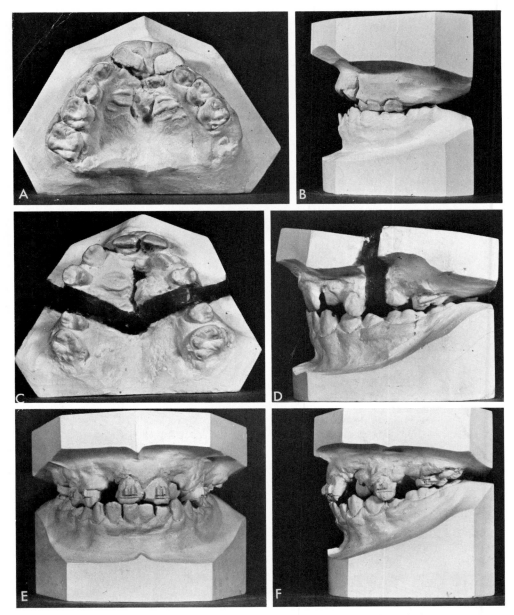

FIGURE 30–169. Use of dental casts in planning the combined orthodontic and surgical treatment to correct the malocclusion associated with bilateral cleft lip and palate (see Fig. 30–168). *A*, Preoperative view showing the lingual inclination of the mobile premaxilla. *B*, Preoperative profile view. *C*, After orthodontic repositioning of the premaxilla, the advancement of the anterior segment of the maxilla is planned by sectioning the study casts. *D*, Profile view of the planned advancement. *E*, *F*, Occlusal relationships following completion of surgical treatment. (From Converse, J. M., Horowitz, S. L., Guy, C. L., and Wood-Smith, D.: Surgical and orthodontic procedures in bilateral cleft lip and cleft palate. Cleft Palate J., *1*:153, 1964.)

FIGURE 30–170. The premolar maxillary advancement osteotomy. *A*, Outline of the interdental osteotomy extending upward to the pyriform aperture. *B*, The general outline of the osteotomy of the dentoalveolar region, hard palate, and septum.

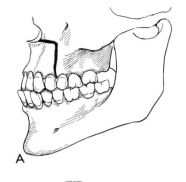

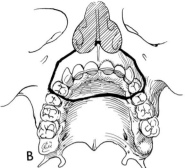

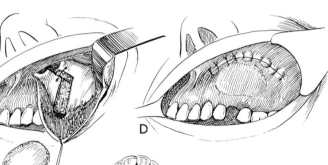

FIGURE 30–171. The premolar maxillary advancement osteotomy. *A*, A mucoperiosteal palatal flap has been raised, and the outline of the osteotomy is indicated. *B*, After the advancement, bone grafts are wedged into the line of osteotomy. *C*, An onlay of cancellous bone is placed over the osteotomy area. *D*, The incision is sutured. *E*, The exposed portion of the anterior hard palate epithelizes spontaneously. The palatal flap is sutured to the buccal mucoperiosteum to cover the bone grafts in the alveolar area.

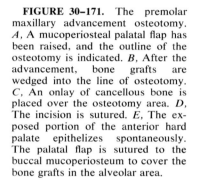

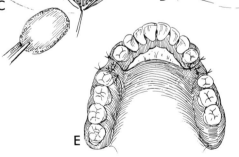

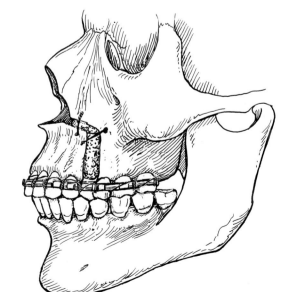

FIGURE 30–172. Monomaxillary fixation. Fixation is based upon the stable posterior teeth. Intermaxillary fixation is not necessary except to adjust the occlusion. It can then be released. An arch bar is represented in the drawing but an orthodontic appliance is preferred.

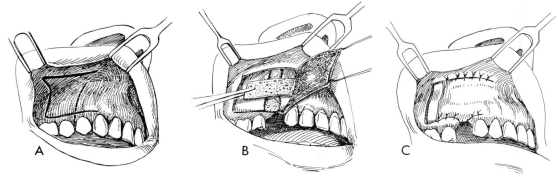

FIGURE 30–173. The premolar maxillary advancement osteotomy. *A,* When the advancement exceeds 1 cm, an anteriorly based mucoperiosteal flap is outlined to release the soft tissue tension and to cover the bone grafts. *B,* Bone grafts are wedged into the gap in the alveolar process. A thin cancellous bone onlay is placed over the area of the osteotomy. *C,* A mucoperiosteal flap free of tension is sutured over the bone grafts. The posterior raw surface epithelizes spontaneously. The drawing shows that a premolar tooth has been extracted; an interdental osteotomy usually obviates the need for the extraction.

The palatal mucoperiosteal flap serves to cover the bone grafts in the palatal defect (Fig. 30–171, *E*). Depending on the amount of maxillary advancement, the palatal flap usually does not cover the anterior portion of the hard palate. The exposed bone, however, epithelizes secondarily. Usually there is sufficient vestibular and alveolar mucoperiosteum to cover the bone grafts in the alveolar defect. When the planned maxillary advancement exceeds 1 cm, an anteriorly based buccal mucoperiosteal flap should be employed to ensure coverage of the bone grafts (see Fig. 30–173). Exposure to the open maxillary sinus does not complicate the healing of the bone grafts; the lining of the maxillary sinus rapidly covers the undersurface of the grafts.

COMPLICATIONS OF MAXILLARY SEGMENTAL OSTEOTOMIES. The most feared complication is the total loss of the mobilized dentoalveolar segment. A labial or palatal mucoperiosteal flap alone will ensure the viability of the fragment. Care must be taken to prevent kinking, compression, and excessive tension on the flap. Because of the excellent blood supply to the maxilla, loss of bone grafts is rare, provided that soft tissue coverage is maintained.

In maxillary set-back osteotomies, excessive compression due to inadequate bone removal must be avoided. The soft alveolar bone is particularly susceptible to pressure necrosis, and loss of teeth adjacent to the osteotomy site can be the consequence of this mistake. While preoperative planning with the dental casts and cephalograms is essential, final estimation of the amount of bone to be removed is made during the operation. If an excess of bone has been resected, some of the removed bone may be replaced between the fragments with impunity.

Hogeman and Sarnäs (1967) studied patients for 14 months following a maxillary set-back procedure. When the final result was achieved, no relapses were noted. Improvement in the lip relationship (contour, profile, and lip seal) was maintained. All of the mobilized fragments were clinically stable despite roentgenographic evidence of incomplete healing in a few of the patients who had undergone a premolar segmental osteotomy and also in patients in whom a paramedian palatal splitting osteotomy had also been performed.

Tooth vitality depends upon two precautions: (1) leaving sufficient bone between the line of osteotomy and the apices of the teeth, and (2) avoiding injury to the teeth adjacent to the interdental osteotomy.

The most vulnerable apices are those of the maxillary cuspids because of their relatively high position and cornerstone location (Leibold, Tilson, and Rask, 1971).

The Surgical-Orthodontic Treatment of Bimaxillary Protrusion: Simianism. The face of modern man is distinguished from his early forebears and living primate relatives by a reduction in the forward projection of the jaws. Relative protrusion of the snout is seen in all simians but only rarely in humans (particularly whites); even when it does occur, it is usually confined to either the lower jaw (mandibular prognathism) or maxilla (skeletal Class II).

In the patient shown in Figure 30–174, *A* and *C*, bimaxillary protrusion caused a severe and unusual facial deformity (Converse and

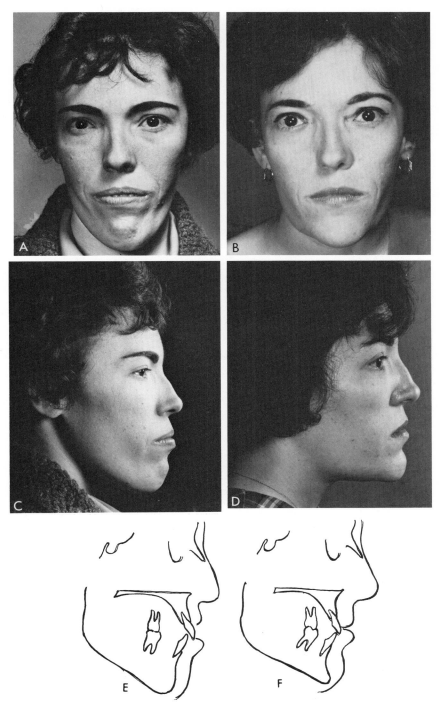

FIGURE 30–174. *A*, Appearance of a patient nicknamed "monkey face." Note the considerable increase in facial height. *B*, Postoperative photograph of the patient after completion of treatment. *C*, Profile view showing bimaxillary protrusion. *D*, Profile view of the patient following surgical-orthodontic treatment. *E*, A cephalometric tracing prior to treatment showing the increased skeletal facial height. *F*, Cephalometric tracing four years following completion of treatment showing changes in the dentoalveolar relationships, diminution in facial height, and adequate protrusion of the mental symphysis. (Figs. 30–174 to 30–177 from Converse, J. M., and Horowitz, S. L.: Simianism: surgical-orthodontic correction of bimaxillary protrusion. J. Maxillofac. Surg., *1*:7, 1973. Georg Thieme Verlag, Stuttgart, Germany.)

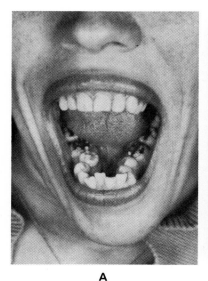
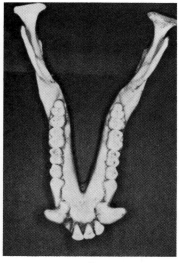

A   B

FIGURE 30–175. Comparing the lower jaw of the patient shown in Fig. 30–174 with that of a primate. *A,* Note the elongated shape of the patient's mandible with restriction in the horizontal dimension reminiscent of the jaw of a primate (*B*).

Horowitz, 1973). The patient's mandible and dentoalveolar arch are elongated, with contraction of the horizontal dimension (Fig. 30–175, *A*), similar to the jaw of the primate (Fig. 30–175, *B*); a simian bony shelf could be felt by digital palpation, immediately behind the incisor area.

Several factors were considered in planning the total corrective program for the patient: (1) the increased skeletal facial height, as shown in the cephalometric tracing (see Fig. 30–174, *E*) and also demonstrated by the location of the chin pad above the mental symphysis (see Fig. 30–174, *A*); (2) dental malocclusion (Class I) with severe crowding (Fig. 30–175, *A*); and (3) protrusion of the upper and lower dentoalveolar areas in relation to other facial structures.

In planning the treatment, the principal objectives were to diminish facial height and to reduce the bimaxillary protrusion. Several staged procedures were used to accomplish these goals.

STAGE I. The first operation consisted of a reduction in the vertical dimension of the body of the mandible by the resection of a predetermined portion of the mandible along its inferior border (horizontal osteotomy) and transplantation of the resected segment anterior to the mental symphysis. The fragment was adapted to the contour of the mandible by burring the cortex of its posterior surface until the horseshoe-shaped graft was accurately fitted to the host bed (see Figs. 30–113 and 30–114). The procedure shortened the total face height and provided adequate protrusion of the mental symphysis. As can be observed on the cephalo-

metric tracing of the patient four years following procedure, a satisfactory contour was maintained (see Fig. 30–174, *F*).

STAGE 2. Orthodontic treatment to relieve the severe dental crowding and to reduce the protrusion of the maxillary and mandibular dentoalveolar areas comprised the second stage of treatment. This required extraction of

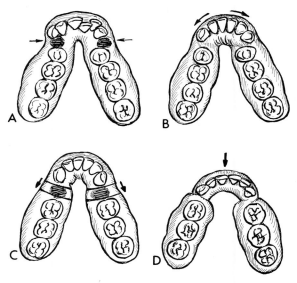

FIGURE 30–176. Drawing made from dental mandibular casts of patient shown in Figure 30–174. *A,* Original dental malalignment of the mandibular teeth. The arrows indicate the extraction of the first premolars. *B,* Result obtained following orthodontic therapy. *C,* The arrows indicate the extraction of the second premolars prior to a dentoalveolar set-back procedure. *D,* Contour of the mandibular arch following the set-back osteotomy.

the maxillary and mandibular first premolar teeth. The spaces thus made available were used to realign the anterior teeth and to retract them as much as possible using upper and lower edgewise arch orthodontic appliances over a period of approximately one year (Fig. 30–176). Since much of the extraction space was required for tooth realignment (particularly in the mandibular dental arch), both the upper and lower dentoalveolar areas were still relatively prognathic following orthodontic therapy. In order to correct this disharmony, a combined surgical-orthodontic approach was planned to correct the remaining bimaxillary protrusion.

STAGE 3. In the third phase, the mandibular second premolars were extracted (Fig. 30–176, *C*); the dentoalveolar process was exposed subperiosteally, and an alveolar set-back osteotomy was performed below the level of the apices of the teeth (see Fig. 30–17). The dentoalveolar block was moved posteriorly virtually the entire width of the extraction space, temporarily producing an overjet of nearly 1 cm between the upper and lower anterior teeth. The edgewise arch orthodontic appliance was used for fixation.

STAGE 4. In order to harmonize the occlusion and complete the reduction of the bimaxillary protrusion, the upper second premolars were removed, and the anterior portion of the maxilla containing the six anterior maxillary teeth and dentoalveolar bone was moved backward (Fig. 30–177, *C, D*) by means of a maxillary premolar segmental set-back osteotomy. Fixation was provided by the edgewise arch orthodontic appliance after resection of the appropriate amount of bone from the hard palate.

As seen from the drawings of the dental casts, the combination of orthodontic alignment and surgical set-back of the anterior dentoalveolar segments resulted in considerable improvement in the general contour of the dental arches, which assumed a parabolic rather than a simian form. Removal of the eight premolar teeth permitted foreshortening of the dental arches, without loss of dental arch continuity, and also provided reduction of the bimaxillary protrusion.

The period of treatment could have been shortened by combining Stages 3 and 4 through careful predetermination of the desired position of the dentoalveolar segments and concomitant maxillary and mandibular dentoalveolar osteotomies.

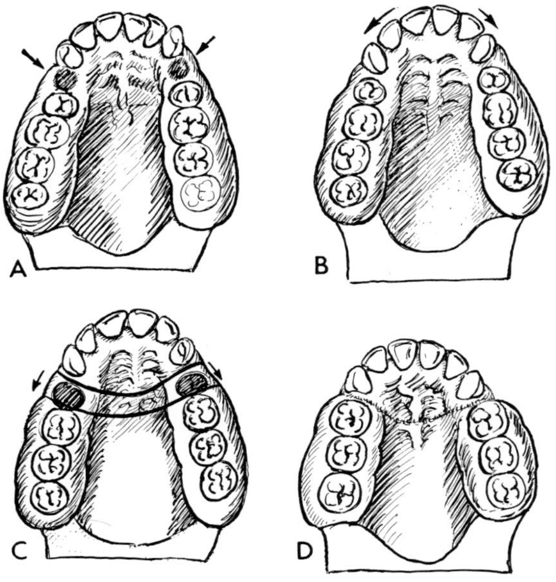

Maxillary Micrognathia

The deformity may involve only the dentoalveolar segment of the maxilla, resulting in malocclusion. Maxillary micrognathia resulting from childhood injury may involve either the entire maxilla or only one side. In Chapter 26, the influence of trauma on the growth of the nasomaxillary complex is reviewed. Because of the intimate relationship of the maxilla and the external nose, the nose is often affected, appearing flat or depressed when the maxilla is maldeveloped; nasomaxillary recession ("dishface" deformity) often results. The zygoma may lack its usual cheekbone prominence; the rim of the orbital floor may be depressed backward, not only in the medial maxillary portion but also in the lateral zygomatic portion.

Hypoplasia is a frequent complication of cleft palate and is a characteristic of craniofacial dysostosis, mandibulofacial dysostosis (Treacher Collins syndrome), and other craniofacial anomalies.

When the entire maxilla is hypoplastic, the condition is referred to as maxillary micrognathia. When a maxilla of normal size is retroposed as a result of malunited fractures, the

FIGURE 30–177. *A*, Drawing of the maxillary arch prior to treatment. The arrows indicate extraction of the first premolars. *B*, Contour of the arch following orthodontic therapy. *C*, The shaded areas indicate the extraction of the second premolars. *D*, Contour of the maxillary arch following the dentoalveolar set-back osteotomy.

term maxillary retrusion, retrognathism, or retromaxillism may be applied. The term retrognathism of the maxilla indicates the backward position of the bone and the lingual position of the maxillary teeth in relation to the mandibular teeth (Class III malocclusion).

Because of malocclusion, whether the maxillary deformity is the result of hypoplasia (maxillary micrognathia) or a posterior displacement (maxillary retrusion), it is essential that adequate interocclusal relationships be reestablished.

CHOICE OF TREATMENT METHODS IN MAXILLARY MICROGNATHIA

Three types of treatment are available to correct maxillary micrognathia: prosthodontic treatment, onlay bone grafts, and osteotomy of the maxilla.

Prosthodontic Treatment. This is the oldest method and was originally used in edentulous or partially edentulous patients. A denture which protrudes under the upper lip will increase the projection and thus improve contour. To obtain further projection, the sulcus is deepened and lined with a skin graft inlay (Fig. 30–178). The denture can then be extended upward as far as the pyriform aperture or even along the sides of the pyriform aperture. In the past the prosthodontic appliance was more extensively applied in patients with a normal complement of teeth; an overlay denture was made over the patient's teeth to improve contour. The nasomaxillary skin graft inlay technique, which was described in Chapter 29 (see Fig. 29–208), involves an even more extensive application of prosthodontic techniques to obtain contour restoration.

Prosthodontic restoration can be combined

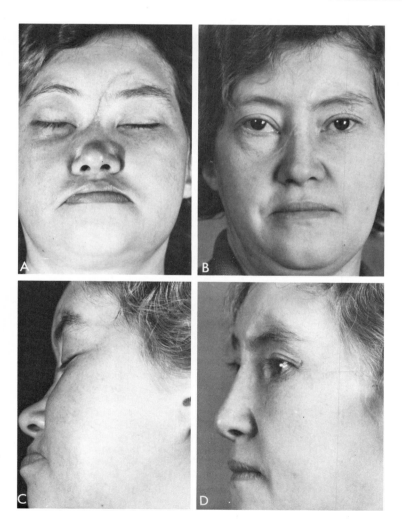

FIGURE 30–178. Contour improvement in an edentulous patient by a denture. *A, C,* Preoperative appearance. The deformity resulted from an automobile accident. Note the saddle-nose deformity and the retrusion of the nasomaxillary area. *B, D,* Appearance following iliac bone graft reconstruction of the nose and a denture with an upward extension into the labiobuccal sulcus deepened by a skin graft inlay.

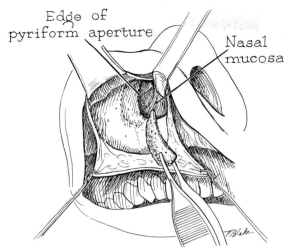

FIGURE 30–179. Crescent-shaped bone grafts are placed around the pyriform aperture and are combined with an iliac graft to the nose to correct saddle nose deformities with nasomaxillary depression. Costal cartilage grafts can also be employed. (From Converse, J. M.: Technique of bone grafting for contour restoration of the face. Plast. Reconstr. Surg., *14*:332, 1954. Copyright 1954, The Williams & Wilkins Company, Baltimore.)

with bone grafting of the alveolar process in edentulous patients to obtain improved retention and contour. In this procedure, an incision is made on the labial aspect of the vestibule to raise a flap of mucosa from the orbicularis oris muscle. The alveolar process is exposed subperiosteally, and a bone graft is placed anteriorly or along the crest of the atrophied alveolar process to increase its projection.

Onlay Bone Grafts. Restoration of contour can be achieved by bone grafts applied through either the intraoral or extraoral route (Converse, 1950; Schmid, 1952; Converse and Shapiro, 1954) (see discussion of routes of approach, p. 1425).

In nasomaxillary deformities with depression not only of the nose but also of the adjacent maxillary portion of the face, bone grafts are placed over the dorsum of the nose and over the maxilla around the edge of the pyriform aperture. The exposure is obtained subperiosteally through the intraoral approach. Crescent-shaped pyramidal pieces of cancellous bone are placed on each side to correct the nasomaxillary depression (Fig. 30–179). Large depressed areas of the maxilla are repaired by a bone graft, which consists of a shell-like segment that is shaped from the medial aspect of the ilium (Fig. 30–180). The onlay bone graft is applied as a bridge over the defect. Small chips of cancellous bone are placed in the intervening crevices beneath

FIGURE 30–180. Contour restoration by onlay bone grafts through the intraoral route. *A,* Profile view of the depression of the anterior maxillary wall. *B,* After an incision is made through the mucosa on the labial aspect of the sulcus, the periosteum is raised from the bone. *C,* The exposed pyriform aperture and infraorbital nerve. *D,* Onlay bone grafts in position filling the depressed areas of the maxilla.

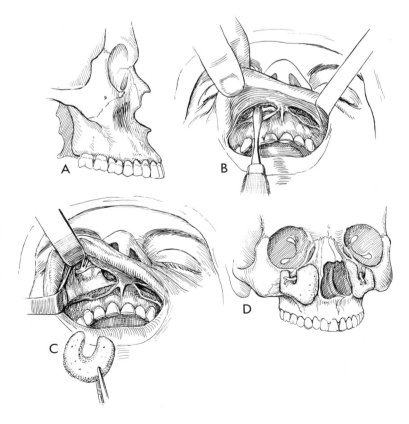

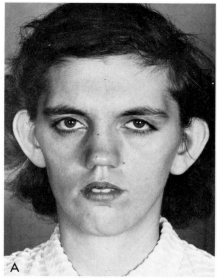
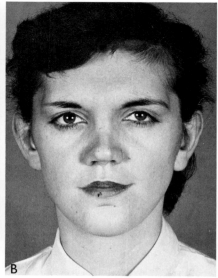

FIGURE 30–181. Contour restoration of the maxilla by bone grafting. *A,* Preoperative appearance showing retrusion of the nasomaxillary area due to hypoplasia. *B,* Restoration of contour obtained by bone grafts applied over the maxilla through the intraoral approach, as illustrated in Figure 30–180. Additional corrective measures included orthodontic treatment, a corrective rhinoplasty, and corrective surgery for protruding ears.

the onlay bone to improve contact with the host bone and to increase the projection of the graft. An overcorrection is necessary to compensate for some degree of bone absorption, particularly if a large quantity of bone is employed. After the vestibular incision is sutured, an external pressure dressing immobilizes the graft and prevents hematoma formation. The eyelids are temporarily sutured to avoid corneal abrasion should the lids be opened under the pressure dressing. Fixation of the graft occurs within one week, and additional dressings are not necessary. A contour restoration obtained by this technique is shown in Figure 30–181. Other techniques of contour restoration by bone grafting are discussed later in this chapter.

Onlay bone grafts are not as reliable in maintaining contour as the actual modification of the facial skeleton by osteotomy combined with bone grafting. Much progress has been made in the treatment of skeletal deformities of the maxilla by the development of selective osteotomies. Midface osteotomies are indicated to correct malunited fractures and congenital malformations.

Maxillary Osteotomies to Correct Skeletal Deformities. When the maxillary deformity extends beyond the dentoalveolar complex,

major osteotomies must often be performed. The choice of the type of osteotomy depends upon (1) the extent of the maxillary deformity; (2) the portion of the maxilla that is affected; (3) the type of malocclusion; and (4) the degree of involvement of the neighboring structures, such as the nose, zygoma, and orbits.

Maxillary osteotomies are generally performed along the classic lines of fracture described by LeFort (1901): the lower maxillary osteotomy (LeFort I), the pyramidal naso-or-bitomaxillary osteotomy (LeFort II); the high maxillary osteotomy (LeFort III), in which the midfacial skeleton is detached from the cranium; and the tripartite midface osteotomy. Variations and combinations of these osteotomies are indicated for a wide variety of malformations, such as maxillary micrognathia or hypoplasia with retrusion, open bite deformities, and craniofacial malformations.

THE COMPLETE HORIZONTAL LOW MAXILLARY OSTEOTOMY (LEFORT I). The complete horizontal low maxillary osteotomy transects the maxilla at the level of a LeFort I (Guérin) maxillary fracture, above the dentoalveolar segment of the jaw and the floor of the nose (Fig. 30–182). Wassmund performed this type of procedure in 1927 for the closure of an open bite malocclusion. Axhausen (1934) was the first to advance the lower portion of the

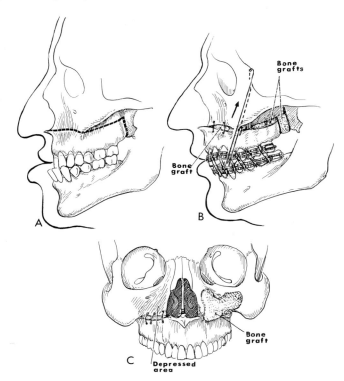

FIGURE 30–182. Advancement of the maxilla by a low horizontal osteotomy (LeFort I). *A,* The broken line represents the line of osteotomy extending above the apices of the teeth and above the level of the floor of the nose. The vertical line indicates the site of osteotomy to separate the tuberosity of the maxilla from the pterygoid plates. *B,* The lower maxillary segment has been advanced. Intermaxillary fixation and frontal bone suspension wiring have been established. Bone grafts assist in ensuring consolidation. A bone graft is wedged between the pterygoid process and the tuberosity of the maxilla to aid in maintaining the forward position of the advanced maxillary segment. *C,* Onlay bone grafts are placed over the lines of osteotomy and lateral to the pyriform aperture for contour restoration.

maxilla using this technique. Schuchardt (1942) applied forward traction by means of a pulley and weight system to produce an advancement of the sectioned maxillary segment. Transection of the pterygoid processes in the LeFort I osteotomy was described by Moore and Ward (1949) and was recommended by Ullik (1970) in adult patients who had been operated upon for cleft lip and palate. Hogeman and Willmar (1967) reported a series of 49 cases of maxillary retrusion treated by a complete low maxillary osteotomy and included the pterygoid processes in the transection. Colantino and Dudley (1970) used a similar complete horizontal osteotomy, including the pterygoid plates, to retroposition the maxilla in the correction of maxillary prognathism.

Willmar (1974), in reviewing the historical aspects of the LeFort I osteotomy, noted that Dingman and Harding (1951) were the first to separate the maxillary tuberosities from the pterygoid processes in performing the operation. Converse and Shapiro (1952), in a different type of operation (see Fig. 30–189), also separated the tuberosities from the pterygoid processes and preserved the posterior portion of the hard palate.

The use of bone grafts over the osteotomy sites was reported by Gillies and Rowe (1954), Cupar (1954), Cernéa, Grignon, Crepy, and Benoist (1955), and Lévignac (1958). In 1969 Obwegeser introduced the technique of wedging a bone graft between the pterygoid process and the tuberosity of the maxilla for stabilization and placing additional bone for the consolidation of the advanced maxillary segment. Dupont, Ciaburro, and Prévost (1974) have advocated sectioning through the tuberosity rather than at the pterygomaxillary interface. There is to date no evidence that this technique offers any advantage over the standard technique.

The LeFort I osteotomy and its modifications are among the most frequently employed procedures in the treatment of maxillary deformities.

Technique of the LeFort I osteotomy. The procedure (see Fig. 30–182) is performed under general anesthesia administered through a nasotracheal tube. An incision is made through the mucoperiosteum of the gingiva; the mucoperiosteum is undermined backward to and around the maxillary tuberosity. The procedure is repeated on the contralateral side. The maxilla is sectioned transversely from the edge of the pyriform aperture back to the max-

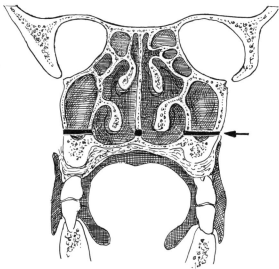

FIGURE 30–183. A frontal section through the maxilla illustrates the level of the osteotomy lines of the LeFort I osteotomy through the lateral and medial walls of the maxillary sinus and the septum at the vomer groove (shown in its anterior portion).

illary tuberosity (Fig. 30–182, *A*) with a sharp osteotome, small round or fissure bur, or the Stryker oscillating saw. The level of the osteotomy should be sufficiently high to leave 3 to 5 mm of bone above the apices of the teeth.

After careful elevation of the mucoperichondrium and mucoperiosteum on each side of the septal framework, the septum is sectioned at the base of the vomer along the entire length of the nasal floor. Despite the presence of the nasotracheal tube, the septal procedure is done without difficulty through the contralateral nasal airway.

The lateral walls of the nasal cavity are now sectioned with an osteotome. The approach is through the nasal cavity or across the maxillary sinus through the previously made osteotomy along the anterior surface of the maxilla. The line of osteotomy is parallel to the line of osteotomy through the maxilla (Fig. 30–183).

The lower maxillary segment is now freed from its adjacent bony attachments except at the junction of the maxillary tuberosities and the pterygoid processes.

The maxillary segment is separated posteriorly from its remaining attachment at the pterygomaxillary suture line (Fig. 30–182, *B*). A curved periosteal elevator is placed beneath the mucoperiosteum to and around the maxillary tuberosity as far back as the pterygo-

maxillary junction. A short vertical incision through the mucoperiosteum anterior to the tuberosity facilitates the insertion of the curved osteotome. The curved osteotome then *gently* severs the connection between the tuberosity and the pterygoid processes (Fig. 30–184). Undue force applied during the disjunction can fracture the pterygoid plates. If the pterygoid plates are fractured, the bone graft placed in the area will be deprived of a posterior buttress.

The remaining resistance to advancement is encountered from the soft tissues and is overcome by slow and careful manipulation with a pair of Rowe disimpaction forceps. One branch of the forceps is placed on the floor of the nose and the other on the hard palate bilaterally. Forward traction and rocking is exerted in a circular motion until the desired position is attained. The lower maxillary segment, once "rocked" loose, can be advanced into position. The new occlusal relationships are maintained by intermaxillary fixation using an orthodontic appliance (Fig. 30–185) or by some other type of intermaxillary fixation if orthodontic collaboration is not available.

Prior to the establishment of intermaxillary wiring, the mandible is recessed so as to place the condyles into the glenoid fossae. Cranial or circumzygomatic fixation by internal suspension wiring is established from the mandibular or the maxillary arch wire (Fig. 30–

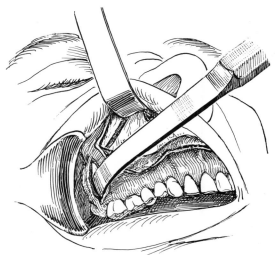

FIGURE 30–184. Pterygomaxillary disjunction. A short posterior incision facilitates the placing of the curved osteotome at the maxillary pterygoid interface. The mucoperiosteum has been elevated from the bone, and the osteotome is placed beneath it.

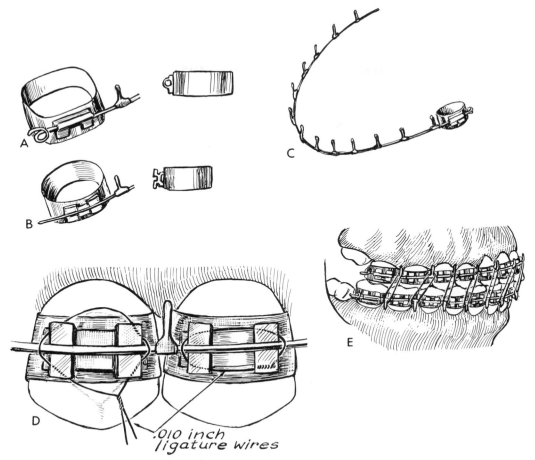

FIGURE 30–185. Edgewise orthodontic and fixation appliance. *A*, A molar band with a rectangular sheath through which the edgewise arch wire is inserted. *B*, Dental bands with "twin brackets" are placed on the remaining teeth. The brackets permit the insertion of the edgewise wire. *C*, Arch wire with spurs soldered to the gingival side as it appears prior to final insertion. *D*, The arch wire has been inserted in the "twin brackets" and is secured in position with wire ligature ties. *E*, The appliance in place with intermaxillary wires (0.028 inch) placed between the arches to fix one jaw to the other.

182, *B*). The maxilla is thus maintained in its advanced position with minimal danger of recession, a complication which can occur when the condyles have been allowed to drift forward during intermaxillary fixation.

Bone grafting is important in ensuring the success of the procedure (Fig. 30–182, *C*). The measured bone grafts wedged into the pterygomaxillary spaces assist in the consolidation of the line of osteotomy and in the maintenance of the forward projection of the detached maxilla. The chances of postoperative recession are thus minimized.

Thin, cancellous, onlay bone grafts are also placed over the line of osteotomy (Fig. 30–182, *C*). The advancement of the maxillary segment produces a step between the repositioned segment and the intact portion of the

maxilla; bone grafts placed over this area improve contour.

The mucoperiosteal incision is sutured, and a pressure dressing is applied. Consolidation is rapid. Intermaxillary fixation and internal wires are usually left in position for six to eight weeks. After removal of the intermaxillary wires, orthodontic surveillance is continued to verify the maintenance of the corrected occlusal relationships.

THE LEFORT 1½ OSTEOTOMY. In patients with pronounced recession in the nasomaxillary area, it is advantageous to advance the retruded portion of the maxilla situated lateral to the pyriform aperture. To accomplish this, Obwegeser (1969) advocated a horizontal maxillary osteotomy at a higher level. The higher level of the osteotomy places it further

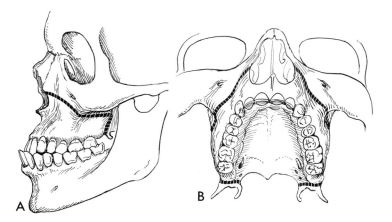

FIGURE 30–186. Advancement of the maxilla by a horizontal osteotomy at a higher level (LeFort 1½ osteotomy). *A*, Outline of the line of section. The anterior portion of the osteotomy is extended up to the lateral rim of the pyriform aperture. *B*, An occlusal view of the osteotomy showing the line of section through the body of the maxilla and at the pterygomaxillary junction.

from the apices of the incisor and canine teeth, with less danger of devitalization through loss of blood supply. The technique is similar to that of the basic LeFort I osteotomy, except that the anterior portion of the osteotomy is performed at a higher level on the lateral rim rather than the base of the pyriform aperture (Figs. 30–186 and 30–187). It is important to recall that the nasolacrimal duct empties into the upper portion of the inferior meatus at the junction of the frontal process of the maxilla and the inferior turbinate.

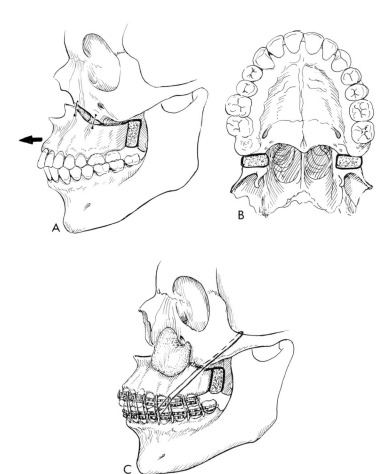

FIGURE 30–187. Completion of the LeFort 1½ maxillary osteotomy. *A*, The maxillary segment has been advanced, and interosseous wire fixation has been applied. Bone grafts are placed in the interstices. *B*, Maintenance of the forward projection of the maxillary segment is assisted by bone grafts placed in the pterygomaxillary gap. Internal wiring looped around the zygomatic arch and the arch wires provide cranial suspension and maintain each condyle in the glenoid fossa. Onlay bone grafts over the line of osteotomy assist bony consolidation and improve contour restoration.

MAXILLARY ADVANCEMENT IN CLEFT PALATE PATIENTS. Maxillary hypoplasia is a complication of unilateral and bilateral clefts. When molar relationships are adequate, a premolar segmental maxillary advancement osteotomy is indicated (see Fig. 30–171). When the maxillary dental arch is in a Class III malocclusion, the LeFort I advancement osteotomy is the operation of choice. After the osteotomy, the advancement is more difficult than in idiopathic maxillary hypoplasia and requires considerable force and forward and downward traction with the Rowe disimpaction forceps.

RETROMOLAR SEGMENTAL ADVANCEMENT OF THE MAXILLA. The operation was designed to preserve the posterior portion of the hard palate and to avoid advancement of the soft palate and consequent velopharyngeal incompetence. It is indicated in those patients in whom velopharyngeal competence is threatened by a LeFort I advancement osteotomy (see p. 1451, Speech Following Maxillary Advancement Osteotomies).

The operation (Converse and Shapiro, 1952) was devised to advance the lower portion of the maxilla with the dentoalveolar component,

to reestablish dental occlusion, and to restore facial contour in a patient who had suffered facial trauma in an automobile accident at the age of 3 years (Fig. 30–188).

Exposure of the maxilla is similar to that employed in the LeFort I advancement osteotomy (see Fig. 30–182); the incision is extended backward toward the maxillary tuberosity on each side. The osteotomy is performed on both sides beyond and around the maxillary tuberosities (Fig. 30–189, *A* to *C*). The mucoperiosteum is then reflected from the hard palate after an incision is made through the gingiva (Figure 30–189, *C*). The hard palate is exposed as far back as the greater palatine foramina; the descending palatine arteries and anterior palatine nerves are preserved. The osteotomy around the maxillary tuberosity extends through the pterygomaxillary interface to a point above the level of the roots of the molar teeth; it extends around the tuberosity and in a forward direction on the palatal aspect of the alveolar process to a point situated anterior to the greater palatine foramen on each side (Fig. 30–189, *C*). The palatine process of the maxilla is sectioned transversely,

FIGURE 30–188. Maxillary hypoplasia with retrusion of the middle third of the face. *A,* Preoperative profile. *B,* Following surgical advancement of the lower portion of the maxilla and an onlay bone graft to the nose. *C,* Preoperative dental relationships. *D,* Improvement obtained following advancement of the maxilla. (From Converse, J. M., and Shapiro, H. H.: Treatment of developmental malformations of the jaws. Plast. Reconstr. Surg., *10*:473, 1952. Copyright 1952, The Williams & Wilkins Company, Baltimore.)

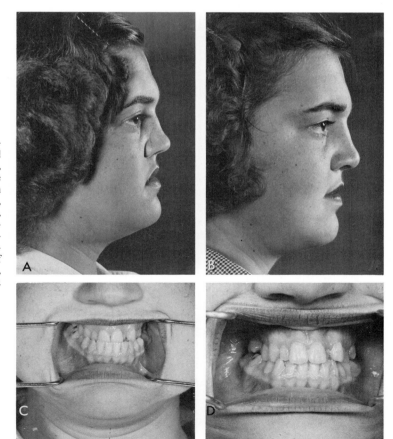

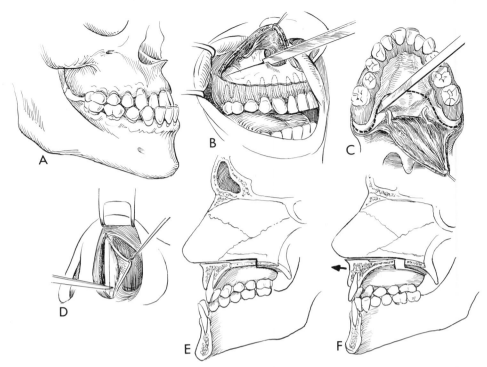

FIGURE 30–189.   Technique of the retromolar segmental advancement osteotomy. *A*, Drawing illustrating the skeletal deformity of the patient shown in Figure 30–188. *B*, The mucoperiosteum is reflected to demonstrate the line of osteotomy. A labiobuccal flap of mucoperiosteum raised from the bone is preserved to maintain blood supply. *C*, The retromolar and transpalatal osteotomies. *D*, The vomer is severed. *E*, Sagittal section illustrating the line of section of the vomer and hard palate. *F*, The maxillary segment is advanced.

including the vomer, leaving intact the attachment of the greater portion of the vomer to the floor of the nose. The septal cartilage is exposed by raising a mucoperichondrial flap and is severed along its insertion into the vomer groove (Fig. 30–189, *D, E*); the incision through the cartilage joins the transverse palatal osteotomy. The severed portion of the maxilla is then mobilized, loosened, and advanced to the planned intermaxillary relationships (Fig. 30–189, *F*). Bone grafts are wedged into the line of osteotomy through the hard palate. Sutures are placed to reapply the mucoperiosteal flap to the gingival tissues. The anterior portion of the hard palate is left exposed, and re-epithelization is spontaneous. Fixation is maintained by intermaxillary wiring. The final phase of the operation consists of maintaining cranial fixation, as previously described.

OTHER VARIATIONS. In malunited LeFort I fractures, the area of malunion is identified, and the osteotomy is done through the healed fracture site.

There are many other variations, depending on the nature of the deformity. Downward rotation of the mobilized segment, as well as advancement, will close an anterior open bite. Bone grafts fill the void produced by the displacement. A lateral deviation deformity requires lateral rotation and correction of the crossbite. In unusual deformities, the mobilized maxillary segment is displaced downward to increase the vertical dimension of the midface, or upward, after resection of a measured segment of bone above the line of osteotomy, to diminish the vertical dimension of the midface.

RESULTS. The results of the LeFort I advancement osteotomy are usually satisfactory when the operative steps outlined in the previous pages are followed. An example of such a result is shown in Figure 30–190. The intraoral views before and after the surgical advancement are shown in Figure 30–191. The preoperative and postoperative cephalograms illustrate the degree of advancement obtained (Fig. 30–192). A mistaken diagnosis of mandibular prognathism could have been made;

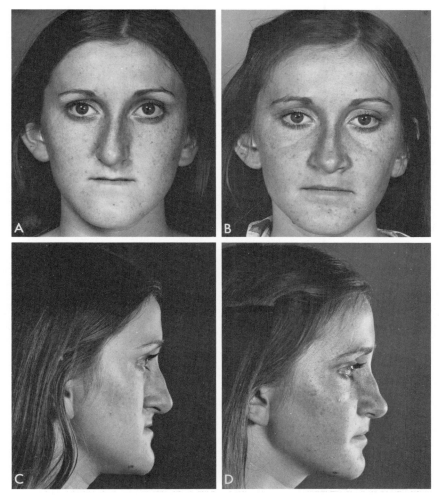

FIGURE 30–190. LeFort 1½ advancement osteotomy. *A*, Preoperative view of a patient with idiopathic maxillary hypoplasia. *B*, Appearance following advancement of the maxilla. *C*, Lateral preoperative view showing pseudoprognathism of the mandible. *D*, Change in the appearance after maxillary advancement. Note the additional projection of the nasal tip.

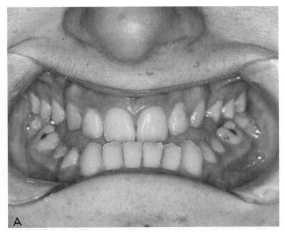

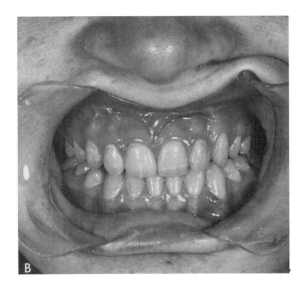

FIGURE 30–191. Intraoral views of the patient shown in Figure 30–190. *A*, Prior to operation. *B*, After completion of treatment.

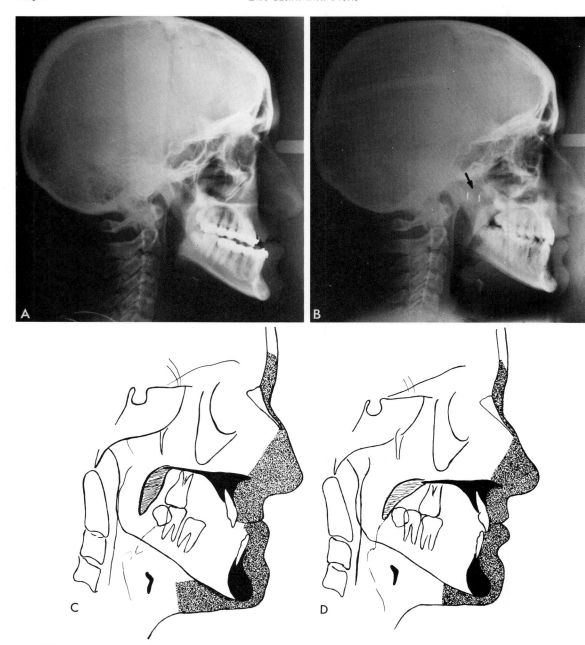

FIGURE 30–192. Cephalograms and tracing of patient shown in Figure 30–190. *A*, Preoperative cephalogram. *B*, Six months after the operation. The bone graft placed at the pterygomaxillary junction is indicated by the arrow. *C*, Preoperative tracing. *D*, Postoperative tracing.

however, cephalometric analysis showed that the patient had pseudoprognathism and that the deformity was the result of maxillary hypoplasia.

Willmar (1974) reported the long-term dentoalveolar and skeletal changes following Le Fort I osteotomies in 106 patients. Metallic implants accurately recorded the positional changes of the maxilla relative to the anterior cranial base. The dentoalveolar relationships were noted to remain stable throughout the observation period of up to three years; small changes were insignificant. The posterior portion of the maxillary skeleton in cleft lip and palate patients shifted upward of 1.0 mm during the first postoperative year and remained stable thereafter. In patients with idiopathic and post-traumatic anterior crossbites, the entire maxilla had a tendency to move upward during the period of intermaxillary fixation. The anterior portion of the maxilla was displaced superiorly 1.8 to 2.3 mm and the posterior portion 0.8 to 1.1 mm. The upward shift was greater in males. Changes in maxillary position did not occur after removal of the intermaxillary fixation. Since the occlusal relationships remained fairly constant, one must assume that the dentoalveolar segment compensated for the skeletal changes.

In our series, a tendency toward retrocession was a problem in the past, particularly in the cleft palate group. Willmar (1974) noted a similar tendency toward a backward horizontal movement of the maxilla in the cleft palate group; the majority of these cases had not been bone grafted. This complication has been minimized since bone grafts have been applied over the lines of osteotomy, over the tuberosity of the maxilla, and as a wedge interposed between the maxillary tuberosity and the pterygoid processes. It would appear *a priori* that bone grafting would be an adjuvant to consolidation during the first postoperative year. Willmar (1974) found that no changes in position occur after one year.

VELOPHARYNGEAL INCOMPETENCE FOLLOWING MAXILLARY ADVANCEMENT. The incidence of velopharyngeal incompetence following maxillary advancement procedures is not known. It is suspected that the patient with a repaired cleft palate incurs a greater risk of this postoperative complication than those patients undergoing maxillary advancements for other causes.

Since these procedures involve forward movement of the palate for distances often ranging between 1 and 2 cm, it is felt that such advancement, carrying as it does the soft palate, might be responsible for the development of postoperative velopharyngeal inadequacy.

In a preliminary communication, Schwartz (1976) has reported a prospective study of nine patients with craniofacial dysostoses who underwent midface (including maxillary) advancement (average of 12.4 mm). The following analyses were made. Preoperative and postoperative recordings were obtained from each patient as he sustained vowels in isolation and uttered monosyllables containing a variety of consonants. These recordings were reviewed by a panel of speech pathologists for evaluation of hypernasality. The method of Equal Appearing Intervals (Guilford, 1954) was used to obtain the scale judgments. The recordings were also subjected to spectrographic analysis, and the spectrograms were analyzed for traces of acoustic correlates of hypernasality (Schwartz, 1968). Finally, aerodynamic studies involving intraoral air pressure and transnasal air flows (Warren, 1964) were used to assess the magnitude of velopharyngeal patency during consonant production (see Chapter 52).

Postoperative hypernasality was observed in none of the patients. All three groups of tests, i.e., listener judgments, acoustic analysis, and aerodynamic analysis, supported this conclusion. For several of the patients, velopharyngeal openings were found for the production of certain non-nasal consonants. In no instance did the openings exceed 5 mm²; thus they were all well below the critical threshold of adequacy of 20 mm² (Warren and Ryan, 1967).

Preoperatively the patients with Crouzon's disease exhibited hyponasality—that is, an absence of the nasal resonance normally found in the consonants /m, n, and ng/. This finding was attributed to the lack of maxillary growth coupled with a normal appearing soft palate which served to occlude the entrance to the posterior nares. Preoperative lateral cephalograms showed that the soft palate obscured

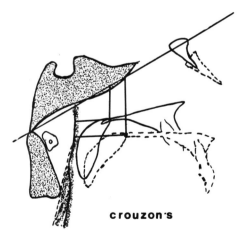

crouzon's

FIGURE 30–193. Lateral preoperative (solid line) and postoperative (dotted line) cephalometric tracings of a patient with Crouzon's disease. Note the anterior and inferior displacement of the maxilla following the maxillary advancement. There is a concomitant change in the position of the velum and its relationship to the posterior pharyngeal wall; the dimensions of the airway have also been increased.

the entrance to the nasopharynx (Fig. 30–193). Postoperative cephalograms showed a more normal position of the soft palate and nasopharynx, thereby permitting passage of sound into the nose and eliminating the preoperative hyponasal condition.

Cephalometric studies have also documented changes in the configuration of the velum and its relationship to the posterior pharyngeal wall following maxillary advancement (Figs. 30–194 and 30–195).

PHARYNGEAL FLAPS AND MAXILLARY ADVANCEMENT PROCEDURES. In planning a maxillary advancement in a patient who has undergone a pharyngeal flap procedure for the correction of velopharyngeal incompetence, the surgeon is faced with several possibilities:

1. If the pharyngeal flap is narrow and tethered and has not improved speech, the flap is divided and inhalation anesthesia can be administered via a nasotracheal route. At a later stage, the velopharyngeal incompetence can be corrected by a lateral port control procedure (see Chapter 52).

2. If the pharyngeal flap is functional and sufficiently large, with only slitlike nasopharyngeal ports, and it is feared that the proposed operation will jeopardize the airway, a temporary tracheotomy is the procedure of choice. Endotracheal intubation is accomplished through an oral route, and the tracheotomy is performed over the endotracheal tube. The latter is withdrawn as the tracheostomy tube is inserted, and an alternative inhalation anesthetic route is provided.

3. If the pharyngeal flap is inferiorly based and is tethered, and it is felt that advancement of the maxillary complex will result in velopharyngeal incompetence, the length of the flap can be augmented by dividing the inferior pedicle, raising a new superiorly based pharyngeal flap, and inserting it into the nasal surface of the velum or the divided flap (Weber, Chase, and Jobe, 1970; McEvitt, 1971; Owsley, Creech, and Dedo, 1972). With a tracheotomy this procedure can be done at the same time as the maxillary advancement. (See also a discussion of maxillary advancement in the presence of a velopharyngeal flap in Chapter 47, p. 2194.)

THE TEETH IN MAXILLARY OSTEOTOMIES. The vitality of a tooth depends upon its blood supply and not upon its nerve supply; pulp testing is invalid in the evaluation of tooth vitality. Instead, color changes, the loosening of the tooth, and the development of periodontal disease are the criteria used to evaluate the return of the blood supply to the tooth.

Tooth damage can occur when an interdental osteotomy is performed. If the lamina propria is penetrated by an instrument in the course of the osteotomy, the tooth may later become loose and require extraction. Revascularization of the maxillary segments or of the entire lower portion of the maxilla (after a LeFort I osteotomy) has been studied experimentally and

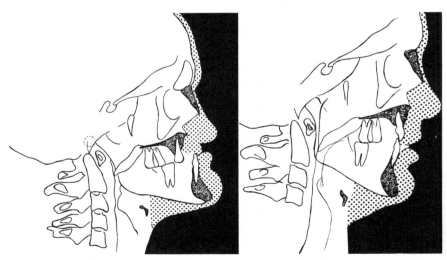

FIGURE 30–194. Patient with a repaired cleft lip and palate and maxillary hypoplasia. Velopharyngeal inadequacy was not observed postoperatively. *Left,* Preoperative cephalometric tracing. *Right,* Postoperative cephalometric tracing. Note change in contour and position of the velum.

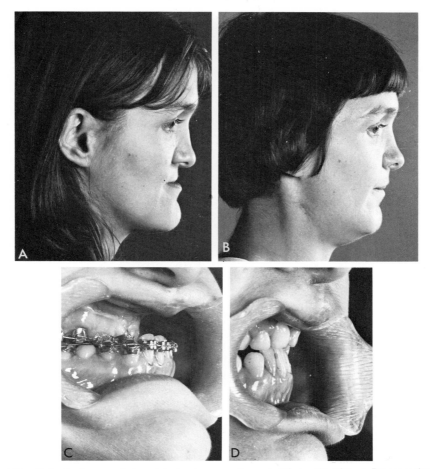

FIGURE 30–195. Patient whose cephalometric tracings are shown in Figure 30–194. *A,* Preoperative profile. *B,* Appearance following a staged LeFort I maxillary advancement and vertical osteotomy (recession) of the mandible. *C,* Preoperative occlusion. *D,* Postoperative occlusion.

clinically by Butcher and Taylor (1951), Bell (1969), Bell and Levy (1970), Rontal and Hohmann (1972), and Bell (1973). Rapid revascularization of the bone, teeth, and mucoperiosteum occurs.

The reinnervation of the teeth after segmental osteotomy of the anterior portion of the maxilla (the set-back premolar osteotomy) has been studied in animal experiments and in patients by Leibold, Tilson, and Rask (1971), Ware and Ashamalla (1971), and Pepersack (1973). While after a LeFort I osteotomy the teeth do not respond to the pulp tester for a variable period of time extending over a period of many months, they usually recover their sensibility. As stated earlier, the vitality of the tooth depends upon its blood supply and not upon its nerve supply. The teeth may therefore be vital but denervated (Mårtensson, 1950;

Poswillo, 1972). Willmar (1976) has observed the return of sensibility in the teeth and gingiva within one year after a LeFort I osteotomy was performed with interposition of bone in the osteotomy line for the purpose of increasing the vertical dimension of the dental alveolar process, indeed a remarkable phenomenon (see p. 1466).

COMBINED OSTEOTOMIES; EXPANSION OSTEOTOMIES. When there is gross disparity in arch form between a constricted maxillary arch and a normal mandible, a sagittal osteotomy through the hard palate with interposition of bone grafts to restore hard palate continuity is indicated.

Lingual crossbite malocclusion of the posterior teeth can be unilateral or bilateral. This type of malocclusion is often seen in patients with idiopathic maxillary hypoplasia and in

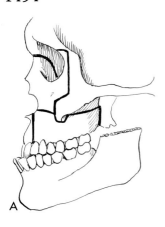
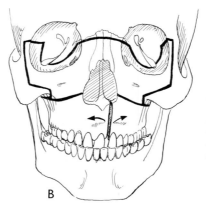

FIGURE 30–196. Maxillary expansion osteotomy combined with the LeFort I and III osteotomies. *A*, Lateral view of the osteotomies. *B*, Frontal view illustrating parasagittal splitting of the alveolar bone and palate. (After Obwegeser.)

cleft palate patients with medial collapse of the posterior segments. It also occurs after malunited fractures of the maxilla.

Axhausen (1934) described the "midline" palatal split to correct a malunited fracture. The sagittal osteotomy of the hard palate actually extends through the bone immediately lateral to the vomer. In cleft palate cases, the maxillary expansion is facilitated by the cleft but may be hindered when the palatal mucosa is excessively scarred.

Obwegeser (1969) has combined the expansion osteotomy with the LeFort I and LeFort III osteotomies (Fig. 30–196). The maxillary fragments are immobilized by fixation appliances. Gaps in the bony skeleton resulting from the expansion are filled with bone grafts for further stabilization.

THE LEFORT II OSTEOTOMY (HENDERSON AND JACKSON, 1973). This is indicated when the patient has nasomaxillary hypoplasia in addition to recession of the lower maxillary segment and Class III malocclusion. The

zygomas are spared. The lines of osteotomy follow the classic LeFort II fracture lines (Fig. 30–197). Through a coronal incision or incisions made over the frontal process of the maxilla on each side of the nose, a subperiosteal dissection exposes the medial wall of the orbit after the medial canthal tendon is detached and the lacrimal sac is raised from the lacrimal groove.

Through an intraoral approach the maxilla is exposed subperiosteally, and the infraorbital nerves are identified. Laterally, the junction of the zygoma with the maxilla on each side is exposed.

The osteotomy across the root of the nose is continued posteriorly along each medial orbital wall until it reaches the lamina papyracea of the ethmoid, posterior to the lacrimal groove. The osteotomy then changes direction, extending vertically downward to the floor of the orbit and lateral to the lacrimal groove (medial to the infraorbital foramen); it curves laterally along the area of junction of the maxilla and zygoma

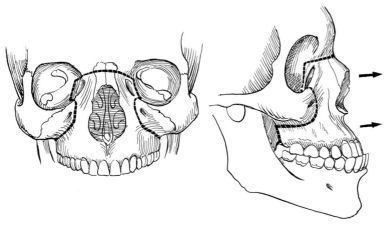

FIGURE 30–197. The LeFort II osteotomy. *Left*, Outline of the LeFort II osteotomy. The osteotomy crosses the upper portion of the nasal bones, extends along the medial orbital wall above and behind the lacrimal groove, medial to the infraorbital foramen downward and laterally, below the zygomatic process of the maxilla to the pterygomaxillary junction. *Right*, Lateral view of the osteotomy.

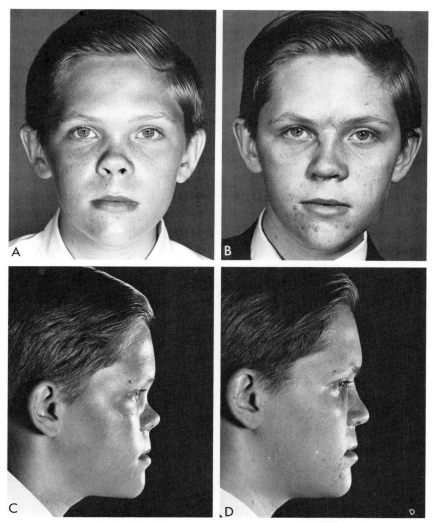

FIGURE 30–198. Correction of nasomaxillary hypoplasia by naso-orbitomaxillary advancement osteotomy. *A,* Preoperative appearance showing the retrusion of the midfacial skeleton. The patient had a septal abscess at age 4 years which destroyed most of the septal cartilage. *B,* Appearance after advancement. *C, D,* Preoperative and postoperative profile views. Note the elongation of the nose and the increased nasomaxillary forward projection. (Figs. 30–198 to 30–203 from Converse, J. M., Horowitz, S. L., Valauri, A. J., and Montandon, D.: The treatment of nasomaxillary hypoplasia. A new pyramidal naso-orbital maxillary osteotomy. Plast. Reconstr. Surg., *45*:527, 1970. Copyright 1970, The Williams & Wilkins Company, Baltimore.)

and backward to the pterygomaxillary junction (Fig. 30–197).

The ethmoid plate of the septum is cut with scissors after the midface has been rocked forward and downward.

The remainder of the operation is similar to the LeFort I osteotomy. Bone is placed in the pterygomaxillary gap and over the lines of osteotomy. Intermaxillary fixation and cranial fixation are established.

THE NASO-ORBITO-MAXILLARY OSTEOTOMY. Maxillary hypoplasia is often characterized by hypoplasia of the nasomaxillary complex. A LeFort I osteotomy is contraindicated, since the nasal deformity is left uncorrected.

The masomaxillary skin graft inlay technique (see Chapter 29, p. 1201) has the disadvantage of obliging the patient to wear a permanent supporting prosthesis.

Converse, Horowitz, Valauri, and Montandon (1970) designed a pyramidal naso-orbito-maxillary osteotomy to correct both the nasal and maxillary deformities. The patient shown in Figure 30–198 had a history of a nasal septal hematoma following injury at the age of 4 years. An abscess and subsequent necrosis of the septal cartilage resulted in failure of growth and development of the nasomaxillary area.

The principles of the procedure include the following: (1) the foreshortened nasal septal framework must be freed, as it will oppose nasal lengthening; (2) a forward and downward repositioning of the underdeveloped nasomaxillary complex is required to correct the maxillary retrusion and to elongate the nose; (3) the nasolacrimal apparatus must not be disrupted; (4) bone grafts are used to restore the nasal contour and to fill in the defects resulting from the advancement of the nasomaxillary complex so as to ensure rapid consolidation and to diminish the chances of relapse; (5) skin coverage and nasal lining must be provided to accommodate the nasal elongation.

Exposure of the nasal framework. The nasal framework and medial orbital skeleton are exposed through a trapdoor incision, triangular in shape with its apex at the glabella (Fig. 30–199); the incision provides additional skin coverage by means of a V-Y advancement. The incision extends downward laterally over the frontal process of the maxilla. Retraction of the flap provides exposure and permits subperiosteal elevation of the soft tissues from the bony framework of the nose and the nasal cartilages. The dissection is extended to the base of the pyriform aperture. The periosteum is reflected from the bone cradling the lacrimal groove, and the medial wall of the orbit is exposed over the lamina papyracea of the ethmoid. The medial canthal tendon and the lacrimal sac are reflected laterally with the orbital contents.

Elongation of the nose. The first phase of the skeletal surgery involves lengthening the cartilaginous nose. A submucous resection of the residual septal framework is done. Released from the restrictive influence of the septum, the cartilaginous portion of the nose becomes more extensible. By reflecting the trapdoor flap downward, the area of junction of the lateral cartilages with the nasal bones is exposed. The lateral cartilages are separated from the undersurface of the nasal bones. The mucoperiosteum underlying the nasal bones is undermined as far upward as possible and incised transversely. At this point, by placing the thumb and index finger on each side of the columella near the tip of the nose, it is possible to draw the nasal structures downward. Further elongation is also obtained by dividing the loose connective tissue joining the alar and lateral nasal cartilages. By these means, the short nose can be appreciably lengthened.

The osteotomy. A horizontal osteotomy separates the nasal bones from the frontal bone (Fig. 30–200). The line of osteotomy is extended laterally along the medial orbital wall, above the lacrimal groove to the lamina papyracea. The osteotomy is directed vertically downward to the medial portion of the floor of the orbit, then anteriorly lateral to the lacrimal groove but medial to the infraorbital foramen to preserve the lacrimal apparatus and the infraorbital nerve. It is continued downward through the anterior wall of the maxillary sinus

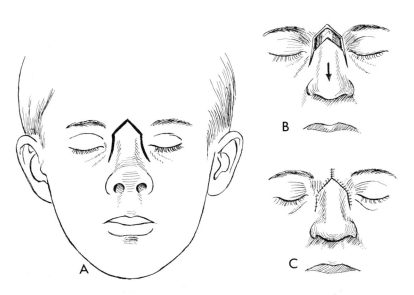

FIGURE 30–199. Exposure of the nasal framework and elongation of the nose. *A,* Incision, outlining the trapdoor flap. *B, C,* V-Y advancement to elongate the skin of the nose.

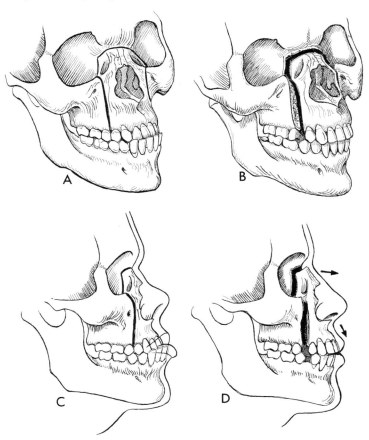

FIGURE 30–200. Naso-orbitomaxillary osteotomy for forward and downward displacement of the nasomaxillary complex. *A,* The line of osteotomy extends across the nasofrontal junction and posteriorly to the lacrimal groove through the rim of the orbit and downward through the maxilla into the premolar area and across the hard palate. *B,* After the posterior portion of the nasal septum is severed, the nasomaxillary block is mobilized. *C,* Lateral view of the line of osteotomy. *D,* Forward and downward displacement made possible by the osteotomy. Bone grafts are wedged into the gaps to maintain the position of the nasomaxillary complex and to ensure consolidation. When the molar relationships are in a Class III malocclusion, the osteotomy is modified and is extended posteriorly as far as the pterygomaxillary junction (see Fig. 30–197).

and through the alveolar process between the first and second premolar teeth.

A posteriorly based mucoperiosteal flap is raised from the palatal vault, exposing the hard palate. The osteotomy is completed by cutting transversely across the palate into the floor of the nose and through the vomer if it has not been resected during the submucous resection of the septum (Fig. 30–201). The undisturbed posterior portion of the maxilla provides a strong

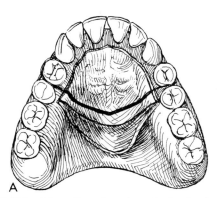
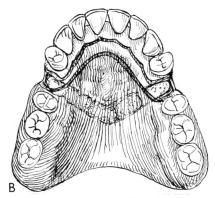

FIGURE 30–201. Line of section through the hard palate in the naso-orbitomaxillary osteotomy. *A,* After the mucoperiosteal palatal flap has been raised, the palatal osteotomy is made as outlined. After the naso-orbitomaxillary segment has been advanced, bone grafts are wedged into the defect in the hard palate, and the palatal flap is returned to cover the bone-grafted area. The denuded anterior portion of the hard palate is left to epithelize spontaneously.

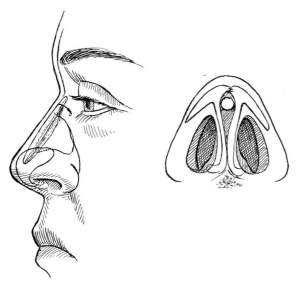

FIGURE 30–202. Nasal contour restoration with an iliac bone graft. The superior end of the bone graft is wired to the nasal bones. The domes of the alar cartilages are sutured over the distal end of the bone graft.

bellar area provides the necessary additional cutaneous cover. The operation is completed by placing a carefully molded dental compound splint over the nose, which is left in position for a period of five days. Cephalometric tracings before and after the pyramidal naso-orbito-maxillary osteotomy are shown in Figure 30–203.

A six-year longitudinal study was completed on the patient shown in Figure 30–204, who also underwent a naso-orbitomaxillary osteotomy. Figure 30–205 shows the dental occlusion before and after treatment.

Psillakis, Lapa, and Spina (1973) have employed a modification of the naso-orbitomaxillary osteotomy in patients whose dental occlusion is adequate. The osteotomy does not include the dentoalveolar segment of the maxilla.

CHOICE OF TECHNIQUE OF MAXILLARY ADVANCEMENT OSTEOTOMY: PREMOLAR SEG-

abutment, and the molar teeth can be used as stable posterior points of fixation. The entire nasomaxillary segment is then advanced the desired distance using the mandibular dental arch as a guide, and the position is maintained by the orthodontic appliance anchored on the posterior maxillary teeth. Intermaxillary fixation is not necessary. The forward movement of the mobilized segment is also accompanied by a downward movement to lengthen the nose.

The bone grafts. The gaps in the facial skeleton are filled with fragments of iliac bone. A thin layer of cancellous bone is placed over the bony voids in the lamina papyracea. Wedges of bone are placed into the bony defect in the nasofrontal area, into the remaining gaps in the medial portion of the orbit, and over the maxillary sinus. The open spaces in the hard palate and the alveolar process are also packed with bone grafts. A carved iliac bone graft is introduced over the dorsum of the nose (Fig. 30–202). The upper portion of the bone graft is maintained by transosseous wire fixation near the nasofrontal osteotomy, and the distal tip of the bone graft is placed between the domes of the alar cartilages, which are sutured to each other over the graft.

A V-Y advancement of the skin in the gla-

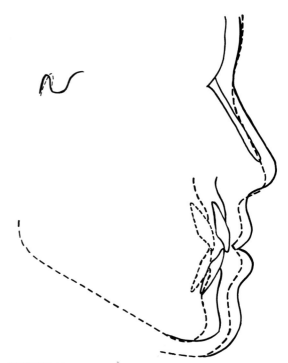

FIGURE 30–203. Cephalometric tracings of the patient shown in Figure 30–198 illustrating the changes in facial contour. The preoperative tracing is indicated by the broken line, and the solid line represents the postoperative change.

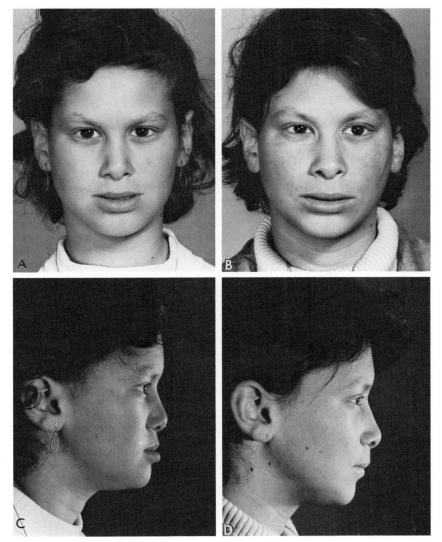

FIGURE 30–204. *A,* A 14 year old female patient with nasomaxillary hypoplasia and Class III malocclusion. *B,* Six years after naso-orbitomaxillary osteotomy. Note the forward projection of the nasomaxillary complex. *C,* Profile view showing the nasomaxillary hypoplasia. *D,* Profile view six years after the osteotomy.

MENTAL OR LEFORT I. One of the principle advantages of the LeFort I osteotomy is that dental arch continuity remains intact; edentulous spaces are not produced by the operation.

The advantage of the premolar segmental osteotomy is that molar relationships are not disturbed when they are satisfactory, a condition which is not infrequent in cleft palate patients.

The premolar osteotomy also offers the advantage of maintaining a stable posterior segment for monomaxillary fixation. Intermaxillary fixation is not necessary, and velo-pharyngeal competence is not jeopardized. Another advantage of the premolar segmental maxillary osteotomy is the relative facility of the advancement, compared with the considerable difficulty in advancing the entire lower portion of the maxilla (LeFort I osteotomy) in cleft palate patients. The disadvantages of this technique are that it cannot be employed when gross disparity between the maxillary and mandibular molar relationships exists and that the continuity of the dental arch is interrupted, resulting in a gap in the maxillary arch.

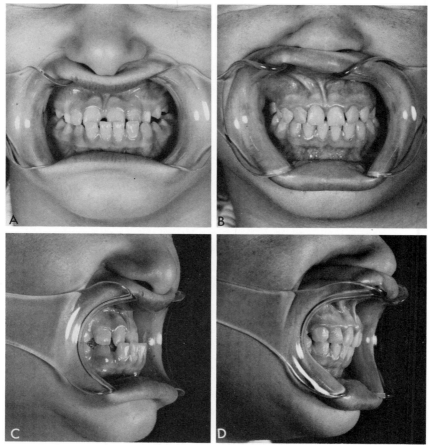

FIGURE 30–205.   Intraoral views of the patient shown in Figure 30–204. *A*, Frontal view prior to surgical correction. *B*, Dental occlusion six years later. *C*, Lateral view of the dental occlusion prior to the osteotomy. *D*, Six years following a naso-orbitomaxillary osteotomy.

The Short Face

This idiopathic deformity of the maxilla was described by Willmar (1974). The deformity was observed in five female patients whose mean age was 19 years. During speaking and smiling the maxillary front teeth were hidden behind the upper lip, resulting in an edentulous appearance. The face in full view demonstrated a square-shaped outline with prominent mandibular angles. When the mandible was maintained in its rest-position, the space between the maxillary and mandibular teeth (freeway space) was found to average more than 10 mm.

Intraoral examination showed adequate dental occlusion and the upper incisor teeth were of normal length and width, but the maxillary alveolar process was unusually short in its vertical dimension.

Cephalometric examination. The skeletal and soft tissue profiles were studied on profile cephalograms before and after operation with dimensions described by Lindegård (1953), Sarnäs (1959), Björk (1960), and Solow (1966). Reference points and lines used by Willmar are illustrated in Figure 30–206.

Preoperative measurements were obtained to investigate and describe the skeletal and soft tissue morphology of this particular deformity in comparison with that of a control group of 172 Swedish female students, aged 19 to 23 years (Sarnäs, 1973). Supplementary studies were done using standardized posteroanterior cephalograms.

The preoperative study of the skeletal and soft tissue profiles was compared with the morphologic data of the control group. The most significant differences between the profiles of the five patients with an idiopathic

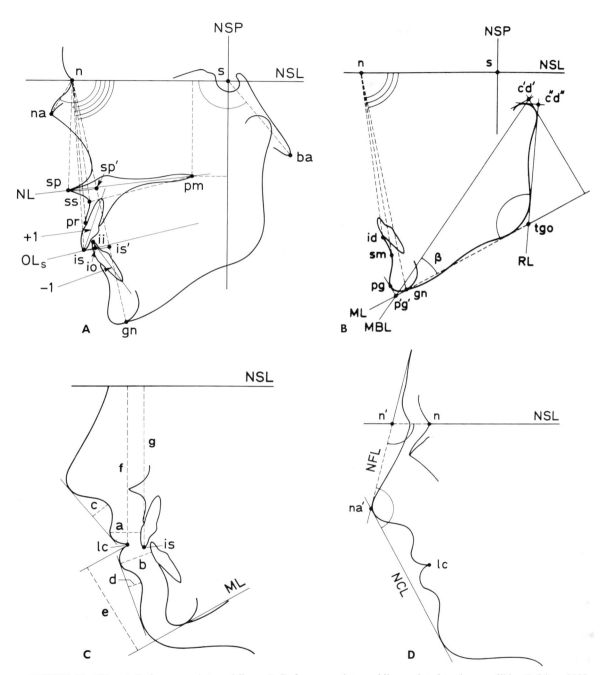

FIGURE 30–206. *A*, Reference points and lines. *B*, Reference points and lines related to the mandible. *C*, Lines NSL and ML. *D*, Construction of the soft tissue lines NFL and NCL. (Figs. 30–206 to 30–212 courtesy of Dr. K. Willmar.)

short face and those of the control group, expressed in mean values, were the following:

The height of the alveolar process, measured as the distance *sp'-is'*, was 8 mm less than that of the control group (P> 0.001), and the ratio between the edges of the upper incisors and the upper lip, expressed as the difference between *s-lc vert* and *s-is vert,* was an average of 0.7 mm, signifying that the upper lip concealed the incisors. In the lower face the gonial angle was smaller, 114.2°, compared with 125.7° in the control group (P> 0.001). The anterior lower face height, expressed as *sp-gn,* was reduced, differing 11.8 mm from that of Sarnäs' group (P> 0.001), mainly because of shortness of the alveolar process of the maxilla. The total face height, *n-gn,* was 12.7 mm (P> 0.001), and the angle NSL/ML° was only half as large as that in the control group, i.e., 16.2° versus 31.8°. The soft tissue profile differed significantly from that of Sarnäs' group. The lower vermilion was thicker (P >0.001), the

lower lip height shorter (P> 0.001), and the facial angle (NFL/NCL) more obtuse (P> 0.01). Clinical and radiographic studies confirmed that the underlying anatomical deficiency was an underdevelopment of the maxillary alveolar process, particularly in its anterior portion. To increase the vertical dimension of the alveolar process and to reestablish the relationship between the maxillary incisor teeth and the upper lip, it was necessary to perform a LeFort I osteotomy, with lowering of the mobilized maxillary segment and filling the defect along the osteotomy sites with bone grafts.

Preoperative planning. Preoperative preparation included an estimation of the amount of necessary lowering of the alveolar process; application of fixation appliances; electrical pulp testing of the maxillary teeth; and insertion of metal indicators in the skeleton of the alveolar process of the maxilla.

Determination of the freeway space was

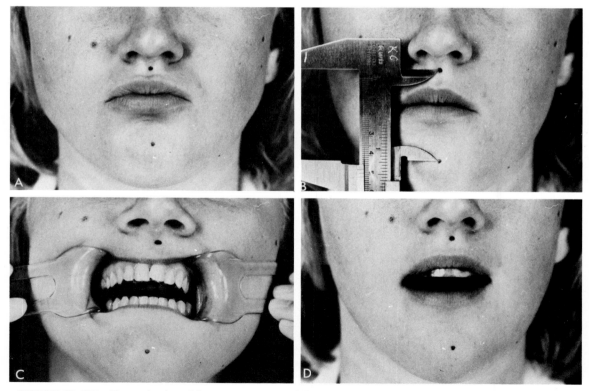

FIGURE 30–207.   Determination of freeway space. *A,* Midline inkmarks on the upper lip and chin serve as reference points. The jaws are held with the teeth in centric occlusion. The distance between the ink marks is measured. *B,* The mandible is in its rest position. The distance between the skin marks is again recorded. *C,* The jaws are closed on the wax wafer to within 3 mm of the distance between the skin marks in *B. D,* The wafer is trimmed to a level corresponding to the border of the upper lip.

done extraorally by using two skin marks in the midline of the upper lip and on the chin. The distance between these points was measured when the jaws were in centric occlusion (Fig. 30–207, *A*) and when the mandible was held in its rest position (Fig. 30–207, *B*). The difference between these two measurements represents the freeway space. A wax wafer was placed between the upper and lower teeth, and the patient was asked to close the jaws until the distance between the skin marks was 3 mm less than the freeway space (Fig. 30–207, *C*). The distance of 3 mm represents the average normal freeway space that must be maintained. In the standing position, the patient was asked to talk, smile, and do other mimic expressions. At this point the wax was trimmed to a level which corresponds to the free border of the upper lip (Fig. 30–207, *D*). The vertical dimension of the wax between the impression of the incisal edges and the cut surface provided an estimation of the amount of cancellous bone required to fill the gap produced by the LeFort I osteotomy when the maxillary teeth were lowered to the desired position.

To confirm the reinnervation of the teeth postoperatively, electrical pulp testing was done with a Bofors pulp tester. Pain reaction to an electric current of less than 125 microamperes was accepted as a normal sensibility reaction of the teeth.

Minute tantalum pins (Björk, 1955) were inserted in the maxilla close to the midline and in the molar regions for postoperative analysis of the maxillary position. Additional profile and posteroanterior cephalograms were obtained with the implants in position prior to surgery.

The position of the maxilla in relation to the anterior cranial base preoperatively and longitudinally was studied as follows: the anterior and posterior metal indicators were designated X and Y, respectively, and were studied in relation to a coordinate system composed by the axes NSL and NSP (Lindegård, 1953). In this way the following measurements were obtained: *s-x hor, s-x vert, s-y hor,* and *s-y vert* (Fig. 30–208).

Surgical technique. The LeFort 1½ osteotomy in Figure 30–187 was performed in 1967 under hypotensive anesthesia by Hogeman in collaboration with Willmar. To avoid the apices of the teeth, the level of the osteotomy was placed to 8 mm above the floor of the nose.

The lower portion of the maxilla was mobilized and brought into the planned occlusal position, where it was maintained in intermaxillary fixation by ligatures. The fixation appliances were secured by transalveolar steel wires for additional reinforcement. The gap resulting from the osteotomy was filled with blocks of cancellous bone grafts from the iliac crest which were fixed with interosseous wires. Additional cancellous grafts were placed over the osteotomy sites to augment the contour. Disk-shaped cancellous bone grafts of appropriate size were inserted into the gap between the pterygoid processes and the maxillary tuberosities to promote fixation and bony union.

Longitudinal cephalometric examinations. The fixation period varied between four and six weeks. Cephalograms were obtained before removal of the fixation appliances to check fixation and the position of the maxilla.

After the fixation period, the patients were examined every second month until sensibility had returned. Further clinical and radiographic examinations were performed one, two, and three years postoperatively.

Follow-up study. The results of the treatment were checked at various intervals up to five years in four patients and two years in one patient and were compared with the preoperative findings.

Healing of soft tissue and bone. The mucoperiosteal incision healed in all the patients with a minimum of scarring. Bony union and stability was clinically assessed by manually pulling and pushing the dentoalveolar portion of the maxilla, after removal of the fixation

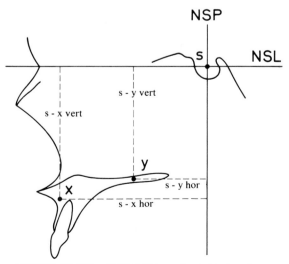

FIGURE 30–208. Horizontal and vertical reference lines of points X and Y.

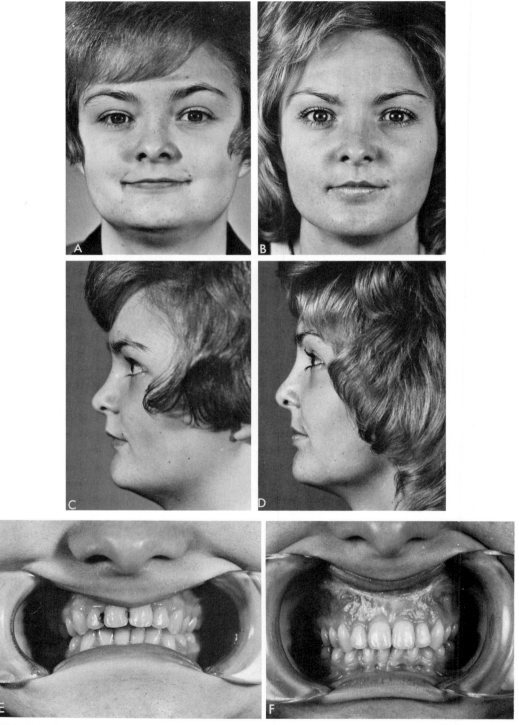

FIGURE 30–209. The short face. *A,* Preoperative full-face view. *B,* Appearance five years after the operation. Note the elongation of the face. *C,* Preoperative profile. *D,* Postoperative profile. *E,* Intraoral view before the operation. *F,* Postoperative view. The increase in the vertical dimension of the maxillary alveolar process is evident.

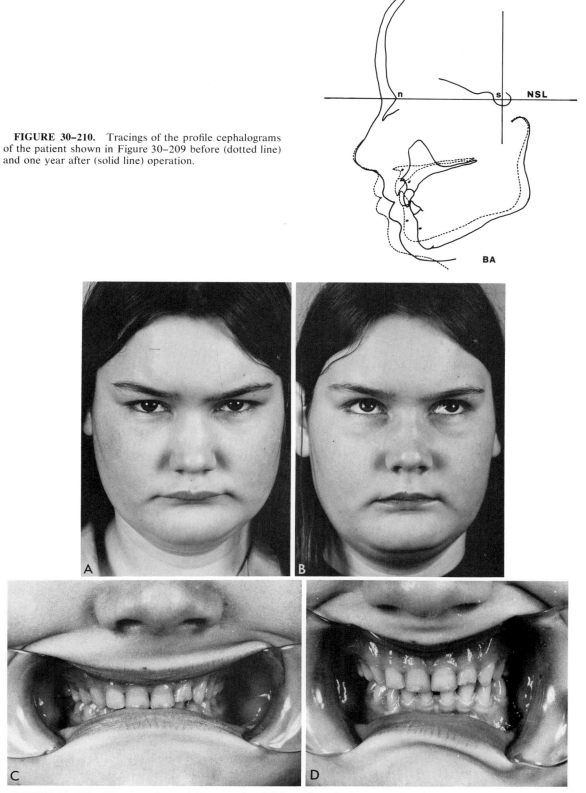

FIGURE 30–210. Tracings of the profile cephalograms of the patient shown in Figure 30–209 before (dotted line) and one year after (solid line) operation.

FIGURE 30–211. The short face. *A*, Preoperative full-face view. *B*, One year after the surgical procedure. Note the elongation of the lower third of the face and the improvement in the lip relationships. *C*, Preoperative intraoral view. *D*, Postoperative view.

appliances; the union was found to be stable within six to eight weeks.

Reinnervation of mobilized upper jaw. As an immediate effect of the operation, a total loss of sensibility to electrical stimulation of the maxillary teeth and anesthesia to pin prick of the labial, buccal, and palatal alveolar gingiva were demonstrated. Return of sensibility to the maxillary teeth and gingiva occurred within one year after operation.

Position of the lower maxillary segment. The position of the maxillary segment was studied with the aid of the metal indicators. Surgical correction in these patients concerned mainly the superoinferior position of the maxilla. Although the operation did not significantly affect the anteroposterior maxillomandibular relationships, this relationship was also studied.

The mean posterior change of point X immediately following operation was due to the downward displacement of the maxilla. Before removal of the fixation appliances, a slight but insignificant forward movement of the maxilla occurred. After one year no further changes were observed.

The average primary change of point X and Y inferiorly was 9.5 mm (P > 0.01) and 3.2 mm, respectively. At the completion of the intermaxillary fixation period, an insignificant

positional change of point X upward was registered with a maximum of 3 mm in one patient. At one and three postoperative years, no further mean changes were observed.

Skeletal and soft tissue profiles. The postoperative position of the mobilized maxilla was studied by clinical examination and profile cephalograms (Figs. 30–209 to 30–212). The increased vertical dimension of the maxilla improved the position of the front teeth in relation to the vermilion border and the facial profile, resulting in a thinner nose and longer lower lip height.

LeFort III Osteotomies. Because these osteotomies are most frequently employed in craniofacial deformities, the history of the development of the LeFort III osteotomy and the variations in technique are described in the chapter dealing with craniofacial surgery (see Chapter 56).

Correction of Maxillomandibular Disharmony

Disparities in size and position between the midfacial skeleton, the maxilla in particular, and the mandible require careful diagnostic evaluation. Mandibular pseudoprognathism, a condition in which the mandible appears protruded because the midface is recessed, was discussed earlier in the text (see p. 1310). The remedial measure in this type of deformity is to advance the maxilla, since backward displacement of the body of the mandible, a compromise procedure, would only mask the true underlying deformity and result in a "flat" face. In the reverse situation, the maxilla appears to be prognathic because the mandible is micrognathic; advancement and increase in size of the mandible are the solution to this type of deformity.

A combination of maxillary micrognathia and mandibular prognathism may also exist. Cephalometric analysis and studies of the dental casts and dentoalveolar relationships are used as guides for a plan of treatment. Tracings made from the cephalogram, modified to outline a suitable profile, and the guide lines furnished by the facial planes are helpful in evaluating such deformities.

Osteotomies of both the maxilla and the mandible performed in the same operative session are feasible. Intermaxillary fixation is required, and obstruction of the airway is a

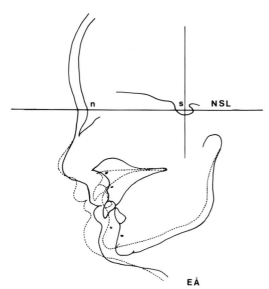

FIGURE 30–212. Tracings of the profile cephalograms of the patient shown in Figure 30–211 before (dotted line) and one year after (solid line) operation.

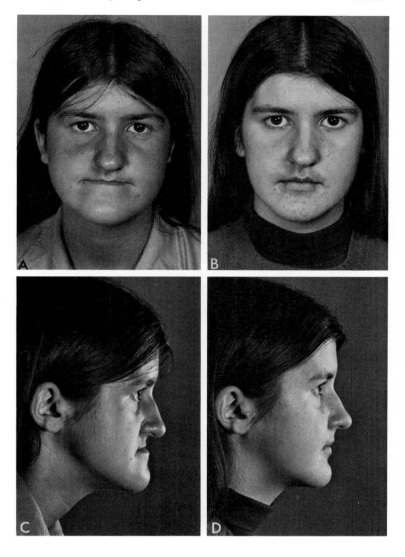

FIGURE 30–213. Consecutive osteotomies of the maxilla and mandible. *A,* Patient showing maxillary hypoplasia and mandibular prognathism. *B,* Postoperative view. The maxilla has been advanced in a first stage, followed by a recession of the mandible. *C,* Preoperative profile view showing the conspicuous maxillary retrusion which accentuates the mandibular prognathism. *D,* Postoperative profile view showing the restoration of facial harmony.

danger. A nasotracheal tube must be left in position postoperatively to maintain the patency of the airway until the patient is fully awake. If necessary, the tube should be left in position overnight; a soft rubber nasopharyngeal tube is then substituted and allowed to remain for a few days until the edema has subsided and the airway is patent.

To achieve optimal results, a two-stage procedure is preferable. In a first stage the maxilla is advanced, and in a second stage the mandible is recessed. The advantage of this plan is that it gives an opportunity to evaluate the result of the first operation; the operation on the opposing jaw can then be done with greater certainty of the final result. If a slight change in the position of the mobilized jaw occurs postoperatively, compensation can be made during the second operation on the opposing jaw, thus achieving optimal dental occlusal relationships.

A patient who underwent operative procedures on both jaws is shown in Figure 30–213. The preoperative cephalogram (Fig. 30–214, *A*) documented the fact that the maxilla required advancement and the mandible recession. At a first stage, a high LeFort I (LeFort 1½) osteotomy was performed (Fig. 30–214, *B*). After an interval during which intermaxillary fixation was released to allow jaw motion, a second operation, bilateral sagittal osteotomy of the ramus, was employed to recess the mandible (Figs. 30–213, *B, D* and 30–214, *C*).

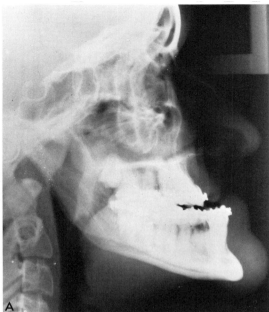

FIGURE 30-214. Cephalogram and tracings of patient shown in Figure 30-213. *A*, Preoperative cephalogram showing the mandibular prognathism and maxillary hypoplasia. *B*, Tracing of cephalogram after maxillary advancement. *C*, Tracing of cephalogram after mandibular recession showing satisfactory occlusal relationships.

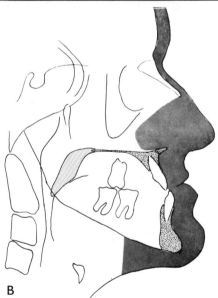

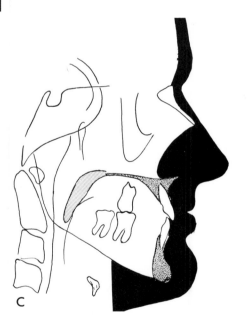

Complications Following Corrective Surgery of the Jaws

Some complications are common to all surgical procedures; others are specific to certain operations. Complications which are common in all procedures include hematoma, infection, and abscess formation; necrosis of bone due to inadequate soft tissue coverage; bony relapse; and malunion, delayed union, and nonunion.

Hematoma, Infection, and Abscess Formation. The protective umbrella provided by antibiotics has allowed the surgeon to take liberties that were not possible in the preantibiotic era. The advent of antibiotic therapy has permitted exposure of the bone to the oral bacterial flora with impunity if the operative site is adequately covered with well vascularized soft tissues. The prophylactic antibiotics should be effective against the gram-negative as well as the gram-positive microorganisms of the oral cavity. Anaerobic streptococci and staphylococci are frequent offending organisms. The rapid healing of intraoral wounds, despite heavy bacterial contamination, can be explained by the rich blood supply of the oral cavity.

On the other hand, the vascularity of the region can be detrimental if it is not controlled. Hematoma is a major complication and should be avoided by careful hemostasis and the use of dependent suction drainage. A hematoma furnishes an excellent culture medium for the bacterial organisms and the potential for abscess formation. The presence of an interosseous wire in an infected area causes continued suppuration, which will usually persist until the wire is removed. Removal of the wire, therefore, is imperative. However, in the absence of infection interosseous stainless steel wires are well tolerated.

Necrosis of Bone Due to Inadequate Soft Tissue Coverage.   Small areas of uncovered bone heal despite being exposed to the oral cavity. Portions of the cortex may be sequestrated, but the main portion of the bone maintains sufficient blood supply to survive. Usually after elimination of some of the cortex of the exposed bone, granulation tissue appears and there is progressive epithelization of the mucosal defect. The healing process is accelerated by resection of obviously necrotic bone. Persistent osteitis and spreading osteomyelitis are rare complications if the patient is maintained under antibiotic therapy during the period of healing. Provision of soft tissue coverage is one of the major concerns in operations to elongate the body of the mandible. The oral vestibular approach usually provides sufficient tissue; in some cases, however, a flap of mucous membrane from the cheek is needed to cover the additional bony surface (see Fig. 30–70).

Relapse.   Minor imperfections in the dental occlusion are not uncommon after fixation has been discontinued, regardless of the type of procedure employed. Individual teeth are constantly subjected to the action of the opposing dentition, the cheeks, the lips, and the tongue and undergo slow migration. Fortunately dentoalveolar readaption frequently results in improved occlusion. It is often necessary to make minor adjustments to equilibrate the occlusion. This can be done by judicious spot grinding of the cusps of the teeth or by orthodontic therapy.

A more serious complication is the development of a skeletal relapse despite apparent consolidation of the bone. This condition occurs mostly in those patients in whom a mandibular ramus osteotomy is performed; the pull of the muscles of mastication tends to cause displacement of the fragments. Minor adjustments can be achieved by orthodontic therapy. The more severe malocclusion may require a secondary surgical-orthodontic procedure.

Malunion, Delayed Union, and Nonunion. Malunion of bone is caused by inadequate planning and fixation. Delayed union and nonunion are the result of the absence of bony alignment, apposition, and impaction of the fragments of bone. Poor fixation of the fragments is the usual cause of these complications.

The pull of the musculature is a leading cause of recurrence of the deformity following surgical intervention. The powerful muscles of mastication, the suprahyoid muscles, and the muscles of the tongue exert traction upon the repositioned osseous segments. Displacement of the ramus fragments by the elevator muscles of the jaw and the recurrence of an open bite as the result of downward pull of the suprahyoid musculature upon the mandibular symphysis are two common complications. The problem has been diminished by wide subperiosteal detachment of the muscles and ligaments, allowing each muscle to seek a new point of insertion upon the bone postoperatively. The muscles thus adapt to the modified skeletal framework. Clinical experience has shown that considerable progress has been made in the surgical treatment of jaw malformations since the principle of disinserting the muscle attachments has been applied. The design of the osteotomy is also an important consideration.

A secondary osteotomy may be required to correct the malunion. Nounion which persists beyond a period of 60 days should be treated by exposing the area of the nonunited bone, excising the fibrous tissue between the fragments, and inserting bone grafts, preferably of the cancellous type.

Loss of Teeth.   Military experience has shown that the teeth retain their vitality in a bone fragment that is detached from the main body of the jaw under two conditions: first, the blood supply must be maintained by the remaining attached mucoperiosteal tissue; second, sufficient bone must cover the apices of the teeth. In performing osteotomies of the body of the mandible or maxilla, one should be careful to avoid exposure of or injury to the roots of the teeth (see p. 1356). Judicious selective extraction of a tooth may be a prerequisite to surgical recession of a segment of the jaw. Dental arch continuity is usually restored by approximation of the segments on either side of the ostectomy site.

Sensory Nerve Loss. When operations on the mandibular body are being performed, injury to the inferior alveolar nerve is avoided by keeping the nerve under direct observation during the procedure. When an osteotomy posterior to the mental foramen is required, the inferior alveolar canal is decompressed, and nerve continuity is maintained. When the mandible is sectioned anterior to the mental foramen, the anterior extension of the inferior alveolar nerve, the incisive nerve, is divided. This results only in the loss of sensibility in the lower incisor teeth, a minor inconvenience to the patient. The other terminal branch of the inferior alveolar nerve, the mental nerve, must be carefully preserved at its exit from the mental foramen. The dissection of the branches assists in avoiding damage to the nerve, a frequent cause of annoying loss of sensibility in the lower lip.

Presently available operative techniques upon the mandibular ramus preserve the integrity of the inferior alveolar nerve. In the vertical or oblique osteotomy of the ramus, the line of section extends posterior to the point of entry of the nerve into the inferior alveolar foramen. When the ramus is split in the sagittal plane, the split should be made in such a manner that the inferior alveolar nerve remains intact within the medial fragment. However, as mentioned earlier in the text, a significant percentage of permanent loss of sensibility of the lower lip has been reported following this operation. The Dautrey modification of the sagittal-split operation (see p. 1330) avoids any direct contact with the inferior alveolar nerve.

Other Complications. The migration or the expulsion of an inorganic implant, the displacement of an advanced lower segment of the mandible following a horizontal osteotomy, or the absorption of an onlay bone graft are occasional, and often unexplained, complications. Inorganic implants appear to be contraindicated in jaw deformities with tight overlying soft tissues. Expulsion or a more serious complication, the gradual incorporation of the implant into the bone, which endangers the roots

of the teeth, should also be kept in mind (see p. 1399).

Acquired Deformities of the Jaws

MALUNITED FRACTURES OF THE JAWS

Malunion of fractured bones of the face occurs when (1) the patient's physiologic condition has been too seriously disturbed to permit optimal management of the facial fracture; (2) the extent of the damage in multiple comminuted facial fractures is such that reduction and fixation of all the bony fragments is not possible; or (3) bone loss has occurred, and the ends of the fragments are drawn together by scar and muscle contraction.

A distinction must be made between the deformities due to loss of bone and those caused by malposition of bony fragments. Malunited fractures are responsible for varying degrees of malocclusion, depending upon the extent of loss of bone or displacement of the fragments. The alterations in facial appearance are also variable, ranging from a conspicuous retrusion of the maxilla, chin, or mandible to a subtle flatness or deviation. To eliminate confusion over deformities due to loss of bone and those caused by rotation, overriding, and displacement of the fragments, a careful preoperative study of the facial contour, dental casts, and roentgenograms of the patient should be made.

The diagnosis is not obvious in some cases; following malunited fractures of both jaws, it is sometimes difficult to determine whether the maxilla or the mandible is in the correct anatomical position.

Disturbances in dental occlusal relationships also span a wide range. Premature contact of a single posterior tooth prevents the occlusion of the remaining teeth. Complete loss of occlusal contact occurs in malunited, impacted, complete horizontal or pyramidal fractures of the maxilla. The lack of occlusal contact is also the result of loss of bone in the region of the mental symphysis, which allows the medial collapse of the remaining portions of the mandible.

Treatment of Malunited Fractures

When treatment of a maxillary or mandibular jaw fracture has been delayed for three weeks and malunion is established, surgical intervention, i.e., secondary osteotomy and realignment of the fragments, is indicated. The decision to perform a secondary osteotomy to replace the malunited fragments in a more satisfactory anatomical relationship depends largely upon the state of the patient's dentition.

When a normal complement of healthy teeth is present, the treatment should be directed toward the restoration of dental occlusion and masticatory function; osteotomy is indicated in these cases.

If the malocclusion is slight, dental restorative procedures alone may suffice to improve the occlusion; these measures include orthodontic therapy, judicious spot grinding of interfering cusps, fixed or removable prosthodontic appliances, and extraction of teeth when indicated. Minor types of malocclusion often undergo self-correction; the cusps of the teeth gradually assume new occlusal relationships.

When the patient is totally edentulous or when the teeth have been lost as the result of injury, the reestablishment of anteroposterior or lateral relationships between the edentulous area and the opposing arch is not essential if the displacement is only moderate. Compensation for moderate malalignment is achieved by prosthodontic restoration. Instability of the denture may result, however, if the disparity between the arches is great. Reestablishment of centric relationships by an osteotomy is necessary in such cases.

Malunited Fractures of the Mandible. Malunion of mandibular fractures results from displacement of the fragments or loss of bone between the ends of the fragments. An osteotomy, a prosthodontic appliance, or bone grafting, alone or in combination, must be selected as the treatment of choice.

When an osteotomy is indicated in malunited mandibular fractures, the prime consideration is reestablishment of dental occlusion and facial contour. Usually, the jaw is refractured at the site of malunion; in some cases, it may be advantageous to perform an osteotomy at a site distant from the line of fracture. A study of the dental casts is helpful in making the decision. Open bite deformities are frequent in malunited fractures. They require osteotomy at the healed fracture sites or a mandibular alveolar osteotomy (see Fig. 30–18) to permit upward displacement into a position of occlusion with the maxillary teeth.

Bone grafting may be required to assist in the consolidation of the osteotomy site as well

as to improve the contour of the jaw. Packed between the fragments, cancellous bone chips promote union. Onlay bone grafts are also placed over the osteotomy lines to accelerate consolidation and to restore contour.

Malunited Fractures of the Maxilla. Early fibrous fixation of maxillary fractures is to be expected; bony union is late in comparison to that in the mandible; non-union in maxillary fractures is unusual. Fractures of less than one month's duration can be reduced by continuous intermaxillary elastic traction. If a greater force must be exerted, external traction by means of a head frame is used. After reduction, intermaxillary wiring immobilizes the maxilla when the mandible is intact. Alternatively, the arch bar can be suspended by a circumferential wire around the zygomatic arch or from the frontal bone above the lateral orbital rim using internal stainless steel wire (see also Chapter 24).

In the patient with an intact dentition who has failed to respond to traction, Dingman and Harding (1951) recommended mobilization of the fractured segment by forced manipulation. The upper dental arch is fixed to a dental impression tray by dental compound. When the compound is set, the segment is firmly manipulated using the tray as a lever. In some patients in whom a greater force is necessary to mobilize the jaw, the tray is struck with a firm blow by a heavy mallet in the direction of the original injury to loosen the fragment. Rowe disimpacting forceps are usually employed in place of the dental tray. The fracture is then treated in a routine manner.

In edentulous patients, treatment by osteotomy is not required if the posterior displacement of the maxillary alveolar arch is not excessive. As previously stated, prosthodontic restoration will compensate for the disparity.

In fractures that have progressed to solid malunion, an osteotomy is necessary to free the fragments to achieve an anatomical restoration. Subperiosteal exposure of the midface is obtained through the intraoral approach and through small, strategically placed, external incisions in the lower eyelid and in the lateral part of the eyebrow. An osteotome sections through the fracture lines, and the mobilized bone is treated as an acute fracture. In long-established, consolidated fractures of the maxilla, one of the various maxillary osteotomies described earlier in the chapter is indicated.

RECONSTRUCTION OF FULL-THICKNESS DEFECTS OF THE MANDIBLE

Introduction

An acquired jaw deformity with associated loss of bone and soft tissue is one of the greatest challenges faced by the reconstructive surgeon. There are few problems that place such a high demand on the combined restorative needs of form, function, and esthetics. The vast majority of the operations performed on other parts of the body require fullfillment of one or two of these requisites, rarely of all three.

Acquired jaw defects are caused by trauma and ablative operations for neoplasia; osteomyelitis and congenital absence of a major portion of the jaw produce similar defects. Gunshot wounds are responsible for most of the severe deformities produced by trauma. In such cases, the initial impression of the damage is dramatic because the apparent defect is greater than the true anatomical deformity. The soft tissue defect appears larger because of the retraction caused by the contraction of the surrounding tissues (Fig. 30–215). The distraction of the remaining bony fragments by the attached muscles adds to the distortion and deceptive magnitude of the problem.

The Importance of Soft Tissue. A basic difference exists in the problems of reconstruction posed by the patient who has a full-thickness defect of the mandible with well-vascularized soft tissues and the patient who has lost both hard and soft tissues. In the patient with sufficient soft tissue, the restoration of the mandible is generally feasible and successful when the defect does not involve a major portion of the mandible. Adequate fixation of the mandible can be established, and the soft tissues will revascularize the bone graft rapidly. In contrast, the compound loss of bone and soft tissue requires procedures for soft tissue replacement which are often complex but are essential if a bone graft is to survive.

The Age of the Patient and the Etiology of the Defect. A basic difference also exists between the young patient who has been the victim of an accident and the older patient whose deformity is the result of cancer. The young patient has well-vascularized soft tissues that favor soft and hard tissue reconstruction, and a satisfactory result is possible. The older patient with cancer may have received radiation treatment, may have a poor prognosis, or may be too debilitated to tolerate complicated restorative operations; palliative procedures are indicated (see Chapters 57 to 64 and Chapter 67).

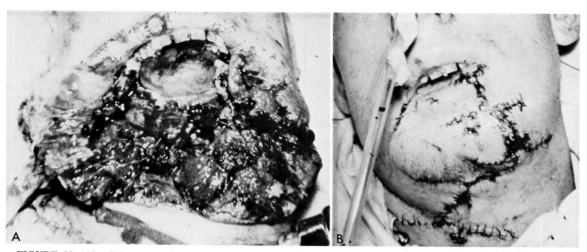

FIGURE 30–215.   Primary reconstruction of a military gunshot wound. *A,* Typical compound wound. Note the retraction of the soft tissues. *B,* After primary suture within hours of the injury. (Courtesy of Colonel L. C. Morgan, U.S. Army Medical Corps.)

Congenital and developmental malformations requiring bone grafting present different problems of treatment. Developmental malformations have been considered in the earlier sections of this chapter. Congenital malformations are also discussed in Chapters 54 and 56.

Restoration of the Continuity of the Mandible: A Brief Historical Review

It is informative to review the history of man's attempt to replace a missing portion of the mandible. The imagination and the ingenuity of the reconstructive surgeon is reflected in the wide variety of techniques and materials used since Claude Martin described the immediate restoration of a resected segment of the mandible with a prosthetic appliance in 1889. Partsch (1897) used a metal band to restore the continuity of the jaw. A pessary made of celluloid material was used by Berndt (1898). White (1909) favored the use of a silver wire. Scudder (1912) reported that Ollier and Martin were replacing segments of the mandible with hard rubber, while König bridged the gap with ivory. Well-tolerated metals, such as vitallium (Castigliano, 1941), stainless steel mesh (Attie, Cantania, and Ripstein, 1953) and ticonium (Walsh, 1954), have been and are occasionally still used. With the introduction of plastic materials, surgeons have looked toward this type of material to reconstruct the jaw. Acrylic was used by Aubry and Pillet (1950) and Edgerton, Ward, and Sikes (1950). Despite the appeal of the inorganic materials, the complications and extrusions that followed their use have led to their abandonment except as temporary prostheses. The method of choice in treating skeletal defects of the jaws remains replacement by bone.

The pioneer work in bone grafting jaw defects is found in the German literature. Delayed autogenous bone grafts from either rib or tibia were transferred to the jaw by Bardenheuer (1892) and Sykoff (1900). World War I gave rise to the need and spurred interest in the bone grafting of jaw defects.

Bone Grafts. Based on the early experimental work of Ollier (1860, 1867) and the clinical experience of Delagénière (1916), tibial osteoperiosteal grafts were favored to bridge bony defects of the jaws during World War I (Imbert and Réal, 1916; DuBouchet, 1917; Lemaitre and Ponroy, 1920). The Germans continued to use ribs and tibia as sources of bone grafts during the early part of the war.

Around 1915 the superiority of cancellous bone was recognized by Lindemann (1916) and Klapp and Schroeder (1917). According to Ivy (1951), the British surgeons adopted the ilium as the osseous donor site when word reached their plastic surgery centers via Dolamore from Holland of the success of the Germans. After an exchange of wounded prisoners, British soldiers returning to the Plastic Surgery Hospital at Sidcup were found to have excellent results following iliac bone grafting by the German surgeons. Waldron and Risdon (1919), Gillies (1920), and Chubb (1920) soon reported the British experience using iliac bone grafts. Chubb was also one of the first to report the use of composite skin–clavicular bone flaps for mandibular reconstruction.

Ivy (1921) reported a case of resection of a part of the mandible with immediate grafting using iliac bone. The bone graft remained in place and functioned well, as noted in a 38-year follow-up report (Ivy and Eby, 1958).

During World War II, Mowlem (1944) reemphasized the importance of cancellous bone. Realizing that cortical bone grafts are almost noncellular, are slowly revascularized, and are a poor source of osteoblasts, Mowlem reconstructed the jaw with cancellous bone chips from the ilium. Fragmentation of the cancellous bone increases the surface of contact with the soft tissue and enhances the opportunity for rapid revascularization of the grafts.

The Use of Trays Combined with Cancellous Bone Chips. During World War II, Converse (1945) used a fenestrated metal tray with bone chips to reconstruct the entire body of the mandible that was destroyed by a gunshot wound. The fenestrated tantalum tray served as an internal splint and as a means of carrying the bone chips (see Fig. 30–234). The tantalum tray was later removed, and iliac bone grafts were added to reinforce the reconstructed mandibular body. The patient and the results achieved using this technique are shown in Figures 30–232 and 30–233. Soderberg, Jennings, and McNelly (1952) employed a perforated vitallium tray and blocks of iliac bone graft to reconstruct the mandible. After consolidation was obtained, the metallic tray was removed.

Renewed interest in this concept was stimulated by Boyne's report (1969) of the use of a chromium-cobalt alloy crib and his later report (1973) of a titanium tray to support particulate cancellous bone grafts and to act as an internal splint. A cellulose acetate micropore filter was recommended to line the crib to prevent connective tissue invasion. The impediment to revascularization of the bone grafts due to the presence of the millipore filters appears to defy the concept that rapid revascularization of a bone graft is as essential as it is for a skin graft (see Chapter 13). Morgan and Thompson (1975) have reported that, on the removal of such trays, a layer of fibrous tissue of varying thickness was found between the graft and the filter.

Swanson, Habal, Leake, and Murray (1973) reported the use of a wire-reinforced silicone tray with windows to hold chips of bone. Repeated aspirations of serous fluid which collected around the silicone trays were required. In a subsequent report, Murray (1976) stated that the method had been abandoned because of a high failure rate. Leake in 1974 described the use of a Dacron mesh impregnated with urethane. The crib formed by this combination is sufficiently rigid to support the bone graft chips and to serve as an internal splint while new bone formation is proceeding. The micropore filter was found to be unnecessary. The use of inorganic trays is not recommended in irradiated tissues because of the high rate of failure under these circumstances.

Despite the early clinical reports of the use of inorganic materials to correct defects of the mandible, only autogenous bone has withstood the test of time. Ivy in 1972 reported a remarkable 49-year clinical and radiological follow-up of an iliac bone graft that was used to reconstruct a mandibular symphysis which was lost due to osteomyelitis of dental origin.

Bone Allografts. Early, and probably premature, encouraging results have been reported with the use of lyophilized decalcified allograft mandibles carved into the shape of a trough into which are packed cancellous bone chips (Pike and Boyne, 1973, 1974). One disadvantage of this technique, based on the earlier work of Urist (1968), is that it is difficult to obtain mandibular cadaver bone in the United States, and it is doubtful whether allografts can replace autografts in major defects.

Orthopedic surgeons were the first to use banked allografts of bone (Inclan, 1942; Bush, 1947; Wilson, 1948). Converse and Campbell (1950) described their experience with banked bone allografts as onlay grafts to restore facial contour. Reidy (1956) and Markowitz (1958) reported the successful application of bone allografts for the restoration of the continuity of the mandible. However, allografts have

not replaced autografts because of the greater reliability of the autograft. It also seems inappropriate to use other than the best, namely bone autografts, for such an important structure as the mandible (see Reconstruction by Composite Flaps and Microvascular Free Transplants, p. 1503).

Indications for Bone Grafting. The goals of mandibular reconstruction are to reestablish the function of the mandible, to permit the wearing of a denture, and to provide for adequate mastication of food; the reconstructed mandible also restores the contour of the lower portion of the face. Bone grafting is indicated in the following types of mandibular defects: (1) nonunion following fractures of the mandible; (2) mandibular reconstruction predicated upon the size of the defect and the age and physical status of the patient.

Cardinal Prerequisites of Successful Bone Grafting. Kazanjian (1952) listed the cardinal prerequisites of successful bone grafting of mandibular defects: (1) bone transplantation into healthy tissues, (2) a recipient area with adequate blood supply, (3) wide contact between adjacent bone and the graft, and (4) positive fixation.

After the recipient site criteria have been satisfied, reconstruction of the supporting structures of the lower jaw can begin. The first step in this process is the return of the remaining bony fragments to their anatomical position. In delayed cases, this may be a difficult task if provision for maintaining the fragments in alignment was not made initially. The musculature must be detached subperiosteally to free the remaining fragments and, by the appropriate means of fixation, maintain them in their corrected anatomical position. When teeth are present, the occlusion of the teeth serves as a guide for the positioning of the fragments.

Methods of Fixation

A wide variety of methods of fixation of the fragments of the mandible is available to provide immobilization during the healing of bone grafts. Depending on the size of the defect, these vary from relatively simple techniques, such as intermaxillary fixation and monomaxillary fixation with a splint, to more complex methods providing cranial fixation by specially constructed external fixation appliances (see Figs. 30–218 to 30–223 and Fig. 30–237).

Intraoral Fixation

TEETH ARE PRESENT ON BOTH SIDES OF THE DEFECT. When teeth are present on both sides of the defect, a splint is made (monomaxillary fixation) and applied prior to the bone grafting. Intermaxillary wiring is advisable to relieve some of the stress placed on the appliance and to prevent breaking or slippage during the operation. In the early postoperative period, the intermaxillary fixation is released and the monomaxillary splint is retained for stabilization. Early movement of the mandible is thus permitted.

In defects of the symphysis, each lateral fragment is provided with a splint; the two splints are joined by a lock-bar. The lock-bar is removed before the operation, and each mandibular fragment is wired to the teeth of the maxilla. The lock-bar is replaced following completion of the operation. The intermaxillary wires are removed a few days later, and fixation of the mandibular fragments is maintained by the splint and lock-bar appliance.

THE RAMUS FRAGMENT IS LOOSE. In patients who have no teeth on the posterior fragment, the fragment is usually displaced forward

and medially by the muscles of mastication after resection of the body of the mandible when provision has not been made to prevent the displacement of the ramus. The masseter and medial pterygoid muscles should be detached subperiosteally from the ramus; the procedure frees the posterior fragment and allows its repositioning. The control of the posterior fragment can be accomplished by a number of methods: (1) the graft is wedged into position between the anterior and posterior fragments to prevent forward displacement of the posterior fragment; (2) an intraoral appliance with a forked wire extension that maintains the retroposition of the edentulous posterior fragment until the bone graft is in place; (3) an acrylic splint maintained by circumferential wire around the mandible (Fig. 30–216) controls the posterior fragment as well as the anterior portion of the mandible during consolidation of the bone graft; (4) an external fixation appliance (see Figs. 30–218 to 30–223 and 30–237).

THE MANDIBLE IS EDENTULOUS: THE MAXILLARY DENTITION IS PRESENT. A bite-block is fitted over the remaining portion of the mandible and is maintained in position by circumferential wires around the mandible (see Fig. 30–216). Holes are drilled through the acrylic bite-block for the passage of the circumferential wires. Hooks are imbedded into the bite-block; these serve to establish intermaxillary fixation with the maxillary teeth.

THE MAXILLA IS EDENTULOUS. A bite-block or the patient's denture is maintained in cranial fixation by wires passed around each zygomatic arch or anchored to the frontal bone. The mandibular fragments are held in intermaxillary fixation with the upper denture either by wiring the teeth or by means of the bite-block described above if the mandible is edentulous.

THE MAXILLA AND MANDIBLE ARE EDENTULOUS. The maxillary bite-block is maintained in cranial fixation by internal wire fixation as described above; intermaxillary fixation is established between the mandibular bite-block, fixed to the mandible by circumferential wiring, and the maxillary bite-block (Fig. 30–217).

The collaboration of an expert prosthodontist is essential in order that the appliances be made with precision, thus avoiding excessive compression and necrosis of the mucoperiosteum, loosening of the fixation appliances, and loss of the bone graft.

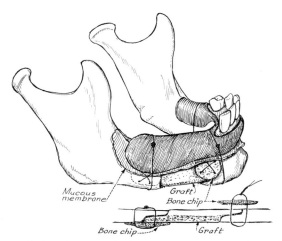

FIGURE 30–216. The loose ramus fragment. Control and fixation of the ramus by a prosthodontic appliance. The patient's denture was relined (in the operating room) and was maintained by circumferential wiring after placing of the bone graft. This type of fixation appliance requires the services of a maxillofacial prosthodontist. Excessive pressure over the mucoperiosteum should be avoided to prevent subsequent necrosis. (Appliance made by Augustus J. Valauri, D.D.S.)

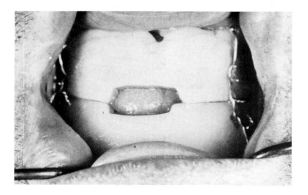

FIGURE 30–217. Fixation when both jaws are edentulous. When both jaws are edentulous, bite-blocks are fabricated. The maxillary bite-block is maintained by cranial fixation. The mandibular bite-block is adjusted and relined in the operating room after the bone grafting. Intermaxillary fixation is established after the mandibular bite-block has been attached to the mandible by circumferential wiring. Note the anterior opening to provide an airway and space for feeding.

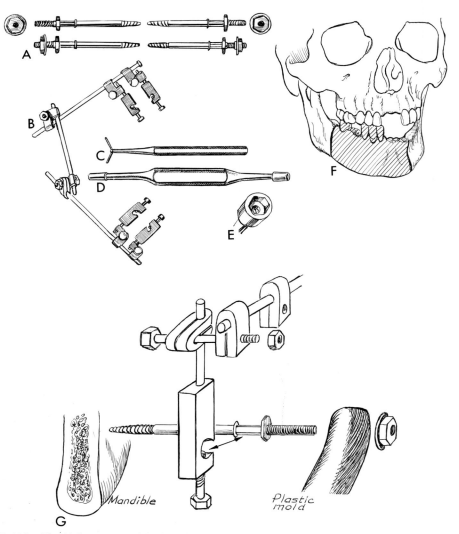

FIGURE 30–218. The biphase external skeletal fixation appliance. *A*, Vitallium bone screws with special heads and washer-faced lock nuts. *B*, Primary assembly of the splint fixation appliance with rods and screw clamps in position for adjustment. *C*, Anti-torque wrench. *D*, The wrench. *E*, The end of the wrench which accepts hexagonal nuts. *F*, The shaded area represents the mandibular bone defect that is to be repaired. *G*, Details of the vitallium bone screw and screw clamp. The hexagonal surface of the screw facilitates positive no-skid fixation. Rod clamps are shown above as they maintain the primary splint rods in position. (From Kazanjian and Converse.)

External Fixation. External fixation is indicated in patients in whom insufficient dentition is present to secure an interdental fixation appliance and when fixation cannot be obtained by means of prosthodontic appliances. An external fixation appliance is particularly useful when the posterior fragment is edentulous and there is a large anterior defect of the mandible.

Anderson in 1936 reported the use of an external appliance in the treatment of fractures of the shaft of the femur. The converging pins technique of the Roger Anderson appliance was applied to fractures of the mandibular angle by Converse and Waknitz (1942). Two pins are placed in each remaining mandibular fragment, each pin converging with its twin at an angle of approximately 70 degrees. The pins are usually inserted side by side along a line parallel with the lower border of the mandible or one above the other in the region of the angle of the ramus. Each pin is carefully passed through the skin and soft tissues and is drilled into the bone, penetrating both the outer and inner cortical plates. After the fragments are returned to their normal position, the connecting portion of the appliance is adjusted, and the joints are locked to secure fixation. In addition to the Roger Anderson twin-pin appliance, other external fixation appliances, such as the Morris appliance (see Fig. 30–218) and precise craniomaxillary external fixation appliances, have been constructed (see Fig. 30–237).

THE TWIN-SCREW MORRIS BIPHASE APPLIANCE. The twin-screw Morris biphase appliance (Morris, 1949; Fleming and Morris, 1969) is highly versatile. The Morris external fixation splint (Figs. 30–218 to 30–223) employs vitallium bone screws 1/8 inch* in diameter. The screws are threaded at both ends; one end is inserted into bone, and the other receives a washer-faced nut which secures an acrylic bar that joins the two units of parallel screws (Fig. 30–218). A stablike soft tissue incision is made over the proposed site of insertion of the screw, and a hole is drilled into the bone with a 3/32 inch* twist drill (Fig. 30–219). A drill of smaller dimension is preferred to place holes into the ramus. The screws are inserted with a distance of at least 2 cm between each screw of the pair. After realignment of the fragments is achieved, the two units of parallel screws are joined by a connecting portion of the apparatus (the first phase), which is designed to maintain the position of the two units (Fig. 30–220) until an acrylic bar (the second phase) assures permanent fixation (Fig. 30–221). The term "biphase" defines this double maneuver. Quick-curing acrylic, while it is in its rubberlike, pliable state (Fig. 30–221), is molded and adapted over the ends of the screws of each unit (Fig. 30–222). After the acrylic bar has

---

*1 inch=2.54 cm.

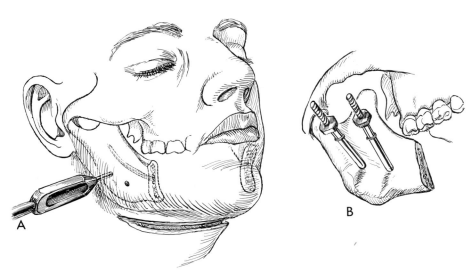

FIGURE 30–219. The biphase external skeletal fixation appliance. *A,* Drill holes are made with a hand drill to receive the bone screws. *B,* The bone screws are threaded into position. (From Kazanjian and Converse.)

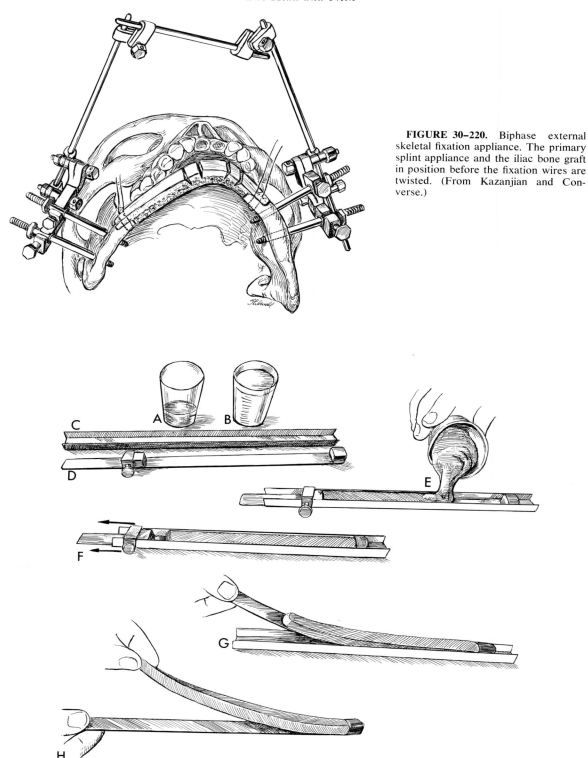

FIGURE 30–220. Biphase external skeletal fixation appliance. The primary splint appliance and the iliac bone graft in position before the fixation wires are twisted. (From Kazanjian and Converse.)

FIGURE 30–221. Fabrication of an acrylic resin bar. *A*, Acrylic liquid monomer. *B*, Acrylic resin polymer powder. The liquid monomer and powdered polymer are mixed in a 1 to 3 ratio. *C, D,* The metallic tray and rod which make up the take-apart mold. *E*, Acrylic mixture being poured into the take-apart mold. *F*, Mold being separated from the "room temperature curing" acrylic splint. *G, H,* The still pliable acrylic bar is carefully removed from the mold without deforming its shape. (From Kazanjian and Converse.)

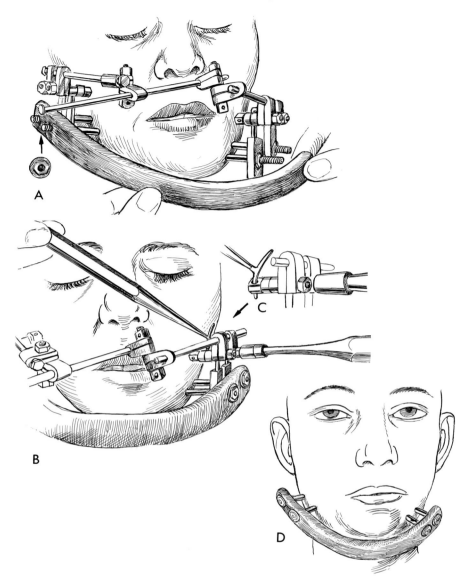

FIGURE 30–222. Adapting the acrylic resin splint. *A*, While still in a semi-putty condition, the acrylic bar is gently pressed onto the machined threads of the bone screws. Washer-faced lock nuts are initially twisted to a position just short of being flush with the end of the screw. *B*, *C*, After the heat of polymerization has dissipated three to five minutes later and the acrylic bar has hardened, final tightening of the lock nuts is performed. To overtighten the lock nut while the acrylic is soft invites weakness in the splint due to excessive thinning of the bar at this site. The primary mechanical splint is removed in the reverse order of its application—that is, first unlock the rod clamps, then release the screw clamp, and finally remove the screw clamp from the bone screw. *D*, The secondary rigid, resilient, light acrylic bar (biphase splint) is relatively unobstrusive as the bone graft heals. When properly placed, this splint can be expected to maintain its mechanical stabilization for periods exceeding nine months. (From Kazanjian and Converse.)

hardened, a washer-faced nut is secured to the exposed thread of each screw. The temporary connecting splint is removed. The Morris apparatus is strong, although light in weight. The vitallium screws are well tolerated and can be left in position for long periods of time (Fig. 30–223).

The external splint controls the remaining mandibular fragments during the consolidation of the bone grafts. Prior to bone grafting, the external fixation appliance is used to retain the edentulous fragments in position. After the bone is transplanted and fastened with interosseous wires to the remaining mandibular seg-

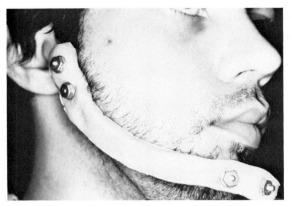

FIGURE 30–223. Morris appliance in position controlling the posterior edentulous fragment. A large portion of the body of the mandible has been reconstructed by a bone graft. (From Kazanjian and Converse.)

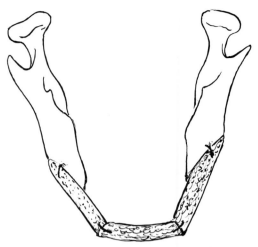

FIGURE 30–224. Reconstruction of the missing portion of the mandibular arch by three bone grafts wired to each other and to the posterior mandibular fragments.

ments, additional fixation methods are not required.

Internal Fixation.   Fixation of the remaining fragments is provided by the bone graft (or grafts), which bridges the gap between the mandibular fragments. In moderate-sized defects, the main bone graft, containing cortical bone, is strong enough to maintain the position of the fragments in the edentulous mandible.

Successful results have been obtained in patients in whom bone grafts were wired to each other and to the mandibular stumps (Figs. 30–224, 30–225). Some type of internal fixation splint (stainless steel, tantalum, ticonium, a Dacron mesh) holding the fragments may be required in larger defects (see Fig. 30–234). Such internal splints are usually removed after the consolidation of the fragments, as they may

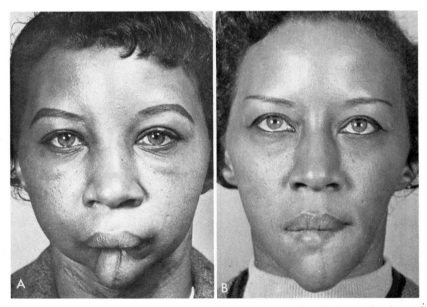

FIGURE 30–225.   Reconstruction of the mandibular arch by three bone grafts wired to each other as illustrated in Figure 30–224. *A*, Appearance after resection of the major portion of the mandibular arch and floor of the mouth for the eradication of carcinoma. *B*, After reconstruction by bone grafts and skin graft inlay procedure (see Figs. 30–251 and 30–252).

interfere with the subsequent restoration of the functional buccal sulcus.

Defects of the Mandible with Little Loss of Soft Tissue

Conditions are favorable for bone reconstruction if there has been no loss or little loss of soft tissue and the bone graft is placed in a well-vascularized bed. The bone graft is placed in contact with the adjacent bone fragments, which have been stripped of their periosteum; thus, a bone-to-bone contact is obtained. Chips of cancellous bone are packed in any interstices

between the ends of the fragments and also over the junction line; the additional grafts promote bony consolidation as they are revascularized rapidly.

If adequate fixation of the mandibular fragments is provided and the defect is not too large, the consolidation of the graft is usually uneventful. Careful hemostasis to avoid hematoma formation (suction drainge when there is any doubt concerning the hemostasis), intermaxillary fixation (which is maintained for a variable period of time if monomaxillary fixation has been established), a pressure dressing, and a figure-of-eight Barton bandage complete the operation. The following factors must also

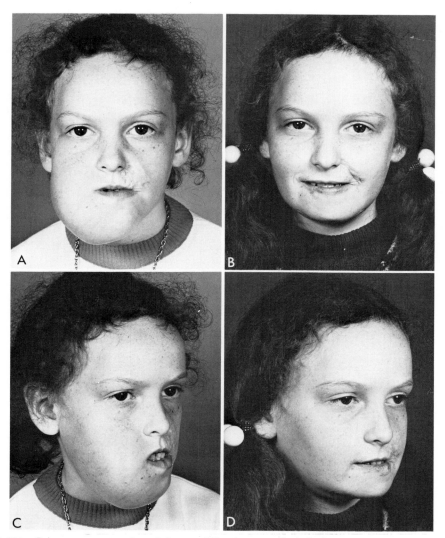

FIGURE 30–226. Primary reconstruction of the mandible after resection of a large area of fibrous dysplasia. *A,* Appearance of a 7 year old child with a giant tumor (see Fig. 30–227). Note radiation scarring in region of left nasolabial fold. *B,* After resection and primary bone grafting through the intraoral approach. *C,* Preoperative view. *D,* Postoperative view.

be considered: (1) as much cancellous bone as possible must be included in the graft for rapid revascularization; (2) cortical bone is required to provide strength to the graft; (3) periosteum, if preserved over the cortex, is a vascular structure and will assist in the revascularization of the graft through the cortical layer (see Chapter 13).

Iliac Bone Grafts Versus Split Rib Grafts. Corticocancellous bone grafts removed from the crest of the ilium, as initiated by Linde-

mann during World War I, were successful in a high proportion of patients during World War II. This procedure remains the favorite technique of reconstruction of the mandible with average size defects.

Whole rib grafts have been less successful because of the absence of exposed cancellous bone and the slow rate of revascularization. Split rib grafts, however, have been highly successful in some extensive defects when their cancellous surfaces are exposed to the soft tissues to encourage rapid revascularization (see Fig. 30–236).

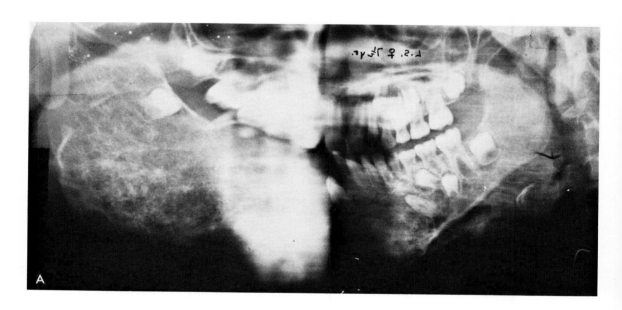

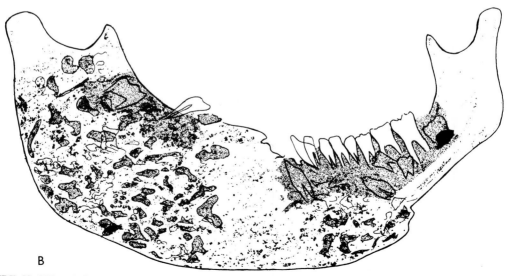

FIGURE 30–227. *A,* Panoramic roentgenogram of the mandible showing the large area of involvement extending from the neck of the right condyle to the premolar area on the left side. *B,* Diagram outlining the extent of the tumor.

Primary Bone Grafting

Primary Bone Grafting Following Tumor Resection. In nonmetastasizing tumors, such as ameloblastomas, primary bone grafting is feasible and has been successful in treating large defects. In the 7 year old child shown in Figure 30–226, the resection of a giant tumor diagnosed as fibrous dysplasia (Fig. 30–227) resulted in a defect extending from the premolar region on the left side of the mandible to the subcondylar area on the right side. The defect was successfully bone grafted after the man-

dible had been "degloved" (see Fig. 30–21) and the tumor exposed and resected (Fig. 30–226). Intermaxillary fixation had been established between the remaining mandibular teeth and the maxillary teeth. A guide plane was placed on the left side to prevent the tendency for deviation to the right after intermaxillary fixation was released. Healing was uneventful except for the extrusion of some bone chips at the area of junction of the bone grafts and the remaining mandibular body (Fig. 30–228). The success of such a procedure can be attributed to the fact that adequate soft tissues

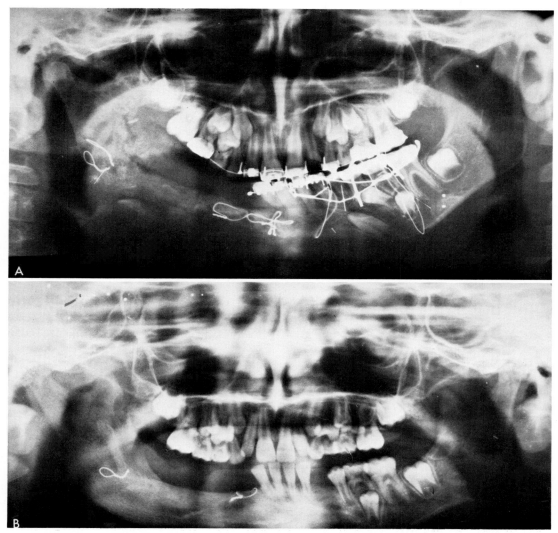

FIGURE 30–228. Radiographic follow-up of the patient shown in Figure 30–226. *A,* Panoramic roentgenogram taken a few days after bone grafting. *B,* One year after the operation, the mandible has been reconstructed with adequate symmetry with the contralateral hemimandible.

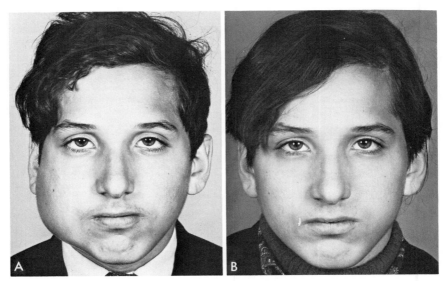

FIGURE 30–229. Preservation of the medial cortex of the ramus after resection of a tumor of the ramus. *A*, Patient in whom a biopsy showed a recurrent granuloma. Note the large mass. *B*, After resection of the mass, the medial cortex remains, preserving the inferior alveolar neurovascular bundle. Spontaneous regeneration of bone precluded the need for bone grafting.

were available to ensure coverage of the transplanted bone.

Primary bone grafting is also indicated when it is possible to preserve one cortex, thus maintaining the continuity of the bone. The patient shown in Figure 30–229 had developed a bony mass extending over the major portion of the right mandibular ramus. A biopsy report indicated that the tumor was a recurrent granuloma. Surgical exposure through a submandibular incision showed an eggshell lateral cortex under which there was a soft bony mass which extended to the medial cortex. The mass was removed by curettage, care being taken to preserve the inferior alveolar neurovascular bundle. Bone grafting was not necessary, as bone regeneration occurred spontaneously in this young patient. This is the type of case in which primary bone grafting can be done in an older patient.

Primary reconstruction should be attempted only when the soft tissue coverage and lining can provide a secure and tension-free wound closure. The advantages of immediate reconstruction are that the bone graft can be placed in a fresh, scarless bed; the distortion produced by the forces of wound contraction on the soft tissue and the remaining fragment of bone is lessened; earlier patient rehabilitation is possible; and the number of operations is decreased. Most surgeons recommend that no

attempt be made to reconstruct the jaw at the time of radical extirpative surgery and prefer to wait until the soft tissue repair has healed. The possibility of recurrence of the cancer and the age of the patient are other considerations discussed earlier in the chapter.

Primary Bone Grafting of Traumatic Defects. In defects caused by trauma, when the soft tissues are intact or can be sutured primarily, primary bone grafting is successful provided that adequate fixation of the fragments is established. Unthinkable before the advent of antibiotics, the intraoral approach is employed for the exposure of the mandibular fragments, the bone grafting, and the soft tissue coverage; the tissues are sutured without tension so as to ensure primary healing.

Technique of Bone Grafting Small and Medium-Sized Defects. When the gap between the two fragments of bone is narrow, as in nonunited fractures, the ends of the fragments are exposed through either a short incision made below the lower border of the mandible or an intraoral approach. The interposed fibrous tissue is removed, and the bone stumps are trimmed with a rongeur or an osteotome. Bone chips from the crest of the ilium are packed between the fragments; an additional bone graft onlay over the fragments bridges the

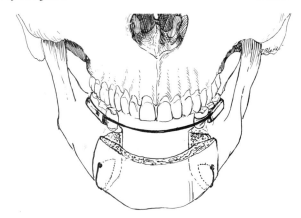

FIGURE 30–230. Large block of iliac bone carved, fitted, and wired to the remaining mandibular fragments. Two molars were present on each posterior fragment and served as a means of anchorage by bands placed around the teeth and an arch bar joining the two mandibular fragments.

gap. Cancellous bone chips are preferable to a single large piece of bone, for it is generally acknowledged that they are more resistant to infection and are revascularized more rapidly.

A larger defect requires a solid piece of bone shaped to overlap the ends of the fragments (Figs. 30–230 and 30–231). The graft is held in place by direct interosseous wiring supplemented by intraoral or external fixation. The surface of contact between the graft and the host bone should be as wide as possible. The interstices between the transplant and the mandible are filled with bone chips. The curvature of the iliac crest supplies a suitable graft, for it simulates the curvature of the mandibular arch.

Iliac bone grafts are successful for the repair of small, medium-sized, and even large defects in a high percentage of patients with mandibular defects. Split rib grafts are rapidly revascularized and can also be used successfully in extensive defects (see Fig. 30–236).

Bone Grafting to Reconstruct the Major Portion of, or the Entire Body of, the Mandible. As stated earlier in the chapter, a defect involving the symphysis and part of the body of the mandible can be reconstructed by the use of three large iliac bone grafts: one median graft in the area of the symphysis, and one on each side (see Fig. 30–224). The bone grafts are wired to each other and to the posterior mandibular fragments. Rigid fixation of the remaining mandibular fragments by intermaxillary fixation is of critical importance for success. Gillies and Millard (1957) used lengths of rib which were notched on the inner aspect and bent to a suitable shape by making a series of greenstick fractures. The degree of success of this technique has not been reported.

When the entire or major portion of the man-dibular arch is absent and no teeth are present for intermaxillary fixation, a method of treatment is the use of an internal splint filled with chips of iliac bone consisting mostly of cancellous bone. The patient shown in Figures 30–232 and 30–233 lost the body of the mandible following severe comminution by a shell fragment. Reconstruction was achieved using a fenestrated tantalum splint filled with bone grafts (Converse, 1945) (Fig. 30–234). Six months after the bone grafts had become consolidated, the splint was removed and onlay bone grafts were added to increase the bulk of the reconstructed mandibular body. At a later stage the buccal sulcus was deepened by the skin graft inlay technique (Fig. 30–251).

Albee (1919) advocated using a U-shaped piece of bone removed from the ilium. A similar U-shaped piece of bone cut from the ilium was used by Seward (1974) for reconstruction of the body of the mandible following resection of an ameloblastoma. To obtain a pattern of the proposed U-shaped bone graft, Seward used a tracing of the outline of the lower border of the mandible from angle to angle as seen in a submental vertex radiograph, together with a dental model cast from an impression of the lower arch. A roll of wax was bent to the shape of the mandible and was tested against the lower border of the patient's jaw. Care must be taken that the shape of the patient's jaw is precisely followed and that the posterior portion of the U has adequate width to fit over the angle of the jaw on each side. This latter precaution is of particular importance, as the ramus normally lies lateral to the occlusal line of the molar dental arch.

Fry (1975) has employed a technique utilizing split ribs. Two symmetrical rib grafts are removed from the region of the posterior ax-

Text continued on page 1490

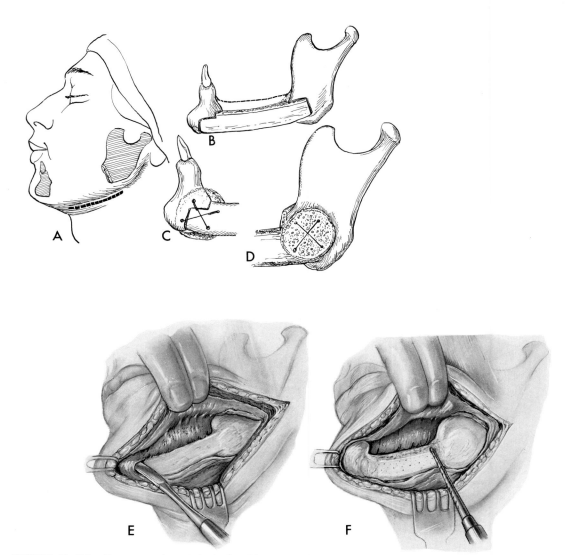

FIGURE 30–231. Reconstruction of the body of the mandible by bone grafting and subsequent addition of bone to increase the vertical dimension of the alveolar ridge. *A,* Extensive defect involving the body of the mandible. *B,* The iliac bone graft in position. Note the overlap between the bone graft and the mandibular fragments. *C,* A piece of cancellous bone has been cross-wired into place on the lingual aspect of the junction between the graft and the anterior mandibular fragment. *D,* Cancellous bone has been placed over the junction of the posterior end of the bone graft and the ramus fragment. *E,* In a second stage, after consolidation of the bone graft, the height of the alveolar ridge was increased to improve retention of the denture. Subperiosteal exposure of the grafted area is shown. *F,* The cortex is removed from the upper portion of the bone graft.

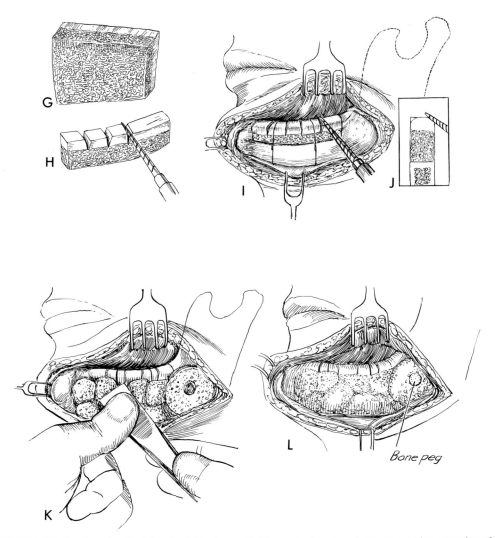

FIGURE 30–231 *Continued.* *G,* A block of iliac bone. *H,* The cortex is cut as shown to permit contouring of the graft to form the new alveolar ridge. *I,* Circumferential wiring is used to secure the added bone graft. *J,* The sharp edges of the upper portion of the bone graft are rounded off. *K,* Cancellous bone is added to the buccal surface of the new alveolar arch to increase the bulk of the mandible. *L,* Note the use of a bone peg for fixation of a piece of cancellous bone.

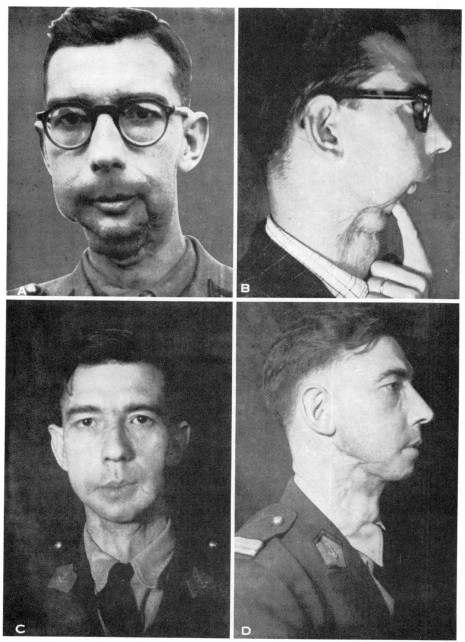

FIGURE 30–232. Reconstruction of the body and symphyseal region of the mandible. *A*, Appearance following loss of a major portion of the mandible as a result of injury by a shell fragment. Although the defect was large, little loss of the soft tissues occurred. *B*, The patient demonstrates the loss of the bony support by pressing the soft tissue backward. *C, D,* Following completion of the mandibular reconstruction according to the technique illustrated in Figure 30–234. The patient is wearing a full denture. (Figs. 30–232 and 30–233 from Converse, J. M.: Early and late treatment of gunshot wounds of the jaws in French battle casualties in North Africa and Italy. J. Oral Surg., *3*:112, 1945.)

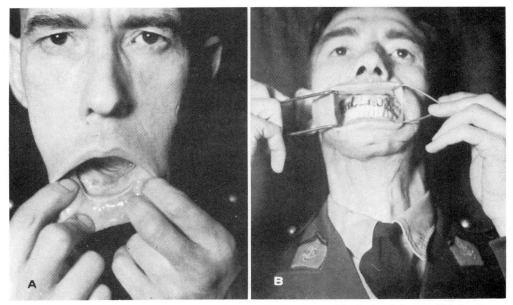

FIGURE 30–233. Intraoral views of the patient shown in Figure 30–232. The body of the mandible has been restored. The tantalum splint (see Fig. 30–234) has been removed. *A*, The sulcus was deepened by the skin graft inlay technique (see Figs. 30–251 and 30–252). *B*, Full denture in position.

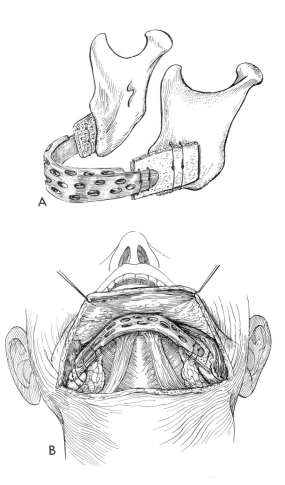

FIGURE 30–234. Internal fixation by a metallic splint. *A*, The fenestrated tantalum splint is wired to a bone graft, which in turn is wired to the ramus stump. Greater stability can be achieved by direct fixation of the metallic splint to the ramus stump. The splint maintains the alignment of the bone grafts, not represented in the drawing, which consist mostly of cancellous bone. *B*, The metallic splint in position. The patient shown in Figure 30–232 was treated by this technique. Six months after the original operation, the metallic splint was removed and additional onlay bone grafts were placed to increase the bulk of the new mandibular arch.

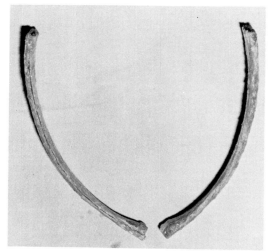

FIGURE 30–235. Fry's technique. Two ribs are removed from the region of the posterior axillary line (ninth and tenth ribs). Each graft is 13 cm long.

illary line where the curvature is greatest. The length of each graft is 13 cm. The ninth or tenth ribs are most satisfactory. The grafts are removed, care being taken to preserve the periosteum, even at the expense of penetrating the pleura (Figs. 30–235 and 30–236, *A*).

Muscle tissue is dissected from the rib grafts, the periosteum being preserved. The ribs are split with an osteotome. Each rib

therefore provides two sections of cortical bone, curved top and bottom, covered by periosteum and enclosing an inner layer of cancellous bone. These sections are light but strong because of the shape of the cortical section itself (Fig. 30–236, *B*).

The medullary cavity of the mandibular remnants is reamed out with a drill (Fig. 30–236, *C*).

The two halves of a split rib are joined together by a halving technique, which entails the removal of cancellous bone (Fig. 30–236, *D*), and are pressed together; the ends of the two halves are inserted as far as possible into the reamed out medullary cavity of the ramus (Fig. 30–236, *E*).

Fixation is secured with a through-and-through wire suture (Fig. 30–236, *E*). The same maneuver is then repeated on the contralateral side, and it will be found that the split ribs cross over naturally in a satisfactory position to re-create the mental symphysis.

The anterior joint is made by slotting one rib unit into the other, as shown in Figure 30–236, *F*. At the anterior joint there is little if any sliding of one rib half over the other, and the joint is secured by a suture which also attaches it to the tissue of the floor of the mouth (Fig. 30–236, *G*). Excess rib projecting beyond the anterior joint is resected (see Fig. 30–236, *E*).

The grafts are carefully covered by soft tissues. The reconstructed jaw is immobilized by pins inserted into the mandibular remnants

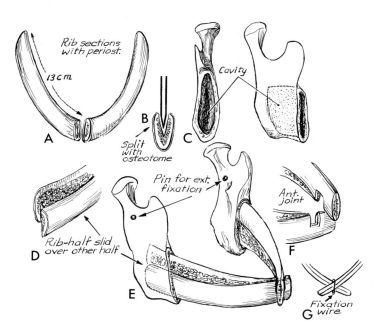

FIGURE 30–236. Osteoperiosteal split rib grafts for mandibular construction. *A*, Two ribs (ninth and tenth) are removed with attached periosteum from the region of the posterior axillary line. *B*, The rib is split. *C*, The medullary cavity of the ramus remnant is reamed out. *D*, The split ribs are joined by a halving technique. Note that a wide surface of cancellous bone is exposed, thus accelerating the revascularization of the grafts. *E*, The grafts have been inserted into the reamed out cavity of the ramus, and fixation is obtained by transosseous wiring. *F*, Technique of joining the grafts anteriorly. *G*, A suture secures the joint and also attaches it to the tissues of the floor of the mouth. (After Fry, 1975.)

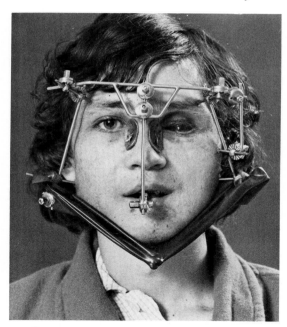

FIGURE 30–237. Technique of fixation of the ramus on each side by the Levant frame. (From Fry, 1975.)

above the grafts and fixed by a Levant frame (Fig. 30–237). The two patients treated with this method were immobilized for eight weeks.

Fry achieved successful reconstruction of the mandibular body in two patients who required angle to angle reconstruction. The first patient had sustained severe multiple injuries, including multiple facial fractures with loss of the mandible from angle to angle, from a traffic accident. The result of the reconstruction some 15 months after the reconstruction is shown in Figure 30–238, *A*. There has been no bony absorption. There was evidence of bony union both clinically and radiologically at the posterior and anterior joints (Fig. 30–238, *B*).

Reconstruction of the Ramus, Angle, and Posterior Portion of the Body of the Mandible. A defect involving the ramus and a major portion of the mandible requires an angular bone graft. Such a graft is obtained from the medial aspect of the anterior superior iliac spine and the iliac table, including the medial portion of the iliac crest (Fig. 30–239). The bone graft is obtained

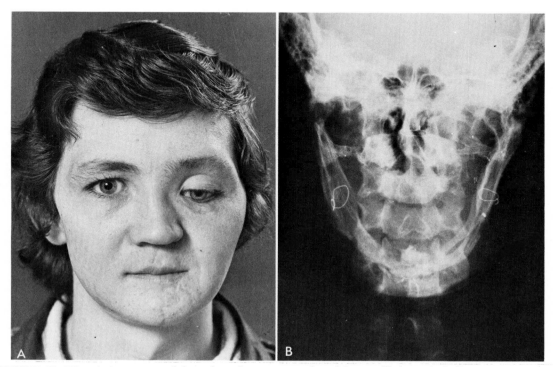

FIGURE 30–238. *A*, Appearance of the patient after reconstruction of the mandibular arch. *B*, Roentgenogram showing the consolidated bone grafts. (From Fry, 1975.)

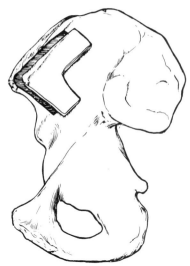

FIGURE 30–239. Angular bone graft removed from the medial aspect of the anterosuperior spine of the ilium for reconstruction of the ramus and body of the mandible.

from the iliac bone on the same side as the defect. The vertical portion of the graft serves as the ramus, and the horizontal portion restores the body; the angle between the two portions of the graft forms the new mandibular angle. The cancellous surface of the graft is placed inward for better revascularization. The graft is outlined at its donor site from a template cut out of a piece of Asche metal and applied over the bone. The template is prepared after the exposure of the mandibular defect. The outline on the iliac bone is marked with a chisel.

A dual approach provides adequate access: (1) a preauricular incision which extends upward into the temporal area and exposes the remaining condylar or ramus fragment; (2) a submandibular incision which exposes the posterior portion of the mandibular body. A cleavage plane, deep to the masseter muscle, the parotid gland, and the facial nerve branches, is sought. The absence of the ramus results in an intimate relationship between the masseter and medial pterygoid muscles. The plane of cleavage for the insertion of the bone graft lies between these two muscles and must be carefully dissected. The bone graft is securely wired to the posterior portion of the body of the mandible and overlies the stump of the ramus, which has been denuded of periosteum. Cancellous bone chips are added around the junction of the graft and the body of the

mandible, and thin, flat pieces are placed between the graft and the remaining portion of the ramus. The soft tissues are sutured. The lower border of the masseter and the medial pterygoid muscles are sutured to each other. For six to eight weeks, positive immobilization must be maintained to ensure consolidation. Figure 30–240 shows photographs and roentgenograms of a patient who was treated in this manner to reconstruct the major portion of the right side of the mandible.

Reconstruction of the Hemimandible. Manchester (1965) has reproduced the anatomy of the hemimandible for immediate reconstruction following resection for tumors that are slow-growing and not aggressively malignant (Fig. 30–241, *A*). In one patient, the resection was performed for the eradication of fibrous dysplasia; in two patients the tumor was a myxoma; and in a fourth patient, the jaw was resected because of a melanoma of the cheek which had invaded the mental foramen and the inferior alveolar canal.

It is important to preserve the meniscus of the temporomandibular joint when the mandible is being resected in order to obtain a satisfactory functioning joint.

A template (Fig. 30–241, *B*) of the resected hemimandible is prepared after intermaxillary fixation is established by silver cast cap splints. The template is then applied over the lateral surface of the ilium on the same side as the defect (Fig. 30–242). The outline of the graft is marked with a chisel, and the graft is partly shaped before it is finally cut free. The graft includes the full thickness of the ilium. Final shaping of the graft is then completed, the precaution being taken to avoid making the condyle too large, as this would interfere with the hinge action of the temporomandibular joint. The graft is then placed in the bed of soft tissues. The condyle is placed against the meniscus. A stainless steel nail (Kirschner wire) is used to fix the anterior end of the graft to the uninvolved hemimandible which is maintained in position by the cast cap splint. An excellent result was obtained (Fig. 30–243). Radiographic studies documented survival of the graft.

At the autopsy of the patient with melanoma performed 11 months after the operation, the graft was grossly normal in appearance. The radiographic examination of the graft, particularly the condyle, showed that architectural changes had begun to occur under the influence of functional stress.

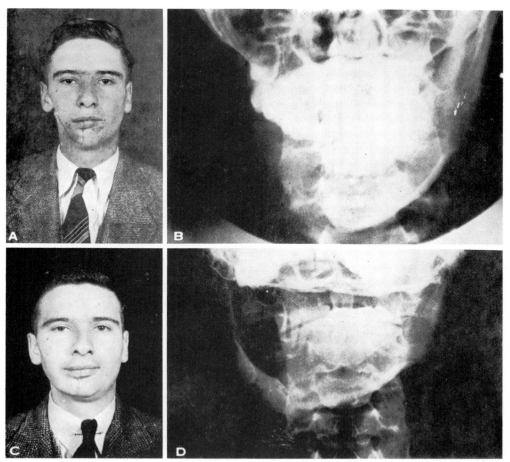

FIGURE 30–240. *A, B,* Absence of the entire half of the mandible. *C, D,* Bone graft extending from the temporomandibular joint to the median line of the mandible, restoring the ramus and half of the body of the mandible.

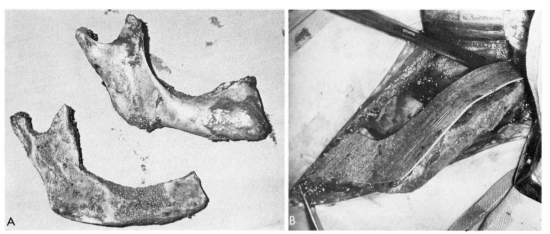

FIGURE 30–241. Immediate reconstruction of the hemimandible. *A,* The resected hemimandible (above) and the sculptured iliac bone (below). *B,* An aluminum template is resting on the hemimandible prior to the resection. It will serve as the pattern for the graft. (From Manchester, W. M.: Immediate reconstruction of the mandible and temporomandibular joint. Br. J. Plast. Surg., *18*:291, 1965.)

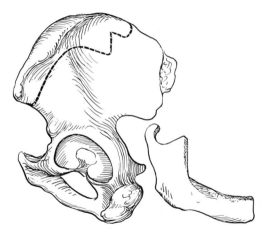

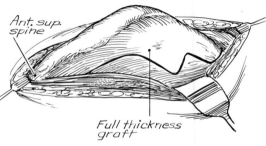

FIGURE 30–242. Removal of the iliac bone graft. The pattern is applied over the lateral portion of the ilium and iliac crest and a full thickness bone graft is removed as illustrated. (Drawn after Manchester, W. M.: Immediate reconstruction of the mandible and temporomandibular joint. Br. J. Plast. Surg., 18:291, 1965.)

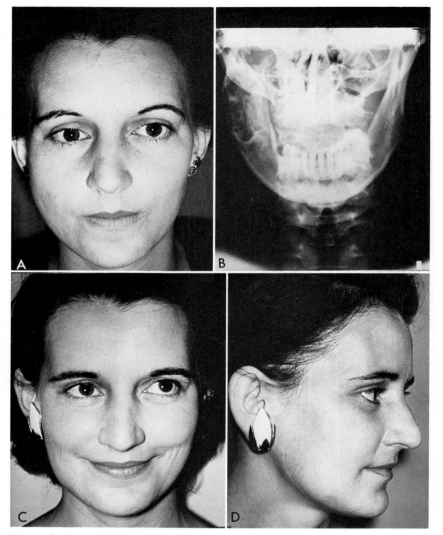

FIGURE 30–243. *A*, Patient, age 27 years, showing a swelling of the right cheek caused by fibrous dysplasia. *B*, The roentgenogram shows the pathologic process extending to the base of the condyle. *C*, *D*, Postoperative result two years later. (From Manchester, W. M.: Immediate reconstruction of the mandible and temporomandibular joint. Br. J. Plast. Surg., 18:291, 1965.)

Bilateral Reconstruction of the Ramus. Reconstruction of both rami is required in bilateral and hemicraniofacial microsomia (see Chapter 54). Kazanjian (1956) reconstructed both rami in a patient with this type of deformity.

The patient shown in Figure 30–244 had a retracted chin and a conspicuous depression on each side of the face; the ramus on the left was represented by a tenuous stemlike structure; the ramus and the angle of the mandible were also absent on the right side (Fig. 30–244, *A, C*). The body of the mandible was "floating" and could easily be manipulated in any direction. The symphyseal region was increased considerably in its vertical dimension, and the cortical border was greatly thickened, giving the external appearance of a transverse shelf across the front of the neck, above the thyroid cartilage. This hypertrophy may have resulted from the overuse of the suprahyoid muscles in achieving opening of the mouth, since the lateral pterygoid muscles appeared to be absent. To construct the ramus, combined preauricular and submandibular incisions were used to introduce iliac bone grafts. Each graft extended from the rudimentary glenoid fossa to the posterior portion of the body of the mandible.

The right iliac crest was exposed, and two

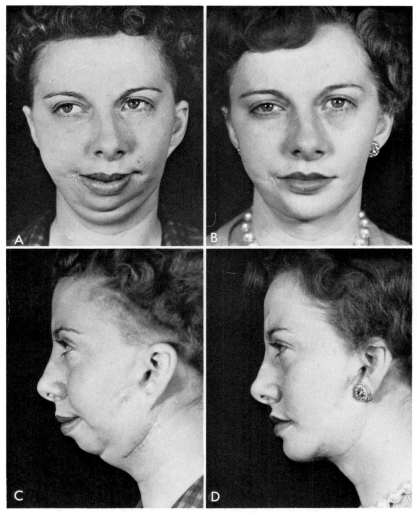

FIGURE 30–244. Congenital absence of the right mandibular ramus and near complete absence of the left ramus. *A, C,* Preoperative views showing pronounced retraction of the chin and retrusion of the mandible. The transverse ridge of soft tissue below the chin is caused by the downward retraction of the mental symphysis. *B, D,* Postoperative appearance. (From Kazanjian, V. H.: Bilateral absence of the ascending rami of the mandible. Br. J. Plast. Surg., 9:77, 1956.)

large sections of bone and several smaller sections were removed from the crest to be used
as "fill." A section of bone was then transplanted into the prepared tunnel, the graft extending from the rudimentary glenoid fossa to
the posterior portion of the right body of the
mandible, where the bone graft was wired firmly to the body with two stainless steel wires.
Several smaller chips of cancellous bone were
placed in strategic areas to reconstruct the
angle of the jaw and to add fullness where
required.

The anomalous conditions found on the right
side were also present on the left. A similar
reconstructive operation was done on the left
side. The lower end of the bone graft was
wired directly to the posterior portion of the
body as on the contralateral side, and cancellous bone chips were also placed where indicated. Both wounds were closed in layers.

The intermaxillary wires were then removed,
and the teeth were retained in satisfactory
temporary occlusion by elastic bands and were
maintained for approximately six weeks. Roentgenograms (Fig. 30–245) showed that the bone
grafts reconstructing each ramus articulated
with the base of the skull and that there was
good union at the points of contact of the bone
grafts with the body of the mandible (Fig. 30–
245, C).

Five months after the initial surgical procedures, the dental occlusion remained satisfactory and the patient could chew food with
no difficulty. Although a slight grinding action of the teeth could be detected during
mastication, the patient could control mandibular motions effectively.

Satisfactory function of the mandible was
achieved, and the depression on each side of
the face was corrected; the retracted appear-

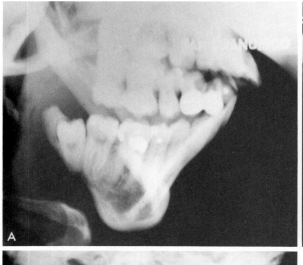

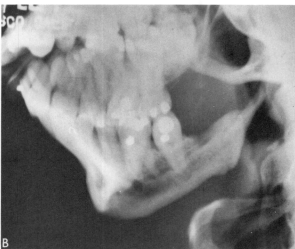

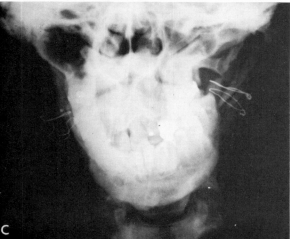

FIGURE 30–245. Roentgenograms of the patient
shown in Figure 30–244. *A*, Absence of the right ramus.
B, Stemlike ramus on the left side. Note the hypertrophy
of the bone of the mental symphysis. *C*, Bone grafts articulating with the base of the skull. (From Kazanjian, V.
H.: Bilateral absence of the ascending rami of the mandible. Br. J. Plast. Surg., 9:77, 1956.)

ance of the chin, however, had not been appreciably altered. Two subsequent operations were peformed to restore facial contour, additional onlay iliac bone grafts being transplanted to the region of the chin and to the lateral aspect of the mandible.

An additional operation was performed to obtain further improvement in contour. Bone was again removed from the ilium; some of this bone was transplanted to the chin to accentuate the mental prominence. Other portions of bone were added to the lateral aspect of the body of the mandible on the left side to achieve symmetry with the contour of the right side (Fig. 30–244, *B, D*).

NERVE GRAFTING FOLLOWING RESECTION OF THE BODY OF THE MANDIBLE AND BONE GRAFT RECONSTRUCTION. After resection of a segment of the mandible, the proximal and distal nerve stumps are tagged by a suture. After the reconstruction of the mandible by an iliac bone graft, a sural nerve graft is placed without tension between the stumps of the inferior alveolar nerve. Hausamen, Samii, and Schmidseder (1973) embed the nerve graft at a distance from the healing bone below the mandibular angle in the midst of well-vascularized soft tissue.

Defects of the Mandible Associated with Loss of Soft Tissue

Trauma and ablative operations for oromandibular cancer are the two major causes of extensive defects of the mandible and adjacent soft tissues.

Injuries of the lower face with loss of varying amounts of soft tissue, including the lip, chin, and sublingual tissue, associated with loss of mandibular bone are usually the result of gunshot wounds or of severe industrial injuries.

After operations for tumor, the loss of tissue is more extensive than that following injury. The retraction of the tissues after trauma, such as a gunshot wound, exaggerates the magnitude of the soft tissue defect, and reconstruction is less involved than that following extensive resection for the eradication of malignancy.

The following stages should be observed in sequence in the late reconstruction of defects of the lower portion of the face involving the lower lip, chin, mandible, and floor of the mouth.

1. Fixation of the remaining mandibular fragment or fragments must be assured. The fixation should maintain the fragments in their anatomical position in adequate occlusal relationship with the teeth of the maxilla.

2. The soft tissues of the floor of the mouth, chin, and lip are reconstructed.

3. Bone grafting is employed to restore the continuity of the mandible.

4. A labiobuccal sulcus must be restored by incising the tissues on the labiobuccal aspect of the bone, surgically deepening the sulcus, and restoring a new sulcus lining by a skin graft inlay (see Figs. 30–251 and 30–252).

5. Completion of the vermilion portion of the lip, the introduction of muscle flaps from the upper lip and adjacent portion of the cheek, and the restoration of hair-bearing cutaneous continuity by rotation flaps of adjacent bearded skin in male patients are final procedures.

Fixation of the Remaining Fragments in Adequate Occlusal Relationships. The initial goal in the correction of such deformities is control of the bony fragments. Although the external wound may give the appearance of almost total destruction of the underlying skeletal framework in traumatic defects, a sufficient amount of bone is usually present to be used as a foundation for future reconstruction. This may include a part of the body of the mandible on each side with or without teeth or may consist of only the ramus on each side.

Following resection of the mandible with the cervical lymph nodes in continuity ("neck dissection"), the soft tissue defect is variable, as it may include a major portion of the cheek, the lips, and the floor of the mouth. The mandibular resection varies according to the extent of the lesion.

It is advisable to establish immediate fixation of the remaining mandibular segments. Unless fixation of the bony segments is provided at an early date, displacement complicates subsequent reconstructive procedures. If stabilization of the mandibular fragments is neglected, the ramus fragments will be displaced forward, upward, and medially by scar contracture and muscle pull; the body remnants will be drawn into a medial position; and the symphyseal fragment will be drawn downward and backward. In addition, a difficult dissection is encountered as attempts are made to locate and liberate the remaining fragments from the scarred tissues at the time of the reconstructive surgery.

The principles established by Kazanjian and Burrows (1917–1918) are valid today: (1) the residual fragments are replaced in occlusal

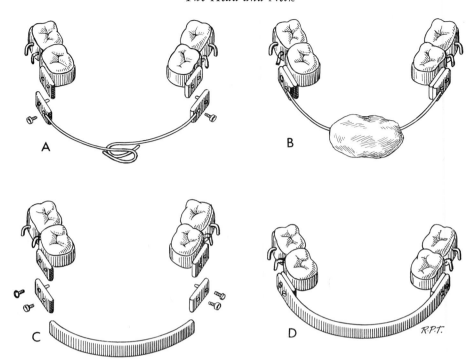

FIGURE 30–246. Type of sectional splint used in the patient shown in Figure 30–248. *A,* Bands or caps are cemented to the abutment teeth. Metal plates have been soldered to the outer surface of the bands. Adaptable arch wires are soldered to additional plates arranged in such a way that they can be bolted to the plates on the bands. *B,* Fragments are manipulated to attain occlusion of mandibular teeth with the opposing teeth of the upper jaw, and the wires are joined in the midline with dental compound or acrylic resin. *C, D,* The adaptable arch wire is replaced by a solid arch bar, and various parts of the sectional splint are assembled. The prosthetic mold shown in Figure 30–247 can be attached to the arch bar.

relationships with the maxillary teeth; (2) the fragments are connected by a sectional splint (Fig. 30–246) to maintain the separated portions in their anatomical positions and to serve as a splint for future reconstruction with a bone graft; (3) a removable prosthetic mold serves as a framework for the reconstruction of the soft tissues.

Kazanjian's original appliance is illustrated in Figure 30–247. An arch wire is soldered to the bands cemented to the remaining molar teeth (see Fig. 30–246). The anterior portion of the arch wire has a wire soldered to it at a right angle, thus forming a T-shaped retention arch bar (Fig. 30–247, *A*). A prosthetic mold is prepared with vertical and horizontal slots on its lingual surface to receive the branches of the T-bar. The prosthetic mold (Fig. 30–247, *B, C*) provides support to the remaining tissues until reconstruction can be undertaken and serves as a supportive framework for the reconstruction of the soft tissues.

When the fragments have not been maintained in fixation but instead have been displaced by a misguided attempt at primary clo-

sure of the soft tissue defect (Fig. 30–248, *A*), surgical replacement of the fragments is indicated. The patient's true soft tissue and bony defects are disclosed by severing the constricting tissues and muscular attachments and replacing the bones and the soft tissues into their anatomical position (Fig. 30–248, *B*). Only then can subsequent successful soft tissue reconstruction and bone grafting of the true mandibular defect be achieved (Fig. 30–248, *C, D*). A strong fixation appliance is required, such as the one illustrated in Figure 30–246, when technical facilities are available. Many variations of this appliance can be made. Bands (or cap splints) are fitted over the remaining molar teeth. Each band has a hook for intermaxillary fixation. The anterior band carries a plate which is soldered to it and includes two holes to receive screws for fixation of an outer plate to which an arch wire is soldered. The outer plates are then held to the inner plates by screws. With the teeth in intermaxillary fixation, the length of the definitive arch bar is measured by fashioning the wires (see Fig. 30–246, *A*), joining them with wax (see Fig.

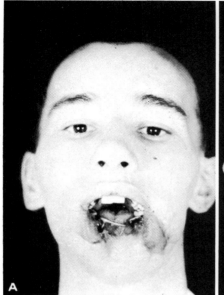
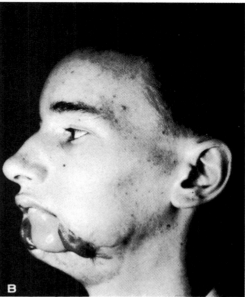

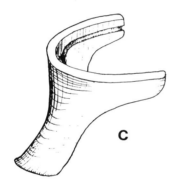

FIGURE 30–247. *A*, Patient who sustained a gunshot injury. The remaining mandibular fragments are controlled by an appliance similar to that illustrated in Figure 30–246. *B*, The prosthetic mold in position. *C*, Diagram of the prosthetic mold. The lingual surface is slotted to receive the horizontal and vertical portions of the arch bar. (From Kazanjian and Converse.)

30–246, *B*), and soldering the arch bar to the outer plates (see Fig. 30–246, *C*). The supporting arch bar is then held to the tooth-bearing fragments by the screws (see Fig. 30–246, *D*).

When teeth are not available for fixation, temporary stabilization of the remaining mandibular arch can be achieved by a stout internal Kirschner wire that is threaded into the divided ends of the bone.

Reconstruction of the Soft Tissues. After fixation of the bone fragments, the second step in the correction of extensive deformities is the reconstruction of the soft tissues. As mentioned earlier in the text, in traumatic deformities such as those resulting from gunshot wounds, the soft tissue defect is not as great as a rapid examination of the patient would indicate. The reconstructive problem is quite different and usually less difficult to solve than in defects resulting from extensive resection for malignant disease; the defect is smaller, the patient is usually in the younger age group, and the problem of dealing with irradiated tissue is not encountered.

Lining tissue must also be provided. This is as essential as the covering tissue. In defects of the symphysis of the mandible and the lower lip, the supportive prosthesis provides a framework for the reconstructed soft tissues and also serves to maintain the mandibular segments in their anatomical position. In traumatic defects, stumps of the lower lip often survive the mutilation and furnish muscular function to the lower lip. Sufficient mucosa is often available to supply additional lining for the upper portion of the lower lip, which is re-reconstructed by rotating cheek flaps. A defect

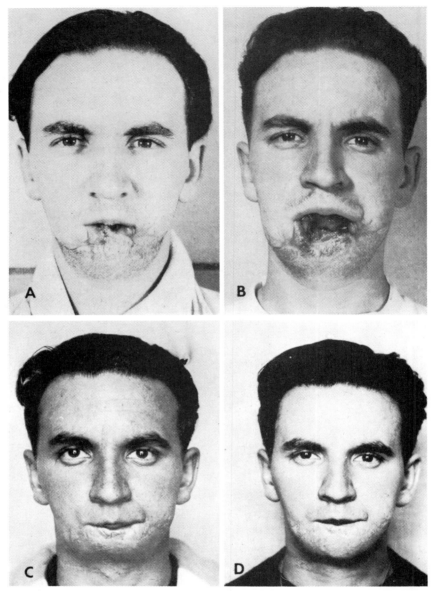

FIGURE 30–248. A gunshot wound which had been neglected, allowing soft tissue contracture and medial displacement of the mandibular fragments. *B*, The cicatricial tissue was incised; the fragments were replaced in their anatomical position and maintained in intermaxillary fixation with an arch bar and band appliance (see Fig. 30–246). The patient had lost most of the mandibular body; two posterior fragments with two molars remained. *C*, A deltopectoral skin tube was employed to furnish tissue for the floor of the mouth and the lining of the lower lip and chin. Large rotation flaps (see Fig. 30–249) restored the lower lip. In male patients it is important to restore the continuity of the bearded areas of the face; such continuity is provided by neck rotation flaps. The patient is wearing the mold attached to the arch bar illustrated in Figure 30–247. *D*, After bone graft reconstruction of the mandible, a skin graft inlay reconstructs the sulcus to permit wearing of a denture.

remains in the lower portion of the lip, the chin, and the anterior portion of the floor of the mouth.

In large defects, a flap from a distance is required. Axial pattern flaps, such as the deltopectoral flap, furnish tissue for the floor of the mouth. The flap can then be folded on itself to reconstruct the lower lip and chin. In traumatic defects, to avoid a beardless patch in the midst of the bearded area of the male face, wide rotation flaps including the remains of the lower lip (Fig. 30–249) can be used to restore continuity of the hair-bearing skin (see Fig. 30–248).

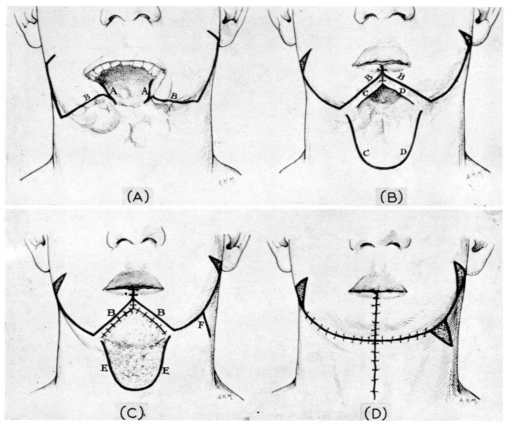

FIGURE 30–249. Large rotation flaps for the reconstruction of the lower lip and chin soft tissue defect. *A,* Outline of Dieffenbach-type full thickness skin flaps. *B,* The flaps have been rotated, and the stumps of the lower lip are approximated. In unusual cases in males, when little hair is present, and in females, a trapdoor flap can be outlined and delayed. *C,* The trapdoor flap is turned in to furnish lining tissue. *D,* The operation is completed by additional rotation of flaps to resurface the mental area. (From Kazanjian and Converse.)

Another technique which can be used on occasion for the restoration of the hair-bearing skin of the face in the male patient is the bipedicle scalp flap (Fig. 30–250). This flap was employed by Dufourmentel (1919) in World War I. The bipedicle flap should be designed to extend obliquely backward toward the vertex to gain sufficient length. Lining tissue is obtained from adjacent scarred skin, as shown in Figure 30–249, *B, C.*

The disadvantage of scalp flaps on the face is their relative rigidity and their color which results from the high density of the hair follicle population. When the hair is allowed to grow, as in the patient shown in Figure 30–250, *B, C,* and is suitably trimmed, a Lincolnesque appearance is achieved.

In the cancer patient with a large defect, a more expeditious method is Bakamjian's non-delayed deltopectoral flap (see Chapter 63). The flap is employed to reconstruct the floor of the mouth and is then detached from the thorax and folded upon itself to form a lower lip. If the upper lip and adjacent cheek tissue is intact, two small Estlander flaps, one on each side, are transposed into the reconstructed lower lip. In the older cancer patient, such a procedure will provide the necessary support to eliminate drooling and to permit oral feeding.

A considerable diminution in the magnitude of the deformities following ablative operations for cancer has resulted from the primary transfer of forehead and deltopectoral flaps for the restoration of the floor of the mouth and major defects of the cheeks (see Chapters 61, 62, and 63). The use of the denuded undersurface of the tongue to cover the floor of the mouth resulted in a severe retrusion of the low-

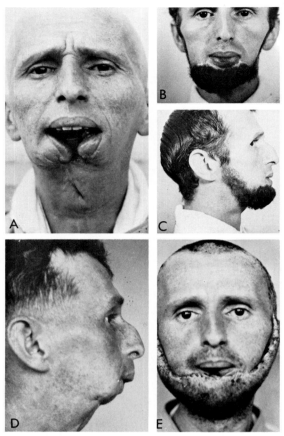

FIGURE 30–250. Reconstruction by a bipedicle scalp flap. *A,* Extensive loss of mandible caused by a gunshot wound. There is considerable loss of soft tissue in the area of the chin. *B,* Result obtained after repositioning the remaining mandibular fragments and retaining them in intermaxillary fixation. Lower lip continuity was restored, and a bipedicle scalp flap taken from the vertex repaired the soft tissue defect. *C,* Postoperative profile appearance. *D,* Profile view showing the extent of mandibular bone and soft tissue loss. *E,* The scalp flap, prior to division, with two vascular pedicles vascularized by the superficial temporal vessels. (From Converse, 1945.)

er face (the Andy Gump deformity); such disfiguring deformities are prevented by the newer techniques, which immediately replace the resected soft tissues.

The opportunity for primary palliative reconstructive procedures following resection of oromandibular cancer is facilitated by the clean-cut edges of the resected site, which contrast with the ragged and damaged edges of the wound following severe trauma. Primary reconstruction of a large cheek defect by the superimposition of forehead and deltopectoral flaps (see Chapter 62), the reconstruction of the floor of the mouth, and the restoration of the

continuity of the lips have eliminated the problem of the disfigured patient who becomes a social outcast, unable to feed himself or to communicate with others.

In cases of trauma, the stumps of lower lip tissue usually survive the destructive injury and provide muscular support for the reconstructed lower lip. After excision of the entire lower lip, the drooping of the lip is a problem. Estlander skin-muscle-mucosal flaps from the upper lip or cheek assist in providing muscular support. In Chapter 32, the techniques of reconstructing and providing support of the lower lip are discussed.

Bone Grafting. Bone grafting is the third step in the reconstruction. The techniques of bone grafting have been described earlier in this chapter.

The success of bone grafting is dependent upon the quality of the soft tissue reconstruction. The vascularity of the soft tissues provides a favorable bed for the revascularization of the bone graft.

In the older cancer patient who has undergone resection of the hemimandible and of the cheek wall, reconstruction is often neither feasible nor successful. The presence of the firm tissues used to reconstruct the soft tissue defect (forehead flap and deltopectoral flap, for example) often obviates the need for reconstruction. The remaining mandible is able to perform its masticatory function without losing occlusal relationships with the maxillary teeth because of the absence of soft tissue contractile forces, which would tend to displace the remaining hemimandible. During the early stages after the resection of the bone and primary reconstruction of the soft tissues, a flange or guide plane based on the maxillary teeth will prevent medial displacement of the remaining hemimandible. In the reconstruction of the body of the mandible with associated loss of soft tissue, internal fixation (see Fig. 30–234) and external fixation appliance are often required to stabilize the remaining ramus fragments (see Figs. 30–218 to 30–223 and Fig. 30–237).

Alternative Techniques of Reconstruction

In addition to the techniques described in the previous pages, other modalities of reconstruction are available. These include (1) composite flaps, (2) microvascular free flaps, and (3) microvascular bone grafts.

Reconstruction with Composite Flaps. The concept of transferring soft tissue and bone in a single step as a composite flap is an attractive one. In 1892, Bardenheuer used a composite flap from the forehead that contained skin, periosteum, and bone to restore the continuity of the mandible. A technique using a composite flap consisting of a portion of the lower part of the adjacent body of the mandible, muscle, and skin to fill an adjacent mandibular gap was described by Wildt (1896) and Krause (1907). Looking for other bony donor sites, Rydigier (1908) transferred the clavicle with the overlying skin to a lower jaw defect. Blair (1918) used a similar clavicle-containing flap, as well as a composite flap which transplanted costal bone. Interest in these procedures remained dormant for over a half century until Snyder, Bateman, Davis, and Warden (1970) reported their experience with a clavicular osteocutaneous flap to restore mandibular continuity. Conley (1972) reported a large series of regional bone-muscle-skin flaps; bone was obtained from the ribs, sternum, clavicle, scapula, zygoma, and temporal bone.

Experimental animal studies by Strauch, Bromberg, and Lewin (1969) showed that the soft tissue portion of the composite flap could be dispensed with and that rib grafts could be transferred as an island flap based on the internal mammary artery. In 1974 Ketchum, Masters, and Robinson applied the island rib flap principle to repair a mandibular defect in a patient.

Reconstruction with Microvascular Free Flaps. The development of microvascular techniques has made it possible to transfer large areas of soft tissue as microvascular free flaps. Harii, Ohmori, and Ohmori (1974) reported their clinical application of these techniques to the face. Free transfers of soft tissue from the scalp, deltopectoral region, and groin have been performed. In addition to the usual prerequisites of a donor site, microsurgical procedures require the following: (1) the presence of one viable artery and vein that are sufficiently large to be anastomosed under the microscope; (2) the mass of the tissue to be transferred should not exceed the vascular network of the main vessels; (3) the blood supply to the donor site should have little anatomical variation. The recipient site must also have suitable vessels for anastomosis. Details of microsurgical techniques are described in Chapter 14.

Reconstruction with Microvascular Bone Grafts. McKee (1971) extended this concept one step further and transplanted the rib as a microvascular free graft. Using microsurgical techniques, he anastomosed the internal mammary artery and vein to either the external maxillary or superior thyroid vessel. Subsequent experimental work along this line has been reported by McCullough and Fredrickson (1973) and Östrup and Fredrickson (1974). Successful transfer of bone into irradiated tissues has also been reported by Östrup and Fredrickson (1975) using microvascular anastomotic techniques.

The advantage of these techniques is obvious: the blood supply to the bone graft is maintained. The risk of bone graft loss is decreased, as is the subsequent absorption of the bone. When the island composite flap or free transfer flap using microsurgical techniques is employed, the need for a second operation to sever the pedicle is eliminated. The disadvantage is the risk of failure and loss of valuable tissue.

In the small to medium-sized mandibular defect with healthy covering soft tissues, the microvascular graft would appear to be a surgical exercise, in view of the high rate of success in bone grafting the mandible. In larger defects, such as loss of the major portion of the body of the mandible, the microvascular techniques are advantageous if suitable arteries and veins are available and can be satisfactorily anastomosed.

Restoration of a Buccal Sulcus and a Functional Alveolar Ridge: The Skin or Mucosal Graft Inlay Technique

Operative procedures which restore the external contour of the face and reestablish the bony continuity of the mandible should be supplemented by artificial dentures which restore masticatory function. Skin or mucosal grafting is often a necessary procedure to provide an adequate sulcus and a retentive alveolar ridge following bone graft reconstruction of the mandible.

The term "epithelial" inlay was used by Esser (1917), who devised the technique of intraoral skin grafting. The term is a misnomer, since the graft, which includes both epidermis and dermis, is composed of more than epithelium alone, as the original term employed by Esser implies. It is preferable to employ the term "skin graft" inlay. Esser conceived the technique for the purpose of establishing a buccal sulcus in patients in whom the mandible had been reconstructed by means of bone grafts. The purpose of restoring a vestibule was to increase the retention of a denture. He made an incision through the skin in the submandibular area, extending the incision to the lower border of the reconstructed mandible, then upward along the buccal aspect of the mandible as far as the mucosa of the floor of the mouth. Into this cavity he molded a piece of softened dental impression compound. Around the mold, a split-thickness skin graft, raw surface outward, was wrapped and the compound mold was placed into the cavity; the submandibular incision was sutured.

In a second-stage operation a number of weeks later, Esser incised through the mucosa of the floor of the mouth into the skin-grafted cavity, removed the dental compound mold, and extended the buccal flange of the patient's denture into the restored sulcus.

Waldron, an American surgeon during World War I, modified the technique by placing the skin graft directly into the new sulcus through an intraoral incision. Since World War I, the skin graft inlay technique has been used extensively to restore an adequate lining in the oral cavity. The typical skin graft inlay technique consists of three parts: the incision, the prosthesis, and the graft (Fig. 30–251).

THE INCISION. The incision is made through the mucosa on the labiobuccal aspect of the alveolar ridge down to the periosteum. The reason for leaving the periosteum intact over the bone is that grafting is more successful over the vascular bed provided by the periosteum. The incision is extended downward along the buccal surface of the mandible, and the mucosal flap thus formed is reflected inferiorly and partially lines the labiobuccal aspects of the new sulcus (Fig. 30–251, *A, B*). This type of incision has the advantage that the cut edges of the oral mucosa are not situated at the same level; thus, a constrictive scar band is not formed at the junction of the skin and the mucosa after the skin graft has healed. Careful hemostasis is obtained by pinching the bleeding vessels with fine forceps and occluding them by electrocoagulation. Complete hemostasis is essential to prevent hematoma, which would interfere with the revascularization of the skin graft.

In order that the revascularization of the graft may occur without interference, two conditions must be met. First, the contact between the graft and host must be as intimate as possible, and there must be no interposition of blood or serum, which would act as a barrier to the ingrowth of host vessels. Second, satisfactory fixation and immobilization (Fig. 30–252) must be provided so that the vessels are not torn during the period of vessel penetration into the graft.

In large skin graft inlays, considerable dis-

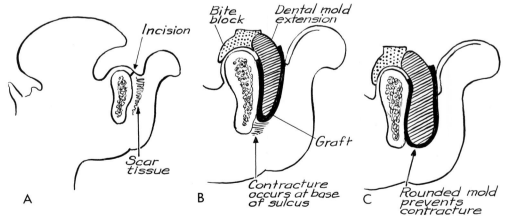

FIGURE 30–251. The skin graft inlay for the restoration of a labiobuccal sulcus. *A,* The incision is made through the mucosa but does not extend through the periosteum. A flap is raised and reflected forward to line the lower lip (see *B*). *B,* The sulcus has been deepened; an impression has been taken with soft dental compound and hardened in situ with cold water. A split-thickness skin graft covers the dental compound mold. Note that the pointed shape of the tip of the mold will result in contracture of the grafted tissues postoperatively. *C,* Correct shape of the mold to maintain the depth of the sulcus. Fixation of the bite-block or denture which maintains the skin-grafted mold is often best obtained by circumferential wiring around the mandible (see Fig. 30–252).

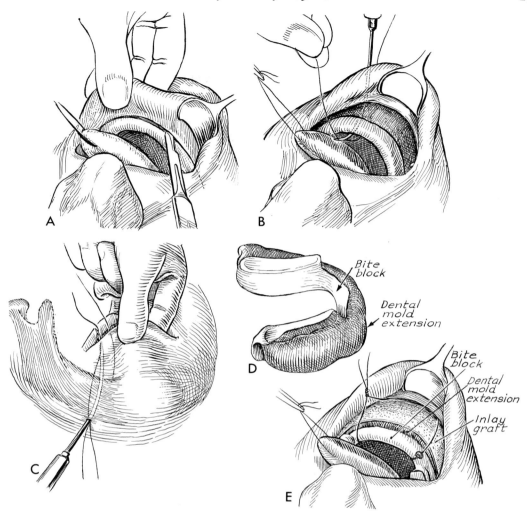

FIGURE 30–252. The skin graft inlay for the restoration of the labiobuccal sulcus in the edentulous patient. *A,* Incision through the mucosa. *B, C,* Passing a circumferential wire. *D,* The bite-block with the skin graft–carrying mold. *E,* Circumferential wires hold the skin graft inlay in position.

tention of the soft tissues in the region of the symphysis is necessary to permit the introduction of a compound mold of sufficient size. In such cases, it may be necessary to sever the lower attachments of the musculature of the lower lip and the platysma to permit adequate stretching of the soft tissues.

THE PROSTHESIS. Two features are essential in the construction of the dental compound mold: (1) It must provide an accurate impression of the new surgical cavity; (2) it must be considerably larger than the cavity in order to distend the tissues in every direction, and be free of sharp edges that would cut into the tis-

sues. One cannot overemphasize the need for considerable distention of the soft tissues, and the construction of a grossly oversize mold, which can be reduced progressively during subsequent weeks. The construction of an oversize mold is important for two reasons. All skin grafts tend to contract during the healing period; thus, if the skin graft is placed over a mold that is oversize, an excess of skin graft will be transplanted, thus counteracting the eventual contraction of the graft. Moreover, hematoma formation, which would interfere with the revascularization of the graft, is prevented.

Newly developed synthetic materials have made possible the fabrication of a definitive prosthesis while the patient is in the operating room. However, this procedure causes considerable delay despite the rapidity of curing of some of the new resins. In most complicated cases, it is more practical to prepare two appliances. The first is a temporary bite-block (occlusal wafer), which serves to anchor the compound mold for the primary skin grafting procedure; the second is a definitive denture with an oversize flange that fills the reconstructed sulcus. The flange is gradually reduced during the weeks subsequent to the operation. The shaping of the flange is important. It should fill the entire cavity and be of a shape that will ensure its retention (Fig. 30–251, C).

THE GRAFT. Grafts of split-thickness skin are the most frequently used tissue to reline the raw surface of the surgically prepared cavity. Their use is especially indicated in the inlay technique when large areas must be resurfaced.

Skin grafts have the disadvantage of lacking pliability, of having a keratin surface that is difficult to "wet," of being malodorous, and of occasionally transferring hair to the oral cavity. The "wetness" is an especially desirable feature when maxillary vestibuloplasties are performed (Steinhauser, 1971).

To provide a more physiologic vestibular lining, a split-thickness graft of oral mucosa can be removed from the inner aspect of the lower lip by a Castroviejo mucotome (a small electric dermatome) (Converse, 1964c; Steinhauser, 1969) (see Chapter 6, Fig. 6–12). The cheeks and the undersurface of the tongue can also serve as donor sites. The entire hard palatal mucoperiosteum has also been used (Hall and O'Steen, 1970). In an effort to increase the area of coverage, Morgan, Gallegos, and Frileck (1973), using the mucoperiosteum of the hard palate, placed the graft through a skin mesher to expand the graft. Thus a greater surface area could be covered by the limited amount of graft. The denuded hard palate reepithelized spontaneously.

Originally, the skin graft inlay was made with very thin split-thickness grafts. The thin graft has the advantage of becoming vascularized rapidly and having what is referred to as an excellent "take." The inconvenience of the thin graft is its contraction during the postoperative healing period. For this reason, thicker varieties of split-thickness grafts are now employed. The usual thickness is 0.014

inches,* as calibrated on American dermatomes. The skin graft should be removed from a hairless area of the body to prevent subsequent growth of hair inside the oral cavity.

FIXATION OF THE SKIN GRAFT–CARRYING PROSTHESIS. The fixation of the appliance which maintains the skin graft in the newly made sulcus varies according to the status of the dentition. When the patient has teeth, it is possible to provide fixation of the partial denture by fixed band and arch appliances. When the patient is edentulous, a complete denture or bite-block (occlusion rim) is maintained by circumferential wiring around the body of the mandible (Fig. 30–252). A denture can be made in patients who have teeth on portions of the adjacent mandible. Clamps keep the denture stabilized to the teeth, and circumferential wires ensure completion of the fixation. Softened dental compound is added to the denture and extended into the deepened sulcus; a definitive appliance can be made immediately in the operating room with quick-curing methylmethacrylate.

POSTOPERATIVE CARE. The skin graft is immobilized for a period of seven days, following which the compound mold is removed under sedation, regional anesthesia, or general anesthesia. Any excess skin graft overlapping the edges of the sulcus and any points where granulation tissue is seen are trimmed and cauterized with a silver nitrate stick. The appliance is *immediately replaced* to prevent contraction of the graft and diminution of the sulcus. At no time during the subsequent months should the prosthesis be left out of the skin-grafted cavity, as contraction of the skin graft will prevent replacement of the prosthesis. The duplicate acrylic resin mold is used to replace the primary mold. This prosthesis is left undisturbed for another four or five days, when it is removed for cleansing. After this, it is removed every few days. As previously emphasized, the prosthetic mold should be grossly oversized for all large skin graft inlays. After a period varying between three and five weeks, the size of the acrylic resin prosthesis is reduced by progressively grinding it down to the desired size and shape. All skin grafts contract; the period of maximum contracture spans several weeks, and the reduction in size should be slow and progressive. The best results are obtained if a period of about eight to ten weeks is spent in developing the final size

---

*1 inch = 2.54 cm.

and shape of the prosthesis. The patient should be instructed to avoid removing the appliance for any length of time to prevent contraction in the skin-grafted area.

Occasionally hair growth in the transplanted skin graft can be troublesome. Fortunately, it is sparse, and usually the simplest way to eliminate the hair is direct excision of the hair follicles.

The Skin Graft Inlay in Mandibular Defects. After bone grafting for the restoration of the continuity of the body of the mandible, a new sulcus must be made so that a denture can be retained in position. It is essential that the surgeon allow for added contour of the denture in planning his reconstruction. This is particularly true in bony restoration of the anterior part of the body of the mandible and the symphysis. After reconstruction of the anterior half of the body of the mandible and the symphysis, an extension of the sulcus downward into the region of the chin is usually necessary to secure good retention of the denture. Thus, the labial flange of the denture contributes to the contour of the chin in these patients. Should the surgeon not allow for the thickness of the denture, the chin might appear to be too prominent and give the patient a prognathic appearance. It is necessary, therefore, not to correct the contour fully by means of the bone grafts and to allow the prosthesis to establish the final contour of the chin.

Final Procedures. These include the replacement of a hairless skin patch by rotating flaps of hair-bearing skin over the area (see Fig. 30–249), the refinement of the contour of the vermilion border by means of a flap from the upper lip (see Chapter 32, Fig. 32–68), and the restoration of muscle continuity, when it is absent in the reconstructed lip, by Estlander-Abbé or fan flaps from the upper lip and adjacent cheek tissues. Restoration of muscle continuity to support the lower lip is important when a major portion of the lower lip is destroyed.

Procedures to Increase the Area of Purchase for the Denture in the Edentulous Mandible

Recession of the Muscular Attachments on the Lingual Aspect of the Mandible and Lowering the Floor of the Mouth. In the edentulous jaws, the attachments of the muscles are closer to the alveolar ridges, thus limiting the depth of the labiobuccal sulcus and the lingual sulcus.

In certain cases it may be advantageous to increase the purchase surface of the denture by increasing the vertical height of the alveolar ridge on the lingual aspect of the transplanted bone. This is accomplished by recessing the attachments of the muscles of the floor of the mouth, thus lowering the floor of the mouth. The technique of lowering the floor of the mouth was first demonstrated by Trauner in 1950 and published by him in 1952; it was later modified by Rehrmann (1953) and Obwegeser (1964). In such cases, deepening the buccal sulcus is not enough; it is also necessary to recess the structures on the lingual aspect of the mandible to establish an adequate ridge (Fig. 30–253).

The procedure consists of detaching the muscles attached to the lingual surface of the mandible, principally the mylohyoid muscle, and recessing the muscular attachments lower down on the bone so as to gain additional vertical dimension for the alveolar ridge and thus extra purchase surface for the prosthesis. The procedure is done without disturbing the periosteum over the alveolar bone. After infiltration with a local anesthetic vasoconstrictor solution, an incision is made from the retromolar region to the retromolar region on the contralateral side, the incision being placed immediately lingual to the crest of the ridge. The entire periosteal surface on the lingual side of the mandible is exposed to a point situated immediately above the lower border of the mandible. In the most posterior portion of the wound, it is necessary to divide the superior fibers of the superior constrictor muscle. Blunt dissection avoids injury to the lingual nerve. Anteriorly, the lateral and superior fibers of the genioglossus muscle are resected. One should avoid, however, complete section of the genioglossus muscle to prevent a backward displacement of the tongue and difficulty in control of eating and of swallowing. The edge of the mucous membrane of the recessed floor of the mouth is then displaced downward, and catgut sutures are passed under the lower border of the mandible, rejoining the depth of the newly constructed vestibule on the buccal surface of the mandible. Fibrous tissue accumulated over the lingual aspect of the mandible is resected down to the periosteum. At this point in the operation, it will be noted that a portion of the crest and the lingual aspect of the mandible are bare of mucous membrane. A split-thickness skin graft is used to resurface the area. An impression is taken using the patient's own denture or a preoperatively prepared acrylic bite-block as a tray. Softened

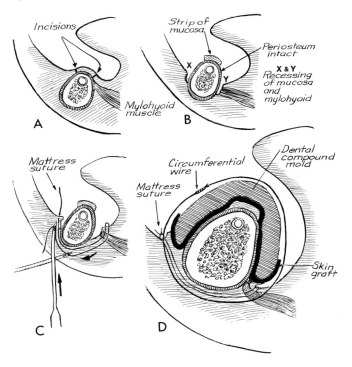

FIGURE 30–253. Technique for increasing the depth of the sulcus on the labiobuccal aspect and also on the lingual aspect of the mandible by muscle recession. *A*, Cross-sectional appearance of the atrophied alveolar process. The buccal sulcus is shallow, and the floor of the mouth is close to the alveolar crest. Incisions are placed below the crest of the alveolar process, and a strip of mucosa is allowed to remain and cover the ridge. *B*, The buccal and lingual mucosa is dissected from the periosteum, as is the attachment of the mylohyoid muscle. The periosteum is left intact. *C*, The buccal and lingual mucosa and the mylohyoid muscle are displaced inferiorly and held by a catgut mattress suture passed below the border of the mandible. *D*, An acrylic splint maintains the molded dental compound and a split-thickness skin graft in position. The appliance is maintained in position by circumferential mandibular wires. (After Trauner.)

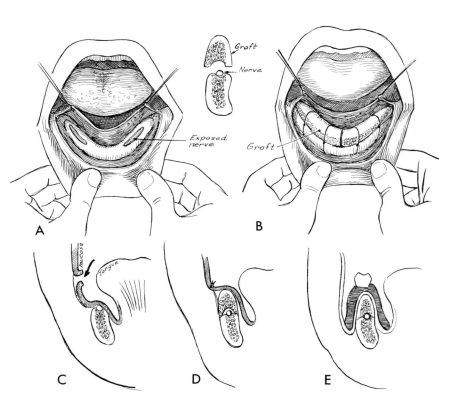

FIGURE 30–254. Increasing the vertical projection of the mandibular arch. *A*, Exposure of the mandible through a labiobuccal incision. The inferior alveolar nerves are exposed. *B*, The bone graft is shaped to fit over the nerves, and is secured by circumferential wires. *C*, The labiobuccal incision is made. *D*, Suture completed. *E*, The denture now has better retention as a result of the increased height of the alveolar process. Often the labiobuccal sulcus must be reconstructed as a secondary procedure.

dental compound is molded over the area and hardened with ice water. A split-thickness skin graft, raw surface outward, is placed over the dental compound, and the skin graft–carrying denture or splint is immobilized by circumferential wires. After the skin graft has healed, a definitive denture with fully extended flanges is inserted.

Increasing the Vertical Projection of the Edentulous Mandibular Arch. Exposure of the alveolar process is obtained preferably through an intraoral or an extraoral approach. A bone graft is fashioned and fitted over the bone and maintained by circumferential wires laid into grooves on the upper surface of the graft (Fig. 30–254). There is usually sufficient mucosa to redrape it over the bone graft and deepen the sulcus.

There is considerable absorption of the grafted bone, but usually sufficient bone remains to protect the inferior alveolar nerve and furnish a retentive alveolar process. While bone resected from the lower border of the mandible is less prone to absorption, the edentulous mandible is often so tenuous that little bone is available for this purpose. Autogenous cartilage grafts have also been successfully employed. Inorganic implants remain in position for a limited period of time before being extruded.

RECONSTRUCTION OF THE MAXILLA

In contrast to the many references in the literature to reconstructive surgery of the mandible, little has been written about reconstruction of the maxilla. Upper jaw defects have been treated by closing the palatal defect with an obturator connected with a denture which is retained by the maxillary teeth on the contralateral side (see Chapter 60). By deepening the buccal sulcus, an upward extension of the denture improves the contour of the middle third of the face.

The forces applied to a prosthodontic appliance have an adverse effect on the remaining teeth that serve as anchoring points. Design of the appliance is critical. Obtaining support and retention for the prosthesis may be difficult. The problem of retention is compounded in the patient with an edentulous maxilla. Nevertheless, a skilled maxillofacial prosthodontist can

overcome many of these problems and provide a valuable service to the facially crippled patient.

Bone grafts are employed in the reconstruction of the maxilla, either as onlay grafts to restore contour or as framework grafts to replace the missing maxillary skeleton.

Reconstruction of the Upper Jaw Skeleton. In 1938, Figi used iliac bone to reconstruct the maxilla after removal of a malignant tumor of the maxillary sinus. Campbell (1948), borrowing from the principles of Figi, reported the successful restoration of half the midfacial skeleton following a resection of the maxilla and the malar bone. In a first stage, the void left by the resection was filled by a flap consisting of the anterior third of the temporalis muscle (Gillies, 1920). Lining was obtained from the remaining half of the palate. Iliac bone grafts were used, according to the technique described by Figi, in a second stage to reconstruct the skeletal defect and to restore contour. The buccal sulcus was restored in a third stage by the skin graft inlay technique (see Figs. 30–251 and 30–252).

When the floor of the orbit has been removed along with the remainder of the maxilla, the periorbita and the orbital fascia, including the suspensory ligament of Lockwood, are undisturbed. A progressive sagging of the orbital contents results in the ocular globe being situated at a lower level than the unaffected eye. Since the extraocular musculature is not appreciably disturbed, diplopia does not usually follow. These patients, however, complain of transient diplopia when fatigued.

Destructive injuries, such as a gunshot wound, or disruption of the floor of the orbit followed by sequestration of bone fragments after wound sepsis can cause extensive loss of the orbital floor. As a result, direct injury of the periorbita and the inferior oblique and inferior rectus muscles can occur. Scar tissue contraction compounds the problem; it may cause downward displacement and rotation of the ocular globe and interfere with the ocular rotary movements. The bony defect can include a major segment of the orbital floor in its maxillary and zygomatic portions and also a large portion of the body of the zygoma.

In 1950 Converse and Smith reported the reconstruction of the upper portion of the maxilla, the zygoma, and the orbital floor with bone grafts. The palatal defect was closed with an obturator, and an upward extension of the ap-

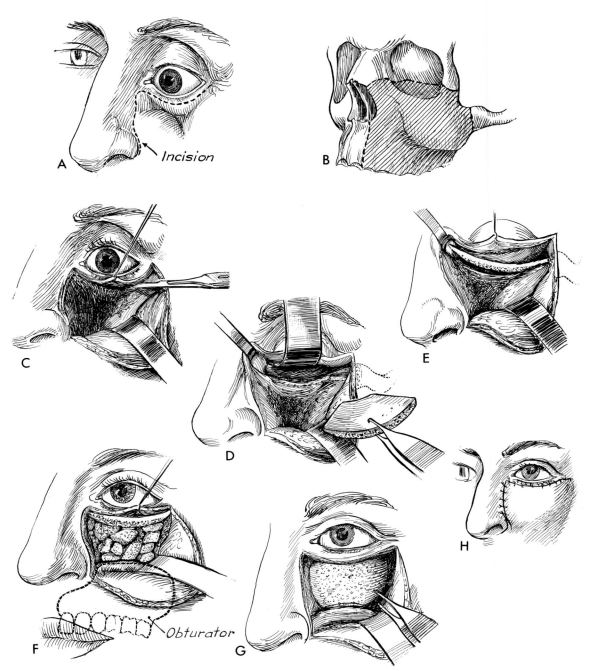

FIGURE 30–255. Technique of reconstruction of the upper portion of the maxilla, the floor of the orbit, and the zygoma by bone grafts. *A,* Line of incision outlining the cheek flap. *B,* The shaded area shows the extent of bone resected. *C,* The cheek flap has been resected. The orbital contents are freed from the binding scar tissue. *D,* The orbital contents are raised. After subperiosteal exposure of the frontal process, the maxilla and the zygomatic arch, a bone graft is prepared for insertion. *E,* Bone graft in position, restoring the floor of the orbit. *F,* The depressed area is filled with cancellous bone chips. *G,* An overlay contour restoring bone graft is placed over the bone chips. *H,* Suture of the edges of the skin flap to the edges of the defect has been completed. In the older patient and in the patient reconstructed following resection for a malignant tumor, closure of the palate is usually contraindicated, since the palatal defect allows clinical observation of the affected area. (From Converse, J. M., and Smith, B.: Case of reconstruction of the maxilla following resection for carcinoma of the antrum. Plast. Reconstr. Surg., 5:426, 1950. Copyright © 1950, The Williams & Wilkins Company, Baltimore.)

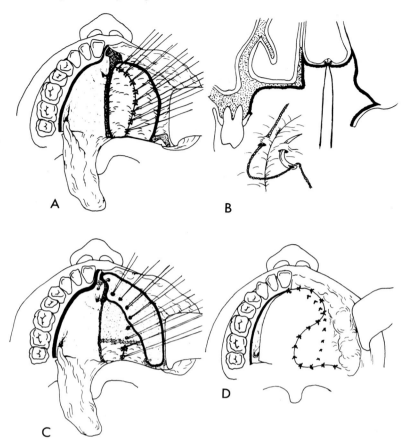

FIGURE 30–256. Technique of reconstruction of the hemimaxilla and alveolar process. *A,* Closure of the nasal cavity is obtained by turned-in flaps of mucoperiosteum from the lateral rim of the defect and of the nasal septum. *B,* Frontal section showing the closure of the nasal layer. Mattress sutures are used to invert the mucosal edges into the nasal cavity. The ends of the sutures are left long. *C,* The hard palate and the alveolar process are restored by bone grafts, which are fixed by interosseous wiring to the remaining hard palate, the anterior portion of the alveolar process, and the pterygoid processes. The long ends of the sutures are passed through the bone grafts and the oral mucosal covering. *D,* Rotation flaps from the remaining hard palate and the buccal mucosa provide the oral lining. The sutures are tied to eliminate dead space. (Figs. 30–256 to 30–259 from Obwegeser, H. L.: Late reconstruction of large maxillary defects after tumor resection. J. Maxillofac. Surg., *1*:19, 1973. Georg Thieme Verlag, Stuttgart, Germany.)

pliance restored the contour of the lower portion of the cheek (Fig. 30–255).

Reconstruction of the hard palate is contraindicated after resection of the maxilla for malignant disease, since the palatal defect permits direct observation of the affected area. Reconstruction of the hard palate and alveolar process is indicated, however, after resection of benign or nonmetastasizing tumors.

RECONSTRUCTION OF THE HARD PALATE AND ALVEOLAR PROCESS (Obwegeser, 1973). The reconstruction is achieved in two stages. In a first stage, a two-layer soft tissue closure is obtained by local flaps; in a second stage, bone grafts restore the bony continuity of the palate and reconstruct an alveolar process.

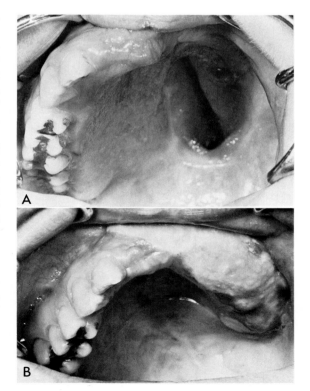

FIGURE 30–257. Reconstruction of a hemimaxillary defect and the alveolar process using the technique shown in Figure 30–256. *A,* A defect of the maxilla and alveolar process 30 years after resection of a malignant tumor. *B,* Postoperative appearance showing the restoration of the maxilla and the alveolar ridge. In a first stage the soft tissue defect was closed, and the bony support was restored. In a second operation, the buccal sulcus was reestablished by the skin graft inlay technique.

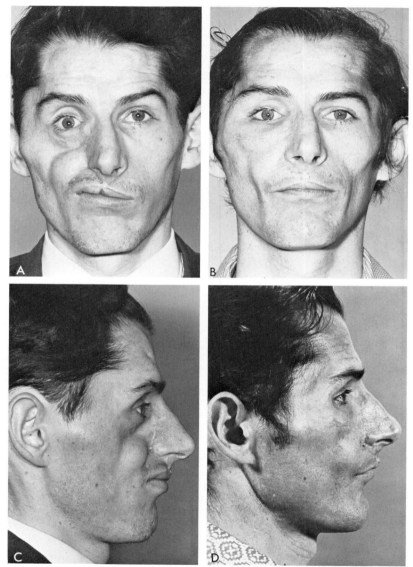

FIGURE 30–258.   *A*, Facial deformity caused by a defect of the major portion of the maxilla resulting from the resection of a tumor in childhood. *B*, Appearance following reconstruction of the hard palate by a skin flap, followed by bone grafting; reconstruction of the alveolar process, floor of the orbit, infraorbital area by iliac bone grafts; posterior recession of the prognathic mandible by a bilateral sagittal split of the mandibular rami. *C*, Preoperative profile appearance. *D*, Postoperative profile appearance.

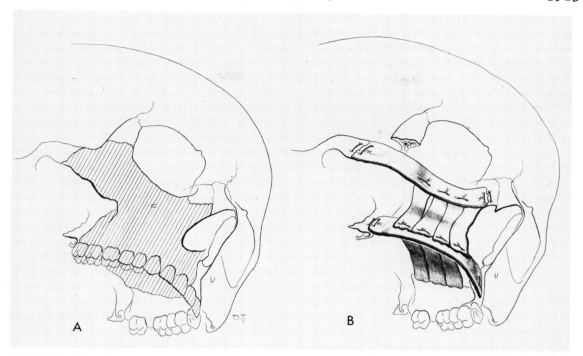

FIGURE 30–259.   Reconstruction of the maxilla, orbital floor, zygoma, hard palate, and alveolar process. *A,* The shaded area represents the extent of the defect. *B,* Placement of costal bone grafts. Undivided rib grafts are used to reconstruct the zygoma, inferior orbital rim, and alveolar process. The hard palate and the lateral wall of the maxilla are restored with split rib grafts.

The nasal lining is obtained by making a circumferential incision around the rim of the defect and freeing the mucoperiosteum from the nasal septum and from the lateral wall of the defect (Fig. 30–256, *A*). The turnover flaps are approximated with inverting sutures that are left long (Fig. 30–256, *B*). Bone grafts are used to reconstruct the hard palate and the alveolar process (Fig. 30–256, *C*). Direct interosseous wiring stabilizes the alveolar bone graft to the remaining alveolar process anteriorly and to the pterygoid process posteriorly. The sutures that had been left long during the closure of the nasal cavity are passed through the bone grafts used to restore the hard palate and the alveolar ridge (Fig. 30–256, *C*). The oral lining and coverage of the grafts are provided by a large rotation flap from the remaining hard palate mucoperiosteum and the labiobuccal mucosa (Fig. 30–256, *D*). The long sutures are then passed through the flaps and tied to help eliminate dead space. Three weeks after the bone grafting, a temporary denture is placed over the reconstructed structures. A skin graft inlay is performed three months later to re-form a sulcus that will aid in the retention of the maxillary denture (Fig. 30–257).

Costal grafts have also been used to correct bony defects produced by resection of half of the maxilla and the infraorbital region (Obwegeser, 1973). The palatal defect is closed, and the alveolar process is reconstructed as shown in Figures 30–258 and 30–259. The Weber-Ferguson incision is reopened to obtain exposure. The exposure facilitates reconstruction of the alveolar process with a section of undivided rib, which is maintained by wire fixation to the alveolar process on the contralateral side and the remains of the pterygoid processes on the same side (see Fig. 30–256).

REFERENCES

Aaronson, S. A.: A cephalometric investigation of the surgical correction of mandibular prognathism. Angle Orthod., *37*:251, 1967.

Abbott, L. C.: The operative lengthening of the tibia and fibula. J. Bone Joint Surg., *9*:128, 1927.

Adams, W. M.: Bilateral hypertrophy of the masseter muscle. An operation for the correction. Br. J. Plast. Surg., *2*:78, 1949.

Albee, F. H.: Orthopedic and Reconstructive Surgery. Philadelphia, W. B. Saunders Company, 1919.

Aller, T. G.: Operative treatment of prognathism. Dent. Cosmos, *59*:394, 1917.

Anderson, R.: An ambulatory method of treating fractures of the shaft of the femur. Surg. Gynecol. Obstet., *62*:865, 1936.

Angle, E. H.: Double resection of the lower maxilla. Dent. Cosmos, *40*:635, 1898.

Angle, E. H.: Classification of malocclusion. Dent. Cosmos, *41*:240, 1899.

Attie, J. N., Catania, A., and Ripstein, C. B.: Stainless steel mesh prosthesis for immediate replacement of hemimandible. Surgery, *33*:712, 1953.

Aubry, M., and Pillet, P.: Sur les implants d'acrylique dans la résection du maxillaire inférieur. Ann. Otol. (Paris), *67*:553, 1950.

Aufricht, G.: Combined nasal plastic and chin plastic; correction of microgenia by osteocartilaginous transplant from large hump nose. Am. J. Surg., *25*:292, 1934.

Axhausen, G.: Zur Behandlung veralteter disloziert geheilter Oberkieferbrüche. Dtsch. Zahn. Mund. Kieferheilkd., *1*:334, 1934.

Babcock, W. W.: Surgical treatment of certain deformities of the jaw associated with malocclusion of the teeth. J.A.M.A., *53*:178, 1909.

Babcock, W. W.: The field of osteoplastic operations for the correction of deformities of the jaws. Items of Interest, *32*:439, 1910.

Babcock, W. W.: Advancement of the receding chin. Ann. Surg., *105*:115, 1937.

Bardenheuer, P.: Ueber Unterkiefer- und Oberkiefer-Resection. Arch. Klin. Chir., *44*:604, 1892.

Barton, P. R.: Segmental surgery. Br. J. Oral Surg., *10*:265, 1973.

Behrman, S. J.: Complications of sagittal osteotomy of the mandibular ramus. J. Oral Surg., *30*:554, 1972.

Bell, H. B.: Biologic basis for maxillary osteotomies. Am. J. Phys. Anthropol., *38*:279, 1973.

Bell, W. H.: Revascularization and bone healing after anterior maxillary osteotomy: A study using adult Rhesus monkeys. J. Oral Surg., *27*:249, 1969.

Bell, W. H.: Correction of skeletal type of anterior open bite. J. Oral Surg., *29*:706, 1971.

Bell, W. H., and Creekmore, T. D.: Surgical-orthodontic correction of mandibular prognathism. Am. J. Orthod., *63*:256, 1973.

Bell, W. H., and Levy, B. M.: Revascularization and bone healing after anterior mandibular osteotomy. J. Oral Surg., *28*:196, 1970.

Berndt: Prosthesis after jaw resection. Arch. Klin. Chir., *52*:210, 1898.

Björk, A.: The Face in Profile: An Anthropological X-ray Investigation of Swedish Children and Conscripts. Lund, Berlingska Boktryckerret, 1947.

Björk, A.: Facial growth in man, studied with the aid of metallic implants. Acta Odontol. Scand., *13*:9, 1955.

Björk, A.: The relationship of the jaws to the cranium. *In* Lundström, A. (Ed.): Introduction to Orthodontics. New York, McGraw-Hill, 1960.

Björk, A.: Variations in the growth pattern of the human mandible: A longitudinal radiographic study by the implant method. J. Dent. Res., *42*:400, 1963.

Björk, N., Eliasson, S., and Sörensen, S.: Relative rotation of fragments during the time of intermaxillary fixation after transverse osteotomy bilaterally in the ascending ramus of the mandible. Sven. Tandlak. Tidskr., *63*:111, 1970.

Blair, V. P.: Operations on the jaw-bone and face; a study of the etiology and pathological anatomy of developmental malrelations of the maxilla and mandible to each other and to the facial outline, and of their operative treatment when beyond the scope of the orthodontist. Surg. Gynecol. Obstet., *4*:67, 1907.

Blair, V. P.: Instances of operative correction of malrelation of the jaws. Int. J. Orthod., *1*:395, 1915.

Blair, V. P.: Surgery and Diseases of the Mouth and Jaws. St. Louis, Mo., C. V. Mosby Company, 1918.

Boldt, H.: Ein Beitrag zur Kenntnis der einfachen Masseter Hypertrophie. Thesis No. 31, Berlin, 1930.

Boyne, P. J.: Restoration of osseous defects in maxillofacial casualties. J. Am. Dent. Assoc., *78*:767, 1969.

Boyne, P. J.: Implants and transplants. Review of recent research in the area of oral surgery. J. Am. Dent. Assoc., *87*:1074, 1973.

Bromberg, B. E., Walden, R. H., and Rubin, L. R.: Mandibular bone grafts, a technique in fixation. Plast. Reconstr. Surg., *32*:589, 1963.

Brusati, R., and Bottoli, V.: L'osteotomia mascellare segmentaria anteriore: Ricerche sperimentali sulla vascolarizzazione del settore osseo osteotomizzato. Riv. Ital. Stomatol., *25*:446, 1970.

Burstone, C. J.: The integumental profile. Am. J. Orthod., *44*:1, 1958.

Bush, L. F.: Use of homogenous grafts. Preliminary report on bone bank. Bone Joint Surg., *29*:620, 1947.

Butcher, E. O., and Taylor, A. C.: The effects of denervation and ischemia upon the teeth of a monkey. J. Dent. Res., *30*:265, 1951.

Caldwell, J. B.: Developmental deformities of the jaws. *In* Kruger, G. O. (Ed.): Textbook of Oral Surgery. 2nd ed. St. Louis, Mo., C. V. Mosby Company, 1964, p. 461.

Caldwell, J. B., and Amaral, W. J.: Mandibular micrognathia corrected by vertical osteotomy of the rami and iliac bone graft. J. Oral Surg., *18*:3, 1960.

Caldwell, J. B., and Letterman, G. S.: Vertical osteotomy in the mandibular rami for correction of prognathism. J. Oral Surg., *12*:185, 1954.

Caldwell, J. B., Hayward, J. R., and Lister, R. L.: Correction of mandibular retrognathia by vertical "L" osteotomy: A new technic. J. Oral Surg., *26*:259, 1968.

Campbell, H. H.: Reconstruction of left maxilla. Plast. Reconstr. Surg., *3*:66, 1948.

Case, C. S.: A Practical Treatise on the Techniques and Principles of Dental Orthopedia. Chicago, C. S. Case Company, 1921.

Casson, P. R., Bonanno, P. C., and Converse, J. M.: The midface degloving procedure. Plast. Reconstr. Surg., *53*:102, 1974.

Castigliano, S.: Massive metallic implant in situ five years after resection of mandible. Am. J. Surg., *88*:490, 1941.

Cernéa, P.: Déviations mandibulaires par hypertrophie condylienne unilatérale et leur traitement chirurgical. *In* Deuxième Congrès International d'Odontostomatologie. Paris, Julien Prélat, 1954.

Cernéa, P., Grignon, J. L., Crépy, C., and Benoist, M.: Les ostéotomies totales des maxillaires supérieurs. Rev. Stomatol., *56*:700, 1955.

Chubb, G.: Bone grafting of the fractured mandible, with an account of 60 cases. Lancet, *2*:9, 1920.

Coccaro, P. J.: Restitution of mandibular form after condylar injury in infancy (a 7-year study of a child). Am. J. Orthod., *55*:32, 1969.

Coffey, R. J.: Unilateral hypertrophy of the masseter muscle. Surgery, *11*:815, 1942.

Cohn-Stock, H.: Die chirurgische Immediatregulierung der Kiefer, speziell die chirurgische Behandlung der Prognathie. Vjschr. Zahnheild., *37*:320, 1921.

Colantino, R. A., and Dudley, T.: Correction of maxillary prognathism by complete alveolar osteotomy. J. Oral Surg., *28*:543, 1970.

Conley, J. J.: Regional bone-muscle-skin pedicle flaps in surgery of the head and neck. Trans. Am. Acad. Ophthalmol. Otolaryngol., *76*:946, 1972.

Converse, J. M.: Early and late treatment of gunshot wounds of the jaw in French battle casualties in North Africa and Italy. J. Oral Surg., *3*:112, 1945.

Converse, J. M.: Restoration of facial contour by bone grafts introduced through the oral cavity. Plast. Reconstr. Surg., *6*:295, 1950.

Converse, J. M.: Masseter muscle hypertrophy. Unpublished case, 1951.

Converse, J. M.: Technique of bone grafting for contour restoration of the face. Plast. Reconstr. Surg., *14*:332, 1954.

Converse, J. M.: Transplantation of the inferior mandibular segment after horizontal osteotomy. In Kazanjian, V. H., and Converse, J. M.: The Surgical Treatment of Facial Injuries. Baltimore, The Williams & Wilkins Company, 1959, p. 867.

Converse, J. M.: Micrognathia. Br. J. Plast. Surg., *16*:197, 1963.

Converse, J. M.: Vertical osteotomy. In Converse, J. M. (Ed.): Reconstructive Plastic Surgery. Philadelphia, W. B. Saunders Company, 1964a, Fig. 23–57, p. 917.

Converse, J. M.: The "degloving" technique. In Converse, J. M. (Ed.): Reconstructive Plastic Surgery. Philadelphia, W. B. Saunders Company, 1964b, p. 897.

Converse, J. M.: Restoration of vestibular sulcus. In Converse, J. M. (Ed.): Reconstructive Plastic Surgery. Philadelphia, W. B. Saunders Company, 1964c, p. 941.

Converse, J. M.: Surgical elongation of the traumatically foreshortened nose: The perinasal osteotomy. Plast. Reconstr. Surg., *47*:539, 1971.

Converse, J. M.: The degloving procedure. In Kazanjian, V. H., and Converse, J. M.: Surgical Treatment of Facial Injuries. 3rd ed. Baltimore, Williams & Wilkins Company, 1974a, p. 1022.

Converse, J. M.: Elongation by sagittal splitting of the body of the mandible. In Kazanjian, V. H., and Converse, J. M.: Surgical Treatment of Facial Injuries. 3rd ed. Baltimore, The Williams & Wilkins Company, 1974b, p. 1061.

Converse, J. M., and Campbell, R. M.: Experiences with a bone bank in plastic surgery. Plast. Reconstr. Surg., *5*:258, 1950.

Converse, J. M., and Campbell, R. M.: Bone grafts in surgery of the face. Surg. Clin. North Am., *34*:375, 1954.

Converse, J. M., and Horowitz, S. L.: The surgical-orthodontic approach to the treatment of dentofacial deformities. Am. J. Orthod., *55*:217, 1969.

Converse, J. M., and Horowitz, S. L.: Simianism: Surgical-orthodontic correction of bimaxillary protrusion. J. Maxillofac. Surg., *1*:7, 1973.

Converse, J. M., and Shapiro, H. H.: Treatment of developmental malformations of the jaws. Plast. Reconstr. Surg., *10*:473, 1952.

Converse, J. M., and Shapiro, H. H.: Bone grafting malformations of the jaws; cephalographic diagnosis in the surgical treatment of malformations of the face. Am. J. Surg., *8*:858, 1954.

Converse, J. M., and Smith, B.: Reconstruction of the floor of the orbit by bone grafts. Arch. Ophthalmol., *44*:1, 1950a.

Converse, J. M., and Smith, B.: Case of reconstruction of the maxilla following resection for carcinoma of the antrum. Plast. Reconstr. Surg., *5*:426, 1950b.

Converse, J. M., and Waknitz, F. W.: External skeletal fixation in fractures of the mandibular angle. J. Bone Joint Surg., *24*:154, 1942.

Converse, J. M., and Wood-Smith, D.: Horizontal osteotomy of the mandible. Plast. Reconstr. Surg., *34*:464, 1964.

Converse, J. M., Horowitz, S. L., Guy, C. L., and Wood-Smith, D.: Surgical and orthodontic procedures in bilateral cleft lip and cleft palate. Cleft Palate J., *1*:153, 1964a.

Converse, J. M., Horowitz, S. L., and Wood-Smith, D.: Deformities of the jaws. In Converse, J. M. (Ed.): Reconstructive Plastic Surgery. Philadelphia, W. B. Saunders Company, 1964b, pp. 869–947.

Converse, J. M., Horowitz, S. L., Valauri, A. J., and Montandon, D.: The treatment of nasomaxillary hypoplasia. A new pyramidal naso-orbito-maxillary osteotomy. Plast. Reconstr. Surg., *45*:527, 1970.

Converse, J. M., Horowitz, S. L., Coccaro, P. I., and Wood-Smith, D.: The corrective treatment of the skeletal asymmetry in hemifacial microsomia. Plast. Reconst., Surg., *52*:221, 1973.

Cotton, W. A., Takano, W. S., and Wong, W. M. W.: The Downs analysis applied to other ethnic groups. Angle Orthodont., *21*:213, 1951.

Crockford, D. A., and Converse, J. M.: The ilium as a source of bone grafts in children. Plast. Reconstr. Surg., *50*:270, 1972.

Cryer, M. H.: Studies of anterior and posterior occlusion. Dent. Cosmos, *55*:683, 1913.

Cunat, J. J., and Gargiulo, E. A.: Changes in mandibular morphology after surgical correction of prognathism: Report of case. J. Oral Surg., *31*:694, 1973.

Cupar, I.: Die chirurgische Behandlung der Formund Stellungs-veränderung des Oberkiefers. Österr, Z. Stomatol., *51*:565, 1954.

Dal Pont, G.: L'osteotomie retromolare per la correzione della progenia. Minerva Chir., *14*:1138, 1959.

Dal Pont, G.: Retromolar osteotomy for correction of prognathism. J. Oral Surg., *19*:42, 1961.

Dautrey, J.: Personal communication, 1975.

Dautrey, J., and Pepersack, W.: Le traitement chirurgical de la proalvéolie supérieure. Acta Stomatol. Belg., *68*:335, 1971.

Delagénière, H.: Les greffes ostéoperiostiques prises au tibia. Bull. Mém. Soc. Chir. Paris, *42*:1048, 1916.

Dingman, R. O.: Surgical correction of mandibular prognathism; an improved method. Am. J. Orthod. Oral Surg., *30*:683, 1944.

Dingman, R. O., and Grabb, W. C.: Surgical anatomy of mandibular ramus of the facial nerve based on the dissection of 100 facial halves. Plast. Reconstr. Surg., *29*:266, 1962.

Dingman, R. O., and Grabb, W. C.: Reconstruction of both mandibular condyles with metatarsal bone grafts. Plast. Reconstr. Surg., *34*:441, 1964.

Dingman, R. O., and Harding, R. L.: Treatment of malunion fractures of facial bones. Plast. Reconstr. Surg., *7*:505, 1951.

Downs, W. B.: Variations in facial relationships; their significance in treatment and prognosis. Am. J. Orthod., *34*:812, 1948.

DuBouchet, C. W.: New method of bone grafting for pseudoarthrosis of the mandible. Bull. Mém. Soc. Chir. Paris, *43*:1328, 1917.

Dufourmentel, L.: Essai de reconstitution totale du massif maxillaire inférieur, Restaur. Maxillofac., *3*:141, 1919.

Dufourmentel, L.: Le traitement chirurgical du prognathisme. Presse Méd., *29*:235, 1921.

Dupont, C., Ciaburro, H., and Prévost, Y.: Simplifying the Le Fort I type of maxillary osteotomy. Plast. Reconstr. Surg., *54*:142, 1974.

Edgerton, M. T., Ward, A. E., and Sikes, T. E.: Fixation and plastic repair after partial mandibular resection. Plast. Reconstr. Surg., *5*:231, 1950.

Egyedi, P.: Evaluation of operations for mandibular protrusion. Oral Surg., *19*:451, 1965.

von Eiselsberg, A.: Ueber Plastic bei Ectropium des Unterkiefers (Progenie). Wien. Klin. Wochenschr., *19*:1505, 1906.

Entin, M. A.: Reconstruction in congenital deformity of temporomandibular component. Plast. Reconstr. Surg., *21*:461, 1958.

Esser, J. F.: Studies in plastic surgery of the face. Ann. Surg., *65*:297, 1917.

Figi, F. A.: Plastic repair after removal of extensive malignancy of the antrum. Arch. Otolaryngol., *28*:29, 1938.

Firmin, F., Coccaro, P. J., and Converse, J. M.: Cephalometric analysis in diagnosis and treatment planning of craniofacial dysostoses. Plast. Reconstr. Surg., *54*:300, 1974.

Fleming, I. D., and Morris, J. H.: Use of acrylic external splint after mandibular resection. Am. J. Surg., *118*:708, 1969.

Friedland, J. A., Coccaro, P. J., and Converse, J. M.: Retrospective cephalometric analysis of mandibular bone absorption under silicone rubber chin implants. Plast. Reconstr. Surg., *57*:144, 1976.

Fromm, B., and Lundberg, M.: Postural behaviour of the hyoid bone in normal occlusion and before and after surgical correction of mandibular protrusion. Sven. Tandklak. Tidskr., *63*:425, 1970.

Fry, H. J. H.: Reconstruction of the mandible from angle to angle. Paper read at the Sixth International Congress of Plastic and Reconstructive Surgery, Paris, France, August, 1975.

Georgiade, N. G., and Quinn, G. W.: Newer concepts in surgical correction of mandibular prognathism. Plast. Reconstr. Surg., *27*:185, 1961.

Gillies, H. D.: Plastic Surgery of the Face. London, Oxford University Press, 1920.

Gillies, H. D., and Millard, D. R., Jr.: Principles and Art of Plastic Surgery. Boston, Little, Brown & Company, 1957.

Gillies, H. D., and Rowe, N. L.: L'ostéotomie du maxillaire supérieur envisagée essentiellement dans les cas de bec-de-lièvre total. Rev. Stomatol., *55*:545, 1954.

Ginestet, G., Frezières, H., and Merville, L.: La correction chirurgicale de l'hypertrophie du masseter. Ann. Chir. Plast., *4*:187, 1959.

Glahn, M., and Winther, J. E.: Correction of unilateral mandibular hypoplasia due to early loss of mandibular condyle. Acta Chir. Scand., *129*:312, 1965.

Goldberg, M. H., Marco, W., and Googel, F.: Parotid fistula: A complication of mandibular osteotomy. J. Oral Surg., *31*:207, 1973.

Gonzalez-Ulloa, M.: Temporomandibular arthroplasty in the treatment of prognathism. Plast. Reconstr. Surg., *8*:136, 1951.

Gonzalez-Ulloa, M., and Stevens, E.: The role of chin correction in profileplasty. Plast. Reconstr. Surg., *41*:477, 1968.

Grabb, W. C.: The Habsburg jaw. Plast. Reconstr. Surg., *42*:442, 1968.

Grant, J. C. B.: An Atlas of Anatomy. Baltimore, The Williams & Wilkins Company, 1951.

Gruca, A., and Meiselles, F.: Asymmetry of the mandible from unilateral hypertrophy. Ann. Surg., *83*:755, 1926.

Guernsey, L. H., and De Champlain, R. W.: Sequelae and complications of the intraoral sagittal osteotomy in the mandibular rami. Oral Surg., *32*:176, 1971.

Guggenheim, P., and Cohen, L. B.: External hyperostosis of the mandible angle associated with masseteric hypertrophy. Arch. Ortolaryngol., *70*:674, 1959.

Guggenheim, P., and Cohen, L. B.: The histopathology of masseteric hypertrophy. Arch. Orolaryngol., *71*:906, 1960.

Guggenheim, P., and Cohen, L. B.: The nature of masseteric hypertrophy. Arch. Otolaryngol., *73*:15, 1961.

Guilford, J. P.: Psychometric Methods. New York, McGraw-Hill, 1954.

Gurney, C. E.: Chronic bilateral benign hypertrophy of the masseter muscles. Am. J. Surg., *73*:137, 1947.

Hall, H. D., and O'Steen, A. N.: Free grafts of palatal mucosa in mandibular vestibuloplasty. J. Oral Surg., *28*:565, 1970.

Hambleton, R. S.: The soft-tissue covering of the skeletal face as related to orthodontic problems. Am. J. Orthod., *50*:405, 1964.

Harii, K., Ohmori, K., and Ohmori, S.: Successful clinical transfer of ten free flaps by microvascular anastomoses. Plast. Reconstr. Surg., *53*:259, 1974.

Harsha, W. M.: Prognathism with operative treatment. J.A.M.A., *59*:2035, 1912.

Hausamen, J. E., Samii, M., and Schmidseder, R.: Repair of the mandibular nerve by means of nerve grafting after resection of the lower jaw. J. Maxillofac. Surg., *1*:74, 1973.

Hayes, P. A.: Correction of retrognathia by modified "C" osteotomy of the ramus and sagittal osteotomy of the mandibular body. J. Oral Surg., *31*:682, 1973.

Heiss, J.: Ueber die chirurgische Unterstuetzung der Dehnung im comprimierten Oberkiefer. Dtsch. Zahnärztebl., *8*:560, 1934.

Hellman, M.: An introduction to growth of the human face from infancy to adulthood. Int. J. Orthod., *18*:777, 1932.

Henderson, D.: The assessment and management of bony deformities of the middle and lower face. Br. J. Plast. Surg., *27*:287, 1974.

Henderson, D., and Jackson, I. T.: Naso-maxillary hypoplasia—the Le Fort II osteotomy. Br. J. Oral Surg., *11*:77, 1973.

Herbert, J. M., Kent, J. N., and Hinds, E. C.: Correction of prognathism by an intraoral vertical subcondylar osteotomy. J. Oral Surg., *28*:651, 1970.

Hinds, E. C.: Surgical correction of acquired mandibular deformities. Am. J. Orthod., *43*:161, 1957.

Hinds, E. C., and Girotti, W.: Vertical subcondylar osteotomy: A reappraisal. Oral Surg., *24*:164, 1967.

Hinds, E. C., and Kent, J. N.: Surgical Treatment of Developmental Jaw Deformities. St. Louis, Mo., C. V. Mosby Company, 1972.

Hofer, O.: Operation der Prognathie und Microgenie. Dtsch. Zahn. Mund. Kieferheilkd., *9*:121, 1942.

Hogeman, K. E.: Surgical-orthopaedic correction of mandibular protrusion. Acta Chir. Scand., Suppl. 159, 1951.

Hogeman, K. E., and Sarnäs, K. V.: Surgical and dental-orthopedic correction of maxillary protrusion or Angle Class II, division 1 malocclusion. Scand. J. Plast. Surg., *1*:101, 1967.

Hogeman, K. E., and Willmar, K.: Die Vorverlagerund

des Oberkiefers zut Korrektur von Gebissanomalien. Fortschr. Kiefer. Gesichtschir., *12*:275, 1967.

Horowitz, S. L., Gerstman, L. J., and Converse, J. M.: Craniofacial relationships in mandibular prognathism. Arch. Oral Biol., *14*:121, 1969.

Hovell, J. H.: Surgical correction of facial deformities. Ann. R. Coll. Surg. Engl., *46*:92, 1970.

Hullihen, S. P.: Case of elongation of the under jaw and distortion of the face and neck, caused by a burn, successfully treated. Am. J. Dent. Soc., *9*:157, 1849.

Hunsuck, E. E.: A modified intraoral sagittal technic for correction of mandibular prognathism. Oral Surg., *26*:249, 1968.

Hunter, J.: Works of John Hunter (with notes by James F. Palmer). London, Longman, Rees, Orme, Brown, Breen and Longman, 1835–1837.

Hutchinson, D., and MacGregor, A.: Tooth survival following various methods of sub-apical osteotomy. Int. J. Oral Surg., *29*:256, 1969.

Imbert, L., and Réal, P.: Le traitement chirurgical des pseudoarthroses du maxillaire inférieur. Marseille Med., *53*:193, 1916.

Inclan, A.: Use of preserved bone grafts in orthopedic surgery. J. Bone Joint Surg., *24*:81, 1942.

Ivy, R. H.: Extensive loss of substance of mandible due to removal of sarcoma, replaced by bone graft from crest of ilium. Int. J. Orthod., *7*:483, 1921.

Ivy, R. H.: Benign bony enlargement of the condyloid process of the mandible. Ann. Surg., *85*:27, 1927.

Ivy, R. H.: Bone grafting for restoration of defects of mandible, collective review. Plast. Reconstr. Surg., *7*:333, 1951.

Ivy, R. H., and Eby, J. D.: Thirty-nine and 38 year followups of mandibular bone grafts in three cases. Plast. Reconstr. Surg., *22*:548, 1958.

Ivy, R. H.: Iliac bone graft to bridge a mandibular defect. 49-year clinical and radiological follow-up. Plast. Reconstr. Surg., *50*:483, 1972.

Jaboulay, M.: Les effets de la resection des condyles du maxillaire inférieur sur la situation de la rangée dentaire et la forme du menton. Lyon Med., *75*:519, 1895.

Jackson, D.: Lip positions and incisor relationships. Br. Dent. J., *112*:147, 1962.

Jacobsen, P. U., and Lund, K.: Unilateral overgrowth and remodeling processes after fracture of the mandibular condyle: A longitudinal radiographic study. Scand. J. Dent. Res., *80*:68, 1972.

Johnson, J. V., and Hinds, E. C.: Evaluation of teeth vitality after subapical osteotomy. J. Oral Surg., *27*:256, 1969.

Kazanjian, V. H.: The treatment of gunshot wounds of the face accompanied by extensive destruction of the lower lip and mandible. Br. J. Surg., *5*:74, 1918.

Kazanjian, V. H.: Jaw reconstruction. Am. J. Surg., *43*:249, 1939.

Kazanjian, V. H.: *In* Kazanjian, V. H., and Converse, J. M.: The Surgical Treatment of Facial Injuries. 1st. ed. Baltimore, The Williams & Wilkins Company, 1949.

Kazanjian, V. H.: Bone transplanting of the mandible. Am. J. Surg., *83*:633, 1952.

Kazanjian, V. H.: The surgical treatment of prognathism: An analysis of 65 cases. Am. J. Surg., *87*:691, 1954.

Kazanjian, V. H.: Bilateral absence of the ascending rami of the mandible. Br. J. Plast. Surg., *9*:77, 1956.

Kazanjian, V. H., and Burrows, H.: Treatment of maxillary fractures. Br. Dent. J., *37*:126, 1917–1918.

Kazanjian, V. H., and Converse, J. M.: Intraoral approach. *In* Kazanjian, V. H., and Converse, J. M.: The Surgical Treatment of Facial Injuries. 2nd ed. Baltimore, The Williams & Wilkins Company, 1959, pp. 838–866.

Kazanjian, V. H., and Converse, J. M.: Open-bite deformities of the jaw. *In* Kazanjian, V. H., and Converse, J. M.: Surgical Treatment of Facial Injuries. 3rd ed. Baltimore, The Williams & Wilkins Company, 1974a, p. 1118.

Kazanjian, V. H., and Converse, J. M.: Intraoral approach. *In* Kazanjian, V. H., and Converse, J. M.: Surgical Treatment of Facial Injuries. 3rd ed. Baltimore, The Williams & Wilkins Company, 1974b, p. 1022.

Kelsey, C. C.: Radiographic cephalometric study of surgically corrected mandibular prognathism. J. Oral Surg., *26*:239, 1968.

Kent, J. N., and Hinds, E. C.: Management of dental facial deformities by anterior alveolar surgery. J. Oral Surg., *29*:13, 1971.

Ketchum, L. D., Masters, F. W., and Robinson, D. W.: Mandibular reconstruction using a composite island rib flap. Plast. Reconstr. Surg., *53*:471, 1974.

Klapp, R., and Schroeder, H.: Die Unterkieferschussbruche. Berlin, Hermann Meusser, 1917.

Knize, D. M.: The influence of periosteum and calcitonin on onlay bone graft survival. Plast. Reconstr. Surg., *53*:190, 1974.

Knowles, C. D.: Changes in the profile following surgical reduction of mandibular prognathism. Br. J. Plast. Surg., *18*:432, 1965.

Koblin, I., and Reil, B.: Die Sensibilität der Unterlippe nach Schonung bzw. Durchtrennung des Nervus alveolar mandibularis bei Progenie Operationen. Vortag auf der XII Jahrestagung der Deutschen Gesellschaft für Kiefer-und Gesichtschirurgie in Berlin, *24*:27, 1972.

Köle, H.: Surgical operations on the alveolar ridge to correct occlusal abnormalities. Oral Surg., *12*:277, 413, 515, 1959a.

Köle, H.: Nouvelles interventions chirurgicales à la hauteur du processus alveolaire en vue de la correction des malformations de l'arcade et des malpositions dentaires. Rev. Belg. Stomatol., *56*:247, 1959b.

Kopp, W. K.: Auriculotemporal syndrome secondary to vertical sliding osteotomy of the mandibular rami: Repair of case. J. Oral Surg., *26*:295, 1968.

Kostečka, F.: Surgical correction of protrusion of the lower and upper jaws. J. Am. Dent. Assoc., *15*:362, 1928.

Krause, F.: Unterfiefer Plastik. Zentralbl. Chir., *34*:1045, 1907.

Kufner, J.: Experience with a modified procedure for correction of open bite. Transaction of the Third International Conference of Oral Surgery. London, E. & S. Livingstone, 1968.

Lane, W. A.: Cleft Palate and Hare Lip. London, London Medical Publishing Company, Ltd., 1905.

Leake, D. L.: Mandibular reconstruction with a new type of alloplastic tray: A preliminary report. J. Oral Surg., *32*:23, 1974.

LeFort, P.: Etude expérimentale sur les fractures de la machoire supérieure. Rev. Chir., *23*:208, 360, 479, 1901.

Legg, W.: Enlargement of the temporal and masseter muscles on both sides. Trans. Pathol. Soc. London, *31*:361, 1880.

Leibold, D. G., Tilson, H. B., and Rask, K. R.: A subjective evaluation of the re-establishment of the neurovascular supply of teeth involved in anterior maxillary osteotomy procedures. J. Oral Surg., *32*:531, 1971.

Lemaitre, F., and Ponroy, J.: Greffes du maxillaire inférieur. Rev. Stomatol., *18*:260, 1920.

Lévignac, J.: Traitement d'un enforcement consolidé du tiers moyen de la face par osteotomies et greffes d'os. Rev. Stomatol., *59*:551, 1958.

Limberg, A. A.: Treatment of open-bite by means of plastic oblique osteotomy of the ascending rami of the mandible. Dent. Cosmos, *67*:1191, 1925.

Limberg, A. A.: A new method of plastic lengthening of the mandible in unilateral microgenia and asymmetry of the face. J. Am. Dent. Assoc., *15*:851, 1928.

Lindegård, B.: Variations in human body-build. Acta Psychiatr. Neurol. Scand., Suppl. 86, 1953.

Lindemann, A.: Bruhn's Ergebnisse aus dem Dusseldorfer Lazarett, Behandlungen der Kieferschussverletzungen. Weisbaden, 1916, p. 243.

Longacre, J. J.: Surgical correction of extensive defects of scalp and cranium with autogenous tissues. Internatl. Soc. Plastic Surgeons, 1st Congress, Stockholm, 1955. Baltimore, The Williams & Wilkins Company, 1957.

Longacre, J. J., and DeStefano, G. A.: Further observations of the behavior of autogenous split-rib grafts in reconstruction of extensive defects of the cranium and face. Plast. Reconstr. Surg., *20*:281, 1957.

Lund, K., and Jacobsen, P. U.: Overgrowth of a hypoplastic mandibular ramus after autoplastic bone grafting: An 18-year longitudinal radiographic study, using metallic implants. Tandlaegebladet, *75*:1279, 1971.

McCullough, D. W., and Fredrickson, J. M.: Neovascularized rib grafts to reconstruct mandibular defects. Can. J. Otolaryngol., *2*:96, 1973.

McEvitt, W. G.: Conversion of an inferiorly based pharyngeal flap to a superiorly based position. Plast. Reconstr. Surg., *48*:36, 1971.

McKee, D.: Microvascular rib transposition for reconstruction of the mandible. Presented at the Annual Meeting of the American Society of Plastic and Reconstructive Surgeons, Montreal, Canada, 1971.

McNeill, R. W., Hooley, J. R., and Sundberg, R. J.: Skeletal relapse during intermaxillary fixation. J. Oral Surg., *31*:212, 1973.

McNichol, J. W., and Rogers, A. T.: An original method of correction of hyperplastic asymmetry of the mandible. Plast. Reconstr. Surg., *1*:288, 1945.

Madritsch, E.: Spätergebnisse nach Korrektur von Dysgnathien und Zahnstellungsanomalien durch Alveolarfortsatzbewegungen und Kortikotomien. Dissertation, University of Zürich, 1968.

Manchester, W. M.: Immediate reconstruction of the mandible and temporomandibular joint. Br. J. Plast. Surg., *18*:291, 1965.

Markowitz, A.: The use of homogenous bone grafts in mandibular reconstruction. Am. J. Surg., *96*:755, 1958.

Mårtensson, G.: Dental injuries following radical surgery on the maxillary sinus. Acta Otolaryngol., Suppl. 84, 1950.

Martin, C.: De la prothèse immédiate, appliquée à la résection des maxillaires; rhinoplastie sur appareil prothétique permanent; restauration de la face, lèvres, nez, langue, voûte et voile du palais. Paris, Masson et Cie, 1889.

Massey, G. B., Chase, D. C., Thomas, P. M., and Kohn, M. W.: Intraoral oblique osteotomy of the mandibular ramus. J. Oral Surg., *32*:755, 1974.

Mayer, R.: Le traitement chirurgical de la prognathie mandibulaire. Acta Stomatol. Belg., *68*:383, 1971.

Meredith, H. V.: Changes in the profile of the osseous chin during childhood. Am. J. Phys. Anthrop., *15*:247, 1957.

Merrifield, L. L.: Profile line as an aid in critically evaluating facial esthetics. Am. J. Orthod., *52*:804, 1966.

Merville, L. C.: The choice of the procedure in surgical correction of mandibular prognathia. *In* Walker, R. V. (Ed.): Transactions of the 3rd International Conference on Oral Surgery. London, E. & S. Livingstone, 1970.

Moore, F. F., and Ward, F. G.: Complications and sequelae of untreated fractures of the facial bones and their treatment. Br. J. Plast. Surg., *1*:262, 1949.

Moose, S. M.: Correction of abnormal mandibular protrusion by intraoral operation. J. Oral Surg., *3*:304, 1945.

Morgan, L. R., and Thompson, C. W.: Mandibular reconstruction. Clinics in Plastic Surgery, 2:561, 1975.

Morgan, L. R., Gallegos, L. T., and Frileck, S. P.: Mandibular vestibuloplasty with a free graft of the mucoperiosteal layer from the hard palate. Plast. Reconstr. Surg., *51*:359, 1973.

Morris, J. H.: Biphase connector, external skeletal splint for reduction and fixation of mandibular fractures. Oral Surg., *2*:1382, 1949.

Moss, M. L.: Functional analysis of human mandibular growth. J. Prosthet. Dent., *10*:1149, 1960.

Mowlem, R.: Cancellous chip bone grafts; report of 75 cases. Lancet, 2:746, 1944.

Murray, J.: Personal communication, 1976.

Neuner, O.: Chirurgische Orthodontie. Schweiz. Monatsschr. Zahnkeilkd., *75*:940, 1965.

Neuner, O.: Surgical correction of mandibular prognathism. Oral Surg., Oral Med., Oral Path., *42*:415, 1976.

New, G. B., and Erich, J. B.: The surgical correction of mandibular prognathism. Am. J. Surg., *53*:2, 1941.

Niederdellmann, H., and Dieckmann, J.: Neurologiache Storungen nach Chirurgischer Korrektur der Progenie und Mikrogenie. Fortschr. Kiefer. Gesichtschir., *18*:186, 1974.

Nordendram, Å., and Waller, Å.: Oral-surgical correction of mandibular protrusion. Br. J. Oral Surg., *6*:64, 1968.

Obwegeser, H. L.: *In* Trauner, R., and Obwegeser, H. L.: The surgical correction of mandibular prognathism and retrognathia with consideration of genioplasty. I. Surgical procedures to correct mandibular prognathism and reshaping of the chin. Oral Surg., *10*:677, 1957.

Obwegeser, H. L.: Surgical preparation of the maxilla for prosthesis. J. Oral Surg., *22*:127, 1964.

Obwegeser, H. L.: Surgical correction of small or retrodisplaced maxilla; the "dish-face" deformity. Plast. Reconstr. Surg., *43*:351, 1969.

Obwegeser, H. L.: Late reconstruction of large maxillary defects after tumor resection. J. Maxillofac. Surg., *1*:19, 1973.

Ollier, L.: Récherches éxperimentales sur les greffes osseuses. J. Physiol., *3*:88, 1860.

Ollier, L.: Traité experimental et clinique de la regénération des os et de la production artificielle du tissue osseux. Paris, V. Masson & Fils, 1867.

Oppenheim, H., and Wing, M.: Benign hypertrophy of the masseter muscle. Arch. Otolaryngol., *70*:207, 1959.

Osborne, R.: The treatment of the underdeveloped ascending ramus. Br. J. Plast. Surg., *17*:376, 1964.

Östrup, L. T., and Fredrickson, J. M.: Distant transfer of free living bone graft by microvascular anastomoses. An experimental study. Plast. Reconstr. Surg., *54*:274, 1974.

Östrup, L. T., and Fredrickson, J. M.: Reconstruction of mandibular defects after radiation, using a free living bone graft transferred by microvascular anastomoses. An experimental study. Plast. Reconstr. Surg., *55*:563, 1975.

Owsley, J. Q., Creech, B. J., and Dedo, H. H.: Poor speech following the pharyngeal flap operation; etiology and treatment. Cleft Palate J., *9*:312, 1972.

Parnes, E. T., and Becker, M. L.: Necrosis of the anterior maxilla following osteotomy. Oral Surg., *33*:326, 1972.

Partsch: Prosthesis of lower jaw after resection. Arch. Klin. Chir., *55*:746, 1897.

Peck, H., and Peck, S.: A concept of facial esthetics. Angle Orthod., *40*:284, 1970.

Pepersack, W. J.: Tooth vitality after alveolar segmental osteotomy. J. Maxillofac. Surg., *1*:85, 1973.

Pepersack, W. J., and Chausse, J. M.: Long term follow up for the correction of prognathism by sagittal split osteotomy. Second Congress, European Association for Maxillofacial Surgery, Zurich, Sept. 16–21, 1974.

Pichler, H.: Unterkieferresektion wegen Progenie. Z. Stomatol., *16*:190, 1918.

Pichler, H., and Trauner, R.: Lehrbuch der Mund- und Kiefer-chirurgie. Wien, Urban and Schwarzenberg, 1948.

Pickrell, H. P.: Double resection of the mandible. Dent. Cosmos, *54*:1114, 1912.

Pike, R. L., and Boyne, P. J.: Composite autogenous marrow and surface decalcified implants in mandibular defects. J. Oral Surg., *31*:905, 1973.

Pike, R. L., and Boyne, P. J.: Use of surface decalcified allogeneic bone and autogenous marrow in extensive mandibular defects. J. Oral Surg., *32*:177, 1974.

Poswillo, D. E.: Early pulp changes following reduction of open bite by segmental surgery. Int. J. Oral Surg., *1*:87, 1972.

Poulton, D. R., and Ware, W. H.: Surgical-orthodontic treatment of severe mandibular retrusion (part II). Am. J. Orthod., *63*:237, 1973.

Poulton, D. R., Taylor, R. C., and Ware, W. H.: Cephalometric x-ray evaluation of the vertical osteotomy correction of mandibular prognathism. Oral Surg., *16*:807, 1963.

Psillakis, J. M., Lapa, F., and Spina, V.: Surgical correction of midfacial retrusion (nasomaxillary hypoplasia) in the presence of normal dental occlusion. Plast. Reconstr. Surg., *51*:67, 1973.

Ragnell, A.: Der Moderna Plastikkirurgien' inklusive den Kosmetiska Kirurgien, dess verksamhetsfalt och arbetsmethoder. Nord. Med. Tidskr., *15*:361, 1943.

Rehrmann, A.: Beitrag zur Alveolarkammplastik am Unterkiefer. Zahnaerztl. Rdsch., *62*:505, 1953.

Reidy, J. B.: Homogenous bone grafts. Br. J. Plast. Surg., *9*:89, 1956.

Ricketts, R.: Planning treatment on the basis of the facial pattern and on estimate of its growth. Angle Orthod., *27*:14, 1957.

Riedel, R. A.: An analysis of dentofacial relationships. Am. J. Orthod., *43*:103, 1957.

Robinson, M.: Prognathism corrected by open vertical condylotomy. J. South. Calif. Dent. Assoc., *24*:22, 1956.

Robinson, M.: Micrognathism corrected by vertical osteotomy of ascending ramus and iliac bone graft. Oral Surg., *10*:1125, 1957.

Robinson, M., and Lytle, J. J.: Micrognathism corrected by vertical osteotomies of the rami without bone grafts. Oral Surg., *15*:641, 1962.

Robinson, M., and Shuken, R.: Bone resorption under plastic chin implants. J. Oral Surg., *27*:116, 1969.

Robinson, M., Shuken, R., and Dougherty, H.: Surgical orthodontic treatment of hemigigantism; report of case. Oral Surg., *27*:744, 1969.

Rontal, E., and Hohmann, A.: Lateral alveolomaxillary osteotomies. Arch. Otolaryngol., *95*:18, 1972.

Rowe, N. H.: Hemifacial hypertrophy. Oral Surg., *15*:572, 1962.

Rusconi, L., Brusati, R., and Bottoli, V.: Indagini elettromiografiche sull'equilibrio muscolare post'operatorio nel trattamento chirurgico del progenismo secondo la techica di Obwegeser-Dal Pont. Riv. Ital. Stomatol., *25*:9, 1970.

Rushton, M. A.: Malformation of the mandibular ramus treated by bone graft. Dent. Rec., *62*:272, 1942.

Rushton, M. A.: Growth of mandibular condyle in relation to some deformities. Br. Dent. J., *76*:57, 1944.

Rydigier, L. R.: Zum osteoplastistischen Ersatz nach Unterkieferresektion. Zentralbl. Chir., *35*:1321, 1908.

Salzmann, J. A.: Practice of Orthodontics. Philadelphia, J. B. Lippincott Company, 1966.

Sanborn, R. T.: Differences between the facial skeletal patterns of class III malocclusion and normal occlusion. Angle Orthod., *25*:208, 1955.

Sarnäs, K. V.: Inter- and intra-family variations in the facial profile. Odontol. Revy, *10*(Suppl. 4), 1959.

Sarnäs, K. V.: The adult facial profile. A radiographic study of 317 male and female students aged 19–23 years. Unpublished data, 1973.

Sassouni, V.: A classification of skeletal facial types. Am. J. Orthod., *55*:109, 1969.

Schmid, E.: Ueber neue Wege in der plastichen Chirurgie der Nase. Beitr. Klin. Chir., *184*:385, 1952.

Schuchardt, K.: Ein Beitrag zur chirurgischen Kieferorthopädie unter Berücksichtigung ihrer Bedeutung für die Behandlung angeborener und erworbener Kieferdeformitäten bei Soldaten. Dtsch. Zahn. Mund. Kieferheilk., *9*:73, 1942.

Schuchardt, K.: *In* Bier, Braun, and Kümmel (Eds.): Chirurgisch Operationslehre, Leipzig, 1954. Johann Ambrosius Barth, Bd. II. Operationen im Gesicht-Kieferbereich, 1954a.

Schuchardt, K.: Die Chirurgie als Helferin der Kieferorthopädie. Fortschr. Kieferorthop., *15*:1, 1954b.

Schuchardt, K.: Formen des offen Bisses und ihre Operativen. Behandlungsmoglichkeiten. Fortschr. Kiefer. Gesichtschir., *1*:22, 1955.

Schuchardt, K.: Erfahrungen bei der Behandlung der Mikrogenie. Langenbecks Arch. Klin. Chir., *289*:651, 1958.

Schuchardt, K.: Personal communication, 1963.

Schwartz, M. F.: The acoustics of normal and nasal vowel production. Cleft Palate J., *5*:125, 1968.

Schwartz, M. F.: Personal communication, 1976.

Scudder, C. L.: Tumors of the jaws. Philadelphia, W. B. Saunders Company, 1912.

Seward, G. J.: Replacement of the anterior part of the mandible by bone graft. J. Maxillofac. Surg., *2*:168, 1974.

Smith, A. E., and Chambers, F. W.: Mandibular prognathism corrected by newly devised osteotomy of the ramus. J. Am. Dent. Assoc., *64*:328, 1962.

Smith, A. E., and Robinson, M.: Surgical correction of mandibular prognathism by subsigmoid notch ostectomy with sliding condylotomy: A new technic. J. Am. Dent. Assoc., *49*:46, 1954.

Snyder, C. C., Bateman, J. M., Davis, C. W., and Warden, G. D.: Mandibulo-facial restoration with live osteocutaneous flaps. Plast. Reconstr. Surg., *45*:14, 1970.

Snyder, C. C., Levine, G. A., Swanson, H. M., and Browne, E. Z.: Mandibular lengthening by gradual distraction. A preliminary report. Plast. Reconstr. Surg., *51*:506, 1973.

Snyder, G.: Personal communication, 1975.

Soderberg, B. N., Jennings, H. B., and McNelly, J. E.: Restoration of the jaw. U.S. Armed Forces Med. J., *3*:1423, 1952.

Solow, B.: The pattern of craniofacial associations. Acta Odontol. Scand., 24(Suppl. 46), 1966.

Spanier, F.: Prognathie-Operationen. Z. Zahnärztl. Orthop. (München), 24:76, 1932.

Steiner, C. C.: Cephalometrics for you and me. Am. J. Orthod., 39:729, 1953.

Steinhauser, E. W.: Free transportation of oral mucosa for improvement of denture retention. J. Oral Surg., 27:955, 1969.

Steinhauser, E. W.: Vestibuloplasty-skin grafts. J. Oral Surg., 29:777, 1971.

Steinhauser, E. W.: Midline splitting of the maxilla for correction of malocclusion. J. Oral Surg., 30:413, 1972.

Steinhauser, E. W.: Advancement of the mandible by sagittal ramus split and suprahyoid myotomy. J. Oral Surg., 31:516, 1973.

Strauch, B., Bromberg, A., and Lewin, M. L.: Artery island composite rib grafts for mandibular replacement. Surg. Forum, 20:516, 1969.

Stuteville, O. H.: Surgical reconstruction of the mandible. Plast. Reconstr. Surg., 19:229, 1957.

Stuteville, O. H., and Lanfranchi, R. P.: Surgical reconstruction of the temporomandibular joint. Am. J. Surg., 90:940, 1955.

Swanson, L. T., Habal, M. B., Leake, D. L., and Murray, J. E.: Compound silicone-bone implants for mandibular reconstruction: Development and application. Plast. Reconstr. Surg., 51:402, 1973.

Sykoff, V.: Zur Frage der Knocken-Plastic am Unterkiefer. Zentralbl. Chir., 27:881, 1900.

Takagi, Y., Gamble, J. W., Proffit, W. R., and Christiansen, R. L.: Postural change of the hyoid bone following osteotomy of the mandible. Oral Surg., 23:687, 1967.

Thoma, K. H.: Oral Surgery. Vol. 2. St. Louis, Mo., C. V. Mosby Company, 1948, p. 1438.

Thompson, N., and Casson, J. A.: Experimental onlay bone grafts to the jaw—A preliminary study in dogs. Plast. Reconstr. Surg., 46:341, 1970.

Toman, J.: Le traitement chirurgical de la progénie par la méthode d'inlay ostectomie. Rev. Stomatol., 67:551, 1966.

Trauner, R.: Alveoloplasty with ridge extensions on the lingual side of the lower jaw to solve the problem of a lower dental prosthesis. J. Oral Surg., 5:340, 1952.

Trauner, R.: The surgical correction of mandibular prognathism and retrognathia with consideration of genioplasty. Part II. Operating methods for microgenia and distoclusion. B. Distoclusion. Oral Surg., 10:899, 1957.

Tweed, C. H.: The Frankfort-mandibular plane angle in orthodontic diagnosis, classification, treatment planning and prognosis. Am. J. Orthod., 32:175, 1946.

Ullik, R.: Erweiterte Osteotomi des Oberkiefers. Osterr. Z. Stomatol., 4:122, 1970.

Urist, M. R.: Surface decalcified allogenic implants. Clin. Orthop., 56:37, 1968.

Van Zile, W. N.: Triangular ostectomy of the vertical rami, another technique for correction of prognathism. Oral Surg., 21:3, 1963.

Waldhart, E., and Lynch, J. B.: Benign hypertrophy of the masseter muscles and mandibular angles. Arch. Surg., 102:115, 1971.

Waldron, C. W., and Risdon, R.: Mandibular bone grafts. Proc. R. Soc. Med., 12:11, 1919.

Walsh, T. S., Jr.: Buried metallic prosthesis for mandibular defects. Cancer, 7:1002, 1954.

Ware, W. A., and Taylor, R. C.: Condylar repositioning following osteotomies for correction of mandibular prognathism. Am. J. Orthod., 54:50, 1968.

Ware, W. H., and Ashamalla, M.: Pulpal response following anterior maxillary osteotomy. Am. J. Orthod., 60:156, 1971.

Warren, D. W.: Velopharyngeal orifice size and upper pharyngeal pressure-flow patterns in normal speech. Plast. Reconstr. Surg., 33:148, 1964.

Warren, D. W., and Ryan, V. E.: Oral port constriction, nasal resistance, and respiratory aspects of cleft palate speech: An analog study. Cleft Palate J., 4:38, 1967.

Wassmund, M.: Fracturen und Luxationen des Gesichtschadels unter Beruksichtigung der Komplikationen des Hirnschadesl. In Klinik und Therapie. Praktischen Lehrbuch. Vol. 20. Berlin, Hermann Meusser, 1927, p. 384.

Wassmund, M.: Lehrbuch der praktischen Chirurgie des Mundes und der Kiefer. Bd. 1, 260, 282, Berlin, Hermann Meusser, 1935.

Weber, J., Jr., Chase, R. A., and Jobe, R. P.: The restrictive pharyngeal flap. Br. J. Plast. Surg., 23:347, 1970.

West, R. A., and Epker, B. N.: Posterior maxillary surgery: Its place in the treatment of dentofacial deformities. J. Oral Surg., 30:562, 1972.

White, R. P., Peters, P. B., Costich, E. R., and Page, H. L.: Evaluation of sagittal split-ramus osteotomy in 17 patients. J. Oral Surg., 27:851, 1969.

White, S.: The employment of silver wire to bridge the gap after resection of a portion of the lower jaw. Br. Med. J., 2:1525, 1909.

Wilbanks, J. L.: Correction of mandibular prognathism by double-oblique intraoral osteotomy: A new technique. Oral Surg., 31:321, 1971.

Wildt: Über partielle Unterkieferresektion und Bildung einer natürlichen Prothese durch Knochentransplantion. Zentralbl. Chir., 23:1177, 1896.

Wilhelm, W.: The surgical treatment of prognathism of the maxilla. Bol. Odontol., 20:146, 1954.

Willmar, K.: On LeFort I osteotomy. A follow-up study of 106 operated patients with maxillo-facial deformity. Scand. J. Plast. Reconstr. Surg., Suppl. 12, 1974.

Willmar, K.: Personal communication, 1976.

Wilson, P. D.: Experiences with a bone bank. Ann. Surg., 210:932, 1948.

Winstanley, R. P.: Subcondylar osteotomy of the mandible and the intra-oral approach. Br. J. Oral Surg., 6:134, 1968.

Wolhynski, F. A.: Qualitative und quantitative Struklurveranderung de M. masseter des Menschen. Anat. Anz., 82:260, 1936.

Wunderer, S.: Die Prognathieoperation mittels frontal gestieltem Maxilla Fragment. Osterr. Z. Stomatol., 39:98, 1962.

Young, R. A., and Epker, B.: The anterior maxillary ostectomy: A retrospective evaluation of sinus health, patient acceptance, and relapses. J. Oral Surg., 30:69, 1972.

Zallen, R. D., and Strader, R. J.: The use of prophylactic antibiotics in extraoral procedures for mandibular prognathism. J. Oral Surg., 29:178, 1971.

CHAPTER 31

DISTURBANCES OF THE TEMPOROMANDIBULAR JOINT

Nicholas G. Georgiade, D.D.S., M.D.

Derangements of the temporomandibular joint are produced by a number of factors, including occlusal disharmony, myofacial spasm, condylar hypermobility, displacement of the meniscus, trauma, arthritic changes, and fibrous and bony ankylosis.

FUNCTIONAL ANATOMY OF THE TEMPOROMANDIBULAR JOINT

The temporomandibular joint involves the articulation between the mandible and the cranium; the articulating surfaces of the bones are lined by a layer of fibrocartilage. The two articulating surfaces constituting this area are (1) the temporal bone (squama), which has a concave fossa (the glenoid fossa); and (2) the condylar process of the mandible. The anterior border of the joint area is the concave articular (tubercular) eminence of the temporal bone. The superior portion of the concave articular temporal fossa constitutes a portion of the floor of the middle cranial fossa. The posterior boundary of the glenoid fossa is the post-glenoid tubercle of the temporal bone. The condylar process of the mandible is convex,

and its transverse diameter may be as wide as 20 mm, approximately twice the size of the condyle in its anterior-posterior dimension. The blood supply to the condyle and the articular capsule is through a branch of the internal maxillary artery, the auricular artery.

The Articular Disc

The temporomandibular joint is divided into two compartments by a meniscus or articular disc, which separates the mandible from the temporal bone of the cranium. The meniscus is composed of dense fibrous tissue with elastic fibers predominating in the posterior portion (the most vascular) and in the socket (Sicher, 1951) (Fig. 31–1, A). Three types of motion are present in this joint: opening and closing, side to side, and a protrusive and retrusive anterior-posterior motion. The gliding motions of the mandibular condyle occur in the superior portion of the joint. The inferior compartment and condyle serve as the hinge joint. The meniscus is advanced as the mandible assumes the open bite position. The medial and superior fibers of the lateral (external) pterygoid muscle are attached to the anteromedial

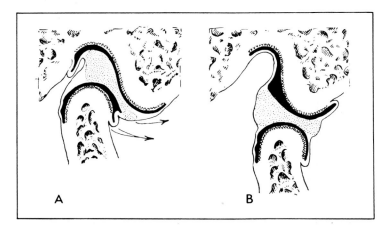

FIGURE 31–1. *A,* The temporomandibular joint, showing the relationship of the condylar head to the articular disc (meniscus), capsule, and surrounding bony structures. *B,* Position of the condylar head in an open bite position.

border of the disc and the fused capsule. Anterior and forward motion of the condyle advances the meniscus as the head of the condyle follows the convexity of the articular eminence. The lateral (external) pterygoid muscle maintains the meniscus in its correct relationship during opening of the bite (Fig. 31–1, *B*). As mentioned, the posterior thick, loose, connective tissue attachment of the meniscus contains considerable elastic tissue. There is therefore a tendency to restrain excessive anterior motion of the meniscus and also to return the meniscus to its normal rest position (Sarnat, 1951).

Radiographic Anatomy of the Temporomandibular Joint

Various views of the temporomandibular joint are obtained, depending on the type of dys-

function suspected. It is often difficult to obtain all the desired information from one type of roentgenogram, and several views may be needed. The basic view consists of an oblique lateral transcranial projection of the joint in both the open and closed bite positions. The closed bite position will show that the condyle is in the glenoid fossa, and the open bite position will show the displacement to and occasionally over the articular eminence (Shore, 1960; Norgaard, 1947) (Fig. 31–2). More recently, panoramic roentgenograms have permitted examination of the entire mandible, including the condylar heads, on one film (Fig. 31–3).

Cineradiographic studies have been useful in the diagnosis of various joint disorders and if available may prove useful in detecting disorders of the temporomandibular joint which cannot be detected by the usual means

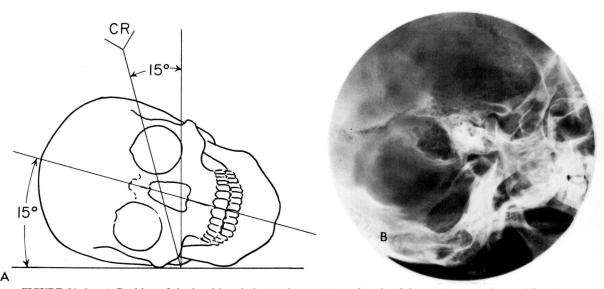

FIGURE 31–2. *A,* Position of the head in relation to the cassette and angle of the roentgen rays in an oblique transcranial projection. CR represents cathode ray. *B,* View of temporomandibular joint and surrounding structures in closed bite position.

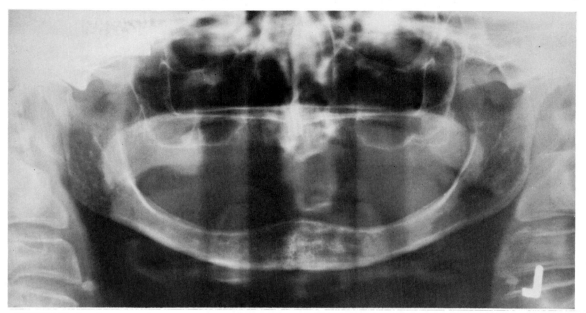

FIGURE 31–3. A panoramic roentgenogram of the entire mandible (edentulous). Note that the condylar heads and the entire body of the mandible are well outlined.

(Cooper and Hoffmann, 1955; Berry and Hoffmann, 1956, 1959; Lindblom, 1956).

Diagnostic problems involving ankylosis or fracture-dislocations of the condylar head necessitate the obtaining of tomograms of the condyle. These are necessary to establish definitely the position of the condylar head, the location and extent of the ankylosis, if present, and its exact relationship to the glenoid fossa and adjacent bony structures (Kieffer, 1938;

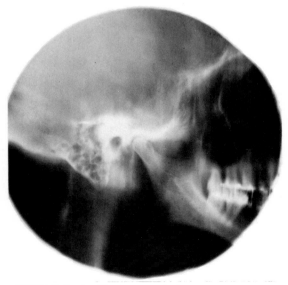

FIGURE 31–4. Tomogram of the temporomandibular joint, showing the condylar head in the glenoid fossa.

Moore, 1938) (Fig. 31–4). A modified Towne view is also usually obtained in patients with fractures of the condyle in order to determine the position of the condyles in a sagittal relationship (Fig. 31–5).

TEMPOROMANDIBULAR JOINT PAIN

Diagnosis

This is a complex problem with many facets; however, investigators have concluded that the most important cause of pain is progressive occlusal disharmony, involving hypersensitive muscle areas, muscle spasm, muscle pain, and associated pain due to limitation of motion (Bonica, 1957). The subsequent findings of limitation of motion with associated pain in the temporomandibular joint area, both during motion and on palpation, and popping and clicking in the joint area, can also be traced to these causes. Clinical evaluation of the patient should include palpation of both joints simultaneously. Disparity in movement and tenderness can be easily ascertained. Pain may also radiate to the ear, the temporal area, and the side of the face.

Clicking in the temporomandibular joint areas is caused by the trapping of the thickened articular disc in the open bite position with

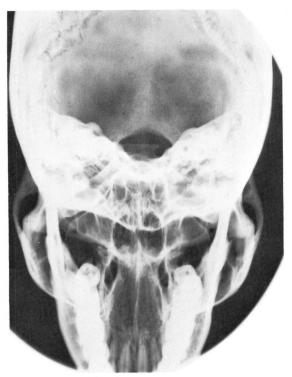

FIGURE 31–5. Modified Towne view, showing the relationship of the condyles to the medial and lateral osseous structures.

advancement of the condylar head over the disc. There is repetition of the clicking when the condylar head returns into the glenoid fossa. The snapping sound in the joint may occur intermittently or at the termination of the opening movements and is directly related to the position of the meniscus.

Changes occurring in the occlusion to which the joint and musculature cannot adjust can produce these symptoms. Disturbance in the muscle balance as a functional unit affects the proprioceptive nerve endings in these muscles, with eventual muscle pain. Any changes occurring in the dentition, such as failure to replace missing teeth, correct a severe overbite or crossbite, or reduce cuspal interference or premature contact, can be the cause of pain manifested in the joint area, muscle, and surrounding facial regions (Georgiade, 1961). Compression of the posterior portion of the disc with its rich blood and nerve supply, which occurs in many of these occlusal disturbances, will trigger and perpetuate the pain.

The common finding of bruxism, the subconscious clenching and gnashing of teeth, is often associated with joint pain in the patient with anxiety, emotional tension, occlusal disharmonies, and areas of periodontal disease (pyorrhea).

A complete oral and facial examination is most important in ascertaining the cause of the joint pain, and any condylar abnormalities should be ruled out by obtaining routine temporomandibular joint roentgenograms both in the open bite and closed bite position.

Treatment

Treatment should be preceded by reassuring the patient that such difficulties can usually be corrected. Muscle pain often is alleviated by an ethyl chloride spray over the affected area. The infiltration of the involved muscle of mastication, which is in spasm, with 2 per cent lidocaine hydrochloride solution with 1:100,000 epinephrine will also serve to reduce the muscle tension.

When present, periodontal disease should be treated. If bruxism is present, equilibration of the occlusion by means of bite plates, particularly at night, should be considered. Bite plates can be constructed with the newer "rapid cure" acrylics with 0.032-inch clasps and 0.030-inch anterior wire for the labial section. The constant clenching of teeth can be relieved by tranquilizing drugs, such as chlordiazepoxide (Librium), 10 mg, or diazepam (Valium), 5 mg, twice a day, in combination with mephenesin, 200 mg three times a day and at bedtime, chlormezanone (Trancopal), 200 mg three times daily and at bedtime, or methocarbamol (Robaxin), 500 mg three times daily and at bedtime. Moist and dry heat applied to the affected areas will often aid in the relief of muscle spasm. Passive use of the jaws with relaxation and maintenance of separation of the teeth and lips relieves any constant pressure on the joint.

Occlusal discrepancies should be corrected by all possible means, including splinting and "bite raising."

The intra-articular injection of triamcinolone acetonide, 0.5 ml (20 mg), has been found to be of value in the treatment of the acute joint-disc pain problem and can be repeated at weekly intervals up to three weeks (Fig. 31–6).

Perhaps the most important thing to do is to reassure these patients and to outline a definite regimen for them to follow as they improve. This consists of showing the patient (in front of a mirror) his subconscious malposition of the mandible and to show him what the normal limi-

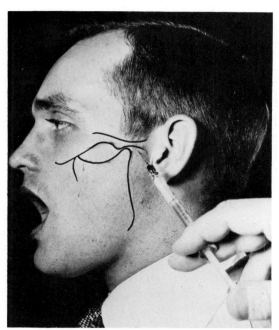

FIGURE 31–6.   Injection of 0.5 ml of steroid into the temporomandibular joint space. Note that the mandible is in the open bite position and the needle is inserted superiorly and slightly anteriorly.

tation of motion should be. Most of these patients will be found to go into a class III (prognathic) occlusal relationship when talking, eating, or yawning. Because of this, undue strain is placed on the condyle-meniscus relationship, thereby setting up an ideal environment for progressive joint disability or complaints. The patients should further be advised to limit the extent of their open-bite to half or less of the usual pattern, and when yawning to place the tongue to the palatal area to restrict the open bite position. A soft diet for four to six weeks should be part of the initial treatment, and lateral mandibular movement should be prohibited to restrict the condyle as close to a "hinge joint" type of motion as possible. At the time of an acute episode, 0.5 ml of steroid (preceded by 0.5 ml of 2 per cent lidocaine) can be injected into the temporomandibular joint space in order to give the patient initial relief of symptoms and to allow the treatment plan to become effective. The intra-articular steroid can be repeated in approximately ten days if desired.

Over a period of six months, the conservative therapy outlined usually results in approximately 90 per cent of these patients responding satisfactorily with relief of symptoms.

SURGICAL APPROACH TO THE TEMPOROMANDIBULAR JOINT

Surgical exposure of the joint capsule, condylar head, and meniscus can be achieved by a number of acceptable incisions (Fig. 31–7). The author prefers the type of incision outlined in Figure 31–7, *E* for routine exploration of the temporomandibular joint, chronic dislocation of the condylar head, ankylosis of the joint, and condylar fractures at the high neck area. Excellent exposure is possible with very little possibility of injury to the facial nerve. The resultant scar is usually not discernible in a relatively few months.

Occasionally the inverted type of incision is used when there is gross displacement of the condylar head medially and into the pterygoid space (Fig. 31–7, *I*). This type of approach will place the incision very close to the branches of the facial nerve, which should be identified and retracted medially prior to locating the displaced condylar head.

The posterior aural approach for exposure of the temporomandibular joint was described by Bocken-Heimer (1920), Axhausen (1931), and Hoopes, Wolfort and Jabaley (1970). This approach offers certain advantages in that no preauricular scars are present and the facial

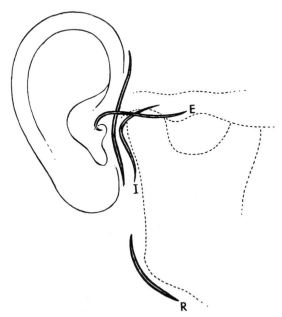

FIGURE 31–7.   The various types of incision for temporomandibular joint surgery. R, Risdon approach; E, endaural approach; I, inverted "hockey stick" approach. Also note the preauricular incision.

nerve does not become a problem in the dissection to expose the joint area. Scarring and stricture of the external auditory canal have been reported following this technique.

HYPERMOBILITY AND DISLOCATION OF THE MANDIBULAR CONDYLE

Acute Dislocation

This condition occurs when the condylar head extends its forward position to the point that its posterior articular surface advances to the articular eminence, even reaching up to and over the projection of the eminence and, on occasion, luxating (dislocating) into the infra-temporal fossa. When this occurs, manual reduction is necessary if spontaneous reduction is not possible. It may be accomplished as follows. Lateral mandibular pressure in both buccal sulci is exerted inferiorly and posteriorly at the angles. Concomitantly, bilateral thumb pressure is applied to the symphysis (Fig. 31–8). Pressure exerted for a minute or two may be necessary to reposition the condyle. The use of meperidine (Demerol) prior to reduction is often advantageous. Restriction of motion for two or three weeks is advisable to allow the traumatized tissues to heal.

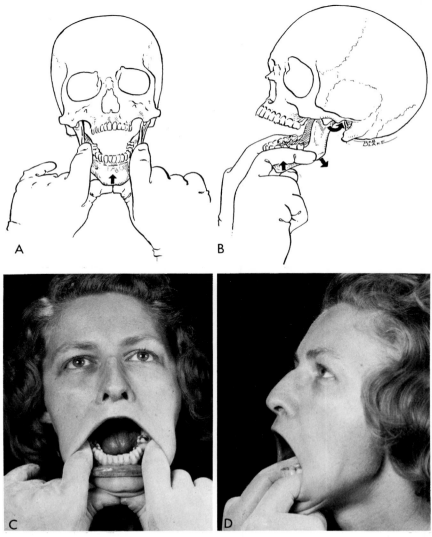

FIGURE 31–8. *A, B,* Diagrams outlining a simple method of replacing the condylar head dislocated anteriorly and slightly inferiorly into the glenoid fossa. Arrows show the direction of pressure being exerted by the operator's fingers. *C, D,* Photographs of a patient undergoing the procedure.

Chronic Dislocation

Recurrent dislocation results in degenerative changes in the meniscus and necessitates removal of the disc.

Exercises should be instituted to strengthen the suprahyoid musculature and to counteract the excessive pull of the lateral pterygoid muscles. The simplest method is to instruct the patient to maintain the tip of the tongue superiorly, touching the anterior palatine vault when the mandible is at rest and when carrying out these exercises. During yawning, the tip of the tongue should be as close to the junction of the hard and soft palates as possible.

Intra-articular injections of sodium psylliate (Sylnasol) were advocated by Schultz and Shriner (1943) in order to produce a moderate fibrosis of the capsular ligaments; however, this has not been found by the author to be an effective method of treatment.

If conservative therapy is inadequate to control the condylar motion, a number of operative procedures are available, as described by Konjetzny (1921), Ashhurst (1921), Nieden (1923), and Foged (1953). Schuchardt (1960) advocated the use of an autograft of bone on the apex of the articular eminence with an intracapsular operation somewhat similar to that described by Mayer (1933), who obtained autogenous bone for the graft from the zygomatic arch. This technique restricts condylar motion without necessitating entry into the joint space.

The method of Myrhaug (1951) and Hale (1972) should also be considered. This technique involves removal of the articular tubercle, thus preventing further "locking" of the condylar head anterior to the articular eminence which has now been removed (Fig. 31–9).

Simple plication of the joint capsule, as suggested by Morris (1930), is also quite satisfactory if there are no complaints referable to the meniscus. Plication of the capsular ligament and reattachment of the overlying fascia decrease the mobility of the condylar head by virtue of the formation of cicatricial tissue and decrease of the capsular size. This procedure may be performed via a transmeatal endaural-zygomatic approach, in which the anterior cartilaginous canal is incised and the tragus is then retracted inferiorly and medially, exposing the temporal artery and vein, which are divided after ligation. The auriculotemporal nerve and the temporal branch of the facial nerve are identified. The articular capsule is exposed over its entire area of coverage from

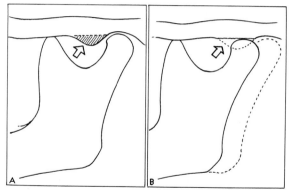

FIGURE 31–9. *A,* The shaded area shows diagrammatically the area and portion of the articular tubercle removed with a high speed bur. *B,* The condylar head can move forward to a more anterior position and still return to the glenoid fossa without being "trapped" anterior to the tubercle.

the condylar neck to the zygomatic arch. A strip of capsule 5 to 7 mm in length may be excised in the anterior-posterior direction, and the capsular edges are plicated with a number of 4–0 white nylon sutures. If there is minimal hypermobility and looseness of the capsule, the condition can be decreased by multiple inverting mattress sutures, which shorten the length of the capsule. Minimal mandibular motion is maintained for approximately ten days, and a gradual increase in opening the bite is continued after that period of time.

Boman (1949) recommended extirpation of the disc and partial detachment of the lateral pterygoid muscle. However, this seems to be a drastic treatment, as the problem is not in the joint itself. A simple procedure which does not involve an opening into the joint is the use of a Dacron mesh strip sling from a drill hole in the zygomatic arch to a hole along the anterior neck of the condyle (Fig. 31–10). Release of the lateral (external) pterygoid muscle from its attachment to the condyle will often be sufficient to prevent excessive forward positioning of the condylar head and subsequent luxation.

When a dislocation has been manually unreducible for a number of months, there is considerable merit in using an intraoral bilateral temporal myotomy in conjunction with release of the lateral pterygoid muscles. One should think seriously of utilizing this simplified technique before attempting more complicated procedures (Laskin, 1973).

Occasionally patients have had chronic dislocations of the mandible (even up to years), either unilateral or bilateral. Operative interven-

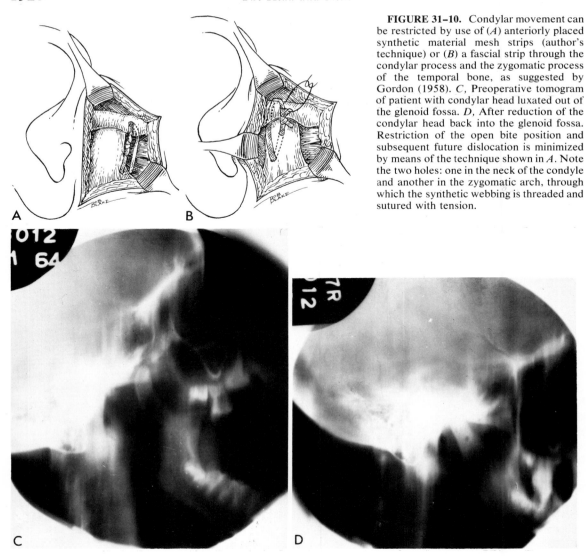

FIGURE 31–10. Condylar movement can be restricted by use of (*A*) anteriorly placed synthetic material mesh strips (author's technique) or (*B*) a fascial strip through the condylar process and the zygomatic process of the temporal bone, as suggested by Gordon (1958). *C*, Preoperative tomogram of patient with condylar head luxated out of the glenoid fossa. *D*, After reduction of the condylar head back into the glenoid fossa. Restriction of the open bite position and subsequent future dislocation is minimized by means of the technique shown in *A*. Note the two holes: one in the neck of the condyle and another in the zygomatic arch, through which the synthetic webbing is threaded and sutured with tension.

tion is necessary to expose the condylar heads while the patient is under general anesthesia by nasal intubation. In order to obtain the maximum traction, to release the fibrosis, and be able to replace the condylar heads back into the fossae, a small hole is drilled at the angle of the mandible through which a 25-gauge wire is inserted, either bilaterally or unilaterally, and strong downward traction is applied. Concomitantly a curare-like drug is administered intravenously during the active phase in order to obtain the maximum relaxation of the musculature. During the downward traction phase, a cupped periosteal elevator is inserted anterior to the condylar head and a backward force is exerted in order to reposition the condylar head. Once the condylar head is back in the fossa, intermaxillary rubber band traction via Ivy type loops or arch bars is used to

minimize the possibility of recurrent condylar dislocation. The traction is usually continued for a period of three to four weeks post reduction. If the capsular ligament is found to be loose, plication of the capsule is done at this time, as described earlier in the chapter. A combination of this technique with the temporal and lateral myotomies or the sling type procedure can also be employed to prevent recurrent mandibular dislocation if the patient still continues to have recurrent dislocations.

INJURY TO THE TEMPOROMANDIBULAR JOINT

Injury to the joint may produce an acute disturbance of the meniscus or the articular surfaces. Daily occurrences, such as yawning or extending the open-bite position, as in eating an apple, may cause injury to the meniscus. The importance of the meniscus as a shock absorber has been stressed by several authors, including Nieden (1923), Goodfriend (1934), Hiltebrandt (1938), and Henny and Baldridge (1957). Some have even advocated replacement of the injured discs by means of polyethylene caps (Gordon, 1955, 1958). In approximately 5 per cent of patients with temporomandibular joint pain, removal of the meniscus has been found to be necessary when all other conservative therapeutic trials have failed (Boman, 1947, 1950; Dingman and Moorman, 1951; Kiehn, 1952; Rongetti, 1954; Rankow and Novack, 1959). Lanz (1909) was the first to describe the removal of the disc for pain and associated symptoms (see also Facial Injuries in Children, Chapter 26).

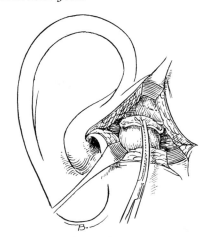

FIGURE 31–11. The meniscus held by a curved clamp just prior to removal. There is continued traction on the meniscus, following which the medial aspect of the meniscus is detached.

Temporomandibular Arthrosis

The author routinely approaches the joint area via the endaural approach previously described. For better exposure the superficial temporal artery and vein are ligated and retracted. The auriculotemporal nerve can be identified and divided in patients with severe preauricular pain. The capsule is incised in a horizontal plane, and the meniscus is exposed and grasped with a small, curved, mosquito clamp. The muscles of mastication are at this time relaxed by the use of one of the curare-like drugs administered by the anesthetist. The meniscus is first incised along its anterior and posterior attachment, and the medial and most vascular attachment is severed along with a portion of the lateral (external) pterygoid muscle (Fig. 31–11). Prior to this it has been found useful to inject the pterygoid space with approximately 5 ml of 1 per cent lidocaine and 1:100,000 epinephrine in order to minimize oozing. Condylar contouring is usually achieved by means of a cross-cutting type (fissure) bur with a Hall air drill, removing any bony irregularities which may be present on the articular surface and recontouring the condylar head, which may be flattened and asymmetrical. The disc may be replaced by a dermal graft, which is draped over the condylar head and acts as a substitute for the removed meniscus (Georgiade, 1962) and also as a covering of the newly contoured condylar head of the mandible.

High condylectomy, with the line of resection at the base of the condyle, has been advocated by some surgeons for the persistently painful temporomandibular joint (Henny and Baldridge, 1957). However, this procedure has been only partially successful and often results in a posterior loss of vertical dimension and shifting of the bite, with a possible resultant permanent open-bite (Smith and Robinson, 1953).

CONDYLAR FRACTURES

The management of condylar fractures has been discussed in Chapter 24.

TEMPOROMANDIBULAR JOINT ANKYLOSIS

Well-adjusted individuals can compensate for many types of physical impairment. The patient with ankylosis of the mandible, however, cannot masticate, enunciate properly, or maintain any semblance of normal oral hygiene (Kazanjian, 1938). Rampant caries with accompanying periodontal disease and abscesses of dental origin are the rule in patients with long-standing ankylosis. The basic requisites for normal everyday living are absent in these unfortunate adults and children.

The cause of ankylosis is usually traced to some traumatic episode in the patient's childhood, often a blow to the chin area, with resultant damage to the condylar head and degeneration of the articular surface, and eventual fibrosis and ankylosis (see Chapter 24). Displacement of the condylar head out of the glenoid fossa is capable of causing ankylosis.

Children with infection involving the mastoid, middle ear, or tonsillar areas with subsequent involvement of the joint area are still seen today with ankylosis; however, they are not as frequent as they were 25 years ago because of the widespread use of antibiotics. Many of the affected children have attained adulthood and have ankylosis resulting from childhood infections. In the older group of patients, progressive ankylosis is seen occasionally in individuals who have generalized arthritis or a post-traumatic history with involvement of the temporomandibular joint.

A rarer form of temporomandibular ankylosis is the congenital type caused by prenatal maldevelopment or intrauterine injury. The congenital form is more severe, the condyle, sigmoid notch, coronoid process, and zygomatic arch forming a solid block of bone. Occasionally the tuberosity of the maxilla and the medial aspect of the ramus are synostosed.

Diagnosis and Type. The principal growth center of the mandible is the condylar region. When downward and forward positioning of the face is altered during development by ankylosis of the condyle, a characteristic facial asymmetry is seen in the growing child, its degree depending on the age at onset. Examination of the patient who has had restrictive motion of the mandible with onset during childhood or of a child with ankylosis of a few years' duration shows considerable disparity between the affected and unaffected sides of the face. Elongation and flatness of the unaffected side contrasts with roundness and fullness of the affected side. The midpoint of the chin is past the midline, deviating toward the affected side. There is an associated deviation of the mandibular dentition toward the affected side as well.

In unilateral ankylosis some motion may occur on palpation of the normal joint area. In bilateral ankylosis of the intra-articular type, no motion or protrusion is possible. In temporomandibular ankylosis affecting one side only, the patient is often able to open his mouth, the distance between the teeth on opening being limited to a few millimeters. A deviation of the mandible toward the affected side is observed. Lateral pterygoid muscle function being abolished on the affected side and active on the unaffected side, the lateral pterygoid muscle on the unaffected side propulses the mandible toward the side of the ankylosis (Kazanjian and Converse, 1974). The best method of diagnosing temporomandibular joint ankylosis (with or without involvement of the coronoid process) is a tomographic examination of the joint area. This technique yields a clear-cut radiographic outline of the temporomandibular joint area without the usual osseous superimpositions (Fig. 31–12).

Treatment. The treatment of temporomandibular ankylosis is surgical. The operative procedure should strive to attain an end result as nearly physiologic as possible. If mandibular bone is removed without interposition of some type of material, recurrence of the ankylosis can be expected. When a wide portion of the mandibular ramus is resected in order to prevent recurrence of the ankylosis, a further derangement of the muscles of mastication

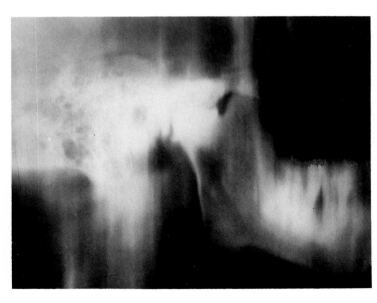

FIGURE 31–12. Tomogram of the temporomandibular joint area, showing the exact area and extent of the bony ankylosis.

occurs on the operated side. As a result there is an increased deviation of the mandible toward the affected side when the mandible goes into the open-bite position. In the case of bilateral ankylosis with too generous removal of the mandibular ramus bilaterally, a permanent open and retrusive bite may occur as a result of the loss of the vertical dimension of the ramus bilaterally.

There has been a gradual evolution and consolidation of the surgical procedures designed to correct temporomandibular joint ankylosis. Humphry (1856) treated ankylosis successfully by resecting the condyle. Esmarch (1860), one of the pioneer surgeons in this field, de-

scribed his procedure, which consisted of resection of a portion of the ramus of the mandible. Verneuil (1872), following a review of the work performed to that date, suggested interposition of muscle and fascia between the newly cut bone surfaces. Blair (1913, 1914), after an evaluation of all available published cases since 1855, advocated an inverted "hockey stick" incision with removal of a wide segment of bone and the interpositioning of temporal muscle or fascia. Murphy (1914) advocated a similar procedure with the interposition of a temporal fat-fascia graft. Phemister and Miller (1918), following an experimental evaluation of ankylosis, found that adequate

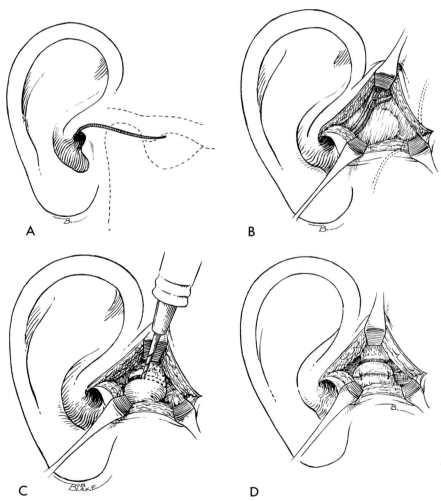

FIGURE 31–13. *A,* The endaural approach to the temporomandibular joint area. *B,* The exposure to the joint area. The temporal vessels are usually ligated and retracted from the field to allow better exposure along the posterior portion of the ankylosis site. *C,* A high-speed, cross-cut fissure bur is utilized for cutting through the ankylosed area and for contouring a new condylar head as close as possible to the anatomical site of the temporomandibular joint. Care is taken to free and locate the medial aspect of the area of bony fusion in order to minimize the possibility of perforating the base of skull in this area. *D,* The newly formed condylar head with a dermal graft completely covering the dome and sides to prevent recurrence of the ankylosis.

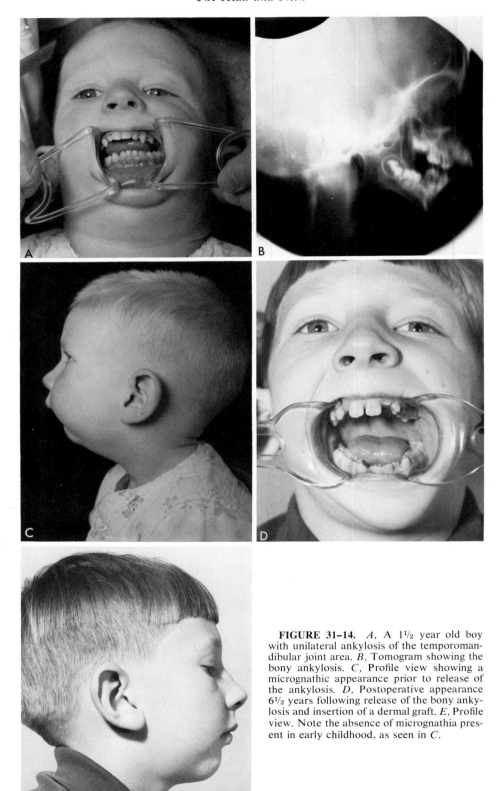

FIGURE 31–14. *A,* A 1½ year old boy with unilateral ankylosis of the temporomandibular joint area. *B,* Tomogram showing the bony ankylosis. *C,* Profile view showing a micrognathic appearance prior to release of the ankylosis. *D,* Postoperative appearance 6½ years following release of the bony ankylosis and insertion of a dermal graft. *E,* Profile view. Note the absence of micrognathia present in early childhood, as seen in *C.*

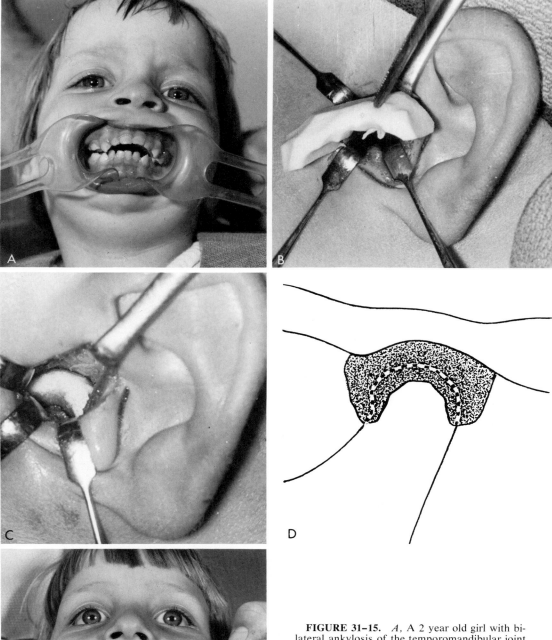

FIGURE 31–15. *A*, A 2 year old girl with bilateral ankylosis of the temporomandibular joint area. *B*, A sculptured Silastic sponge prior to insertion over the condylar head. *C*, The Silastic sponge is in position, separating the newly cut bone ends. *D*, Positioning of the Silastic sponge over the newly created condylar head. *E*, Same patient four years later. Note the ample open bite position and the absence of mandibular deviation.

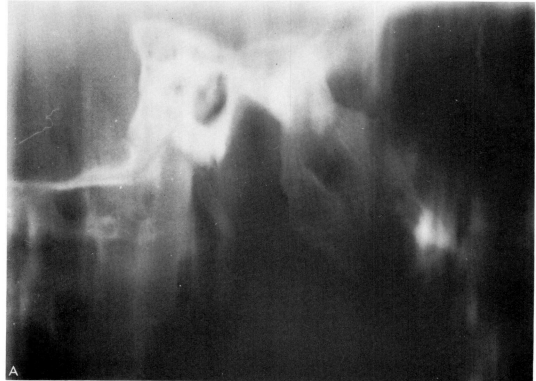

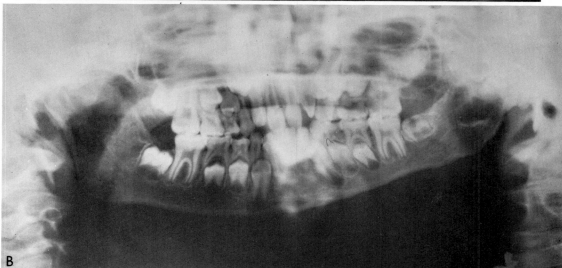

FIGURE 31–16. *A*, Preoperative tomogram of temporomandibular ankylosis. *B*, Preoperative roentgenogram of patient showing a small left ramus and ankylosed joint.

excision of obstructing tissues and early and active postoperative motion were important.

Approaches to the joint area were usually through a preauricular incision (Kazanjian, 1938; Parker, 1948) or a submandibular approach to the ramus of the mandible, as described by Risdon (1934) (see Fig. 31–7, *R*).

ENDAURAL APPROACH. At present the author's procedure of choice for surgical correction of temporomandibular joint ankylosis consists of a modified endaural approach (see Fig. 31–7, *E*), which gives an excellent exposure to the ankylosed joint area. The incision can be extended anteriorly if the ankylosis extends to

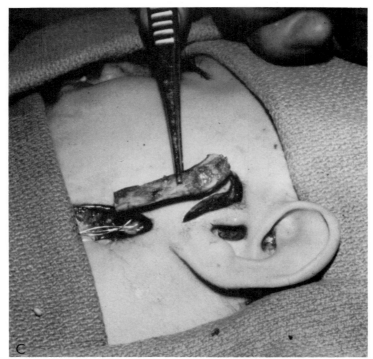

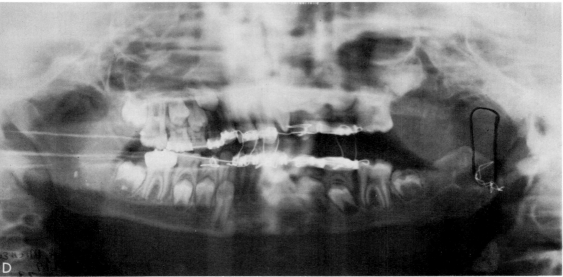

FIGURE 31–16 *Continued.* *C,* Photograph of the rib graft (eighth) and cartilaginous portion prior to insertion, with the cartilaginous portion being placed to create a new condylar head. A distance over 2 cm in length was obtained in this manner. *D,* Postoperative panoramic roentgenogram of the mandible with outline of the cartilage and bone graft used to reestablish the deficient posterior vertical dimension.

the coronoid process. Following exposure of the ankylosis site, a cut is made through the bone. High-speed, cross-cutting bone burs utilizing a Hall air drill are employed. A cut of approximately 4 mm in width is made. Between the newly cut edges of the bone, autogenous material, such as a dermal graft or a Silastic closed-pore sponge, may be interspaced (Figs. 31–13 and 31–14). Removal of as much as 1 to

2 cm of bone from the ramus, as suggested by some authors, is unnecessary and unphysiologic. Autogenous cartilage (Longacre and Gilby, 1951; Stuteville and Lanfranchi, 1955; Hinds and Sills, 1959), muscle fascia (Blair, 1913, 1914; Dingman, 1946), or dermal grafts (Georgiade, Pickrell and Altany, 1957) have been used. Fine, closed-pore, Silastic sponge (Robinson, 1968) shaped to fit around the newly

contoured condylar head has been used for the past six years and has been found to work quite satisfactorily. One must keep in mind that inorganic materials entail a greater risk of infection (Fig. 31–15).

Release of bilateral ankylosis of the mandible can be achieved in one stage with insertion of autogenous cartilage, muscle fascia, dermal grafts, or Silastic sponge, if only about 4 mm of bone is removed. Minimal bone removal will also minimize the occurrence of a retrusive bite in adulthood, as described by some of the earlier surgeons as occurring after bilateral ankylosis was corrected in one stage (Loewe, 1913).

When the ramus is short on the affected side (Fig. 31–16, *A*), surgical release of the ankylosis alone will not be sufficient to overcome the reduced vertical dimension (Fig. 31–16, *B*). If the ramus of the mandible is of sufficient length and width, bilateral sliding osteotomies (in a sagittal plane) or vertical osteotomies (in a frontal plane) may correct the deformity. Bone grafts are inserted in the interstice between the fragments in the ramus in order to provide increased length and to advance the mandible. Unilateral or bilateral release of the ankylosis is done.

An alternate plan is to resect the eighth rib, including a portion of the chondral area (Fig. 31–16, *C*). The cartilaginous portion of this chondro-osseous costal graft is then inserted into the glenoid fossa, and the additional length of the mandible is obtained by the rib graft, which is wired to the ramus after establishing the desired occlusal relationships (Fig. 31–16, *D*); this technique can be applied either unilaterally or bilaterally in one stage.

Deformity with shortening of the ramus and generalized hypoplasia of the mandible (micrognathia) require reconstructive procedures, which have been described in Chapter 30.

Other Types of Temporomandibular Ankyloses

Ankylosis of the mandibular coronoid process or fusion of the ramus to the maxilla, which is usually a post-traumatic complication, may also be diagnosed. Surgical correction may be achieved by an intraoral approach if the ankylosis is produced by bony union between the anterior aspect of the ramus and the maxilla. Removal of the fused coronoid process can be accomplished in the same manner by an intraoral approach. During the postoperative man-

agement, progressive increase in motion of the mandible is encouraged over a period of days following release of the ankylosis. Occasionally, this is not possible when bone grafting is done concomitantly. In these instances the jaws are maintained in intermaxillary fixation for a period of approximately five weeks; active and passive motion is then started. Oral dilators can be used postoperatively, as indicated in the less complicated ankylosis release procedures. In most postoperative patients, tongue blades stacked on each other, usually starting with five or six tongue blades and gradually adding

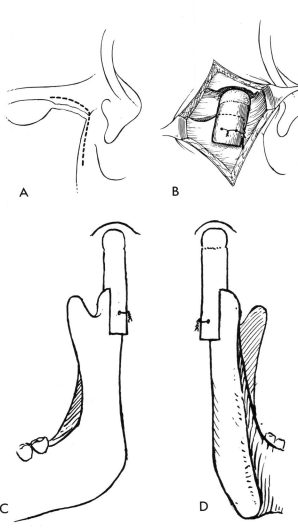

FIGURE 31–17. *A*, The type of incision for approach to the area of ankylosis. *B*, The chondro-osseous costal graft, with the technique of wiring the graft to the ramus. *C*, *D*, Lateral and posteromedial views of the bone and cartilage graft, which can be varied in length depending on the desired increase in length.

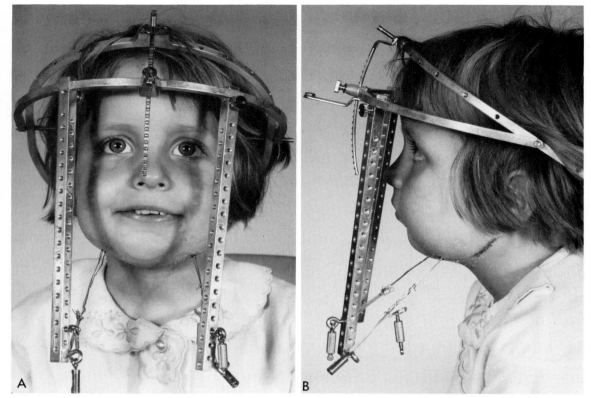

FIGURE 31–18. The halo frame. It is employed in order to obtain maximum forward and downward traction of the mandible, allowing greater flexibility in the early orthodontic treatment phase. *A*, Full face. *B*, Lateral view.

up to 12 or 14, are inserted three times a day for a minimum of four to five months and are kept in place for at least $\frac{1}{2}$ hour at a time. Regardless of the surgical approach or type of material interposed, the arthroplasty should be done as close to the anatomic joint as possible in order to minimize disturbance to the condylar growth center of the mandible, particularly in the child. Muscle imbalance and resultant occlusive disharmony will occur to a degree commensurate with the surgical defect. The less bone removed, the less loss of vertical dimension of the ramus will result.

Complications and Causes of Failures in Surgical Procedures in the Temporomandibular Joint Area

The appropriate surgical approach is of paramount importance (Fig. 31–17). If the incision is extended too far anteriorly, the temporal branch of the facial nerve may be severed; if it is extended too far inferiorly, the main branch of the facial nerve may be injured.

Postoperative infection involving the joint area will cause extrusion of any substance previously inserted, and inorganic materials will be more subject to extrusion. During the operative procedure and postoperative period, patients are continued on broad-spectrum antibiotics, which should be started prior to the surgical procedure.

Ankylosis will recur in joints that have become infected, particularly in small children who are difficult to instruct and whose deciduous dentition does not allow the use of extensive dilating appliances. The use of the Halo head frame with inferiorly based traction works well in children requiring extensive continuous traction (Fig. 31–18).

REFERENCES

Ashhurst, A.: Recurrent unilateral subluxation of the mandible. Ann. Surg., *73*:712, 1921.

Axhausen, G.: Die Operative Freilegung des Kiefergelenks. Chirurg, *3*:713, 1931.

Becker, W. H.: Transosseous wiring fixation of condylar fractures with infrafacial incision. Oral Surg., *3*:284, 1950.

Berry, H. M., Jr., and Hoffmann, F. A.: Cinefluorography with image intensification for observing temporomandibular joint movements. J. Am. Dent. Assoc., *53*:517, 1956.

Berry, H. M., Jr., and Hoffmann, F. A.: Cineradiolographic observations of temporomandibular joint function. J. Prosthet. Dent., *9*:21, 1959.

Blair, V. P.: Operative treatment of ankylosis of the mandible. South. Surg. Gynecol. Tr., *26*:435, 1913.

Blair, V. P.: Operative treatment of ankylosis of the mandible. Surg. Gynecol. Obstet., *19*:436, 1914.

Bocken-Heimer, P.: Eine Neue: Methode zur Freilegung der Kiefergelenkeohnezicht Bare Narben und ohne Verletzung. Des Nervus Facialis. Zentralbl. Chir., *47*:52, 1560, 1920.

Boman, K.: Temporomandibular joint arthrosis and its treatment by extirpation of the disc. Acta Chir. Scand., *95*(Suppl. 118):1, 1947.

Boman, K.: A new operation for luxation in the temporomandibular joint. Acta Chir. Scand., *99*:96, 1949.

Boman, K.: The functioning of the temporomandibular joint after extirpation of the disc. Acta Chir. Scand., *100*:130, 1950.

Bonica, J. J.: Management of myofascial pain syndromes in general practice. J.A.M.A., *164*:732, 1957.

Brussell, I. J.: Temporomandibular joint diseases. J. Am. Dent. Assoc., *39*:532, 1949.

Chasens, A. I.: Occlusal disharmony and temporomandibular joint disturbances as a source of pain. J. Dent. Med., *12*:107, 1957.

Choukas, N. C., and Sicher, H.: The structure of the temporomandibular joint. Oral Surg., *13*:1203, 1960.

Cooper, H., and Hoffmann, F. A.: The application of cinefluorography with image intensification in the field of plastic surgery, dentistry and speech. Plast. Reconstr. Surg., *16*:135, 1955.

Copland, J.: Diagnosis of mandibular joint dysfunction. Oral Surg., *13*:1106, 1960.

Costen, J. B.: A syndrome of ear and sinus symptoms dependent upon disturbed function of the temporomandibular joint. Ann. Otol. Rhinol. Laryngol., *43*:1, 1934.

Costen, J. B.: The present status of the mandibular joint syndrome in otolaryngology. Trans. Am. Acad. Ophthalmol., *55*:809, 1951.

Dingman, R. O.: Ankylosis of the temporomandibular joint. Am. J. Orthod., *32*:120, 1946.

Dingman, R. O., and Moorman, W. C.: Menisectomy in the treatment of lesions of the temporomandibular joint. J. Oral Surg., *9*:214, 1951.

Esmarch, F.: Traitment du resserrement cicatriciel des machoires par la formation d'une fausse articulation dans la continuité de l'os maxillaire inférieur. Arch. Gén. Med., V Serie, *44*, 1860.

Findlay, I.: Operation for arrest of excessive condylar movement. J. Oral Surg., *22*:110, 1964.

Foged, J.: Habitual dislocation of the jaw treated with Konjetzny's operation. Acta Chir. Scand., *105*:78, 1953.

Georgiade, N. G.: Temporomandibular joint dysfunction and facial pain. J. North Carolina Dent. Soc., *44*:110, 1961.

Georgiade, N. G.: The surgical correction of temporomandibular joint dysfunction by means of autogenous dermal grafts. Plast. Reconstr. Surg., *30*:165, 1962.

Georgiade, N. G., Pickrell, K., Douglas, W., and Altany, F.: Extraoral pinning of displaced condylar fractures. Plast. Reconstr. Surg., *18*:377, 1956.

Georgiade, N. G., Pickrell, K., and Altany, F.: An experimental and clinical evaluation of autogenous dermal grafts used in the treatment of temporomandibular joint ankylosis. Plast. Reconstr. Surg., *19*:1633, 1957.

Goodfriend, D. J.: Abnormalities of the mandibular articulation. J. Am. Dent. Assoc., *21*:204, 1934.

Gordon, S.: Recurring dislocation of the temporomandibular joint. Br. J. Plast. Surg., *3*:244, 1951.

Gordon, S.: Subluxation of the temporomandibular joint. Plast. Reconstr. Surg., *16*:57, 1955.

Gordon, S.: Surgery of the temporomandibular joint. Am. J. Surg., *95*:263, 1958.

Hale, R.: Treatment of recurrent dislocation of the mandible. J. Oral Surg., *30*:527, 1972.

Henny, F. A.: A technic for the open reduction of fractures of the mandibular condyle. J. Oral Surg., *9*:233, 1951.

Henny, F. A., and Baldridge, O. L.: Condylectomy for the persistently painful temporomandibular joint. J. Oral Surg., *15*:24, 1957.

Heurlin, R. J., Jr., Gans, B. J., and Stuteville, O. H.: Skeletal changes following fracture dislocation of the mandibular condyle in the adult rhesus monkey. Oral Surg., *14*:1490, 1961.

Hiltebrandt, C.: Die Unterkiefer-Bewegungen und ihre Beziehungen zum Kiefergelenk. Zahnaerztl. Rundschau, *47*:942, 1938.

Hinds, E., and Sills, A.: Cartilage block arthroplasty for correction of temporomandibular joint disturbances. Am. J. Surg., *98*:787, 1959.

Hoopes, J., Wolfort, F., and Jabaley, M.: Operative treatment of fractures of the mandibular condyle in children. The post auricular approach. Plast. Reconstr. Surg., *46*:357, 1970.

Hudson, H.: Operation for recurrent subluxation of temporomandibular joint. Br. Med. J., *2*:354, 1945.

Humphry, G. M.: Excision of the condyle of the lower jaw. Assoc. Med. J. (Lond.), *160*:61, 1856.

Kazanjian, V. H.: Ankylosis of the temporomandibular joint. Surg. Gynecol. Obstet., *67*:333, 1938.

Kazanjian, V. H., and Converse, J. M.: Temporomandibular ankylosis. *In* Kazanjian and Converse's Surgical Treatment of Facial Injuries. Baltimore, The Williams & Wilkins Company, 1974.

Kieffer, J.: The laminagraph and its variations. Am. J. Roentgenol., *39*:497, 1938.

Kiehn, C. L.: Meniscectomy for internal derangement of the temporomandibular joint. Am. J. Surg., *83*:364, 1952.

Kiehn, C. L., and DesPrez, J. D.: Meniscectomy for internal derangement of the temporomandibular joint. Br. J. Plast. Surg., *15*:199, 1962.

Konjetzny, G.: Die operative Behandling der habituellen Unterkieferluxation. Arch. Klin. Chir., *116*:680, 1921.

Lanz, J.: Discitis mandibularis. Zentralbl. Chir., *9*:289, 1909.

Laskin, D.: Myotomy for the management of recurrent and protracted mandibular dislocation. Trans. 4th Internatl. Conf. on Oral Surg. Copenhagen, Munksgaard, 1973, p. 264–268.

Lindblom, G.: A cineradiographic study of the temporomandibular joint. Sven. Tandlak. Tidskr., *49*:324, 1956.

Loewe, O.: Ueber Hautimplantation an Stelle der freien Fraszienplastik. Munch. Med. Wochenschr., *60*:1320, 1913.

Longacre, J. J., and Gilby, R. F.: The use of autogenous cartilage grafts in arthroplasty for true ankylosis of temporomandibular joint. Plast. Reconstr. Surg., *7*:271, 1951.

Mayer, L.: Recurrent dislocation of the jaw. J. Bone Joint Surg., *15*:889, 1933.

Messer, E.: A simplified method for fixation of the fractured mandibular condyle. J. Oral Surg., *30*:442, 1972.

Moore, S.: Body section roentgenography with the laminagraph. Am. J. Roentgenol., *39*:514, 1938.

Morris, J.: Chronic recurring temporomaxillary subluxation. Surg. Gynecol. Obstet., *50*:483, 1930.

Murphy, J.: Arthroplasty for intraarticular bony and fibrous ankylosis of the temporomandibular articulation. J.A.M.A., *62*:1783, 1914.

Myrhaug, H.: New method of operation for bilateral dislocation of mandible. Acta Odont. Scand., *9*:247, 1951.

Nieden, H.: Neber operative Behandling habitueller Kieferluxation. Dtsch. Z. Chir., *183*:358, 1923.

Norgaard, F.: Temporomandibular arthrography. Copenhagen, Einar Munksgaard, 1947.

Parker, D. B.: Ankylosis of the temporomandibular joint. J. Oral Surg., 6:42, 1948.

Phemister, D., and Miller, E.: The method of new joint formation in arthroplasty. Surg. Gynecol. Obstet., *26*: 406, 1918.

Rankow, R. M., and Novack, A. J.: Transmeatal condylectomy and meniscectomy. A.M.A. Arch. Otolaryngol., *70*:703, 1959.

Rehn, E.: Das kutane und subcutane Bindegewebe als plastiches Material. Munch. Med. Wochenschr., *60*:118, 1914.

Rehn, E.: Zur den Fragen der Transplantation. Arch. Klin. Chir., *112*:622, 1919.

Risdon, F.: Ankylosis of the temporomandibular joint. J. Am. Dent. Assoc., *21*:1933, 1934.

Robinson, M.: Temporomandibular ankylosis corrected by creating a false Silastic sponge fossa. J. South. Calif. Dent. Assoc., *36*:14, 1968.

Rongetti, J. R.: Meniscectomy. A.M.A. Arch Otolaryngol., *60*:566, 1954.

Sarnat, B. G.: The Temporomandibular Joint. Springfield, Ill., Charles C Thomas, Publisher, 1951.

Schuchardt, K.: Fortschritte der Kiefer und Gesichts-Chirurgie. Stuttgart, Georg Thieme Verlag, 1960.

Schultz, L. W., and Schriner, W.: Treatment of acute and chronic traumatic temporomandibular arthritis. J. Florida Med. Assoc., *30*:189, 1943.

Schwartz, L.: Disorders of the Temporomandibular Joint. Philadelphia, W. B. Saunders Company, 1959.

Shore, N. A.: The interpretation of temporomandibular joint roentgenograms. Oral Surg., *13*:341, 1960.

Sicher, H.: Functional anatomy of the temporomandibular articulation. Aust. J. Dent., *55*:73, 1951.

Silagi, J.: Temporomandibular joint arthroplasty. J. Oral Surg., *28*:920, 1970.

Smith, A. E., and Robinson, M.: Mandibular function after condylectomy. J. Am. Dent. Assoc., *46*:304, 1953.

Stuteville, O. H., and Lanfranchi, R. P.: Surgical reconstruction of the temporomandibular joint. Am. J. Surg., *90*:940, 1955.

Thilander, B.: Innervation of the temporomandibular joint capsule in man. Trans. Royal School of Dentistry, Stockholm, No. 7, 1961.

Thoma, K. H.: Oral Surgery. 3rd Ed. St. Louis, M., C. V. Mosby Company, 1958.

Verneuil, A. A. S.: De la création d'une fausse articulation par section ou résection partielle de l'os maxillaire inférieur. Arch. Gen. Med., V Série, *15*:284, 1872.

CHAPTER 32

DEFORMITIES OF THE LIPS AND CHEEKS

JOHN MARQUIS CONVERSE, M.D.,
DONALD WOOD-SMITH, F.R.C.S.E.,
W. BRANDON MACOMBER, M.D.,
AND MARK K. H. WANG, M.D.

This chapter is divided into two major sections: congenital deformities and techniques for the repair of defects of the lips and cheeks. Cleft lips are discussed separately in Chapters 38 to 44; reconstruction of massive lip and cheek defects following ablative surgery is discussed in Chapters 61 to 63.

Congenital Deformities

MARK K. H. WANG, M.D.,
AND W. BRANDON MACOMBER, M.D.

CONGENITAL LIP SINUSES

Congenital lip sinuses are among the rarest congenital anomalies recorded. Demarquay reported the first case in 1845. A total of 280 cases have been reported in the literature (Phillips, 1968).

Congenital sinuses of the lip usually appear as a symmetrically placed pair of dimples on the vermilion border of the lower lip, one on each side of the midline. The dimple, either a circular depression or a transverse slit, is often situated at the apex of a nipple-like elevation (Fig. 32–1). Each dimple represents the orifice of a blind sinus extending downward and backward, penetrating the orbicularis oris muscle and ending blindly just beneath the mucosal surface of the lower lip. The orifice may be so small as to barely admit a hair probe, or it may be as large as 2 mm in diameter. The sinus tract ranges from 5 mm to 2.5 cm in length. The mucus secreted from the sinus may be sufficiently copious to require occasional wiping, especially during mastication.

The sinuses may have an asymmetric appearance. This can be due to a difference either in the size of the opening or in their location. The sinuses may be single and occur in either a midline or paramidline location (Fig. 32–2). Everett and Wescott (1961) and Baker (1966) reported lip pits at the commissure of the mouth, either unilateral or bilateral (Fig. 32–3). Lastly, congenital sinuses may occur in the upper lip and frenulum, though they are extremely rare. Kriens (1968) reported two cases of median sinuses of the upper lip, the opening of which, however, was on the skin surface of the philtrum.

On histological examination, the tract is lined by squamous cell epithelium, similar to that of lip vermilion. Near the blind end there are numerous mucous glands in the surrounding tissue whose ducts empty into the lumen of the fundus.

Congenital lip sinuses are asymptomatic and cause no pain. There is no tendency to obstruction or infection. Besides the mild deformity and occasional dripping of mucous secretion from the opening, the patient experiences no inconvenience or discomfort.

Congenital lip sinuses are rare. Coccia and Bixler (1967) cited an incidence of one to 100,000 births. Phillips (1968) quoted the incidence as one to 200,000. Females are more often affected than males. The most common associated malformations are cleft lip and palate. Taylor and Lane (1966) and Coccia and Bixler (1967) stated that between 70 to 80 per cent of all cases of lip sinuses had associated cleft lip or palate. Heredity is apparently an important factor. The deformity not only is often manifested in several members of the same generation but also usually can be traced back through several generations of the same family. There is no sex linkage or sex limitation. The affected person is capable of transmitting the anomaly to approximately one-half

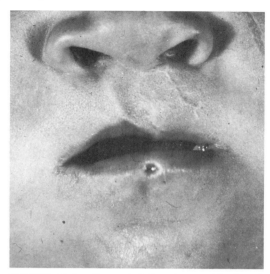

FIGURE 32–2. Congenital lip sinus, with the sinus opening situated at the midline of the lower lip. Note the associated unilateral cleft on the left side previously repaired.

of his offspring. Any member of such a family, even without the anomaly, may transmit the anomaly. Baker (1964) reported one family of three generations with eight cases of lip sinuses. The authors (1956) have encountered a family in which congenital lip sinuses were present in 18 members spread over four generations.

Etiology. The etiology of congenital lip si-

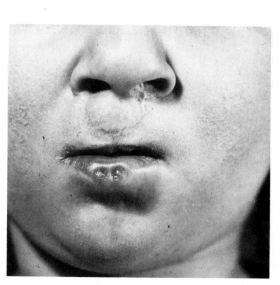

FIGURE 32–1. Congenital lip sinuses. Bilateral, symmetrically situated sinus openings at the apices of a pair of nipple-like protrusions of the lower lip. Note the associated bilateral cleft lip previously repaired.

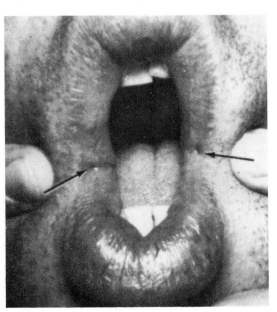

FIGURE 32–3. Bilateral lip pits of the commissures. (From Baker, B. R.: Pits of the lip commissures in Caucasoid males. Oral Surg., *21*:56, 1966.)

nuses is not yet known. Keith (1909) suggested the phylogenetic theory, based upon the findings of mucous canals in each side of the lower lip of sharks. Demarquay (1845), Murray (1860), and DePaul (1891) attributed the deformity to abnormal development of the labial glands in the embryonic stage following intrauterine diseases, such as inflammation or obliteration. Rose (1868), Hamilton (1881), Woollcombe (1905), and Hilgenreiner (1924) advocated the theory that the sinuses with their associated nipple-like protrusions represent an effort on the part of the lower lip to occlude, or to compensate for by excessive growth, defects in the cleft upper lip.

The most widely accepted theory, however, is based upon defective embryonic development. Stieda (1906) first mentioned the possible relationship between the embryonic sulci lateralis labii inferiores of the lower lip and lip sinuses. Sicher and Pohl (1934) and Warbrick, McIntyre and Fergusson (1952) examined the ventral portion of the mandibular arch of human embryos of different stages. They noticed the presence of such sulci as a secondary notch, one on each side of the median groove of the lower lip, in 6.5-mm embryos. In 7.5-mm embryos, the lateral sulci can be traced across the entire ventral surface of the globular process. As growth proceeds, the sulci are gradually obliterated, beginning at the cephalic end. It is normally completed in 12.5-mm embryos (Fig. 32–4). When normal development is retarded or inhibited, the lateral sulci, either as a whole or in part, may persist and produce a furrow which becomes deeper as growth proceeds. The edges of the furrow become more prominent and ultimately meet, fuse, and convert the furrow into a tubular canal open at its upper end.

If such embryonic retardation is the result of a defective gene, transmitted as either a dominant or a recessive factor, and if such a defective gene is also responsible for the formation of a cleft lip or palate, the importance of heredity and the common association of the lip sinuses with cleft lip and palate can be explained. Cervenka, Cerný and Cisařová (1966), however, proposed that the two conditions are caused by two different genes, both linked to the ABO blood group system and located in chromosome 21.

Treatment.   The treatment of congenital lip sinuses is surgical. As these sinuses are asymptomatic, excision can be deferred until the child reaches school age. Rose (1868) suggested an intraoral window that would open

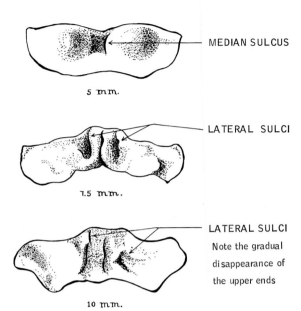

EMBRYONIC DEVELOPMENT of LOWER LIP

MEDIAN SULCUS

5 mm.

LATERAL SULCI

7.5 mm.

LATERAL SULCI

Note the gradual disappearance of the upper ends

10 mm.

FIGURE 32–4. Diagrammatic representation of the developmental changes in the lateral sulci of the lower lip.

the fistula into the oral cavity. Baxter (1939) advocated electrocoagulation of the entire tract. The most effective treatment is a complete excision of the mucosal tract, in association with the attached glandular tissue. The tract is identified by the instillation of methylene blue. A metal probe is inserted as a guide. A transverse incision, parallel to the vermilion border, is made around the orifice of the tract, and the entire tract is isolated and excised. All of the attached mucous glands whose ducts drain into the sinus must be removed with the tract. The closure should be effected in layers with special regard for reapproximation of the muscle.

Complications

FORMATION OF MUCOID CYSTS.   When any of the mucous glands attached to the sinus are left behind, a mucoid cyst may form. This usually occurs four to eight weeks after the operation. For such cysts, additional excision is usually required.

LOOSENING OF THE LIP MUSCLE.   The sinus penetrates and stretches the orbicularis oris muscle, and occasionally the latter will remain in a relaxed state for a considerable time, even after complete excision of the sinuses and reapproximation of the muscle fibers. This may cause drooling of saliva or a mild eversion of the lower lip. Such a deformity is usually mild and temporary; no specific treatment is indicated.

CONGENITAL DOUBLE LIP

Congenital double lip is another clinical rarity. Ascher (1920) described a patient with double lip associated with blepharochalasis and struma. Dorrance (1922) reported a patient with simple double lip without other associated pathology. Calnan (1952) stated that there are only approximately a dozen cases recorded in the literature. Guerrero-Santos and Altamirano (1967), however, in reporting their own 13 cases, believe that the deformity is not as uncommon as recorded.

Congenital double lip occurs most frequently in the upper lip. When the mouth is open, a double vermilion border is seen with a transverse furrow of varying depth between two borders. The buccal portion of the double vermilion border is rather loose and redundant (Fig. 32–5). The deformity is not obvious when the mouth is closed, since the furrow corresponds to the normal line of closure of the mouth. Though the deformity can occur at birth, it usually becomes evident after the eruption of the permanent teeth.

On microscopic examination, the buccal portion consists of normal mucosa overlying prominent, hyperplastic, racemose mucous glands scattered in a normal dermal layer without evidence of inflammatory reaction. The orbicularis oris muscle is normal, and no muscle fibers are found in the buccal portion of the double lip.

In the fetus, the mucosa of the lip is divided into two transverse zones: an outer zone, which is smooth and similar to skin, the pars glabra; and an inner zone, which is villous and similar to the oral mucosa, the pars villosa. Neustaetter (1895) and Warbrick, McIntyre and Fergusson (1952) believed that the furrow dividing the double lip represents an exagger-

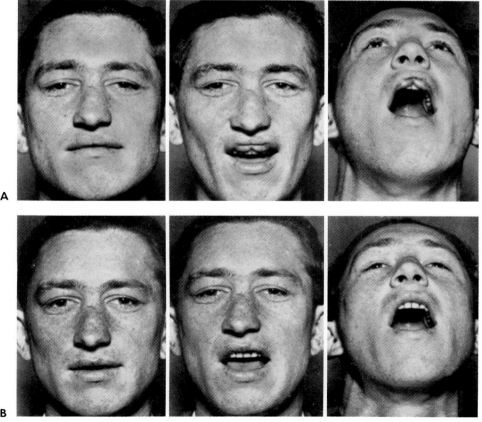

FIGURE 32–5. Congenital double upper lip. *A,* Preoperative photographs. *B,* Postoperative photographs, three months after excision of the double lip. (Courtesy of J. Calnan, F.R.C.S.)

ated boundary line between these two zones, and the buccal portion a hypertrophy of the pars villosa.

Clinically, double lip needs to be differentiated from other types of chronic enlargement of the lip. Macrocheilia may be neoplastic in nature (such as that produced by hemangiomas or lymphangiomas), circulatory (from elephantiasis), or inflammatory (such as cheilitis glandularis). All of these conditions, however, are associated with a uniformly enlarged lip with no transverse furrow dividing the vermilion portion of the lip. Hemangioma of the lip commonly has a purplish or bluish coloration, is compressible, and increases in size when dependent. Lymphangioma produces a diffuse enlargement, making the lip translucent when the overlying mucosa is stretched thin. Elephantiasis is often associated with a thickened mucous membrane and hypertrophic folds on the skin and mucosa. Though cheilitis glandularis represents hyperplasia of the labial salivary glands, chronic inflammatory changes can usually be demonstrated in the dermal and subcutaneous layers.

The treatment is surgical. The buccal fold is excised by transverse elliptical incisions extending from one commissure to the other. The mucosal edges are reapproximated after minimal undermining. Minor adjustments may be necessary to assure a symmetrically smooth and normal vermilion portion of the lip. Guerrero-Santos and Altamirano (1967) advocated the use of W-plasty for the excision of the buccal folds, as the multiple flaps permit the surgeon to make last minute realignment during suturing to avoid asymmetry or "dog-ear" formation.

Techniques for the Repair of Defects of the Lips and Cheeks

John Marquis Converse, M.D., and Donald Wood-Smith, F.R.C.S.E.

In this section a review is made of the various techniques for the repair of defects of the lips and cheeks. Defects of the lips and cheeks due to congenital malformations, to injuries and burns, or to the excision of tumors are varied in type, and each type requires individual consideration. Age and sex are also important factors, since patients in the older age group have looser soft tissues, permitting the use of advancement, transposition, or rotation flaps to greater advantage than in the younger patient. The scars also tend to be less conspicuous in the older patient, thus permitting wider selection of donor sites. Male patients require restoration, whenever possible, of their hair-bearing skin of the face; female patients may apply cosmetics, an artifice not usually possible in the male patient.

DEFORMITIES OF THE UPPER LIP

Superficial Deformities

The contour of the upper lip is easily distorted by contraction of simple linear scars which pull the vermilion border out of line or result in notching. Excision of the scar and Z-plasty is an especially useful method of repair (Fig. 32–6).

Loss of skin of the upper lip results in severe distortion of the lip because of the looseness of the tissue; it may be corrected by skin grafting, local flaps, or the use of flap tissue from a distant site. In the male, attention must be directed to the use of local hair-bearing flaps whenever possible; when this is not feasible, it

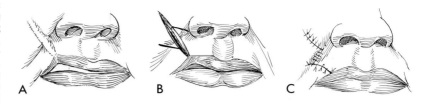

FIGURE 32-6. *A,* Ectropion of the upper lip and contracture from a vertical scar extending through the nasolabial fold. *B,* Excision of the scar with the outline of the limbs of the Z-plasty. *C,* Transposition of the Z flaps completed. The central line of the Z lies in the line of the nasolabial fold.

is often preferable to use an esthetic unit graft to preserve side-to-side symmetry.

The true defect is apparent after the scar tissue is resected and the wound edges have retracted. The type of repair is dependent upon the location of the defect, the amount of tissue loss, and the age and sex of the patient.

Skin Grafts. Full-thickness postauricular skin grafts may be used for small skin defects or for larger defects when local flaps are not available because of surrounding scarring (Fig. 32-7).

Local Flaps. For surface defects other than small defects in the midline of the upper lip, local flaps are the method of choice. A rectangular or triangular nasolabial skin flap is an ex-

cellent method of closure for laterally placed defects; the secondary defect is closed by direct approximation with minimal tension, resulting in a relatively inconspicuous scar (Fig. 32-8).

When a scar crosses the nasolabial fold, a transposed cheek flap parallel to the scar may be used, as illustrated in Figure 32-9.

Skin flaps may be raised in the nasolabial areas on both sides if the skin loss is bilateral or when the entire skin of the lip requires replacement.

Webster (1955) has described an advancement flap for the closure of small upper lip defects which involves excision of a crescentic area lateral to the alar base (Fig. 32-10).

In skin contractures distorting the angle of the mouth, the operation of Serre (1842) may be employed, involving switching of a skin and subcutaneous tissue flap from one lip to the other (Fig. 32-11). When the deformity is

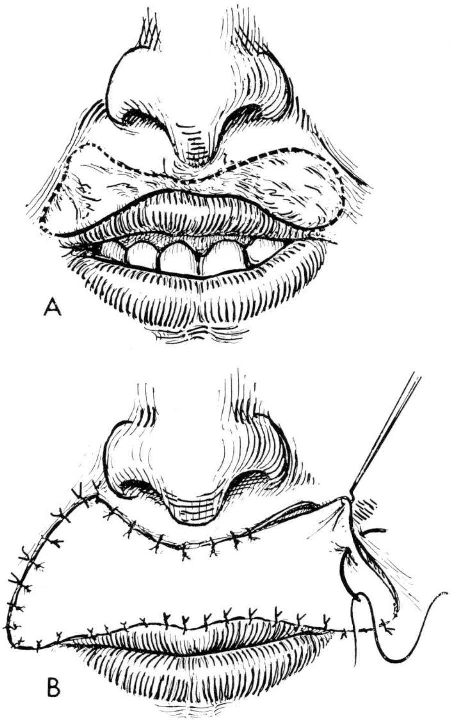

FIGURE 32-7. *A,* A burn scar contracture of the upper lip is excised as far laterally as the nasolabial folds. *B,* A full-thickness skin graft covers the defect and is fixed in position by a "tie-over" (bolus) dressing.

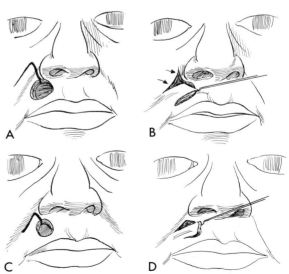

FIGURE 32-8. *A,* A defect of the lateral portion of the upper lip is repaired by a transposition flap raised from the nasolabial area. *B,* The nasolabial flap transposed. The secondary defect is closed after undermining the skin of the cheek. *C,* A smaller defect is repaired by a flap medial to the nasolabial fold. *D,* The flap is transposed, the secondary defect is closed. In older patients the looser skin facilitates this procedure.

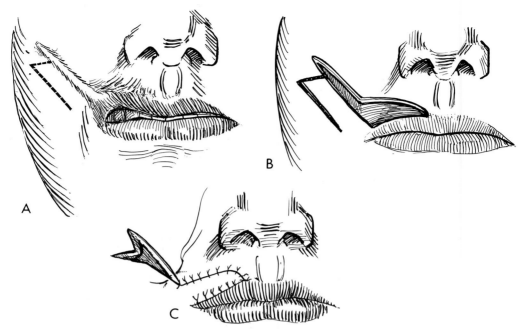

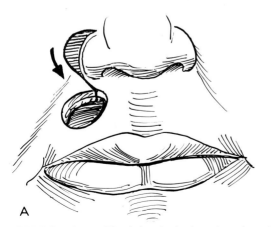

FIGURE 32–9. *A,* Ectropion of the upper lip with a scar transgressing the nasolabial fold, preventing the use of a nasolabial flap. *B,* The scar has been excised and a transposition cheek flap outlined. *C,* The flap is transposed and the secondary defect closed by direct approximation. (Redrawn from Kazanjian and Converse.)

more pronounced, a transposition flap must be raised from a more lateral and inferior portion of the lower lip (Fig. 32–12).

Distant Flaps.   Large areas of the upper lip may be resurfaced by distant flaps, especially when the defect involves adjacent structures. The forehead is utilized in a temporal (Gillies, 1920) or bitemporal flap as a source of hairless skin. Alternatively, in the male, hair-bearing skin from the scalp as a unipedicle or bipedicle flap may be transferred to the patient's upper

lip to provide the basis for a mustache (Fig. 32–13). In this flap, a portion of the forehead skin without hair may be used to cover a philtral defect; if this is not necessary, a narrow strip of hair-bearing skin is left to preserve the hairline.

Full-Thickness Defects of the Upper Lip

Full-thickness loss of lip tissue results from trauma or excision for malignant disease. In

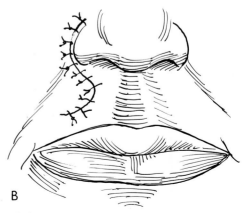

FIGURE 32–10.   *A,* The defect in the lateral portion of the upper lip is closed by excision of a perialar crescent and an advancement flap. *B,* The primary and secondary defects are closed. (Redrawn from Webster, 1955.)

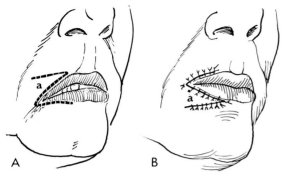

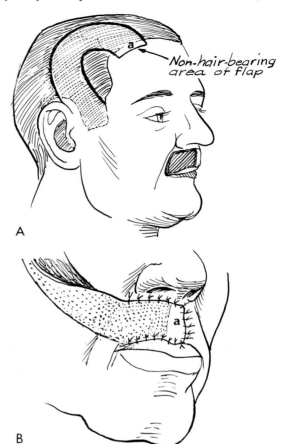

FIGURE 32–11. *A,* Distortion of the corner of the mouth, with a Z-flap incision outlined. *B,* The flap (a) is brought down and sutured into the defect produced by the upward replacement of the corner of the mouth.

the latter case, a segment of definite size is removed and the repair is often completed at the same procedure. Tissue loss following trauma is often difficult to estimate because of

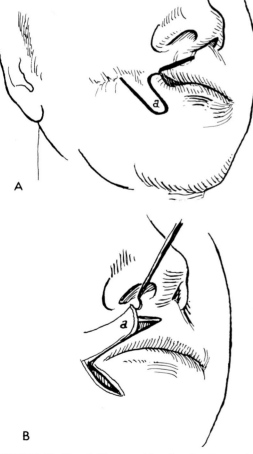

FIGURE 32–12. *A,* Transposition flap for the repair of a contracture of the angle of the mouth and a defect of the upper lip. *B,* The flap (a) is transposed to fill the defect resulting from the repositioning of the corner of the mouth.

FIGURE 32–13. *A,* A full-thickness defect of the upper lip is covered by a sickle flap of hair-bearing skin based on the superficial temporal vessels. *B,* The flap is transferred without tubing and a non–hair-bearing area (a) is used to simulate the philtrum. (After New, 1945.)

the variable amount of retraction of the wound edges. Particularly when treatment has been delayed, the effects of contracting scar tissue in enlarging the size of the defect are maximal.

It may be necessary, as a primary procedure, to excise scar tissue which interferes with the success of subsequent operative procedures. The avoidance of raw tissue areas in reconstructive surgery of the lips is a factor of prime importance; Serre first emphasized this principle in 1842.

Kazanjian and Converse (1959, 1974) stressed the importance of the following principles in planning the reconstruction of the lip: (1) The remaining portions of the injured lip should be utilized. (2) If this is not possible, tissue should be borrowed from the opposing lip. (3) When sufficient lip tissue is not available, flaps are rotated from the sides of the defect. (4) The design of such flaps is often dic-

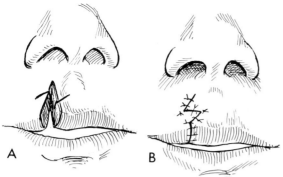

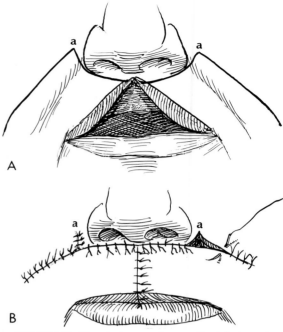

FIGURE 32–14. *A,* A defect following wedge excision of a lesion of the upper lip may be closed with a Z-plasty to prevent distortion of the vermilion border due to contracture of the line of repair. *B,* The Z-flaps are transposed and the repair completed.

tated by the presence of preexisting scars, and it may be necessary to resort to the use of distant flaps. There is no advantage in using distant flaps that shrink and curl inward owing to a lack of muscular action, and every effort should be made to utilize local flaps.

FIGURE 32–16. *A,* A central upper lip defect repaired by two quadrilateral full-thickness flaps (von Bruns). *B,* The repair completed.

The best result is achieved by reconstructing the lip defect with composite skin-muscle-mucosal flaps which become reinnervated and show a high degree of functional restitution.

Median Defects of the Upper Lip. Celsus, in 25 B.C., first described wedge excision of lesions of the upper lip with approximation of the margins of the defect. This procedure is useful only in smaller defects. Because of the linear contraction of a straight line of approximation, breaking the straight line by a Z-plasty procedure is recommended by some surgeons but is not necessary as a routine procedure (Fig. 32–14).

A moderate sized median defect of the upper lip may be closed by direct advancement of the remaining portions of the lip; curved perialar excisions from the upper portion of the naso-labial fold facilitate such closure (Fig. 32–15).

For large median defects a quadrilateral flap is transposed from each side to correct the deformity. A modification of the flap described by Blasius (1839) and by von Bruns (1859) is employed. A diagonal full-thickness incision is made along the alar base to the nasolabial groove, and a slightly curved incision in the line of the nasolabial fold is extended inferiorly to below the corner of the mouth (Fig. 32–16). The two full-thickness flaps are mobilized and

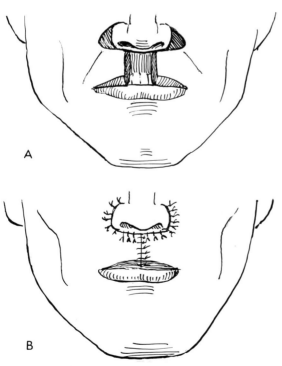

FIGURE 32–15. *A,* A central defect of the upper lip is closed by advancement of the lateral portions, which is facilitated by perialar excisions from each nasolabial area. *B,* The repair completed.

approximated. The flaps should be freed by wide incision of the mucosal attachments in the oral vestibule.

Gillies (Gillies and Millard, 1957) has successfully used a modified form of quadrilateral flap, called by him the "fan flap" and illustrated in Figure 32–17.

Rotation of a portion of the lower lip through 180 degrees to replace a loss in the upper lip was first performed in 1837 by Sabattini in Italy. The next reported use of cross-lip flaps was in 1848 by Stein, who used double flaps in the upper lip turned inferiorly to fill defects in the lower lip (see Fig. 32–49).

THE ABBÉ OPERATION. In moderate sized defects of the upper lip, the Abbé operation is the most useful procedure. A triangular full-thickness flap is taken from the median portion of the lower lip and is left attached to a pedicle near the vermilion border; the labial artery lying close to the labial mucosa provides an adequate blood supply (Fig. 32–18). The flap is swung upward to fit into the defect of the upper lip and accurately sutured into position

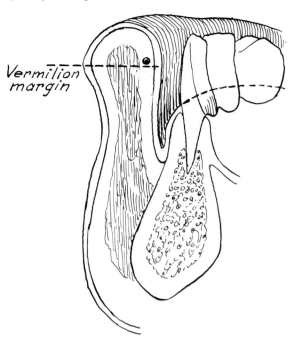

FIGURE 32–18. The position of the labial artery at the lip margin. (Redrawn from Smith, 1961.)

(Fig. 32–19). Smith (1961) stated that the pedicle may be sectioned and the mucocutaneous line reestablished as early as eight days after transplantation; ten days is probably a safer time interval. Recent experience has shown that the repair is just as safe with only the vessels in the pedicle; this allows for a more accurate repair at the time of transposition and an easier division of the pedicle (Fig. 32–19, *E*).

Dufourmentel and his associates (1967) have successfully grafted composite grafts from the lower lip to repair a defect of the upper lip. In our experience, success is achieved when relatively small grafts are transplanted. A similar technique has also been used for the repair of lower lip defects. Microvascular surgery could ensure the success of these procedures. Unless contraindicated, the narrow vascular pedicle from the opposing lip is a relatively simple and safe technique for the rapid revascularization of the transplanted lip tissue.

When the anterior portion of the maxilla has been destroyed, a prosthodontic appliance should be fabricated and placed in position prior to the reconstruction of any major defect of the lip. The appliance restores skeletal contour, is a guide to indicate the true defect, and supports the reconstructed lip.

The Abbé operation combined with transposed flaps. In large median defects, especially when tissue in the lower lip is abundant,

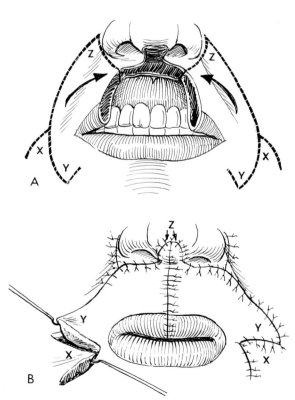

FIGURE 32–17. *A,* A large median defect of the upper lip and the outline of the fan flaps (Gillies). *B,* After transposition of the nasolabial flaps, the secondary defect is closed at the angle of the mouth by transposition of the two flaps X and Y.

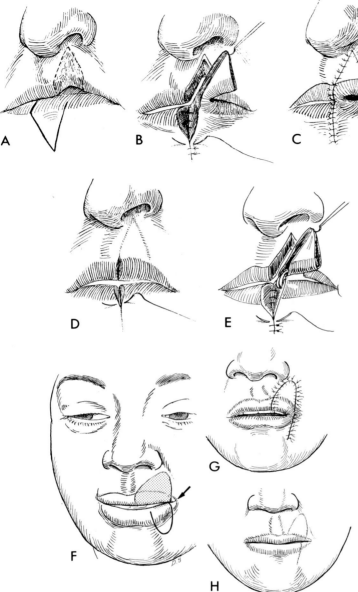

FIGURE 32–19. The Abbé operation. *A*, The defect outlined as well as the flap for repair. *B*, The defect excised and the flap transposed. *C*, The repair completed. *D*, The pedicle is divided and the lip separated with repair of the vermilion borders. *E*, Modified operation with the pedicle consisting of the artery and vein, allowing an immediate closure of the vermilion defect. *F*, A more laterally located defect. Note that the flap is smaller than the defect. The arrow indicates the corner of the mouth which is preserved. *G*, Intermediate stage. *H*, Final result.

the Abbé flap may be combined with transposed local flaps of the type described by von Bruns and Blasius (Fig. 32–20). Use of the Abbé flap in this instance avoids undue tension on the repaired upper lip.

Variations of the Abbé flap. Cannon (1941, 1942) advocated the use of an Abbé flap split in its distal portion to provide for the repair of a large defect of the upper lip (Fig. 32–21).

An Abbé flap may be complemented by an Abbé flap of similar design to repair a bilateral defect of the upper lip (Fig. 32–22).

In the design of the Abbé flap, the outline of the flap may be extended down to the upper

border of the fat pad of the chin and laterally to each side of the pad. The secondary defect may be closed with little tension, especially if there is abundant loose tissue. The pedicle of the flap should be placed at a point opposite the middle of the defect. The height of the flap should equal the height of the defect.

The site of the flap with relation to the defect has been discussed by Smith (1961), who recommended that when the defect lies adjacent to the commissure the pedicle should be placed directly opposite the defect, since otherwise the more mobile medial portion of the lip will be drawn toward a rather fixed corner,

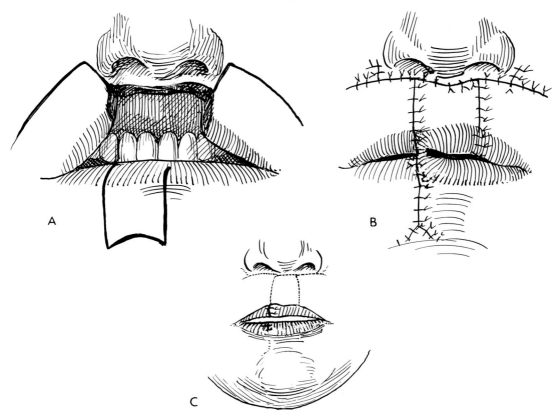

FIGURE 32–20. Large central defect of the upper lip repaired by a modified Abbé technique. *A*, Bilateral full-thickness rectangular flaps are outlined together with an Abbé flap in the lower lip. *B*, Repair completed with closure of the central defect by a square Abbé flap. *C*, Second stage: the pedicle of the Abbé flap is divided and the donor areas are closed. (Modified from Kazanjian and Converse.)

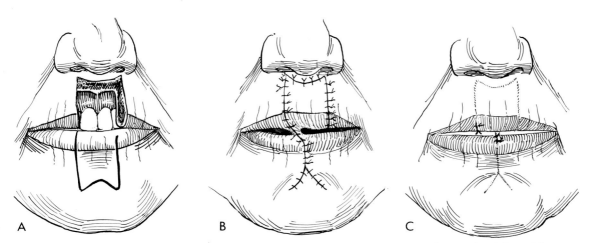

FIGURE 32–21. Modified Abbé operation. *A*, Large, prong-shaped Abbé flap prepared to repair a defect of the upper lip. *B*, The flap after transposition. *C*, After completion of the operative procedure and division of the pedicle in a second stage. (From Kazanjian and Converse.)

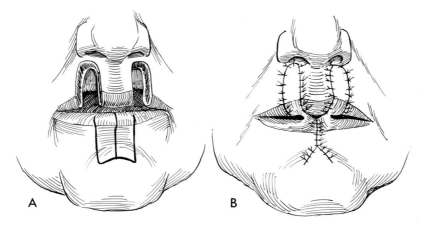

FIGURE 32–22. Modified Abbé operation. *A,* The large, rectangular Abbé flap is split into two halves. *B,* The two tongues of the Abbé flap are employed to repair bilateral full-thickness defects of the upper lip.

and abnormal torsion of the pedicle will result. In defects of the midportion of the lip, he recommends that the flap "straddle" the defect so that after rotation the pedicle will be in the proper position.

Smith (1960) demonstrated in Abbé flaps return of motor function by electromyographic study and also return of pain, temperature, touch, and sudomotor activity to near normal levels within 6 to 12 months.

Lateral Defects of the Upper Lip. In small lateral defects of the upper lip, the nasolabial flap provides a satisfactory method of repair (Fig. 32–23).

Larger defects may require a procedure based on the principles outlined by Sédillot (1848) and Denonvilliers (1863), in which the uninjured section of the upper lip is mobilized through a full-thickness diagonal incision from the medial edge of the lip tissue toward the area lateral to the nose and a wide incision curving downward and laterally into the nasolabial fold (Fig. 32–24). A second rectangular flap from the opposite side of the lower lip is transposed to form the other half of the upper lip and sutured to the flap on the opposite side. There is

little difficulty in closure of the secondary defects by direct approximation.

CHEEK FLAPS. A rectangular full-thickness flap with the base of the flap at the corner of the mouth and the lower portion of the nasolabial fold is raised and rotated through almost 180 degrees to be sutured to the border of the lip defect on the contralateral side. The secondary defect is closed by direct approximation (Fig. 32–25). Care must be taken to avoid sectioning Stensen's duct by cannulation and injection of methylene blue and careful identification. The distortion of the corner of the mouth following this procedure may be corrected at a later date.

THE FERRIS SMITH TECHNIQUE (1942). This procedure involves mobilizing two delayed skin flaps: a short horizontal flap is taken from the side of the defect, raised, and turned back with skin surface inward to form the inner lip surface (Fig. 32–26), and a long vertical flap extending from the distal end of the horizontal flap is raised, transposed through 90 degrees, and sutured over the donor area of the horizontal flap and the new raw lip surface. The presence of hair follicles on the lining flap is an

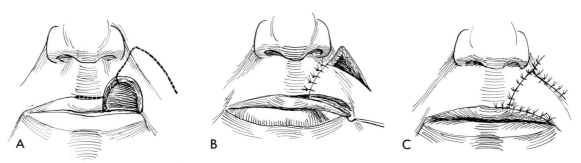

FIGURE 32–23. *A,* Lateral defect of the upper lip with a nasolabial flap outlined for a repair of the defect. *B,* The nasolabial flap is transposed and the vermilion border of the upper lip is advanced laterally to the corner of the mouth. *C,* The repair completed.

inconvenience. The blood supply of the horizontal flap may be tenuous, particularly when much scar tissue exists in the region of the junction between skin and mucosa at the border of the defect.

THE ESTLANDER OPERATION (1872). This procedure also utilizes the labial artery in a labial pedicle, and the reader is referred to an English translation of the original report (Estlander, 1968). It is useful in moderate sized defects of the upper lip near the corner of the mouth and consists of rotation of a triangular shaped flap from the side of the lip to cover a defect (Fig. 32–27). Revision of the rounded angle of the mouth is necessary as a secondary procedure (Fig. 32–27, *D*).

Variations of the Estlander flap. A modification of the Estlander flap has been employed by Converse for defects involving the upper portion of the lateral aspect of the upper lip (Fig. 32–28, *A*). It is also used to replace scar tissue which causes an upward contraction of

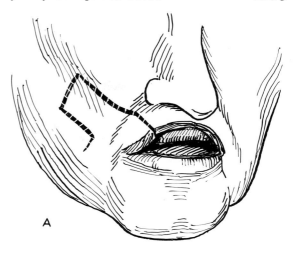

A

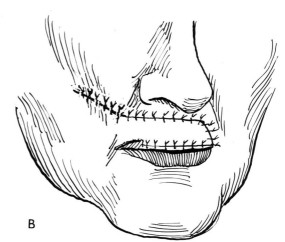

B

FIGURE 32–25. *A*, Full-thickness defect of the upper lip with the outline of a full-thickness cheek flap for repair. *B*, The full-thickness flap is transposed and the secondary defect is closed by direct approximation. (Redrawn from Kazanjian and Converse.)

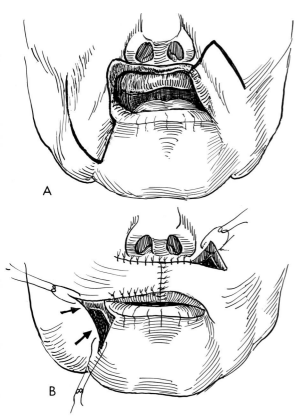

A

B

FIGURE 32–24. *A*, Large central and lateral defect of the upper lip showing the outline of two full-thickness flaps, a nasolabial and a superiorly based lateral flap. *B*, The flaps are approximated and sutured. The secondary defects are closed by direct approximation. (Redrawn from Kazanjian and Converse.)

the lip and a lateral displacement of the alar base. In the repair of such defects, the postoperative tension on the lower lip is greatest at the vermilion border.

Reconstruction of the defect is begun by an incision in the vermilion border, as shown in Figure 32–28, *B*. The incision is made 0.5 cm from the border of the defect to break the straight line extending through the lip. The vermilion border flap is tubed (Fig. 32–28, *B*, *C*). The flap from the lower lip is outlined and incised, avoiding the fat pad of the chin. A mucosal vestibular flap is raised medially to facilitate subsequent advancement of the flap. Additionally, a mucosal vestibular flap is raised

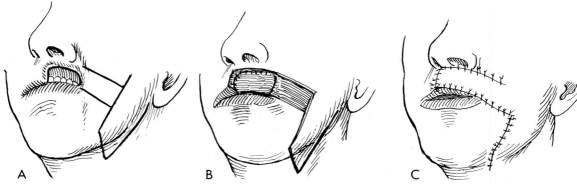

FIGURE 32–26. The Ferris Smith technique for repair of upper lip defects. *A,* Lines of incision for the delayed flaps. *B,* The horizontal flap is turned in as a hinge flap to form the inner lining of the lip. *C,* The vertical flap is transposed and sutured and the secondary defect is closed by direct approximation. This type of repair devoid of muscle can be performed for defects of the upper lip. Defects of the lower lip should have muscle control whenever possible.

to provide sufficient lining for the Estlander flap (Fig. 32–28, *D, E*). The flap from the lower lip is transferred to the defect in the upper lip (Fig. 32–28, *F, G, H, I*). If the anterior portion of the floor of the nose is missing, the mucosa is sutured to the skin along the upper margin of the flap to form a new rim for the nasal floor (Fig. 32–28, *H, I*). The defect of the lower lip is closed by direct approximation, and the edges of the Estlander flap are sutured to the edges of the upper lip defect (Fig. 32–28, *H, I*).

Two weeks later the flap is incised at the

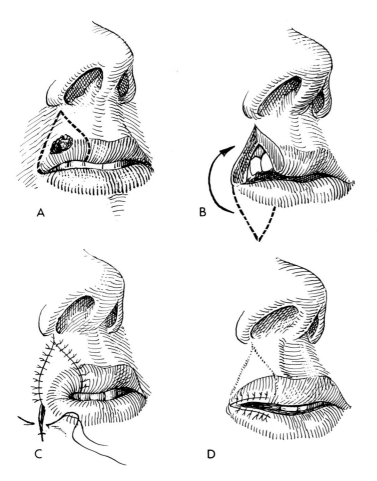

FIGURE 32–27. *A, B, C,* The Estlander operation. A triangular section of the lower lip is shifted to repair a defect of the lateral portion of the upper lip. *D,* Correction of the rounded corner of the mouth is required as a secondary procedure.

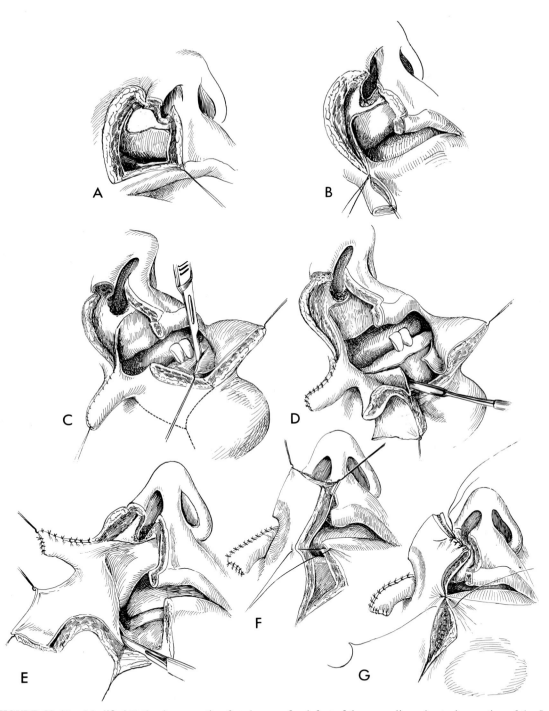

FIGURE 32–28. Modified Estlander operation for closure of a defect of the upper lip and anterior portion of the floor of the nose (Converse). *A*, Defect of the upper lip and anterior portion of the floor of the nose. *B*, Bone is resected from the border of the pyriform aperture. The vermilion border flap is tubed. *C*, The outline of the Estlander flap in the lower lip is indicated by a dotted line. An incision has been made through the lower lip, and a mucosal flap is raised from the lower portion of the oral vestibule on the left side. *D*, The Estlander flap has been incised, and an additional mucosal flap is raised from the lower vestibule on the right side to provide sufficient lining for the flap. *E*, The tissues are retracted, demonstrating the Estlander flap. *F*, *G*, Transfer of the lower lip flap to the upper lip defect.

Illustration continued on following page.

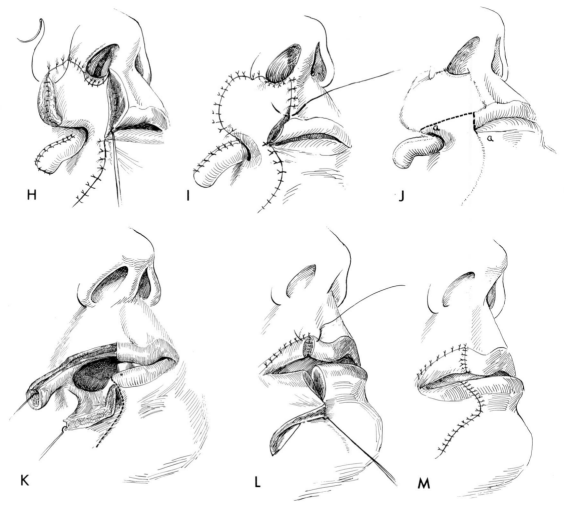

FIGURE 32–28 *Continued.* The modified Estlander operation. *H*, The mucosa is sutured to the skin edge along the upper margin of the Estlander flap. Closure of the lower defect is begun. *I*, The edges of the Estlander flap are sutured to the edges of the defect. Suturing is completed. *J*, The second stage operation. Two to three weeks later the flap is incised along the dotted line. *K*, The tubed upper vermilion flap is incised and opened. *L*, The remaining portion of the Estlander flap comprising the vermilion border is replaced in the lower lip. Suturing of the upper vermilion border flap is completed. *M*, The second stage is completed. (From Kazanjian and Converse.)

second stage of operation (Fig. 32–28, *J*). The tubed vermilion border of the upper lip is opened and inserted; the remaining portion of the Estlander flap is fitted into the lower lip (Fig. 32–28, *L*, *M*).

If the vermilion border of the upper lip can be preserved, Converse (1976) has described a bridge flap for the reconstruction of full-thickness defects (Fig. 32–29).

Complete Loss of the Upper Lip. Muscle function of a reconstructed lip is derived from contraction of the facial muscle fibers. The problem is providing an adequate quantity of suitable tissue to reconstruct the lip. This may

be done by the use of local tissues in the form of lateral flaps combined with an Abbé flap or by the use of local flaps alone. The use of a flap from a distance should be considered only as a last resort and reserved for patients in whom the surrounding tissues are scarred and of deficient vascularity. In the presence of unilateral scarring of the face, the use of a flap such as the temporal forehead flap combined with a nasolabial flap on the unscarred side may make possible a relatively satisfactory repair, or alternatively a compound forehead flap may be used (Fig. 32–30). Flaps lined by skin grafts, however, have an inherent rigidity.

Lateral flaps may be combined with an Abbé

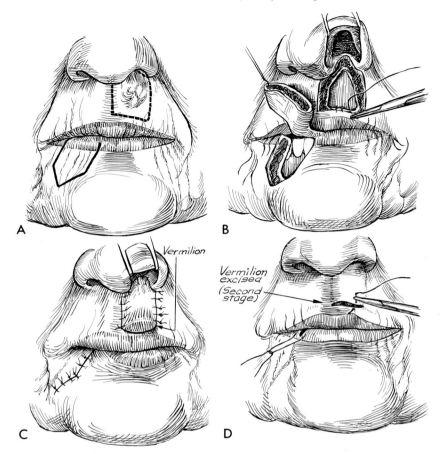

FIGURE 32–29.   Bridge flap technique. *A*, Outline of area to be excised and the proposed full-thickness flap in the lower lip. Note the vermilion border is preserved. *B, C*, Transposition and insetting of the flap under the remaining portion of the upper lip. *D*, The vermilion border of the bridge flap is excised, and the pedicle is divided at a second stage. (From Converse, J. M.: The bridge flap for reconstruction of a full-thickness defect of the upper lip. Plast. Reconstr. Surg., *57*: 442, 1976.)

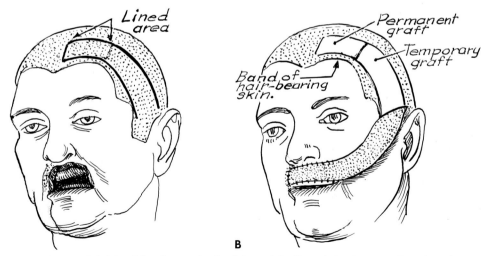

FIGURE 32–30.   Temporal forehead flap for repair of a defect of the lip and cheek. *A*, Outline of the flap. The upper portion of the flap, composed of scalp, is lined by a graft of oral mucous membrane. A narrow strip of hair-bearing skin is left to maintain the hair line. *B*, The hair-bearing scalp portion of the flap forms the outer covering and the mucous membrane-lined portion the inner lining of the defect. (From Kazanjian and Converse.)

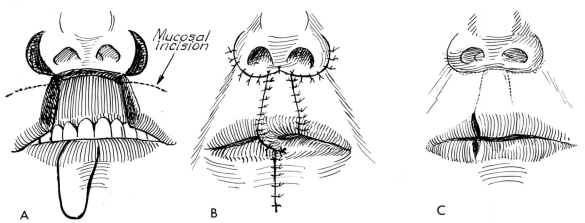

FIGURE 32–31. *A,* Repair of a large central defect of the upper lip facilitated by excision of perialar crescents, allowing advancement of the lateral portions of the upper lip and closure of the central defect by an Abbé flap. *B,* The repair completed. *C,* Readjustment of the vermilion borders after division of the pedicle of the Abbé flap in a second stage 10 to 12 days later. (Redrawn from Webster, 1955.)

flap to form a satisfactory upper lip, and this is the method of choice (see Fig. 32–20).

Webster (1955) described a similar technique; bilateral flaps involving crescentic perialar excisions are combined with an Abbé flap (Fig. 32–31).

Another technique involves the use of rectangular full-thickness flaps transposed from the side of the lower lip (Fig. 32–32). This technique disturbs the normal contour of the mouth and lower portion of the face. However, restoration of the lip is the primary consideration and may justify the resulting secondary deformity, particularly in the older patient in whom tissue laxity facilitates closure of the secondary defects.

The procedure of Ferris Smith previously described (see Fig. 32–26) may be combined with a full-thickness rectangular Sédillot-type flap raised from one side of the lower lip (Fig. 32–33).

Lengthening the Upper Lip. Teale in 1857 described a procedure to increase the height of the upper lip. Diagonal incisions are made through the full-thickness of the upper lip (Fig. 32–34), and the two flaps are imbricated until the desired increase in lip height has been obtained. The procedure may be reversed to diminish the height of the lip.

Webster (1955) described the use of lateral advancement flaps aided by crescentic perialar excisions and a **V-Y** closure to increase the vertical dimension of the upper lip (Fig. 32–35).

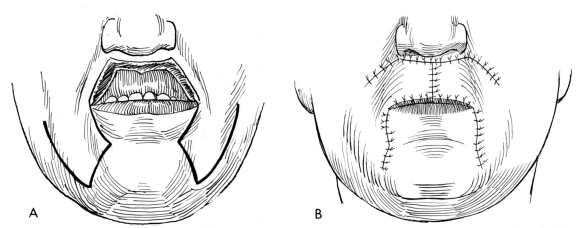

FIGURE 32–32. *A,* Two rectangular full-thickness flaps are removed from the area lateral to the lower lip and chin. *B,* The flaps are raised and approximated and the secondary defects closed. (After Kazanjian and Converse.)

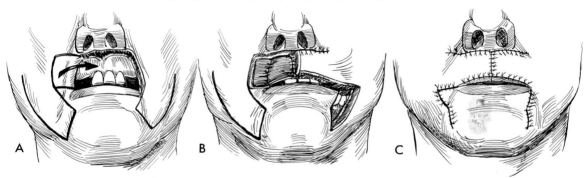

FIGURE 32–33. Reconstruction of the entire upper lip with a full-thickness flap from one side and skin flaps from the other. *A,* The outline of the flaps. *B,* A full-thickness flap is raised from the patient's left side and a skin flap turned in to provide lining on the patient's right side. *C,* The procedure is completed by transposition of a skin flap from the patient's right side.

DEFORMITIES OF THE LOWER LIP

Superficial Deformities

The operative procedures previously discussed for the correction of superficial deformities of the upper lip may be applied in principle to su-

perficial defects of the lower lip. However, care must be taken in the planning and mobilization of lower lip flaps based below the chin, since in the absence of adequate supporting tissue they tend, by the influence of gravity, to retract downward. Lallemand (1824), Blasius (1839), and Langenbeck (König, 1898) realized the necessity for the provision of supporting tissue.

Kazanjian (1949) used supporting flaps, illustrated in Figure 32–36, to prevent retraction and ectropion of the reconstructed lip. Johanson, Aspelund, Breine and Holmström (1974) have used a stepping technique which is based on a similar principle.

Distortion of the Corner of the Mouth. Procedures similar to those employed in the correction of distortion of the corner of the mouth with reference to the upper lip are employed in the lower lip, of course with due attention paid to the effect of gravity and lack of support.

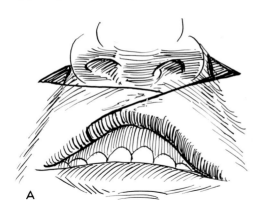

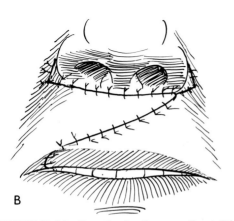

FIGURE 32–34. Lengthening the upper lip. *A,* Diagonal incisions are made in the upper lip. *B,* The flaps are slid across one another and sutured in position. (Modified after Teale, 1857.)

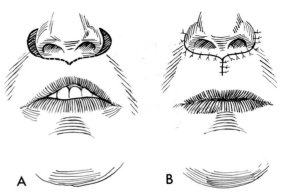

FIGURE 32–35. Lengthening the upper lip. *A,* Outline of the perialar crescents and the lines of incision. *B,* Advancement of the lateral lip flaps and closure medially by the V–Y method, thus achieving lengthening. (Redrawn from Webster, 1955.)

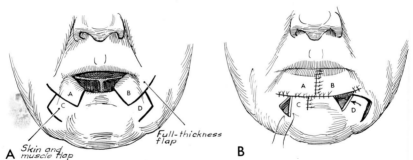

FIGURE 32–36. Supporting flaps used in the reconstruction of the lower lip. *A*, Two supporting flaps are outlined. *B*, The lower lip is repaired by approximation of the two superior flaps. The supporting flaps are rotated superiorly and medially to prevent downward retraction of the reconstructed lip. (Redrawn from Kazanjian and Converse.)

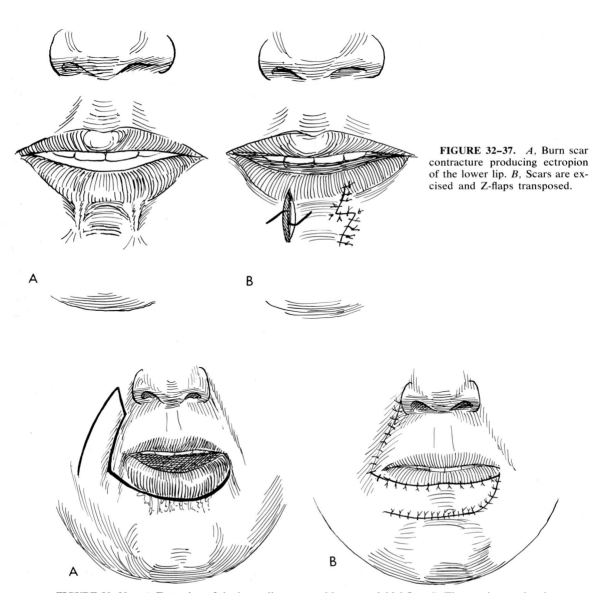

FIGURE 32–37. *A*, Burn scar contracture producing ectropion of the lower lip. *B*, Scars are excised and Z-flaps transposed.

FIGURE 32–38. *A*, Ectropion of the lower lip corrected by a nasolabial flap. *B*, The repair completed.

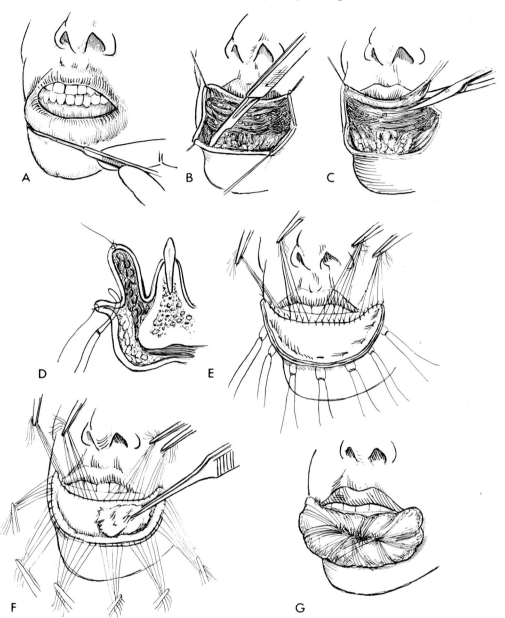

FIGURE 32–39.   Ectropion of the lower lip following burn scar contracture. *A,* Incision along the vermilion border. *B,* Resection of scar tissue and replacement of the distorted structures into their anatomical position. *C,* Excision of scarred wound edges. *D,* Fixation of the thick split-thickness skin graft with excess of graft to allow for shrinkage. *E,* Method of fixation of the graft. *F, G,* Immobilization of the graft by a "tie-over" dressing.

Ectropion of the Lower Lip.   Ectropion of the lower lip commonly follows contraction of burn scars and is more common than in the upper lip. In this deformity there is an eversion of oral mucosa. Correction of the deformity, if caused by linear bands of scar tissue, may be accomplished by a Z-plasty with satisfactory results (Fig. 32–37). In the presence of moderate sized defects, the area of scar tissue is excised to a healthy tissue base, and the defect is closed by a skin graft after the tissues have been allowed to retract into their normal anatomical position; a full-thickness retroauricular skin graft is the graft of choice. A nasolabial flap is another suitable means of closing such a defect; an outline delay may be required if the flap is long and is designed with a narrow base. Figure 32–38 illustrates the

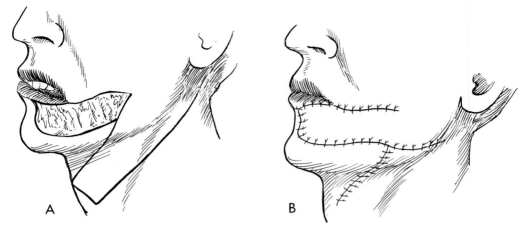

FIGURE 32–40. *A*, Burn scar contracture with distortion of the left corner of the mouth. Excision of the scarred area and outline of the cervical flap. *B*, Transposition of the flap and closure of the secondary defect by direct approximation.

correction of an ectropion of the lower lip by this technique.

In more extensive superficial tissue losses, the defect may be closed either by a skin graft (Fig. 32–39) or by rectangular cervical transposition flaps, if the cervical skin has been spared the effects of the causative injury (Fig. 32–40).

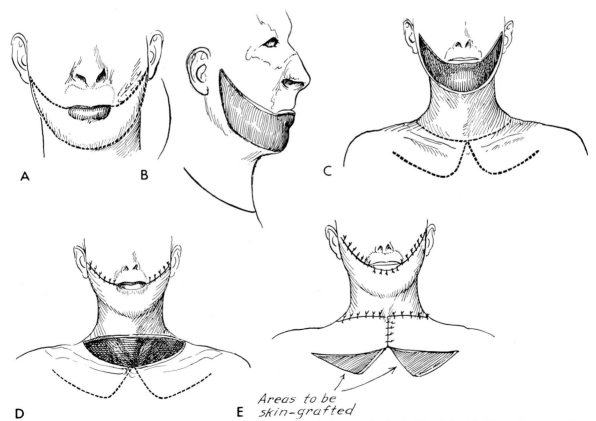

FIGURE 32–41. *A, B,* Extensive skin defect of the chin and adjacent cheek. *C,* Bipedicle skin flap and transposition flaps are outlined. *D, E,* The flaps are transposed and the secondary defects will be skin-grafted. (Figs. 32–41 and 32–42 redrawn from Converse, J. M.: Burn deformities of the face and neck. Reconstructive surgery and rehabilitation. Surg. Clin. North Am., *47:*323, 1967.)

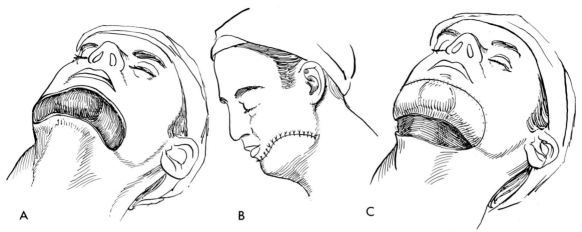

FIGURE 32–42. The 1–2 advancement flap (Converse). *A, B,* Straight advancement flap of the cervical skin to cover the defect of the lower portion of the face. *C,* In the second stage, a submandibular incision severs the pedicle of the flap. The resultant defect is covered with a thick split-thickness skin graft.

In larger defects, bipedicle skin flaps from the neck have been resorted to with adequate results (Fig. 32–41).

The 1-2 Advancement Flap (Converse, 1964). In extensive loss of the skin of the mental region, cover may be achieved by use of the 1-2 advancement flap. In a first stage (1), the skin of the cervical region is raised and the patient's neck is flexed to allow the upper limit of the cervical skin to reach the upper border of the defect

(Fig. 32–42). At a second stage (2) operation 14 to 21 days later, the flap is divided by a submental incision and the cervical skin allowed to retract to its original level. The cervical defect is resurfaced by a thick split-thickness skin graft. The technique is indicated in young patients who can tolerate the flexed cervical position.

Entropion of the Lower Lip. Lacerations and other trauma to the buccal mucosa occa-

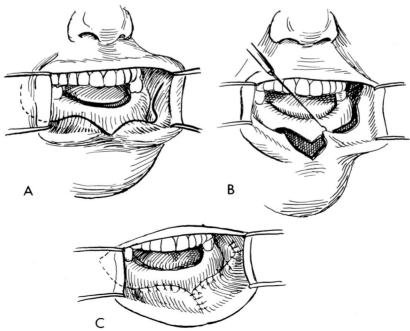

FIGURE 32–43. *A,* Outline of incisions in the buccal sulcus for release of a contracture causing entropion of the lower lip. *B,* Mucosal flaps are raised. *C,* Suture of the mucosal flaps by the V-Y method releasing the contracture. (From Kazanjian and Converse.)

sionally produce entropion of the lower lip; live socket electric burns in children and the ingestion of corrosive fluids, such as sodium hydroxide, are classic causes of this deformity.

When the area of contraction is localized, lateral advancement flaps of mucosa may be utilized, as shown in Figure 32–43. Defects of a more extensive nature require the use of the skin graft inlay technique after excision of the scar. The technique of the skin graft inlay is discussed more fully in Chapter 30.

Full-Thickness Defects of the Lower Lip

The close proximity of a double row of sharp teeth to the lip makes it particularly vulnerable to trauma in sport, transportation, and war. Particular care must be exercised at the time of primary repair to sacrifice a minimum of tissue and yet achieve complete debridement of the wound. In defects too large for immediate reconstruction, or when the patient's condition precludes the performance of a prolonged and complicated operative procedure, marginal skin should be sutured to mucous membrane and the definitive repair postponed until the patient's condition permits operative intervention.

Excision of scars and adhesions must be done in a manner similar to that in the upper lip, together with intelligent use of the Z-plasty technique in order to prevent retraction and vermilion border notching.

Median Defects. A small median defect of the lower lip may be closed by direct approxi-

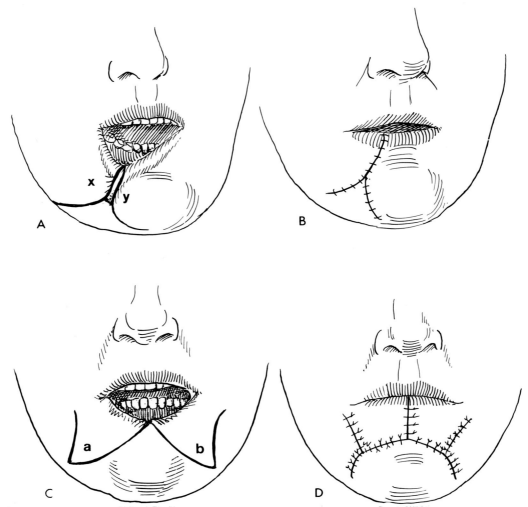

FIGURE 32–44. *A*, Scar with distortion of the lower lip. *B*, Correction by full-thickness flaps advanced by the V-Y method. *C*, *D*, Similar technique employed in the repair of a midline retraction of the lower lip.

mation, care being taken to incorporate a Z-plasty in the closure.

The **V-Y** advancement procedure advocated by Gillies and Millard (1957) tends to prevent linear contraction (Fig. 32–44).

Defects of moderate size are repaired by the rectangular flaps shown in Figure 32–45, and still larger defects by rotation of flaps, as shown in Figure 32–46.

Gillies' fan flap represents a further extension of this principle and is indicated when little of the lower lip remains for the repair (Fig. 32–47). Mucosal lining is easily obtained because of the elasticity and mobility of the oral mucosa. Incisions may be made along the buccal sulcus to the region of the third molar tooth on either side, and the incision is then extended vertically through the mucosa of the cheek for a distance of 2 to 3 cm (see Fig. 32–43). Defects that cannot be closed in this manner may be closed by a split-thickness skin graft in the form of a skin graft inlay by one of the techniques described in Chapter 30.

Free composite lip grafts have been advocated (Flanagin, 1956; Walker and Sawhney, 1972) but are not recommended because of size restrictions and the precariousness of vascularization.

THE STEIN OPERATION (1848). Two full-thickness triangular flaps from the philtrum of the upper lip are employed to repair the defect of the lower lip (Fig. 32–48). Each flap remains attached to a small vermilion pedicle containing the labial vessels. This procedure results in the loss of the normal philtrum contour, and a modification by Kazanjian and Roopenian (1954), preserving the philtrum, is preferred (Fig. 32–49).

THE ESTLANDER OPERATION (1872). For the repair of *lateral* defects of the lower lip,

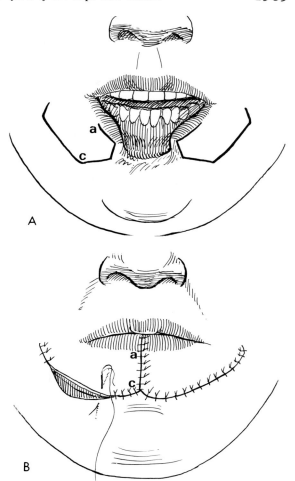

FIGURE 32–46. Median defect of the lower lip. *A,* Outline of incisions for rotation flaps. *B,* Flaps rotated medially to repair the lip.

Estlander described an operation using the corner of the mouth and a narrow labial artery pedicle (Fig. 32–50). This procedure results in a rounded corner of the mouth which must be corrected by a secondary procedure such as the type depicted in Figures 32–61 to 32–64.

Modification of the Estlander operation for median defects. An Estlander type of flap may be utilized in the repair of a large median defect of the lower lip. The median defect is closed by transposition flaps from the lateral half of the lower lip; an Estlander flap is raised and rotated into the lateral secondary defect (Fig. 32–51).

A further modification, similar in principle to the Estlander flap, but in exact definition an Abbé type of flap, is used in the repair of smaller defects. The flap includes only a portion of the upper lip and does not involve

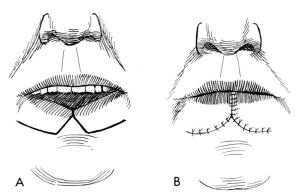

FIGURE 32–45. *A,* Median defect with retraction of the lower lip. *B,* Correction of the retraction by advancement and closure by the V-Y principle.

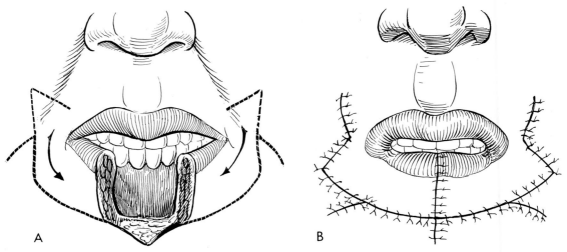

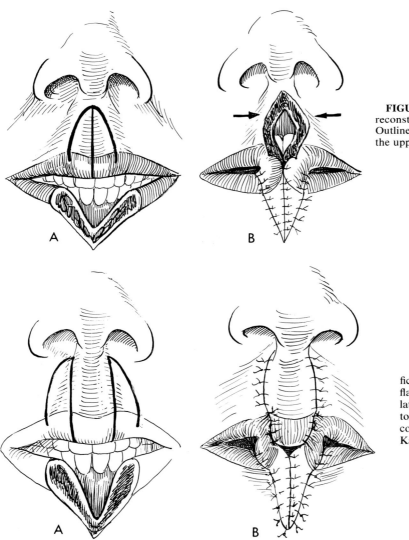

FIGURE 32–47. Reconstruction of a median defect of the lower lip. *A*, Outline of incisions for Gillies' fan flap. *B*, Flaps after transfer.

FIGURE 32–48. Stein's technique for reconstruction of the lower lip (1848). *A*, Outline of flaps taken from the center of the upper lip. *B*, Transfer of flaps.

FIGURE 32–49. Kazanjian modification of the Stein operation. *A*, The flaps are taken from the upper lip lateral to the philtrum to avoid distortion. *B*, Position of the flaps after completion of the operation. (From Kazanjian and Converse.)

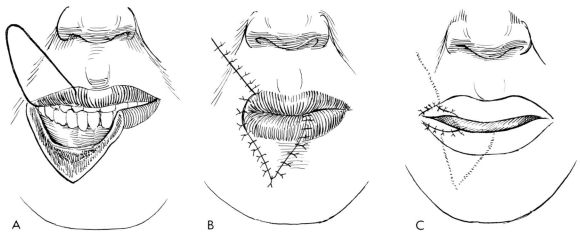

FIGURE 32–50. *A, B,* The original technique described by Estlander for reconstruction of a lower lip defect. *C,* Secondary correction of the angle of the mouth is necessary.

the corner of the mouth; the secondary defect of the upper lip is closed by direct approximation (Fig. 32–52). After division of the flap and realignment of the vermilion border, the presence of the normal commissure of the mouth obviates the need for revision, as with the rounded Estlander-type commissure. Since these operative procedures involve the formation of a relative degree of microstomia, it is obvious that the procedure is of value only in the repair of a relatively small defect.

THE ASHLEY OPERATION (1955).   In the

FIGURE 32–51. Modified Estlander operation for repair of a large median defect of the lower lip including the corner of the mouth. *A,* Median defect and outline of incisions. *B,* The median defect is closed by shifting the remaining lateral lip tissue into the defect. *C,* An Estlander flap which includes the corner of the mouth is rotated into the defect in the lower lip. *D,* Appearance at the conclusion of the operation. A secondary procedure illustrated in Figure 32–63 is necessary to restore the angle of the mouth. (From Kazanjian and Converse.)

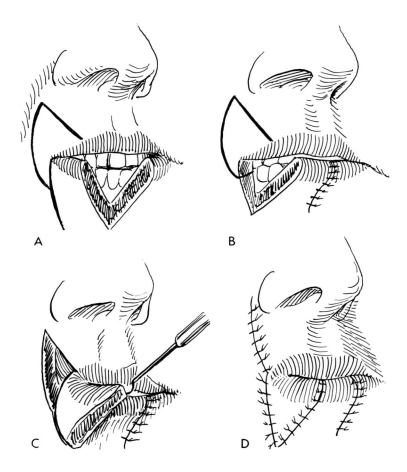

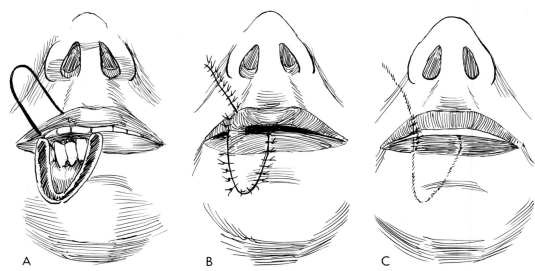

FIGURE 32–52.   The modified Estlander operation. The base of the flap does not include the angle of the mouth, thus avoiding distortion of this structure.

older patient with marked arteriosclerotic vascular changes, Ashley advocated a procedure employing two flaps, one mucosal and one full-thickness. The procedure is illustrated in Figure 32–53. A full-thickness flap is outlined on the upper lip below the nasolabial fold and above the vermilion border. The angle of the mouth is spared in the excision of the lower lip

segment. After the flap is placed in the defect, the remaining vermilion border is utilized to cover the edge of the flap.

THE BERNARD OPERATION (1853).   Camille Bernard applied the principle of lateral advancement flaps facilitated by the excision of Bürow triangles. He preserved the oral mucosa in the area of excision of the Bürow triangles,

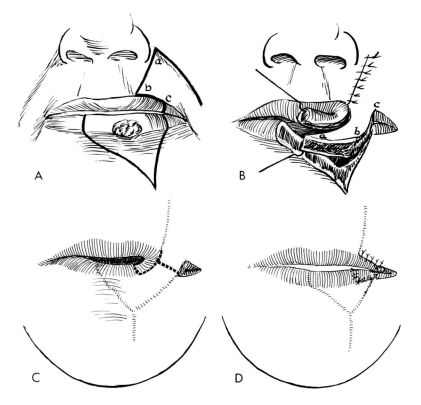

FIGURE 32–53.   The Ashley operation. *A*, The segment to be removed is outlined on the lower lip. The flap is also outlined on the upper lip, sparing the angle of the mouth and the vermilion border in its inferomedial aspect. *B*, The flap is raised and transposed through 90 degrees into the lower lip defect. The vermilion flap is rotated through 180 degrees to line the superior aspect of the lower lip defect. *C*, At a second stage the base of the flap is incised. A vermilion flap is rotated laterally from the lower lip to form the upper lateral vermilion border, and mucosa is advanced from the buccal sulcus to form the inferior vermilion border. *D*, The procedure completed. (Redrawn from Ashley, 1955.)

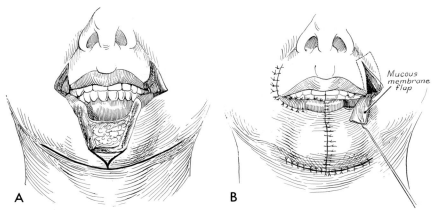

FIGURE 32–54. The Camille Bernard operation (modified). *A,* Bürow triangles removed from the lateral portions of the upper lip above the corner of the mouth. *B,* Position of the flaps after closure of the median defect of the lower lip. Note the use of the mucous membrane flap from the excised Bürow triangle to provide the vermilion border of the lateral portion of the reconstructed lip. (From Kazanjian and Converse.)

and the triangular mucosal flap, based inferiorly, restored the vermilion border in the lateral portion of the reconstructed lip (Fig. 32–54). The procedure illustrated is Martin's (1932) modification of the Bernard operation. Additional modifications of the Camille Bernard technique have been proposed by Fries (1973).

Lateral Defects

NASOLABIAL FLAP. An alternate procedure to the use of the Estlander operation in the repair of lateral defects of the lower lip is the nasolabial flap described in 1859 by von Bruns. This flap comprises the full-thickness of the cheek (Fig. 32–55). An incision is made in the nasolabial fold from the lateral commissure of the mouth toward the alar base for an appropriate distance, curving laterally and finally inferiorly to terminate at the level of the lateral commissure. The flap is raised and rotated through 90 degrees to reconstruct the lower lip, and the secondary defect is closed by direct approximation. The closure of the donor site lies in the line of the nasolabial fold and presents a relatively inconspicuous scar.

LATERAL ROTATION FLAP. This flap differs from the nasolabial flap in that it is obtained from the cheek by a horizontal full-thickness incision lateral to the commissure of the mouth and is based on a labial artery pedicle. Advancement of the flap into the defect aids materially in the closure of the secondary defect. Scars left by this procedure are often inconspicuous (Fig. 32–56). This flap is of particular use when the greater part of the lower lip has been destroyed and results in maximum utilization of available lip tissue.

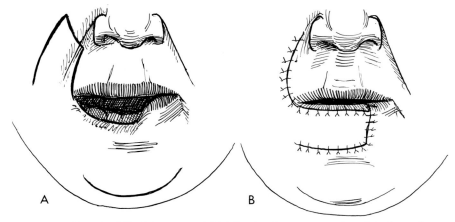

FIGURE 32–55. *A,* Outline of a full-thickness nasolabial flap for the reconstruction of the lower lip. *B,* The lip reconstructed.

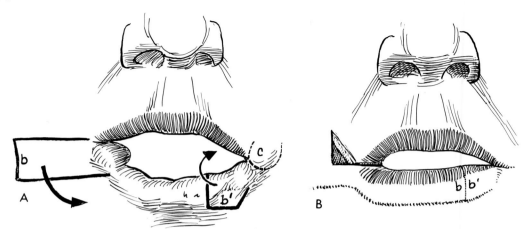

FIGURE 32–56. Full-thickness lateral rotation flaps for reconstruction of the lower lip. *A*, Flap b is rotated through 180 degrees to meet its opposite flap, b′, which is rotated through 90 degrees. Each flap contains muscle tissue and a blood supply from the labial artery. *B*, Flap c is used to reconstruct the angle of the mouth. (Redrawn from Kazanjian and Converse.)

Complete Loss of the Lower Lip

Nasolabial Flaps. Two full-thickness nasolabial flaps of the type described by von Bruns may be raised from each side of the upper lip (Fig. 32–57). Although this procedure provides adequate lip tissue, it has a tendency to tense the upper lip and has the disadvantage of a bilateral section of both muscle and motor nerve fibers of the upper lip. Reinnervation and restoration of muscle function occur after a variable time lapse. Further, vascular insufficiency of the flap may result when the bases of the flaps are scarred. Pierce and O'Connor (1934) modified this technique by employing two flaps of skin only. One flap is folded down to provide the skin lining and the other the covering of the new lip. The lining flap must be raised from an area of non-hair-bearing cheek lateral to the nasolabial fold. This technique suffers from the obvious disadvantage of failure to incorporate muscle tissue into the lower lip. A further modification is the elevation of a flap comprising the full-thickness of the cheek wall from the nasolabial area on one side and a horizontal full-thickness cheek flap from the opposite side (Fig. 32–58). This procedure has the advantage of sparing the function of the orbicularis oris and the levator labii superioris muscles on one side.

The Owens Operation (1944). Owens used a quadrilateral flap of skin and the superficial musculature of expression based on a labial arterial pedicle, raised from a point inferior and lateral to the commissure of the mouth and rotated through 90 degrees to meet a similar flap from the opposite side (Fig. 32–59). Mucosal flaps are raised in a similar fashion from the mucous membrane of the cheek and rotated anteroinferiorly to line the muscle and skin flaps. The mucosal flaps are raised from a slightly

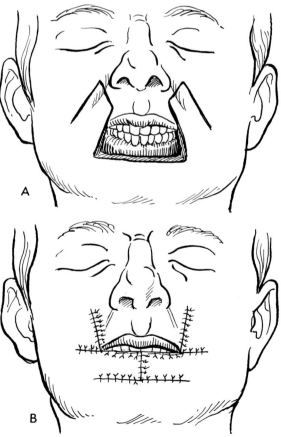

FIGURE 32–57. *A*, Lines of incision for the full-thickness nasolabial flaps. *B*, The flaps sutured to each other in the midline.

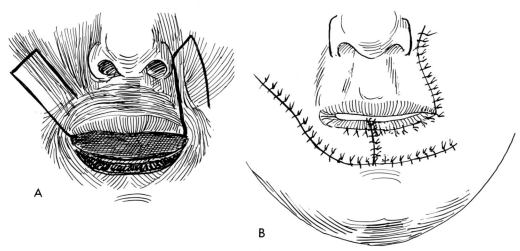

FIGURE 32–58.   *A,* A mucocutaneous flap is raised from the cheek on the right side, and a nasolabial flap is elevated on the left side. *B,* The flaps are sutured to reconstruct the lower lip.

high level, which facilitates covering the superior border of the skin muscle flap to form the new vermilion border of the reconstructed lip.

The Modified Dieffenbach Operation.   Dieffenbach in 1834 described a technique for reconstruction of the entire lower lip, using large, rectangular, full-thickness cheek flaps

advanced from each side of the face. This technique was modified by Adelmann (Szymanowski, 1858), Nélaton and Ombrédanne (1907), and May (1941).

An incision is made from the lateral commissure of the mouth through the skin and the superficial muscles of expression extending toward a point 1.5 cm anterior to the tragus of

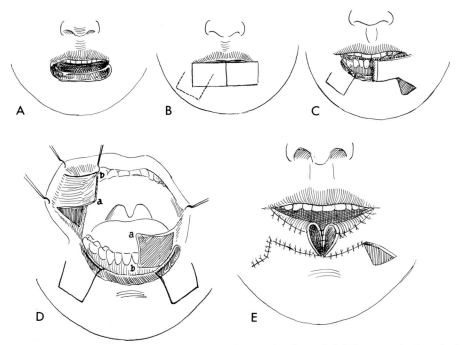

FIGURE 32–59.   The Owens operation. *A,* Lower lip defect. *B,* Sections of tinfoil cut to simulate the lower lip; the right section is rotated inferolaterally. *C,* The left flap containing skin and orbicularis muscle is raised into position. *D,* Mucous membrane flaps, a and b, outlined on the inner aspect of the upper cheek by the pattern and rotated medially to form the inner lining of the reconstructed lip (*E*). (Redrawn from Owens, 1944.)

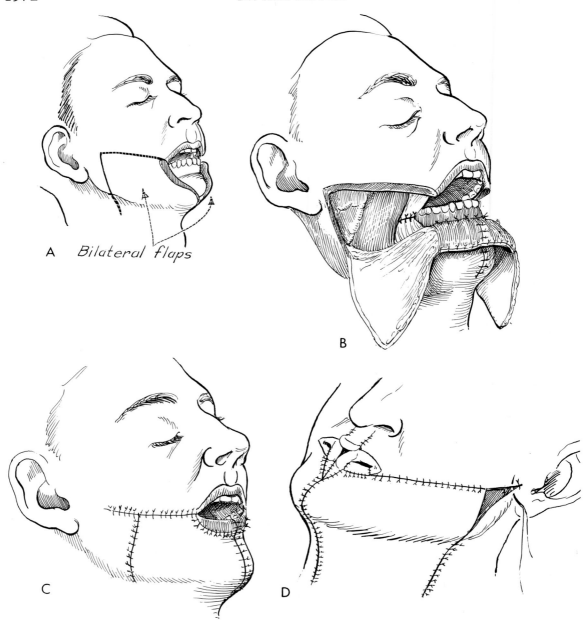

FIGURE 32-60.   The Dieffenbach operation (modified). *A*, Outline of the incision through the cheek wall. *B*, The position of the flaps after suture in the midline. *C*, The operation completed. *D*, Modification of the Dieffenbach operation employing Stein-Kazanjian flaps (Converse).

the ear (Fig. 32-60). The incision extends to but not through the oral mucosa and when it reaches the anterior border of the masseter muscle extends to but not through the parotid-masseteric fascia. The external maxillary artery and anterior facial vein are ligated and sectioned; the incision lies inferior to Stensen's duct, which is easily identified and preserved after cannulation. The incision is extended ver-

tically downward from its posterior end to a point below the angle of the mandible. The flap is raised from the parotid-masseteric fascia, and two small flaps of oral mucosa are dissected from the inner aspect of the cheek above a level parallel to the horizontal line of incision for a distance of approximately 1 cm. This mucosa is everted and provides the vermilion border for the reconstructed lip.

A vertical incision is made through the oral mucosa parallel to the anterior border of the masseter muscle, the lower end of the incision reaching the buccal sulcus, and is extended forward through the mucosa and periosteum overlying the mandibular body immediately below the gingival margin in order to raise as much mucoperiosteum as possible for a lining for the cheek flap. The obliterated oral vestibule may be restored at a later date by a skin graft inlay procedure.

The flap is completely freed from the parotid-masseteric fascia at its posterior limits; the submaxillary gland is exposed in this area.

After a similar procedure on the opposite side of the face, the two flaps are sutured in the midline, restoring the lower lip. The triangular muscle and mucous membrane defect anterior to the masseter muscle is closed by mobilization of the mucous membrane and transplantation of a flap consisting of the lower anterior half of the masseter muscle (May, 1941).

This procedure results in a functionally poor lower lip; however, the result obtained is usually more satisfactory than those following reconstruction by the use of distant flaps. The procedure is particularly useful in the older patient in whom the looseness of the facial tissue and the limited prognosis make this rapid form of repair attractive to the surgeon.

Converse has modified this procedure by the use of Stein flaps (Fig. 32–60, *D*).

Distant Flaps. The use of distant flaps in reconstruction after complete loss of the lower lip should be employed only as a last resort. The procedure is lengthy and generally results in a poor cosmetic and functional result. Owens (1955) has described the use of a compound flap in the repair of such defects (see Fig. 32–90).

O'Brien (1970) employed a sternomastoid compound muscle flap for total lower lip reconstruction.

Defects of the Lower Lip and Chin with Loss of a Section of the Mandible

The repair of defects of this type is intimately associated with restoration of continuity of the mandible and is best accomplished by the use of large rotation flaps combined with lining by local tissues or, if these are not available, the use of distant tissues. Further aspects of this problem are dealt with in Chapters 30 and 61 to 63.

RECONSTRUCTION OF THE CORNER OF THE MOUTH

Severe deformities of the corner of the mouth often result from electrical and thermal burns. The "live socket" burn is a classic example of this deformity. The deformity may be limited

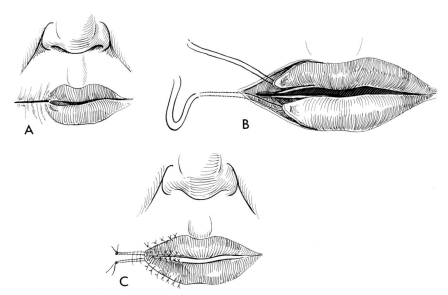

FIGURE 32–61. Technique of elongation of the oral fissure and restoration of the angle of the mouth. *A*, Incision through the area of adhesion. *B*, Mattress sutures placed through the flaps of vermilion. *C*, The flaps of vermilion have been advanced over the deficient area. (Redrawn from Kazanjian and Converse.)

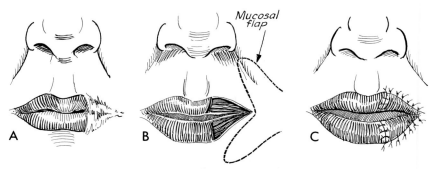

FIGURE 32-62. Technique of elongation of the oral fissure and restoration of the angle of the mouth. *A,* Scarred areas joining the lips. *B,* The scarred area excised; design of the mucosal flaps. *C,* After transposition of the mucosal flaps.

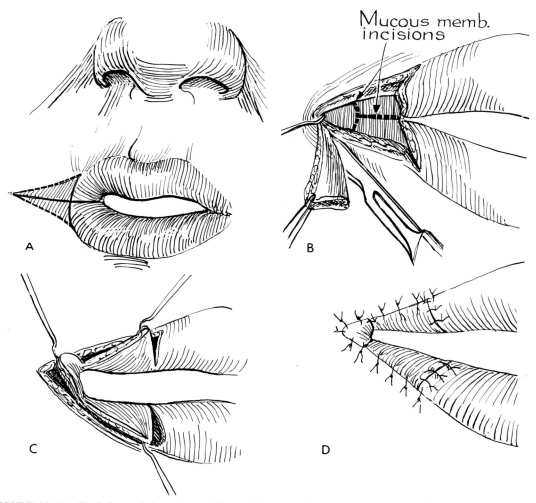

FIGURE 32-63. Technique of elongation of the oral fissure and restoration of the angle of the mouth. *A,* Outline of the skin incision. *B,* Excision of skin and subcutaneous tissue exposing the oral mucosa. Outline of incisions through the mucosa. *C,* After incision, the three mucosal flaps are available. *D,* The mucosal flaps are sutured to the skin edges. Note the mucosal flap at the angle of the mouth. (After Converse, 1959.)

to the corner of the mouth or be complicated by the loss of a portion of the lip.

Kazanjian and Roopenian (1954) described two methods of repair, the choice depending upon the amount of mucosa remaining at the vermilion border.

The First Method. This method is applicable when the upper and lower lips are adherent in the lateral quarter to third of the lips. The adherent avascular scars are excised, and if the raw areas are not more than 1 to 1.5 cm in length, an advancement flap from the vermilion border of the adjacent lip may be used to restore the area adequately (Fig. 32–61). A horizontal incision is extended medially along the mucocutaneous junction for a sufficient length to allow adequate advancement of the vermilion to the commissure of the mouth.

The Second Method. When the loss of the vermilion is more extensive, mucosal flaps must be raised on the inner aspect of the cheek to replace the missing vermilion border (Fig. 32–62). Donor sites are easily closed by direct approximation. The new angle of the mouth is maintained by mattress sutures brought out in a fashion similar to the first method.

Elongation of the Oral Fissure

For the rounded angle of the mouth, the following procedure has been employed by Converse (1959). The position of the new angle of the mouth is determined by comparison with the opposite side, if the commissure is normal (Fig. 32–63). A triangular segment of skin and orbicularis muscle is removed immediately lateral to the vermilion. A horizontal incision is made through the oral mucosa to a point approximately 1 cm from the lateral extremity of the skin incision. A curved incision lying in the vertical axis, with the concavity of the curve directed laterally, is made at this point. The oval flap of mucosa lateral to this incision is sutured laterally to form a new angle of the mouth, an important factor which prevents contraction and shortening of the oral fissure during the healing stages. The inferior and superior mucosal flaps are undermined for a short distance and advanced to form the new vermilion border, suturing the mucosa to the skin edges of the upper and lower lip.

Gillies (Gillies and Millard, 1957) excised a triangular segment of skin lateral and inferior to the corner of the mouth and rotated a vermilion flap laterally, as shown in Figure 32–64. The secondary defect is closed by mucosal advancement.

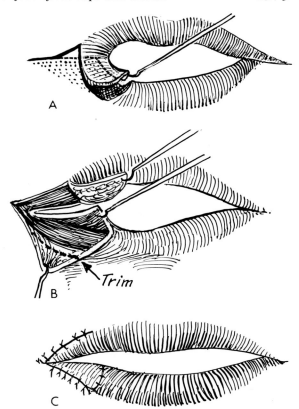

FIGURE 32–64. Technique of elongation of the oral fissure and restoration of the angle of the mouth. *A*, A triangular segment of skin is excised lateral to the rounded corner of the mouth. A vermilion flap is raised from the lower lip. *B*, Mucosa is advanced from the inner aspect of the lower lip to form the vermilion of the lower lip. *C*, The vermilion flap is rotated laterally and sutured in position. (Redrawn from Gillies and Millard, 1957.)

DEFECTS OF THE VERMILION BORDER

The Abbé Procedure. Central defects of the vermilion border may be corrected by the Abbé vermilion procedure (Gillies and Millard, 1957). The principal use of this procedure is when a central scar has been released in the region of the cupid's bow and the lateral portion of the lip has been allowed to resume its normal anatomical position, leaving a central vermilion defect (Fig. 32–65). A horizontal vermilion flap of the lower lip is rotated through 90 degrees and attached to the upper lip as an Abbé vermilion flap. After seven to ten days the flap is divided and the vermilion border readjusted. The donor site is closed by

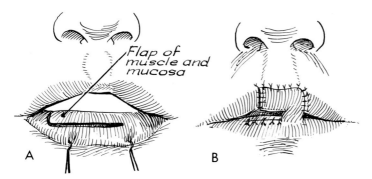

FIGURE 32–65. *A*, A vermilion defect of the central portion of the upper lip. A lower vermilion flap is outlined. *B*, Transfer of the lower vermilion flap to the upper lip defect; the flap consists of both mucosa and a varying portion of muscle. (Redrawn from Gillies and Millard, 1957.)

advancement of mucosa from the anterior buccal sulcus.

The Mucosal Apron Flap (Gillies and Millard, 1957). The vermilion border of the lower or upper lip may be closed by the use of a mucosal apron flap from the inner aspect of either lip in the manner indicated in Figure 32–66.

The Mucous Membrane Tube Flap. When it is difficult to close the vermilion defect by advancement of the mucosa, or if additional bulk is required to close the defect, a tube flap may be raised from the labial sulcus (Fig. 32–67). A bipedicle flap is raised and the defect closed either by direct approximation or by a skin or mucous membrane graft. At a second stage one end of the tube flap is divided and transferred to one end of the defect, and finally after two additional weeks the other end of the tube flap is divided and the tube finally laid in place to fill in the vermilion defect.

The Bipedicle Mucosal Flap. Large defects of the vermilion border may be restored by the use of a large bipedicle mucosal flap from the undersurface of the lower or upper lip. This is an excellent method of reconstruction when the adjacent mucosa is scarred (Fig. 32–68).

Notching of the Vermilion Border. Defects which involve notching of the vermilion border may be corrected by a number of methods; the most frequently employed are shown in Figure 32–69.

A recent development in resurfacing vermilion defects has been the use of tongue flaps (Bakamjian, 1964; McGregor, 1966; Zarem and Greer, 1974). The technique is illustrated in Figure 32–70 and is discussed further in Chapter 63.

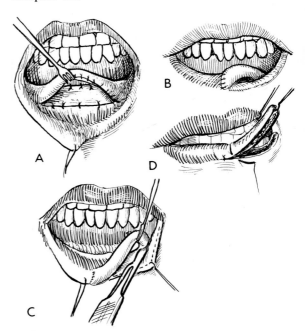

FIGURE 32–67. *A*, A mucosal tube flap is raised on the labial aspect of the sulcus. *B*, After seven to ten days one end of the flap is divided and sutured to the medial end of the vermilion defect. *C*, After an additional interval of seven to ten days, the remaining end of the tube flap is divided. *D*, The tube flap is opened and sutured in position along the vermilion border defect. (Redrawn from Gillies and Millard, 1957.)

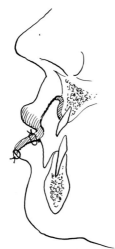

FIGURE 32–66. The mucosal apron flap. A defect of the vermilion border of the lower lip is closed by a mucosal apron flap from the inner aspect of the upper lip. (Redrawn from Gillies and Millard, 1957.)

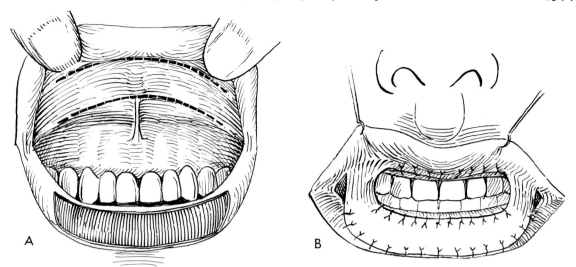

FIGURE 32–68.   Restoration of the vermilion border by a bipedicle mucosal flap from the undersurface of the upper lip. *A,* The design of the bipedicle flap and the vermilion border defect. *B,* The bipedicle mucosal flap is transferred from the upper to the lower lip. (Redrawn from Kazanjian and Converse.)

RESTORATION OF MUSCULAR FUNCTION OF THE RECONSTRUCTED LOWER LIP

The procedure of choice in reconstruction of the lower lip is one that will provide a func-

tioning muscular flap to enable some degree of lip seal and function of the lip.

Orbicularis Muscle Advancement Flap Technique (Converse, 1972).   When it is impossible because of adjacent scar tissue to utilize Estlander type flaps, the vermilion borders are

FIGURE 32–69.   The application of Z-plasty techniques to the correction of vermilion border notching. (Redrawn from Dufourmentel and Mouly, 1959.)

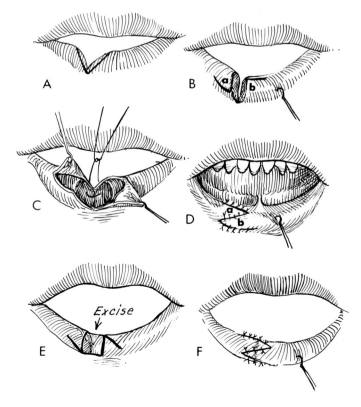

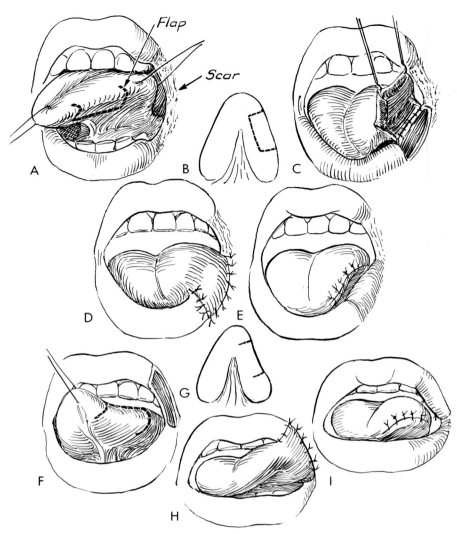

FIGURE 32–70.   Tongue flap for reconstruction of the vermilion border following a live socket burn. *A,* Tongue flap. *B,* Undersurface of the tongue. The dotted line indicates the amount of tissue comprised in the flap. *C,* The flap has been raised. It includes mucous membrane and underlying muscle tissue. *D,* The flap has been sutured into position. *E,* In a second stage, the pedicle of the flap is severed. *F,* A second flap is outlined on the undersurface of the tongue, as illustrated in *G,* and will serve for the reconstruction of the upper lip defect. *H,* The tongue flap in position. *I,* After section of the pedicle of the flap and suture of the wound. (Technique of José Delgado, M.D.)

tubed, and the upper lip muscle tissue is advanced. The vermilion of the upper and lower lips in the lateral third of the lips on the appropriate side is raised as two tube flaps (Fig. 32–71). The opposing skin edges, orbicularis muscle, and oral mucosa are united.

After an interval of 21 days, an incision is made at an appropriate level to the medial point of origin of the vermilion flaps, through skin, orbicularis, and oral mucosa. This incision lies above the previous level of skin union, and the tube vermilion flaps are incised

at the previous line of union and used to form the new vermilion borders. Edwards (1955) has employed a similar procedure.

When this is not possible, some function may be obtained by swinging down a short nasolabial flap or by using a fascia lata sling, in which the fascia lata is passed from the nasolabial region through the upper border of the reconstructed lip in an attempt to obtain some degree of lip seal and function. It should be stressed, however, that even at best the results of these procedures are poor.

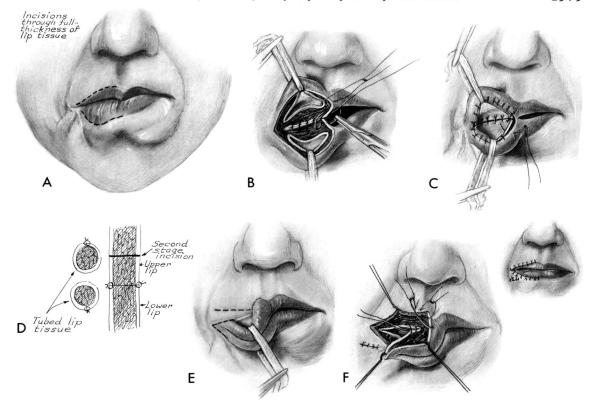

FIGURE 32–71. The muscle advancement flap technique (Converse). *A*, The distorted and scarred angle of the mouth showing the vermilion border incisions. *B, C*, The vermilion border is raised and formed into two tubed flaps; skin and orbicularis muscle are united. *D*, Cross section of the lips at this stage. *E*, Fifteen to 20 days later an incision is made through skin, orbicularis oris muscle, and mucosa at a higher level. *F*, The angle of the mouth is raised and the tubes opened, reinserted at the new site of the angle of the mouth, and employed to restore the vermilion border. (From Converse, J. M.: Orbicularis advancement flap for restoration of the angle of the mouth. Plast. Reconstr. Surg., *49*:99. Copyright 1972, The Williams & Wilkins Company, Baltimore.)

DEFORMITIES OF THE CHEEKS

Superficial Defects

Superficial deformities of the cheek may be repaired in a variety of fashions; the type of repair is dependent upon the etiology, the site, and the size of the deformity. Xeroderma pigmentosum, for example, may require resurfacing of the entire face; burn scars of the face may present an even greater problem with the need for resurfacing a large portion of the face together with the inevitable distortion resulting from scar contracture (see Chapter 33).

In resurfacing the cheeks, care must be taken to establish the size of the true defect in a manner similar to that illustrated (Fig. 32–72), so that the alar base, lips, and angle of the mouth may resume their normal anatomical position. The face is divided into a number of esthetic units, and, whenever possible, an area corresponding to one esthetic unit must be resurfaced at one stage in order to produce the best result (Fig. 32–73).

Use must be made of the facial creases, such as the nasolabial fold, in placing the edges of flaps or skin grafts and in the design of excision and flap donor sites. The parotid-masseteric region is generally more suitable for the application of split-thickness and full-thickness skin grafts because of the lesser mobility of this region and the relative ease of immobilization of skin grafts.

Skin Grafts. Split-thickness skin grafts should be used to cover superficial defects of the cheek only when no other method of repair is feasible. The split-thickness skin graft is cosmetically inferior to the full-thickness graft, and this in turn is inferior to local flaps. The use of the split-thickness graft in this region should be confined to the resurfacing of burns or of large defects where, because of the likeli-

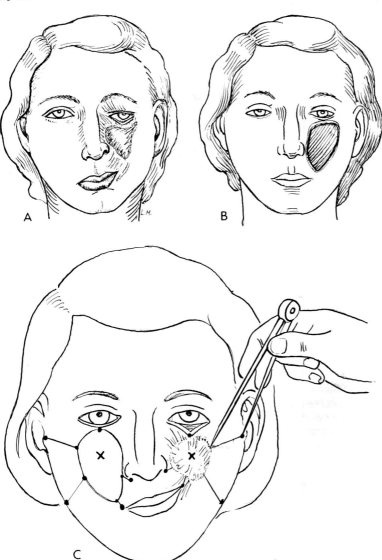

FIGURE 32-72. The apparent defect and the true defect. *A*, The apparent defect due to contracted scar tissue on the left side of the face. *B*, The true defect becomes evident after release and excision of scar tissue. *C*, The dimensions of the true defect may be determined prior to excision by plotting the distance from the surrounding fixed points of the face to the edges of the defect and comparing the distances to those of the opposite normal side of the face. (From Kazanjian and Converse.)

hood of recurrence of malignant disease, a period of clinical observation is desirable before definitive repair becomes safe.

Full-thickness skin grafts, especially those from postauricular or supraclavicular sites, are an excellent method of repair of smaller superficial defects when it is undesirable to use a local flap. The cosmetic appearance of the repair is generally satisfactory with respect to color match, texture, and functional properties. However, full-thickness skin grafts in the male patient suffer the distinct disadvantage of leaving an area of hairless skin, which may be obvious in the heavily bearded individual. For this reason, in the male, use of a local transposition or rotation flap is preferred, with the

application, if necessary, of a full-thickness skin graft to close the secondary defect, which may often be placed in a relatively inconspicuous position, as shown in Figure 32–74.

Overgrafting. Overgrafting is a satisfactory procedure when full-thickness skin grafts or local rotation flaps are not indicated and is a satisfactory method of improving the esthetic appearance of the skin grafted area in the cheek (Hynes, 1957). For further information on this subject refer to Chapters 6 and 33.

Local Flaps. A scar, nevus, or other lesion of moderate size may often be excised and the defect closed by local advancement flaps with undermining of the skin edges. However, in

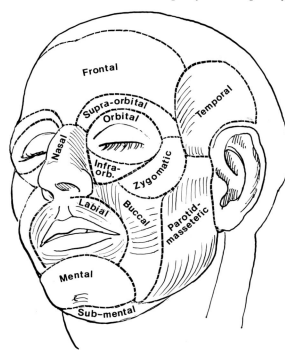

FIGURE 32–73. The esthetic units of the face.

larger nonmalignant lesions, repeated partial excision with undermining of the surrounding skin and approximation of the edges may allow removal of all or the greater part of the lesion. Larger defects may be closed by a transposition flap, such as that shown in Figure 32–75, where the **V-Y** technique is used to close the secondary defect. If this approximation is not possible without undue tension, a full-thickness retroauricular skin graft is applied in a fashion similar to that shown in Figure 32–74.

A larger defect of the center of the cheek may be repaired effectively by two transposition flaps, as in Figure 32–76, or by a transposition and a rotation flap, as illustrated in Figure 32–77.

In a defect with its anterior border parallel to the nasolabial fold, and especially when there is laxity of the neighboring skin, a large flap may be transposed from the cervical area and the donor site closed by the **V-Y** procedure (Fig. 32–78).

Large defects in the region of the angle of the mandible and adjacent parotid-masseteric region may be repaired by postauricular flaps rotated anteriorly; direct closure of the postauricular defect is usually possible (Fig. 32–79).

Larger defects in this region are repaired by large rectangular flaps extending downward in the line of the sternocleidomastoid muscle and terminating by an anterior extension toward the symphysis menti (Fig. 32–80). The donor site is closed by the **V-Y**

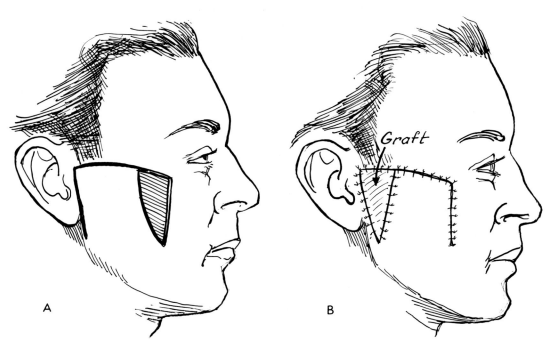

FIGURE 32–74. Use of a transposition flap to close a skin defect in the cheek with closure of the secondary defect in the preauricular region by a full-thickness skin graft.

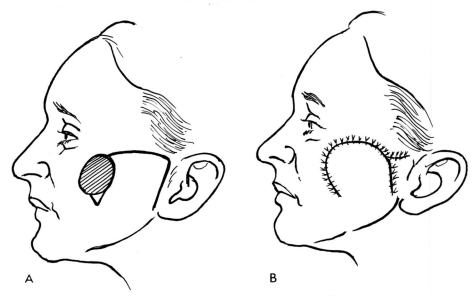

FIGURE 32–75. Use of a transposition flap to close a cheek skin defect. The donor site is closed by the V-Y method.

method, which is especially suitable in the older patient with lax neck skin.

Larger defects of the cheek are closed by large flaps transposed from the cervical area, with closure of the secondary defect by transfer of a second flap from the sternoclavic-ular region, by the **V-Y** method or alternatively by a skin graft (Fig. 32–81).

The Arterial Island Flap. A cheek defect of moderate proportions may be closed by transfer of a portion of the forehead skin based on an arteriovenous temporal pedicle and

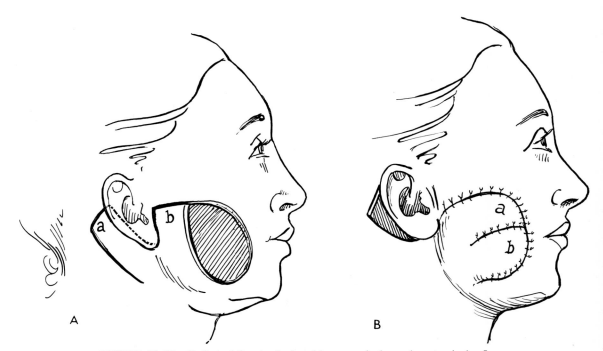

FIGURE 32–76. Defect of the cheek closed by preauricular and postauricular flaps.

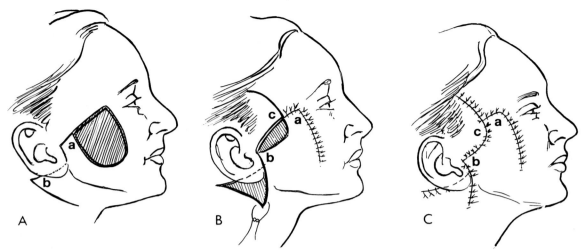

FIGURE 32–77.   Closure of a skin defect of the cheek by the combined use of a transposition flap and a temporal rotation flap.

drawn through a subcutaneous tunnel. The secondary defect, if small, may often be closed by undermining and direct approximation or by a full-thickness retroauricular skin graft, as shown in Figure 32–82.

The Bi-lobed Flap.   The bi-lobed flap, first described by Esser in 1918 and later popularized by Zimany (1953), offers a means of closure of relatively large cheek defects with little distortion of the donor site. An angle of 90

degrees between the two lobes of the bi-lobed flap is an optimum figure, but it may be varied from 45 to 180 degrees or more. The technique is illustrated in Figure 32–83.

Tube Flaps.   Tube flaps may be used to cover extensive surface defects of the cheek. Because of the long period of time involved in the making and the transfer of the tube flap (Fig. 32–84) and because full-thickness skin grafts will often give almost as good cosmetic

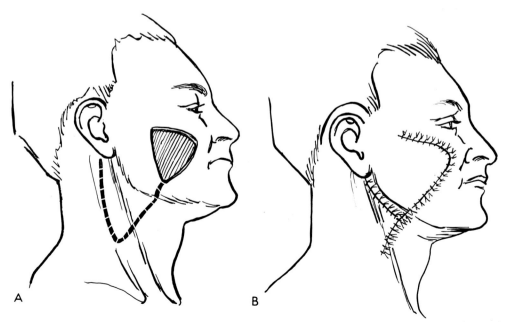

FIGURE 32–78.   Large skin defect of the cheek repaired by a transposed flap from the side of the face and neck.

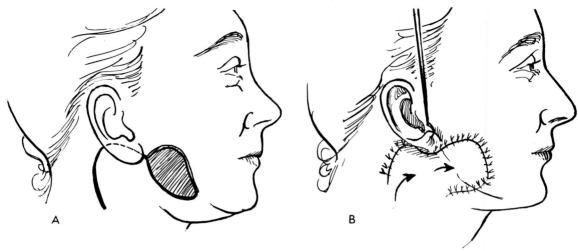

FIGURE 32–79. *A,* Outline of a postauricular flap for the repair of a defect of the angle of the jaw. *B,* The postauricular flap rotated into the defect.

results, it is impossible to present a dogmatic statement on the covering of large surface defects of the cheek.

Tube flaps should be reserved for surface defects with loss of subcutaneous tissue. Deep thermal or radiation burns, hemifacial atrophy, and congenital maldevelopment of the first and second arches are examples of conditions more suited to flap repair than to skin grafting.

Jump Flaps (Cannon and Coworkers, 1947). The jump flap, also known as the closed carried flap (Converse, 1948), is a more rapid method of transfer of a large flap. To en-

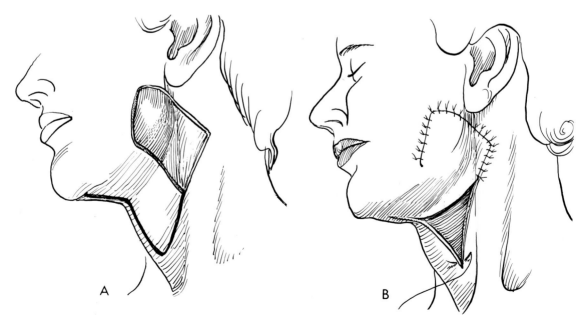

FIGURE 32–80. Large skin defect of the angle of the jaw and side of the face repaired by a rectangular flap from the cervical region and closure of the donor area accomplished by the V-Y method.

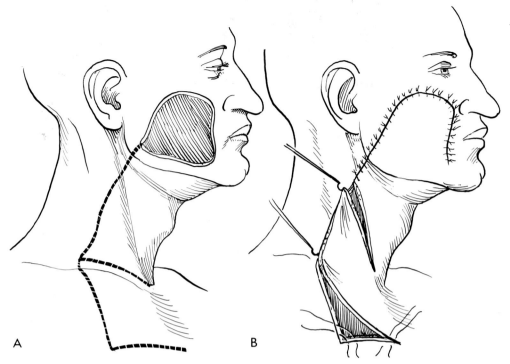

FIGURE 32–81. Closure of a cheek skin defect by a flap transposed from the cervical area. *A*, Outline of cheek defect and design of the flaps. *B*, The superior flap is transferred to the cheek defect. The secondary defect is closed by the inferior flap and the V-Y method.

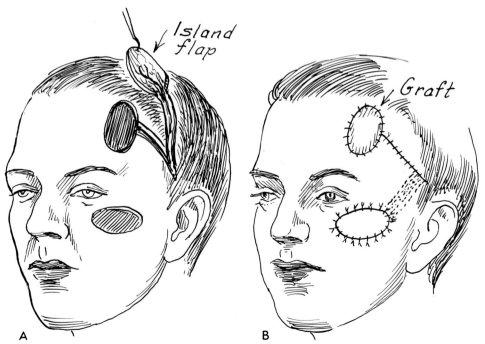

FIGURE 32–82. Closure of a cheek skin defect by an arterial island flap. The flap and its pedicle are drawn through a subcutaneous tunnel to the defect; the donor site is closed by a skin graft. (Redrawn from Gillies and Millard, 1957.)

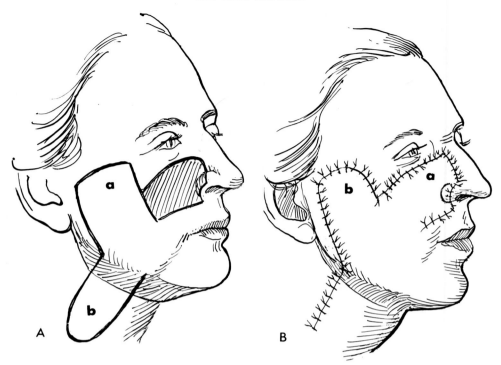

FIGURE 32–83.   The bi-lobed flap. Closure of a large cheek skin defect by transposition of a flap (a) into the defect. The donor area is closed by flap b, the donor area of which is in turn closed by direct approximation. This flap is of value in aged patients with lax tissue. (After Zimany.)

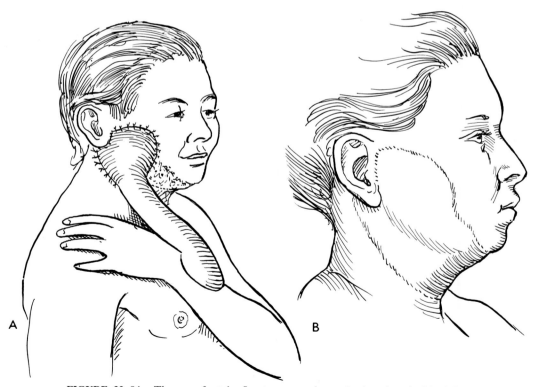

FIGURE 32–84.   The use of a tube flap to cover a large cheek and neck skin defect.

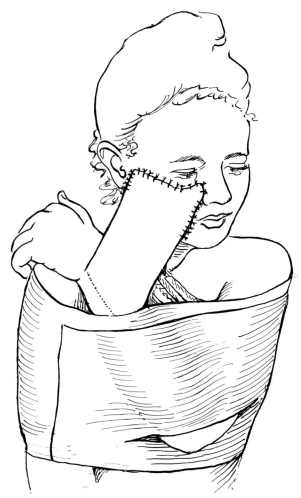

FIGURE 32–85. The jump flap used to repair a large defect of the skin of the cheek.

sure survival of the flap, the proportions should be such that the length does not exceed 1½ to two times the width. Figure 32–85 shows a typical application of the flap.

Full-Thickness Defects

Reconstruction of full-thickness defects of the cheek presents a complex problem because both the surface cover of the cheek and its inner or mucosal aspect must be restored.

Large full-thickness defects of the cheek, usually following ablative surgery, are amenable to repair by temporal flaps (McGregor and Reid, 1966) or simultaneous temporal and deltopectoral flaps (McGregor and Reid, 1970). The subject is further discussed in Chapter 62. However, with less extensive loss

of tissue of the cheek and because of the elasticity of the oral mucosa, it is often possible to advance sufficient mucosa from the areas adjacent to the defect for mucosal closure to be effected (Fig. 32–86). The outer aspect of the cheek may then be repaired by the use of local skin flaps.

Gillies and Millard (1957) have stressed the importance of initial repair of the angle of the mouth. They believe that in all cases in which cheek defects involve the angle, it should be restored as an initial procedure with repair of the cheek defect at a later date (Fig. 32–87).

Wood-Smith (1975) has modified the Converse technique (see Fig. 32–63) by utilizing vermilion advancement flaps in the elongation of the oral aperture. This repair may be com-

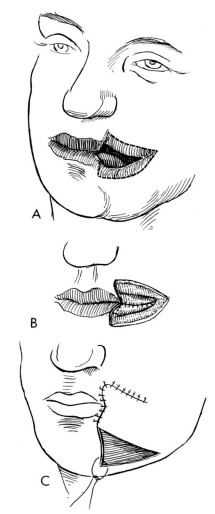

FIGURE 32–86. Closure of a full-thickness defect of the cheek. *A,* An incision is made around the mucocutaneous junction, and mucosal flaps are raised. *B,* The mucosal flaps are united to form the lining of the defect. *C,* The skin defect is closed by a local flap.

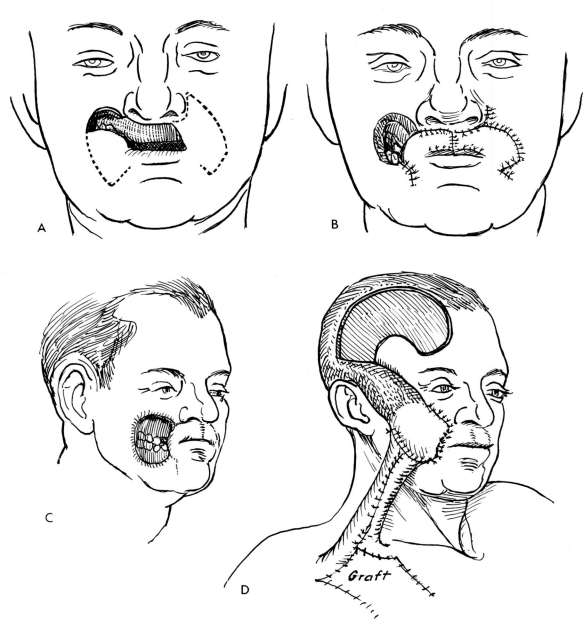

FIGURE 32–87.   Defect involving the cheek and upper lip. *A,* The defect and the outline of flaps designed to reconstruct the upper lip. *B,* The upper lip is reconstructed and mucosa united to skin in the cheek defect. *C, D,* After an interval of 20 to 30 days, the cheek defect is repaired by the combination of a tube flap to provide inner lining and a forehead flap based on the temporal artery to provide skin cover. (Redrawn from Gillies and Millard, 1957.)

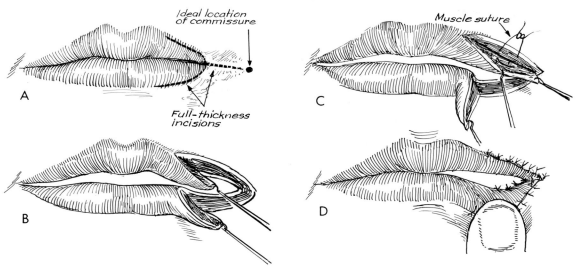

FIGURE 32–88. *A, B,* Incisions and advancement flaps of vermilion, muscle, and mucosa to reconstruct the commissure. *C,* Reapproximation of the muscle. *D,* Completion of the procedure.

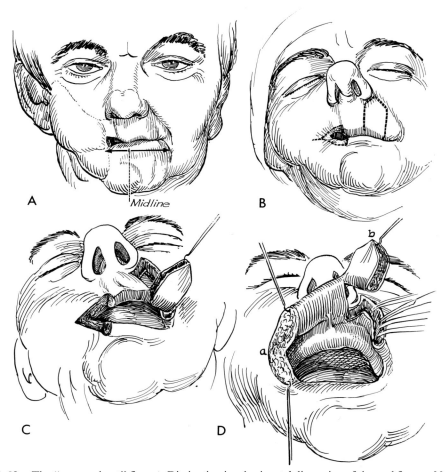

FIGURE 32–89. The "over and out" flap. *A,* Diminution in a horizontal dimension of the oral fissure. Note the defect in the right oral commissure. *B,* Outline of areas of excision to elongate the oral commissure and outline of flap from the contralateral side of the upper lip. *C,* The scar tissue has been resected from the right oral commissure and the oral fissure elongated. The flap from the contralateral portion of the upper lip has been outlined and raised. *D,* The "over and out" flap prior to transfer.

Illustration continued on following page.

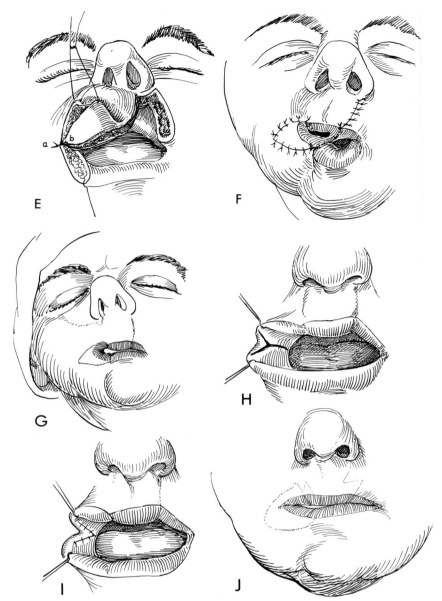

FIGURE 32–89 *Continued.*   *E*, Introduction of the flap into the oral commissure. *F*, The flap has been sutured into position. *G*, After transfer and division of the flap, adjustments are required. *H*, *I*, The adjustment of the excess mucous membrane is achieved by a V-Y advancement into the inner lining skin flap. *J*, At a later stage, additional realignment of tissues may require Z-plasty procedures. (From Converse, J. M.: The "over and out" flap for restoration of the corner of the mouth. Plast. Reconstr. Surg., 56:575. Copyright 1975, The Williams & Wilkins Company, Baltimore.)

bined with restoration of the continuity of the orbicularis muscle when an electrical burn or excision has interrupted continuity. The vermilion and subjacent orbicularis oris muscle are raised and advanced laterally to fill the new fissure margins (Fig. 32–88).

Converse (1975) has restored orbicularis oris continuity in a patient who had undergone resection of the cheek, the angle of the mouth, and the lateral portions of the lips by means of an "over and out" flap. The full-thickness flap was removed from the contralateral side of the upper lip and swung on a narrow pedicle into the corner of the mouth. By suturing the muscle of the flap to the adjacent orbicularis oris muscle, circumoral continuity was restored, a new commissure was formed, and the patient regained muscle control.

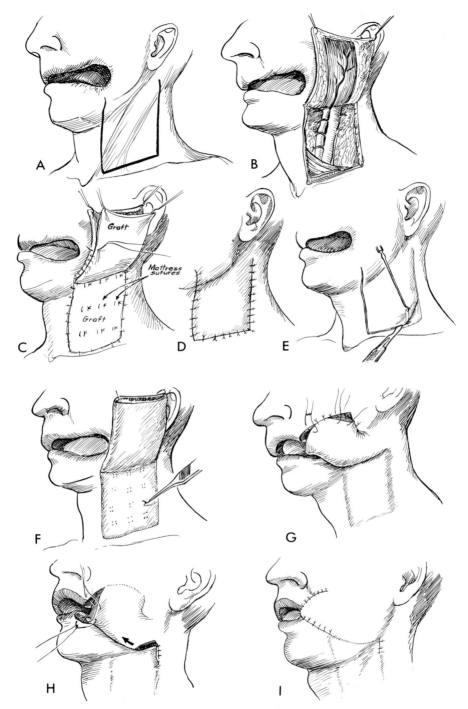

FIGURE 32–90. The Owens technique. *A*, The cheek defect and the outline of a large square cervical flap. *B*, The flap includes the sternocleidomastoid muscle and its blood supply. *C*, A split-thickness skin graft covers both raw areas. *D*, The flap is resutured in position. *E, F, G*, Ten to 14 days later the flap is raised, then rotated anterosuperiorly to close the posterior portion of the cheek defect. *H*, At a later stage, the flap is partly divided at its base to allow for further anterior and superior advancement. *I*, The completed procedure. (After drawings by E. M. Freret.)

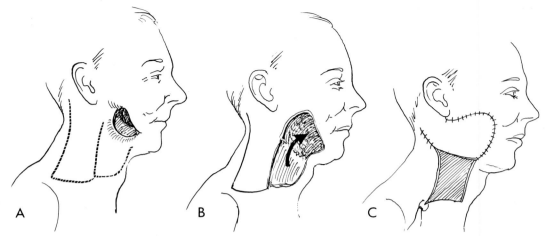

FIGURE 32–91. *A,* Repair of a full-thickness defect of the cheek with two delayed flaps. *B,* Fourteen days following the delay procedure, the anterior flap is turned inward to form the lining. *C,* The posterior flap is placed over the anterior flap and the neck defect closed by a skin graft. (Redrawn from Kazanjian and Converse.)

The Owens Technique. Owens (1955) designed a compound neck flap for the repair of massive facial defects. A large square flap of suitable proportions is dissected from the lateral aspect of the neck; it includes all soft tissues down to the carotid sheath (Fig. 32–90, *A*). The sternocleidomastoid muscle is included, and care is taken to preserve its blood supply (Fig. 32–90, *B*). A split-thickness skin graft is used to cover both raw areas, and the flap is sutured back into its original position by interrupted tacking sutures (Fig. 32–90, *C* and *D*).

After ten days to two weeks the original incisions are opened and the compound flap is raised with the skin graft lining its undersurface (Fig. 32–90, *E*).

The flap is advanced into the defect, and because of the relationship of the base of the pedicle to the defect, a series of staged advancements may have to be performed (Fig. 32–90, *F, G*). In this manner at a second stage a partial severance of the pedicle along its inferior border will allow a further anterior rotation of the compound flap (Fig. 32–90, *H, I*). The advantage claimed for this method of flap repair is that it provides the transfer of a large mass of tissue with a relatively intact blood supply, which will presumably allow the future insertion of a bone graft to restore the continuity of the mandible if a portion of this bone has been removed. This technique has now been superseded by the combined temporal and deltopectoral flaps.

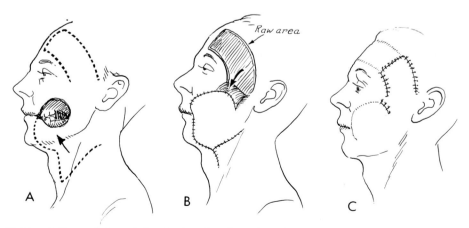

FIGURE 32–92. *A,* Large defect of the cheek and outline of the forehead and cervicofacial flaps. *B,* The temporal flap is brought down to form the lining of the defect; the flap from the lower part of the face furnishes the outer covering of the defect. *C,* Two weeks later the unused portion of the forehead flap is replaced. The forehead defect is covered by a full-thickness postauricular skin graft, and the upper border of the cheek defect is closed. (Redrawn from Kazanjian and Converse.)

Other Methods. Another method of repair of a large defect is by rotation of two delayed flaps from the neck, as shown in Figure 32–91. This procedure is unsuitable in the male patient because of the presence of hair follicles which will be transferred to the inner aspect of the cheek. The use of a forehead flap based in the temporal region to provide the inner lining and a neck flap for cover is a method of obviating this disadvantage (Fig. 32–92). As mentioned previously, a deltopectoral flap combined with a temporal flap (see Chapter 62) can be used in preference to a neck flap. Microvascular free flaps offer an alternate method (see Chapter 14).

REFERENCES

Abbé, R.: A new plastic operation for the relief of deformity due to double hairlip. Med. Rec., *53*:477, 1898.

Adelmann: Quoted by Szymanowski, J.: Handbuch der Operativen Chirurgie. Braunschweig, F. Vieweg und Sohn, 1870.

Ascher, K. W.: Blepharochalsis mit Strauma und Doppellippe. Klin. Monatsbl. Augenheilkd., *95*:86, 1920.

Ashley, F. L.: Reconstruction of the lower lip. Plast. Reconstr. Surg., *15*:313, 1955.

Bakamjian, V.: Use of tongue flaps in lower lip reconstruction. Br. J. Plast. Surg., *17*:76, 1964.

Baker, B. R.: A family with bilateral congenital pits of the inferior lip. Oral Surg., *18*:494, 1964.

Baker, B. R.: Pits of lip commissures in Caucasoid male. Oral Surg., *21*:56, 1966.

Baxter, H.: Congenital fistulae of lower lip: Report of a case. Am. J. Orthod., *25*:1002, 1939.

Bernard, C.: Cancer de la lèvre inférieure opéré par un procédé nouveau. Bull. Mém. Soc. Chir. Paris, *3*:357, 1853.

Blasius, E.: Gaumennaht, Staphylorraphie. *In* Handbuch der Chirurgie. Vol. 2. Halle, E. Anton, 1839–1843.

Bruns, V von: Handbuch der praktischer Chirurgie. Tuebingen, H. Laup, 1859.

Bürow, A.: Zur Blepharoplastik. Monatsschr. Med. Augenheilkd. Chir., *1*:57, 1838.

Calnan, J.: Congenital double lip: Record of a case with a note on the embryology. Br. J. Plast. Surg., *5*:197, 1952.

Cannon, B.: The split vermilion bordered lip flap. Surg. Gynecol. Obstet., *73*:95, 1941.

Cannon, B.: The use of vermilion bordered flaps in surgery about the mouth. Surg. Gynecol. Obstet., *74*:458, 1942.

Cannon, B., Lischer, C. E., Davis, W. B., Chasko, S., Moore, A., Murray, J., and McDowell, A.: The use of open jump flaps in lower extremity repairs. Plast. Reconstr. Surg., *2*:336, 1947.

Cervenka, J., Cerný, M., and Cisařová, E.: Heredity of fistulae to the lower lip and their relation to cleft lip and palate. Cesk. Pediatr., *21*:109, 1966.

Coccia, C. T., and Bixler, D.: Cleft lip, cleft palate, and congenital fistulas of the lower lip. Report of a familial occurrence. Oral Surg., *24*:248, 1967.

Converse, J. M.: Plastic repair of the extremities with nontubulated pedicle skin flaps. J. Bone Joint Surg., *30*:163, 1948.

Converse, J. M.: Technique of elongation of the oral fissure and restoration of the angle of the mouth. *In* Kazanjian, V. H., and Converse, J. M.: The Surgical Treatment of

Facial Injuries. Baltimore, The Williams & Wilkins Company, 1959, p. 795.

Converse, J. M.: 1-2 advancement flap. *In* Converse, J. M., (Ed.): Plastic Reconstructive Surgery. Chapter I. Philadelphia, W. B. Saunders Company, 1964.

Converse, J. M.: Burn deformities of the face and neck. Reconstruction and rehabilitation. Surg. Clin. North Am., *47*:323, 1967.

Converse, J. M.: Orbicularis advancement flap for restoration of angle of the mouth. Plast. Reconstr. Surg., *49*:99, 1972.

Converse, J. M.: The "over and out" flap for restoration of the corner of the mouth. Plast. Reconstr. Surg., *56*:575, 1975.

Converse, J. M.: The bridge flap for reconstruction of a full-thickness defect of the upper lip. Plast. Reconstr. Surg., *57*:442, 1976.

Demarquay, M.: Quelques considérations sur le bec-de-lièvre. Gaz. Méd. Paris, *13*:52, 1845.

Denonvilliers, M.: States that he performed operation in 1854. Bull. Gén. Thérap., *65*:257, 1863.

DePaul, J. A. H.: Case presentation. Séance du 6 Juin, Présidence de M. Laborie. Bull. Soc. Chir., *2*:349, 1891.

Dieffenbach, J. F.: Chirurgische Erfahrungen, besonders ueber die Wiederherstellung Zerstoerter Theile des menschlichen Koerpers nach neuen methoden. Berlin, T. C. F. Enslin, 1829–34.

Dieffenbach, J. F.: Die operative Chirurgie. Leipzig, F. A. Brockhaus, 1845–48.

Dorrance, G. M.: Double lip. Am. Surg., *76*:776, 1922.

Dufourmentel, C., and Mouly, R.: La Chirurgie Plastique. Paris, Les Editions Flammarion, 1959, pp. 709–730.

Dufourmentel, C., Mouly, R., Préaux, J., and Marchac, D.: La greffe composée libre de lèvre à lèvre. Ann. Chir. Plast., *12*:119, 1967.

Edwards, B. F.: A method of lower lip lengthening in chin reconstruction. Case Report. Plast. Reconstr. Surg., *15*:122, 1955.

Esser, J. F. S.: Die Rotation der Wang... u.s.w. Leipzig, F. C. V. Vogel Verlag, 1918.

Estlander, J. A.: Méthode d'autoplastie de la joue ou d'une lèvre par un lambeau emprunté à l'autre lèvre. Rev. Mens. Med. Chir., *1*:344, 1877.

Estlander, J. A.: Classic Reprint. Eine Methode aus der Einen Lippe Substanzverluste der Anderen zu Erstetzen. (A method of reconstructing loss of substance in one lip from the other lip.) Translated from the German by Dr. Borje Sundell: Arch. Klin. Chir., *14*:622, 1872. Plast. Reconstr. Surg., *42*:360, 1968.

Everett, F. S., and Wescott, W. R.: Commissure lip pits. Oral Surg., *14*:202, 1961.

Flanagin, W. S.: Free composite grafts from lower to upper lip. Plast. Reconstr. Surg., *17*:376, 1956.

Fries, R.: Advantages of a basic concept in lip reconstruction after tumor resection. J. Maxillofac. Surg., *1*:13, 1973.

Gillies, H. D.: Plastic Surgery of the Face. Henry Frowde, London, Oxford University Press, 1920.

Gillies, H. D., and Millard, D. R., Jr.: Principles and Art of Plastic Surgery. Boston, Little, Brown and Company, 1957.

Guerrero-Santos, J., and Altamirano, J. T.: The use of W-plasty for the correction of double lip deformity. Plast. Reconstr. Surg., *39*:478, 1967.

Hamilton, E.: Congenital deformity of the lower lip. Dublin, J. Med. Sci., *72*:1, 1881.

Hilgenreiner, H.: Die angeborenen Fisteln Beziehungsweise Schleimhauttaschen der Unterlippe. Dtsch. Z. Chir., *188*:273, 1924.

Hynes, W.: The treatment of pigmented moles by shaving and skin graft. Br. J. Plast. Surg., *9*:47, 1957.

Johanson, B., Aspelund, E., Breine, U., and Holmström, H.: Surgical treatment of nontraumatic lower lip lesions with special reference to the step technique. Scand. J. Plast. Reconstr. Surg., *8*:232, 1974.

Kazanjian, V. H.: Supporting flaps used in reconstruction of the lower lip. *In* Kazanjian, V. H., and Converse, J. M. (Eds.): The Surgical Treatment of Facial Injuries. Baltimore, Williams & Wilkins Company, 1949.

Kazanjian, V. H., and Converse, J. M.: The Surgical Treatment of Facial Injuries. Baltimore, The Williams & Wilkins Company, 2nd Ed., 1959; 3rd. Ed., 1974.

Kazanjian, V. H., and Roopenian, A.: The treatment of lip deformities resulting from electric burns. Am. J. Surg., *88*:884, 1954.

Keith, A.: On congenital malformations of the palate, face, and neck. Br. Med. J., *2*:363, 1909.

König, F.: Lehrbuch der speciellen Chirurgie Für Aerzte und Studierende. Berlin, A. Hirschwald, 1898.

Kriens, O.: Median upper lip sinus. Report of 2 cases. Dtsch. Zahnaerztl. Z., *23*:1425, 1968.

Lallemand, M.: Plaie à la face avec perte de substance, guérie par l'application d'un lambeau détaché des parties voisines. Arch. Gén. Méd., *4*:242, 1824.

McGregor, I. A.: The tongue flap in lip surgery. Br. J. Plast. Surg., *19*:253, 1966.

McGregor, I. A., and Reid, W. H.: The use of the temporal flap in primary repair of full-thickness defects of the cheek. Plast. Reconstr. Surg., *38*:1, 1966.

McGregor, I. A., and Reid, W. H.: Simultaneous temporal and delto-pectoral flaps for full-thickness defects of the cheek. Plast. Reconstr. Surg., *45*:326, 1970.

Martin, H. E.: Cheiloplasty for advanced carcinoma of the lip. Surg. Gynecol. Obstet., *54*:914, 1932.

May, H.: One stage operation for closure of large defects of lower lip and chin. Surg. Gynecol. Obstet., *73*:236, 1941.

Murray, J.: Contributions to teratology: Undescribed malformations of the lower lip occurring in four members of one family. Br. & Foreign Medico-Surg. Rev., *26*:364, 1860.

Nélaton, C., and Ombrédanne, L.: Les Autoplasties. Paris, G. Steinheil, 1907.

Neustaetter, O.: Ueber den Lippensaum beim Menscher, seinen Bau, seine Enwickelung und seine Bedeutung. Jena Z. Naturwissensch., *29*:345, 1895.

New, G. B.: Sickle flap for nasal reconstruction. Surg. Gynecol. Obstet., *80*:597, 1945.

O'Brien, B.: A muscle-skin pedicle for total reconstruction of the lower lip. Plast. Reconstr. Surg., *45*:395, 1970.

Owens, N.: Simplified method of rotating skin and mucous membrane flaps for complete reconstruction of the lower lip. Surgery, *15*:196, 1944.

Owens, N.: A compound neck pedicle designed for the repair of massive facial defects: Formation, development and application. Plast. Reconstr. Surg., *15*:369, 1955.

Phillips, R. M.: Congenital fistulas of the lower lip: Report of case. J. Oral Surg., *26*:604, 1968.

Pierce, G. W., and O'Connor, G. B.: A new method of reconstruction of the lip. Arch. Surg., *28*:317, 1934.

Rose, E.: Ueber die angeborene Lippenfistel und den Unterlippenruessel. Monatsschr. Geburtsk. Frauenkr., *32*:99, 1868.

Sabattini, P.: Genno storico dell'origine e progressî della rinoplastica e cheiloplastica seguito della sescrizione di queste operazioni sopra un salo individuo. Bologna, Bell'Arti, 1838.

Sédillot, C.: Nouveau procédé de cheiloplastie. Gaz. Méd. Paris, *3*:7, 1848.

Serre, M.: Traité sur l'art de restaurer les difformités de la face, selon la méthode par déplacement ou méthode française. Montpellier, L. Castel, 1842.

Sicher, H., and Pohl, L.: Zur Entwicklung des menschichen Unterkiefers. Z. Stomatol., *32*:552, 1934.

Smith, F.: Some refinements in reconstructive surgery of the face. J.A.M.A., *120*:352, 1942.

Smith, J. W.: The anatomical and physiologic acclimatization of tissue transplanted by the lip switch technique. Plast. Reconstr. Surg., *26*:40, 1960.

Smith, J. W.: Clinical experiences with the vermilion border lip flap. Plast. Reconstr. Surg., *27*:527, 1961.

Stein, S. A. W.: Laebedannelse (Cheiloplastik) udført paa en ny methode. Hopsitalsmeddelelser (Cophenhagen), *1*:212, 1848.

Stieda, A.: Die angebornen Fisteln der Unterlippe und ihre Entstehung. Arch. Klin. Chir., *79*:293, 1906.

Szymanowski, J. von: Zur plastichen Chirurgie. Vrtljschr. Prakt. Heilk., *60*:152, 1858.

Taylor, W. B., and Lane, D. K.: Congenital fistulas of lower lip. Arch. Dermatol., *94*:421, 1966.

Teale, T. P.: On plastic operations for the restoration of the lower lip. M. Times Gaz., *35*:561, 1857.

Walker, J. C., and Sawhney, P.: Free composite lip grafts. Plast. Reconstr. Surg., *50*:142, 1972.

Wang, M. K. H., and Macomber, W. B.: Congenital lip sinuses. Plast. Reconstr. Surg., *18*:319, 1956.

Warbrick, J. G., McIntyre, J. R., and Fergusson, A. G.: Remarks on the aetiology of congenital bilateral fistulae of the lower lip. Br. J. Plast. Surg., *4*:254, 1952.

Webster, J. P.: Crescentic peri-alar cheek excision for upper lip flap advancement with a short history of upper lip repair. Plast. Reconstr. Surg., *16*:434, 1955.

Wood-Smith, D.: Personal communication, 1975.

Woollcombe, W. L.: Mandibular process associated with double harelip and cleft palate. Lancet, *1*:357, 1905.

Zarem, H. A., and Greer, D. M.: Tongue flap for reconstruction of the lips after electrical burns. Plast. Reconstr. Surg., *53*:310, 1974.

Zimany, A.: The bi-lobe flap. Plast. Reconstr. Surg., *11*:424, 1953.

CHAPTER 33

FACIAL BURNS

JOHN MARQUIS CONVERSE, M.D.,
JOSEPH G. MCCARTHY, M.D.,
MARIO DOBRKOVSKY, M.D.,
AND D. L. LARSON, M.D.

Burn-related deaths and injuries constitute one of the major health problems in the United States today. According to the report of the National Commission on Fire Prevention and Control, 12,000 Americans die each year as a result of burn injury. In addition, 300,000 sustain serious burns (more than 25 per cent of body surface area) and require prolonged hospitalization (Phillips, 1975). The groups most vulnerable to burn injury are the very young, the elderly, and the physically handicapped. Almost one-half of this country's burn victims are under 15 years of age. The death rate each year from burn injury is more than double the death rate during the poliomyelitis epidemic during the 1950's.

Although the causes of burn injury are numerous, certain patterns appear in nearly every epidemiologic study. Flame burns involving clothing ignition are especially apparent in the data. Feller (1975) reported a series of 4596 cases, 3946 of which involved clothing ignition, as opposed to 650 cases in which clothing was not ignited. Moreover, the severity and extent of the injury involving clothing ignition was dramatic. The mortality rate for victims whose clothing ignited was four times higher than that for patients whose clothing was not ignited; the area of total burn was nearly 100 per cent greater; the percentage of full-thickness injury was six times greater; and the number of days of hospitalization was 60 per cent greater for clothing ignition victims. Most of these accidents occur in the home, the common ignitors including open space heaters, kitchen ranges, and matches. Among elderly victims, the ingestion of alcohol or prescription medications is often a causative factor.

Flammable liquids are another frequent cause of burn injury in this country. Both young and adult males are inclined to use gasoline for cleaning items such as paint brushes, automobile parts, and bicycle parts. In many cases, the gasoline vapors are ignited by the pilot light of a hot water heater or a spark from a metal object. These injuries are generally quite severe and often involve facial areas.

Industrial burn accidents often involve acid, chemicals, or molten metals, and facial burns are common in this type of accident. The intense heat of a flash burn may injure only the exposed parts of the body, most often the hands and face. Ordinary clothing often provides surprisingly effective protection in flash burn situations.

In many automobile accidents, the gas tank will rupture and the fuel may explode, turning what might have been a quite minor accident into a roaring holocaust. Facial and hand burns almost invariably result. Pontèn (1968) studied burn injuries in 94 automobile accidents and showed that the incidence and severity were greater when the fuel tank was located in the front rather than the rear of the vehicle.

Facial burns represent between one-quarter and one-third of all burns (Roper-Hall, 1962;

Skoog, 1963; Tubiana, 1967). In a review of a large burn unit, Dowling, Foley, and Moncrief (1968) reported that almost 60 per cent of all patients admitted to their burn unit had facial burns.

ELECTRICAL BURNS

Accidents associated with the use of various mechanical and electrical devices are fairly common in the contemporary household. Baldridge (1954) and Dale (1954), discussing the electrophysical aspects of electrical burns, described two general types: arc and contact. In the former, the involved area is heated by an electrical arc to a temperature of 2500° to 3000°C, resulting in a charring of the soft tissues and bone. In the latter type, an electric current passes through the body from the point of contact to the point of "grounded" exit, with burns at both sites; death may ensue if the current traverses vital cardiac or cerebral centers.

Electrical burns usually seen by plastic surgeons are of the arc type, due to contact with live electrical sockets, and the tissue injury is confined to the immediate area of the burn. Most electrical burns occur in the perioral region of children ranging in age from 9 months to 4 years; most of the accidents are in the 1- to 2-year age group. That the mishap occurs more frequently in the younger child is quite understandable, for while the child is creeping or playing, the live electrical cord left carelessly on the floor becomes an object of curiosity which must be tasted. The moisture of the mouth completes the electrical circuit, and the resulting arc burns the tissues. If the child is wet or is touching a ground object (i.e., a radiator), the current may pass through the body, even resulting in electrocution. Although it is generally believed that voltages of 110 to 120 volts are not fatal, the authors know of one child who was electrocuted by contact with a live Christmas tree light socket and a radiator.

Examination usually discloses a third degree burn with a centrally depressed charred crater and a slight, pale grayish elevation of the surrounding skin. Pathologic examination shows extensive coagulation necrosis extending for a considerable distance beyond the apparent limits of the wound. The media of the blood vessels is disintegrated, occasionally leading to secondary hemorrhage during the sloughing process. Sensory nerves are widely destroyed,

possibly accounting for the painless nature of the injury. The devitalized tissues slough slowly, with a minimum of surrounding tissue reaction and associated tardy repair. Injured bone is also slow to sequestrate.

WOUND HEALING FOLLOWING BURN INJURY

Contractures and hypertrophic scars are two frustrating sequelae of thermal injury. The former is the end result of contraction, a phenomenon associated with the healing of any granulating or full-thickness wound.

Contraction

Contraction is not limited to the full-thickness burn wound. The second degree burn wound which involves only the partial thickness of the skin also contracts during healing. The re-epithelization of second degree burns originates from the epidermal inclusions in the dermis: remnants of the rete pegs between the dermal papillae, hair follicles, sebaceous glands, sweat glands, and their excretory ducts. On the surface of the dermal wound, islands of epidermis, which originate from the remaining epithelial elements, appear. Each island enlarges in size through a process of multiplication, enlargement, and migration of its epidermal cells. This outburst of epidermal mitotic activity has been attributed by Bullough and Laurence (1960a, b) to a reduction in the concentration of mitotic inhibitors presumed to be present in undamaged skin.

All wounds contract during healing, and dermal wounds are no exception. Contraction of the wound tends to approximate the islands of epithelium to facilitate their eventual coalescence (Fig. 33–1). This phenomenon has been called *interisland contraction* (Converse and Robb-Smith, 1944; Converse, 1967). It is this contraction which explains the tightening of the skin following a burn involving an appreciable thickness of the dermis. Epidermal continuity is restored, but there results a generalized shortness of skin in the area, and invisible skin loss. Thus contractures occur, despite the fact that the full thickness of the skin was not destroyed, especially in the mobile areas of the face—eyelids, nares, lips, cheek, and cervical area.

The mechanisms responsible for wound con-

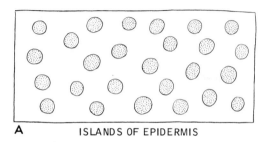

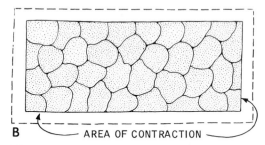

A ISLANDS OF EPIDERMIS

B ── AREA OF CONTRACTION ──

FIGURE 33–1. Mechanism of interisland contraction. *A,* Islands of regenerating epidermis on the surface of a dermal burn wound. *B,* Islands have coalesced by dual process of epithelial spread and contraction between the epidermal islands. The result is contraction and diminution of the healed surface area. (From Converse, J. M.: Burn deformities of the face and neck. Surg. Clin. North Am., *47*:323, 1967.)

Whatever the exact mechanism of wound contraction, the fact is that wounds in which an appreciable surface area of the skin has been destroyed are submitted to an inexorable contraction if the surrounding tissues are sufficiently lax to permit the contraction (e.g., eyelids, lips, and cheeks). In the forehead and scalp areas, where the cutaneous tissues are relatively tightly adapted to the underlying cranial vault, wound contraction is limited.

Intrinsic and Extrinsic Contracture. Four areas characterized by mobility and flexibility are susceptible to contracture: the eyelids, the cheeks, the lips and perioral tissues, and the cervical area (Fig. 33–2). Contracture is *intrinsic,* the result of loss of tissue in the structures themselves, or *extrinsic,* caused by the pull of a healing contracting wound in the periphery.

The upper eyelid is submitted to extrinsic contracture from the healing tissues of the brow and forehead, the lower eyelid from contracture exerted by the cheek tissues. The upper lip, through intrinsic contracture, is pulled up toward the columella, while the lat-

traction have been the subject of considerable investigation. According to Watts, Grillo, and Gross (1958), the potential for the major part of contraction lies in the wound margins (the "picture frame" hypothesis), and the central granulation tissue is not required in the process of contraction. Abercrombie, Flint, and James (1956) cast doubt on the role of preformed collagen or newly formed collagen fibers when they demonstrated unimpaired wound closure in scorbutic guinea pigs, despite almost complete absence of new collagen synthesis. The work of Abercombie, James, and Newcome (1960) also suggests that the "picture frame" hypothesis cannot be held to be generally applicable. Gabbiani and associates (1971) have demonstrated in a contracting wound the presence of a cell (the myofibroblast) with the characteristics of a fibroblast and a smooth muscle cell (see Chapter 3). Larson and his associates (1975) have confirmed an increase in the number of myofibroblasts present in the healed burn wound; the cells have also been identified by antiserum with a fluorescent tag to human muscle cells.

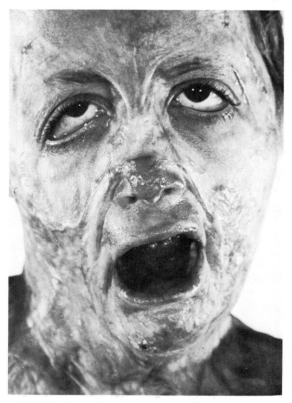

FIGURE 33–2. Burn contractures. Note the pull of scar tissue on the lower eyelids and lower lip.

eral portions of the upper lip are subjected, in addition, to the extrinsic contracture exerted from the cheeks; the lower lip and chin are pulled downward by intrinsic contracture and also by the downward pull of the contracting cervical area.

The healing of the burned tissues in the temporal area may result in the formation of vertical cicatricial bands around the lateral canthus of the eye (cicatricial epicanthus), which interfere with elevation of the upper eyelid and shorten the horizontal dimension of the palpebral fissure. Extrinsic contracture may also affect the medial canthus following burns over the dorsum of the nose. The medial canthal tissues are pulled forward, tending to ride up to the level of the dorsum of the root of the nose. The lacrimal puncta are pulled away from the conjunctival sac and lacrimal lake; the functional disturbance of the lacrimal apparatus is the consequence of this anatomical disruption, and acute dacryocystitis is not an infrequent complication.

Circumferential contracture around the oral fissure has a purse-string–like effect, diminishing its horizontal dimension and limiting the patient's ability to open his mouth (see Fig. 33–11, *A*). Burning of the narial border and of the perinarial portion of the nasal vestibule may cause destruction of part of the naris itself and a circular intranarial contracture resulting in stenosis. The tip of the nose tends to be pulled down into the lip. The base of the columella disappears in a large mass of hypertrophic scar involving the upper lip. When skin is destroyed over the dorsum of the nose, the alae are retracted in a cephalic direction and the alae are everted, exposing the interior of the vestibules. Loss of tissue in the cheek tends to obliterate the nasolabial folds.

Contracture is exerted not only in the cervical area itself but also in the adjacent lower portion of the face; the lower lip and the soft tissues of the chin are contracted down toward the sternal notch (see Chapter 34). The profile contour of the neck and the lower part of the face tends to be a straight line, with a disappearance of the suprahyoid mandibular-cervical angle; the lower lip is in ectropion; the labiomental fold has disappeared, and the chin pad occupies a submandibular position.

Concerning the burn wound, two observations are made: (1) the position of comfort is the position of contracture; (2) the burn wound contracts until it meets an opposing force. The first is readily seen by the flexed position

the burn patient assumes for comfort and the flexion contractures that follow (Fig. 33–3). The second observation indicates that the burn wound will shorten by the force exerted by the myofibroblasts and the flexion of muscles until the surrounding tissue equals this force. These wound shortening mechanisms can be combatted in clinical practice by traction, splinting, and exercise. Exercise may be very effective; however, during rest and sleep, the shortening proceeds rapidly, and consequently some

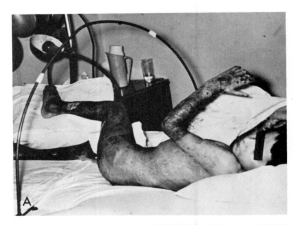

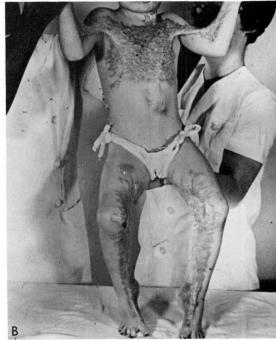

FIGURE 33–3. Burn contractures. *A,* Position of comfort. *B,* Resulting contractures. (From Larson, D. L., and coworkers: Contracture and scar formation in the burn patient. Clinics in Plastic Surgery, *1*:653, 1974.)

method of positioning and splinting is necessary to hold the part in optimum position during this period.

Hypertrophic Scars

The burn patient is frequently discharged from the hospital with a satisfactory result only to return in three to four weeks with severe hypertrophic scars. The latter are seen in areas of contracture after the healing of full-thickness burns and also in areas of deep dermal burns; at the junction line between skin grafts; and between skin grafts and the surrounding skin. Similar scars occur in the donor areas following the removal of split-thickness skin grafts of excessive thickness. They are particularly frequent in children. The propensity of children to hypertrophic scar formation is well known.

In burn wounds with loss of skin, hypertrophy of the burn scars occurs when the long axis of the wound traverses the lines of minimal tension (see Chapter 1). In the course of contraction of the healing wound, hypertrophic scar tissue is laid down. The push and pull and alternating tension and relaxation to which the scar is subjected promote the proliferation of fibroblasts, which continues long after clinical evidence of wound healing has been completed. Thick, contractile cords and bands are formed, which consist of longitudinally arranged bundles of collagen fibers between which are flattened fibroblasts. Proliferating endothelium is seen in histological sections of the fibrous bands; a manifestation of their vascularity is their turgescent appearance in the early stages. Microscopic tears and hemorrhages from forceful exercise produce additional fibroblastic proliferation in the repair process of these tears.

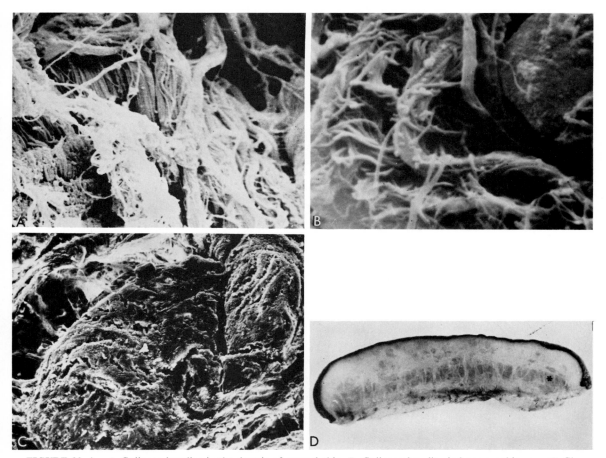

FIGURE 33–4. *A,* Collagen bundles in the dermis of normal skin. *B,* Collagen bundles in hypertrophic scar. *C,* Characteristic nodules of hypertrophic scar. *D,* Full-thickness biopsy through a hypertrophic scar. The asterisk denotes nodules of collagen in the dermis. (From Larson, D. L., and coworkers: Contracture and scar formation in the burn patient. Clinics in Plastic Surgery, *1*:653, 1974.)

Pathophysiology of Hypertrophic Scars.
Normal dermal collagen has a loose, three-dimensional arrangement of fibers (Fig. 33–4, *A*), whereas the burn wound collagen fibers are in disarray, demonstrating twists, turns, and finally the typical whorl-like and nodular arrangement of the hypertrophic scar (Fig. 33–4, *B*, *C*). This may be the result of a centripetal pull (Fig. 33–5, *A*) of the fibroblasts and/or myofibroblasts and the flexion creases (Fig. 33–5, *B*) resulting from voluntary flexion of the underlying muscle. The newly formed collagen fibers thus become compact and disorganized, maintaining the wound in a shortened position. Following normal resolution of the scar, the collagen is less compact, and individual collagen fibers are apparent (Fig. 33–5, *D*). However,

the wound is maintained in a shortened position.

Linares and his associates (1973) examined histologically the granulation tissue in 24 burn wounds which ranged from 26 days to 3 months after burn injury. In 23 biopsies there was a whorl-like arrangement of collagen and fibroblasts; one biopsy failed to show this finding. Patients in the former group developed hypertrophic scarring, while the patients without this finding did not develop hypertrophic scarring. Because of these observations, the Burn Unit at the Shriners Burn Institute in Galveston has initiated a program of manipulation in the early phase of wound healing following thermal burns (Larson and his coworkers, 1971). The technique, which consists of pres-

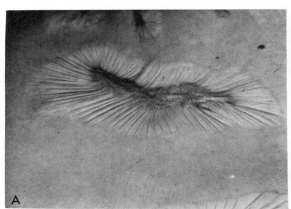
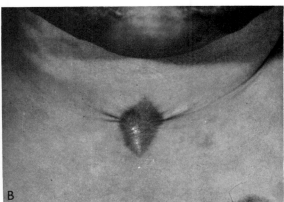
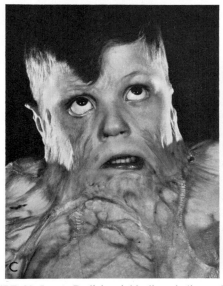
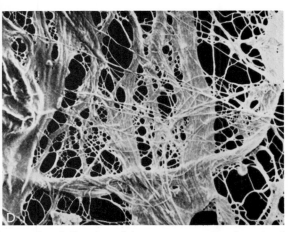

FIGURE 33–5. *A*, Radial wrinkle lines indicate the centripetal direction of the contracture, thought to be the contractile force of fibroblasts. *B*, A hypertrophic scar forms a bridge across the crease lines. *C*, Scars on the flexor surfaces may result in severe contractures. *D*, The dermis in a mature scar shows loosening of the compact collagen. The "holy" pattern is characteristic of a mature scar. (From Larson, D. L., and coworkers: Contracture and scar formation in the burn patient. Clinics in Plastic Surgery, *1*:653, 1974.)

sure and splinting (Fig. 33–6), will be described later in the chapter. Collagen metabolism and hypertrophic scars are also discussed in Chapter 3.

TREATMENT

In the treatment of facial burns, there are several successive stages:
1. Acute period
    a. Pregrafting phase
    b. Skin grafting phase
2. Chronic period
    a. Waiting phase
    b. Early reconstructive phase
    c. Final reconstructive phase

Acute Period

The acute period is defined as that time from occurrence of the burn to complete coverage of the wound.

The Pregrafting Phase. As in most major burns, the initial treatment is concerned with the physiologic resuscitation of the patient and control of the burn wound, as discussed in Chapter 18.

RESPIRATORY TRACT INVOLVEMENT. Respiratory tract damage must be considered in the initial evaluation of all facial burns. Phillips and Cope (1962) indicted respiratory tract damage as a principal killer of the burned patient. Of 100 consecutive patients admitted to a major burn unit, 22 had major respiratory problems (average body surface involvement was 67 per cent). Nineteen of the 22 patients succumbed to their burns (Furnas, Bartlett and Achauer, 1973).

Respiratory tract involvement is usually secondary to chemical injury from the inhalation of products of incomplete combustion. Direct thermal injury is uncommon. Zikria and his associates (1975) have emphasized the role of asphyxia and carbon monoxide poisoning. The latter type of injury, usually unassociated with cutaneous burns, can be confirmed by measuring carboxyhemoglobin saturation (HbCO).

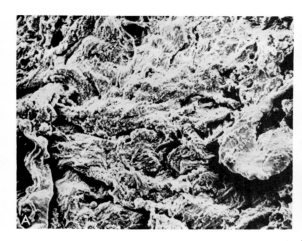
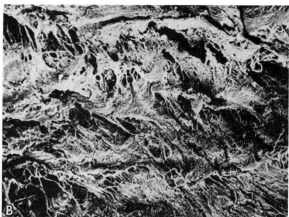
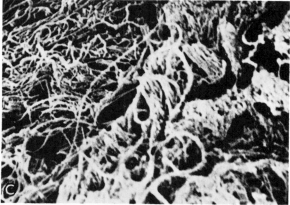

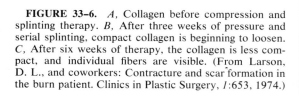

FIGURE 33–6. *A,* Collagen before compression and splinting therapy. *B,* After three weeks of pressure and serial splinting, compact collagen is beginning to loosen. *C,* After six weeks of therapy, the collagen is less compact, and individual fibers are visible. (From Larson, D. L., and coworkers: Contracture and scar formation in the burn patient. Clinics in Plastic Surgery, *1*:653, 1974.)

Patients with inhalation injuries have usually been exposed to heavy smoke or a gaseous chemical in a closed space. Wheezing, hoarseness, and dyspnea may be the principal symtoms. There can be burns of the face, neck, and upper chest. The sputum may be carbonaceous and the vibrissae singed; erythema and blisters may be evident over the pharynx, palate, cheeks, and tongue. Tachypnea, hoarseness, rales, rhonchi, and hemoptysis are often associated findings.

While early chest radiographs are usually unremarkable, there is evidence of pathology by the third to fifth day. With time, sputum cultures become positive. Initial arterial blood gas determinations show hypoxemia, and serial studies serve as an index of the patient's improvement and/or deterioration. Carboxyhemoglobin saturation should also be determined to rule out carbon monoxide poisoning. A level exceeding 60 per cent indicates the need for immediate treatment with high inspired oxygen content.

The major pulmonary complications include pneumonia, pulmonary edema, bronchiectasis, and tracheobronchitis.

Capillary-alveolar block syndrome is one of the most common pulmonary problems seen in the burn patient. This defect is an increased interstitial fluid accumulation in the alveolar wall, resulting in decreased oxygen diffusion; the carbon dioxide diffuses so rapidly it is unaffected. Blood gas studies therefore show a decrease in Po_2 with a near normal Pco_2. The fluid accumulation may be prevented by maintaining susceptible patients on the dry side. If the defect occurs, a diuretic (e.g., Lasix) is the treatment of choice, together with routine therapeutic measures such as oxygen administration and encouragement of coughing, deep breathing, etc.

Initial treatment should consist of coughing exercises and intermittent positive pressure breathing (IPPB) with mucolytic agents. A humidified environment and nasotracheal suction facilitate removal of thick, tenacious sputum. Bronchoscopy and temporary endotracheal intubation are additional aids to the clearing of tracheobronchial secretions.

If the above aids are unsuccessful and serial arterial blood gas studies and chest radiographs show continued clinical deterioration, tracheotomy and mechanical ventilation are indicated. In the series of respiratory burns reviewed by Di Vincenti, Pruitt, and Recklar (1971), 72 per cent of the patients required tracheotomies, the vast majority of which were performed by the fourth postburn day.

The role of steroids remains controversial. Zikria and his associates (1975) feel that patients with smoke poisoning and peripheral (alveolar) respiratory injury benefit from the early use of intravenous steroids to reduce interstitial edema and release bronchial and bronchiolar spasm. Conversely, in respiratory burns in which the injury is more central (pharynx, larynx, trachea, and proximal major bronchi), the drug may be contraindicated because of possible disruption of the mucosal barrier against invasive infection.

DIAGNOSIS OF THE DEPTH OF THE BURN. It is difficult, if not impossible, to make an immediate diagnosis of the depth of the burn in the burned face. Analgesia to pinprick, helpful in the diagnosis of depth in the remainder of the body, is unreliable in the face. The burned areas may be red, white, or black, and the burn may be only of partial thickness. Early excision and grafting are not advisable in facial burns for these reasons.

THE EXPOSURE TECHNIQUE. Early treatment of facial burns includes gentle cleansing with saline, removal of debris and loose epithelium, and evacuation of blisters. The eyes should be carefully examined for possible corneal damage, and the corneas should be protected by instillation of ophthalmic ointment. The patient's head is kept elevated, and emergency tracheotomy equipment is maintained at the bedside. Within 24 hours, the burned face and neck are the site of increasing edema, the facial and cervical tissues being ballooned out and the eyelids closed (Fig. 33-7).

Bulky dressings are not indicated in facial burns. The dressings are uncomfortable, cause mechanical irritation of the burned area, and tend to encourage bacterial proliferation. The exposure method (Wallace, 1949) is preferable. The formation of a dry crust or scab is encouraged by placing the patient in a dry air environment, if such facilities are available, or by blowing warm dry air on the burn with an electric hairdryer. Loose, wet dressings may be employed after several days in order to assist in the cleansing of the sloughing wound. The removal of loose tissue and the separation of scabs and sloughs are assisted with forceps and scissors. The edema subsides, and devitalized tissues become apparent. In partial thickness burns, the devitalized scab of the superficial burn separates itself from the subja-

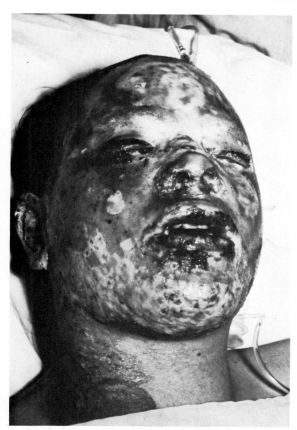

FIGURE 33–7. Third degree facial burn at 72 hours. Note the severe swelling with secondary closure of the eyelids.

nosa, preventing further destruction of surviving epithelial islands, it has been claimed that this topical agent favors spontaneous re-epithelization (Lindberg and his coworkers, 1965).

According to Scapicchio, Constable, and Opitz (1968), silver nitrate used as a topical agent appears to have no effect on the rate of epidermal regeneration when compared with saline solution used in experimental work done in rabbits, or with untreated wounds. Sulfamylon acetate appears to retard epithelization. These findings were confirmed by Flagg, Converse and Rapaport (1969), who concluded that the exposure method remains an effective technique for the treatment of the burn wound. These investigators confirmed the observations of Scapicchio and his associates (1968) that Sulfamylon retarded the rate of wound healing. Silver sulfadiazine appeared to have no effect on the rate of epidermal regeneration. Bacitracin ointment is another topical medication which can be applied to the facial burn wound during this period.

Additional initial care of the burned face includes daily debridement during tubbing in a Hubbard tank. Commercially available porcine skin xenografts are also employed in full-thickness facial burns to prepare a granulating bed for skin autografting.

LYE BURNS. Lye burns of the face are not unusual among some ethnic groups and often are secondary to marital problems. The usual offending agents are caustic potash (potassium hydroxide) and caustic soda (sodium hydroxide).

Bromberg, Song, and Walden (1965) have advocated water irrigation therapy. The patient sits under a running shower; in addition, the corneas can be continuously irrigated with saline through modified scleral lenses. It was emphasized that the therapy must be prolonged because of the progressive nature of alkali burns, residual uncombined alkali in the burn wound, hygroscopic action of alkali, and the length of the destructive capacity of the hydroxide ion.

BURN INVOLVEMENT OF THE EYELIDS AND GLOBES. The thinness of the skin of the eyelids and the intimate relationship of the pretarsal portion of the orbicularis oculi muscle with the skin explains the high frequency of ectropion, not only in burns with full-thickness skin loss but also in partial-thickness burns. The looseness of the eyelid tissues also predisposes them to retraction and ectropion when skin is destroyed in areas in the vicinity of the orbit (extrinsic contracture).

cent healed integument within ten days. A thicker scab separates more slowly in deep dermal burns, revealing alternating areas of healing epithelium and granulation tissue characteristic of the burn of mixed depth. The thick, rigid black eschar of full-thickness burns begins to separate slowly and with difficulty, usually within a period of 15 days, the deep hair follicles of the male face tending to retain the sloughing tissue. The wound becomes rapidly covered with healthy-appearing granulation tissue in subsequent days and should be skin grafted as soon as feasible.

The introduction of techniques involving topical application of 0.5 per cent silver nitrate (Moyer and his coworkers, 1965), 10 per cent *p*-aminomethyl-benzenesulfonamide (Sulfamylon), and silver sulfadiazine (Fox, 1968) has raised the question of their indication in burns of the face and neck. Because Sulfamylon cream appears to suppress bacterial growth, particularly of *Pseudomonas aerugi-*

Full-thickness defects of the lid rarely occur in flash or flame burns; in chemical burns, however, it is not infrequent to see an area of full-thickness destruction of the lid. The structures behind the lids are usually not injured in flash or flame burns. Corneal and conjunctival burns occur in chemical burns, however, and are particularly serious, because spreading infection to the globe from a corneal ulcer may result in enucleation. The cornea was destroyed by acid in a number of our patients who had suffered such an attack, and infection led to endophthalmitis resulting in loss of the eye.

Corneal ulceration and scarring are seen in long-standing ectropion, following flash or flame burns, from exposure, drying, and subsequent infection. Most corneal lesions in burn patients are preventable if precautions are taken to protect the cornea from exposure.

Burn contractures may involve eyelid tissue alone when the remainder of the face has suffered only a superficial burn. Because the eyelid skin is thin and the eyelids are composed of loosely bound tissues, contraction during healing results in ectropion.

The eyelids are often spared in flash burns if the patient is wearing glasses, but the skin of the remaining portion of the face may be burned, and scar contraction of the surrounding tissue may cause extrinsic ectropion.

Even in deep burns of the eyelids with full-thickness destruction of the skin, a sufficient number of orbicularis oculi muscle fibers usually remain to ensure closure of the eye. Function of the levator palpebrae superioris muscle is rarely affected. Also, when the eyelids have been involved in full-thickness burns of the skin, although the eyelashes and eyebrows are scorched, the eyelid margins are usually spared and the tarsal plates remain intact.

Deep burns which involve the full thickness of the eyelid or chemical burns with penetration of the burning agent into the conjunctival sac result in symblepharon, an adhesion between the eyelid and eyeball; complete obliteration of the conjunctival sac is known as ankyloblepharon.

Approximately 7.5 per cent of burn patients admitted to the U.S. Army Institute of Surgical Research (Brooke Army Medical Center) had associated ocular complications (Asch and his coworkers, 1971). Of the 104 patients, 60 had involvement of the globe, including corneal ulcer, corneal laceration, corneal burns, and globe penetration. Another 69 patients had adnexal complications, including conjunctivitis and ectropion. Ectropion was the most common ocular complication.

Corneal exposure following thermal or chemical injury is secondary to (a) inability to blink normally; (b) lack of adequate lid coverage; and (c) disturbances in tear physiology (Constable and Carroll, 1970). Tears are composed of three components: the aqueous from the lacrimal glands; the mucous from the goblet cells of the conjunctiva; and the lipid from the meibomian glands of the lid. Following a burn there is an inordinate decrease in the lipid component, which is needed to reduce the rate of tear evaporation from the surface of the cornea (Mishima and Maurice, 1961). In this way exposure of the cornea is further aggravated.

In the acute management of the exposed cornea, a tarsorrhaphy should be avoided because of associated tearing of the lid and residual deformity of the eyelid margin. Destruction or distortion of the eyelid margin complicates subsequent reconstruction.

During the acute period, local conservative measures such as frequent application of ophthalmic ointment and taping of the eyelids suffice. Temporary lid occlusal sutures can also be employed. Bell's phenomenon protects the eye with a partial ectropion. Constable and Carroll (1970) have advocated the use of scleral lenses to tide the patient over until definitive skin grafting can be performed.

BURN INVOLVEMENT OF THE EARS. The thin skin and subcutaneous layer of the helix provide little protection to the underlying cartilage following burn injury.

Over 90 per cent of patients with facial burns have associated burns of the ears (Dowling, Foley and Moncrief, 1968). Among these patients, approximately 25 per cent of those who survive the burn develop a suppurative chondritis and cellulitis of the auricle.

In a review of 147 patients with post-thermal chondritis, two modes of auricular injury were described (Dowling and his coworkers, 1968). The first is secondary to direct thermal injury involving all helical layers. Autoamputation can occur, and infection is rarely a problem. In the second type, the patient must survive the initial burn period to develop a suppurative chondritis usually three to five weeks after burn injury. When auricular chondritis develops, the patient often complains of local pain. The helix is red, swollen, tender, and protruding, with an increase in the auriculocephalic angle. Abscess formation and drainage may be present.

The best treatment is preventive. Curling of the helix should be prevented by an elastic net dressing; pressure against the external ear should be avoided. Topical ointments should also be applied.

Treatment by incision and drainage with resection of involved cartilage has been recommended once the diagnosis of suppurative chondritis has been established (Spira and Hardy, 1963). If tenderness and induration persist, the helix is bivalved by establishing anterior and posterior helical skin flaps, and cartilage is resected until healthy cartilage is reached (Dowling and his coworkers, 1968). The flaps are then reapproximated. However, the contracting circular scar results in a cup deformity.

If the overlying skin is destroyed, escharectomy and immediate split-thickness skin grafting within the first 48 hours and not later than the fifth postoperative day have been recommended (Grant, Finley and Coers, 1969).

Because of residual auricular cicatrization, distortion, and loss of contour following traditional methods of treating auricular chondritis, local instillation of antiboitic solution combined with warm compresses has been advocated (Apfelberg and his coworkers, 1974). This technique, which involves the insertion of a needle or small polyethylene catheter directly into the auricle, may obviate the need for cartilage debridement.

The Skin Grafting Phase. In full-thickness burns, skin grafting should be done as soon as the granulations have appeared after the separation of the eschar. Relatively thick split-thickness skin grafts of 0.014 to 0.018 inch* in thickness are satisfactorily revascularized and provide a cutaneous surface of better quality than the thinner split-thickness variety (Fig. 33–8). Skin grafting in facial burns should be done not only in the areas of obvious full-thickness loss but also over areas of mixed deep dermal burns as soon as granulations appear. Skin grafting of the burn of mixed depth will greatly reduce the amount of subsequent hypertrophic scar formation which is characteristic after the healing of such areas.

If skin grafting has been delayed because of concern for the general clinical status of the patient, the granulations may have become excessively hypertrophic. In such cases removal of the granulation tissue by scraping the soft superficial layer from the deeper, more resistant layer provides a firm, well-vascularized base for the skin graft.

The dressing used on the face consists of one layer of medicated fine mesh gauze held in place by an elasticized netting. The elasticized netting not only maintains the dressing on these movable parts but also helps to maintain the lips and facial features in proper position. The ears are covered in the same fashion, and this keeps the ears flat against the head and prevents bending of the auricle. As mentioned earlier, it has been our experience that chondritis of the ear is often secondary to curling of the external ear. Chondritis of the ear is rarely seen as long as the ear is kept flat against the head; pillows should be avoided on the beds of patients who have thermal injuries to the ears.

During the early period of treatment, rapidly increasing ectropion of the upper eyelid leading to corneal exposure and possible ulceration requires the application of thin split-thickness skin grafts to overcome the eyelid retraction; usually these early grafts require later replacement because of recurrent ectropion. If danger to the cornea is not present, skin grafting of the eyelids should be postponed until the contractile process is completed and until all areas around the orbit have been grafted.

Early skin grafting has reduced the number of monstrous deformities formerly encountered when face and neck burn wounds were allowed to heal spontaneously (see Figs. 33–2 and 33–5, C).

In applying skin grafts, the surgeon should keep in mind the esthetic units of the face (Fig. 33–9) and should endeavor to resurface each esthetic unit with a single sheet of skin graft.

The Chronic Period

The chronic period has been arbitrarily defined as that period from the completion of wound coverage through the following six months or until the wounds have matured, as evidenced by the fading of the redness and softening of the scar.

The Waiting Phase. As soon as the grafts are sufficiently stable, usually at approximately

---

*1 inch = 2.54 cm metric.

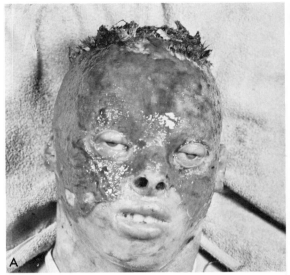

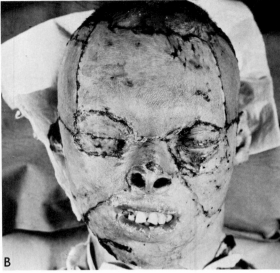

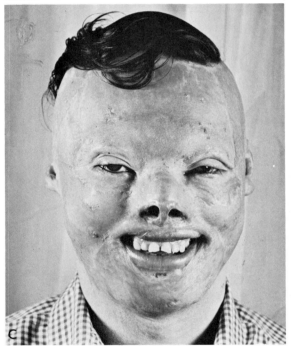

FIGURE 33–8. Skin grafting following a full-thickness facial burn. *A,* Granulation tissue prior to grafting. *B,* Following split-thickness skin grafting of the forehead, cheek, and orbital esthetic units. *C,* After healing of the skin grafts and prior to additional reconstructive surgery. (From Kazanjian and Converse.)

three weeks, an elasticized face mask* is applied (Fig. 33–10) and worn continuously to reduce hypertrophic scarring. As the elasticized face mask does not maintain pressure in the lateral nasal and adjacent cheek areas, a form-fitting Orthoplast nasal splint may be

applied beneath the elastic face mask (Fig. 33–10). Additional aid in maintaining pressure on the grafts is obtained by the use of a silicone sponge face mask (face pad), which is worn under the elastic hood. The custom-made face pad was developed in the Shriners Hospital sculpture department by Mr. Joseph Paderewski. Worn continuously, it not only decreases the amount of scar formation but also

---

*Available from the Jobst Company, 133 East 58th St., New York, NY 10020.

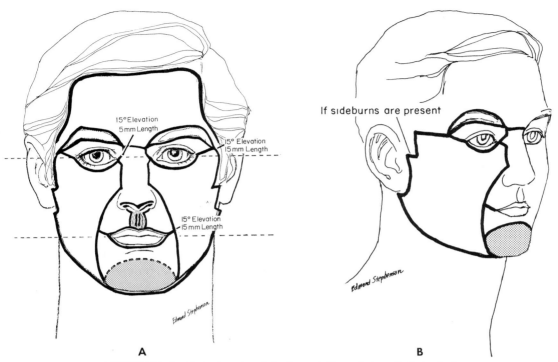

FIGURE 33–9. Esthetic units of the face. *A,* Frontal view. *B,* Lateral view.

keeps the facial features in their anatomical position and prevents contractures of the lips and other facial elements.

Another common site of contractures in the face is the area around the mouth. As the scars about the mouth contract, the opening of the mouth is severely limited. A useful appliance has been developed which fits into the corners

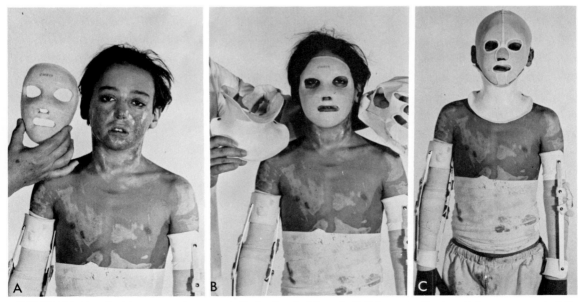

FIGURE 33–10. Facial pressure therapy. *A,* Orthoplast facial mask. *B,* Prior to application of the custom-made Jobst hood of elasticized material (left side) and the cervical collar (right side). *C,* All elements in place. In addition, the patient is wearing elbow splints.

of the mouth; it has a rubber band that causes continuous pull to force the corners of the mouth laterally. A similar device is available from the H. Buccker Dental Laboratory in Iowa City, Iowa. A similar principle is applied, but rather than an elastic push, a fixed device with a metallic spring spreads the corners of the mouth (Fig. 33–11).

To prevent the development of contractures about the nares, vestibular inserts are made and worn almost continuously as splints to keep the nares from being either obliterated or severely narrowed (Fig. 33–12).

If there is coexisting contracture of the neck, the associated pull on the facial structures distorts the latter. Consequently, any therapy to prevent facial scarring and contractures must also include similar therapy to the neck. During the acute phase of burn therapy, a form-fitting Orthoplast splint is applied continuously over the dressing to maintain the neck in a corrected position (see Fig. 33–10, *B, C*). Following grafting of the neck, a form-fitting splint is reapplied as soon as possible. It has been our experience that the cervical contractures can be dramatically diminished by this type of therapy. The Orthoplast neck conformers should be fashioned in such a way that they do not extend to the lower lip, as the resulting pressure influences the inclination of the teeth. The lower lip is maintained in its proper position by the Jobst face mask. The management of thermal injury of the cervical region is discussed in Chapter 34.

During the waiting phase, the patient is encouraged to exercise the periorbital area by frequent opening and closing of the eyelids. This can be done under the supervision of the physical therapist. Similar exercises are helpful in the perioral (lip) region (Fig. 33–13). Contractures of the eyelids and lips will be reduced with such therapy, just as those of the different joints are reduced by exercising.

The return of a patient to his home after a long period of hospitalization may be a traumatic experience. It is essential that the patient be forewarned of the reaction of members of his family, friends, and neighbors. A thorough understanding on the part of the patient's spouse and other members of the family is important. One of our patients recalls that when he returned home his two small children recoiled, screaming at the sight of their disfigured father.

This furlough is essential to allow the patient to regain his psychological balance after the often long ordeal he has been through during the period of hospitalization. It is also necessary to allow metabolic and immunologic stabilization, to provide for a change in the bacterial environment, and to allow time for the maturation of scar tissue. The surgeon must resist the pressure placed upon him by both the patient and the family to undertake early reconstructive procedures. Such operations present technical difficulties because of the activity of the scar tissue and the rapid recurrence of hypertrophic scars, which may be larger and more hypertrophic than the original scars. The recently healed tissues are inadequately vascularized, and latent pathogenic microorganisms in the area may cause local sepsis and contribute to the failure of the skin grafts. In addition, patients do not tolerate anesthesia as well as they do later in convalescence, and there is considerably more bleeding

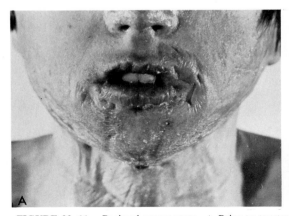 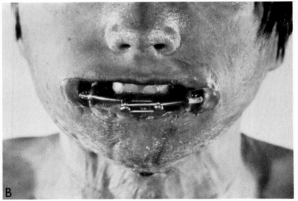

FIGURE 33–11. Perioral contracture. *A*, Prior to treatment. *B*, Degree of expansion obtained by the labial appliance.

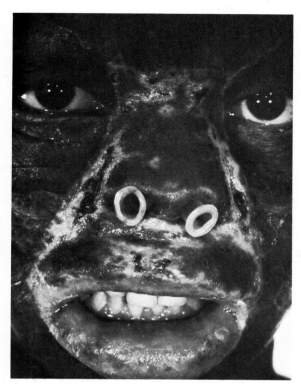

FIGURE 33–12. Nasal vestibular insert splints.

during the operations if they are performed at an early stage.

Unless eyelid ectropion menaces the integrity of the cornea, a waiting period should be allowed before attempting definitive reconstructive procedures.

Frequent psychosocial interviews are necessary during this period. The patient is interviewed alone and with one or more members of his family. While reassurance is necessary, the patient should be brought to the realization that rehabilitation will, of necessity, be prolonged and that he must keep himself usefully occupied during this period. Discussions should be held with the patient about the possibility of his returning to work on either a part-time or a full-time basis during the intervals between operations. Serious consideration should be given at this stage to the vocational problems posed by serious facial disfigurement; the patient must be made to realize that, despite successful reconstructive surgery, his face will still show some of the ravages of the burn and evidence of the surgeon's knife. Consideration may even have to be given to a change in the patient's occupation.

Visits every six weeks permit establishing a rapport between the surgeon and his patient and give the surgeon an opportunity to observe the progress of the convalescing tissues, to study his patient, and to make plans for future reconstructive surgery.

The Early Reconstructive Phase. McIndoe (1949) emphasized the tediousness and difficulty involved in the rehabilitation of the patient with the burn-deformed face. For the patient, the numerous and repeated operations may represent a test for the most courageous; for the surgeon, the results obtained, often satisfactory from a functional standpoint, are frequently disappointing from an esthetic standpoint.

During the early reconstructive phase, a palliative skin graft may be necessary to protect the cornea by releasing a severe ectropion

FIGURE 33–13. Facial exercises of the perioral region under the supervision of a physical therapist.

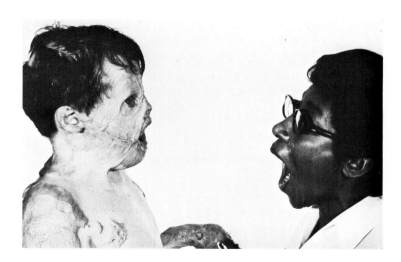

of the upper eyelid. A Z-plasty or a skin graft may be an emergency reconstructive procedure to relieve contracture of the corner of the mouth. These are two examples of early reconstructive surgical procedures. All surgery, other than essential procedures, is postponed until the final reconstructive phase.

The Final Reconstructive Phase. Reconstructive surgery should not be undertaken until the hypertrophic scars have begun to show signs of becoming paler in color and softer in texture and of regressing in size. The development of a slight degree of mobility of the hypertrophic scar over the underlying tissues, due to the formation of a subcicatricial plane of loose connective tissue, is also important (Tumbush, 1962). Excision along this plane of loose connective tissue is facilitated; bleeding is more easily controlled; and skin grafting and other reconstructive surgical procedures are more satisfactorily performed. Mathews (1964) stated that the best results were often obtained in repatriated prisoners of war who had had a delay of approximately two years forced upon them prior to surgical reconstruction.

Planning the surgical reconstruction requires analysis of the deformities, diagnosis of the size of the tissue loss and resultant defect, and choice of the techniques of repair and of the donor sites for the tissues to be transplanted.

In the severely scarred, total-face burn patient, the tight, contracted tissues are "hungry for skin." After each procedure—whether a skin graft, a skin flap, or a Z-plasty—it becomes evident that additional skin is needed to restore an adequate cutaneous surface until the tightness disappears and the functional and expressive facial movements are restored.

GENERAL PRINCIPLES OF TREATMENT. The techniques of surgical reconstruction in extensive burn deformities of the face and neck are so numerous that they could fill the contents of an entire textbook. Certain principles of treatment can be outlined, however, in the general approach to this difficult problem.

1. The relief of contractures is the first objective of treatment, with priority to the eyelid region. The correction of extrinsic contracture should precede that of intrinsic contracture.

2. Skin grafts should be employed in preference to skin flaps whenever possible.

3. Local flaps, transposed or rotated from the neighboring tissue, are employed whenever flap coverage is indicated. The Z-plasty technique is an invaluable aid in the course of treatment.

4. Skin flaps are indicated in deep tissue defects and in the nose, chin, and cervical areas under certain conditions. Local flaps are also useful for the repair of small areas of burn scars.

5. Skin replacement should be done in stages in the various regional esthetic entities of the face: forehead, upper eyelids, lower eyelids, nose, upper lip, anterior cheek area, posterior or parotid-masseteric cheek area, and chin (see Fig. 33–9).

6. The treatment of the burn-scarred skin of the face includes replacement of the full thickness of the skin by skin grafting; surgical abrasion of the burn scar with or without dermal overgrafting; and the use of triamcinolone acetonide to prevent and to soften postoperatively hypertrophic scars.

7. Additional measures include improvement of the chin contour by horizontal osteotomy of the mandible (see Chapter 30); cosmetics to remedy the color disparity of the grafted skin; a hairpiece to replace the destroyed hair-bearing scalp; and a prosthetic ear, in cases of total destruction of the auricle.

RELIEF OF CONTRACTURES: FROM THE EXTRINSIC TO THE INTRINSIC. The extrinsic contracture should always be corrected prior to releasing the intrinsic contracture. This order of treatment is particularly important in contractures involving the mobile areas of the face, i.e., the eyelids and the lips and perilabial tissues. A contracture in the forehead or temporal area may exert a pull on the upper eyelids; contracture of the cheek pulls the lower eyelid into ectropion or exerts upward traction on the corner of the mouth; the lower lip and chin may be pulled downward by a neck contracture. These sites of extrinsic contracture should be remedied first by a suitably indicated technique. After an adequate time interval following healing, the intrinsic contracture should be corrected. The best results are obtained when this order of procedure is followed. As previously mentioned, however, there are exceptions to the rule which may require earlier palliative measures, such as a skin graft to an upper eyelid which is everted in ectropion and is endangering the cornea by exposure. Another example is an extreme contracture involving the corner of the mouth, which can be partially relieved by a skin graft or Z-plasty.

LOCAL FLAPS AND Z-PLASTIES. Local

flaps and Z-plasties are reserved for relatively minor burn contractures or other deformities. They are also employed as adjuncts to skin transplantation procedures in the more major deformities.

The Z-plasty is the plastic surgeon's best friend (and the patient's) in correction of the innumerable linear contractures which must be relieved in the course of the restorative treatment of the burned face. Linear contractures distorting the eyebrows and medial and lateral epicanthal folds; linear contractures at the lateral portions of the bony bridge of the nose, at the base of the alae, at the junction of the lateral nasal wall with the cheek; contractures distorting the vermilion borders of the lips; contractures at the angles of the mouth—all of these require correction by the Z-plasty technique. In contractile bands of the neck, the Z-plasty must often be associated with a skin graft, as the Z-plasty is often inadequate to elongate the contracted tissue sufficiently, and the skin graft will remedy the deficiency of skin (see Chapter 34).

When the linear contracture is surrounded by healthy tissue, wide-limbed Z-flaps can be employed. The larger the flaps, the greater the elongation and the more efficient the correction (see Chapter 1). Often, however, the Z-plasty must be done in burn-scarred skin, which shows a diminished vascularity as compared to normal skin. Large flaps of undermined scarred skin jeopardize the survival of the distal portion of the flap through avascular necrosis.

The double-opposing Z-plasty technique (Converse, 1964b) permits elongation of a contractile band with relatively small flaps. Another useful application of the double-opposing Z-plasty technique is in areas where the anatomy of the region limits the size of the flaps—for example, in the medial canthal region. Double-opposing Z-plasties have been efficient in the correction of the medial epicanthal fold which often occurs in conjunction with burns of the eyelids and naso-orbital region (see Fig. 33–32).

The breaking up of the scar contracture and the relaxation of the scarred area have a beneficial effect on the scar itself. Davis (1931), in his classic article on the use of Z-plasty for the relaxation of scar contractures, noted, "The character of the scar itself often changes materially for the better after relaxation." He also reached the following conclusions: "As we use Z-type incision the scar is not removed, but the contraction is relieved by the transposition of flaps which are usually composed of scar or

scar infiltrated tissue in such a way as to break the line of scar pull. The suture line after transposition of the flaps in a general way is the reverse of the original incision."

Longacre (1972) has performed Z-plasties within scar tissue 3 to 4 cm thick and has noted a softening of the scar, beginning within a few days after the interpolation of the Z-plasty flaps, and the consequent relaxation of the scar. The softening and thinning continue for a long period of time, so that when healing is complete, there appears to be a complete change in the scar-infiltrated tissue. Qualitative and quantitative chromatography studies have shown large amounts of polypeptides I and II, proline, and hydroxyproline excreted in the urine immediately following Z-plasty and for a period thereafter until the resolution of the scar is complete. Only traces of these substances were found in the urine of these patients prior to Z-plasty. Following surgery the amount eliminated was directly proportional to the amount of scar operated upon and was greater following Z-plasty on the young immature scar than on the older mature scar.

SKIN GRAFTING. Progress in restorative surgery for burn deformities of the face and neck has been associated with the increased use of skin grafts.

The thin split-thickness (or Thiersch) skin graft was found to wrinkle and shrink after transplantation. For this reason skin flaps were then favored in preference to skin grafts, particularly in burn contractures of the cervical area (Dowd, 1927; Mixter, 1933; Kazanjian, 1936; MacCollum, 1938; Coughlin, 1939; Aufricht, 1944; Smith, 1950). It was also noted that the full-thickness graft resisted the tendency to shrink and remained smooth, and this type of graft was advocated in preference to skin flaps by Padgett (1932), Brown and Blair (1935), Sheehan (1939), and Blocker (1941). Brown, Blair, and Byars (1935) showed the advantages of the thicker split-thickness graft over the thinner variety; Padgett (1939) removed a thick split-thickness graft with his dermatome, which he called a "three-quarter thickness graft."

After the development of the dermatome, successful results using thick split-thickness skin grafts in resurfacing the burn wound were reported by Greeley (1944), Kazanjian and Converse (1949), McIndoe (1949), and Frankelton (1957). These authors emphasized the need for the postoperative support of the grafted cervical area by means of bandages. A great advance in the treatment of burn contractures in the neck was made by Cronin (1957), who stressed the importance of precise postoperative splinting in order to avoid secondary contracture (see Fig. 33–10).

The thick split-thickness or three-quarter thickness skin graft has the advantage of the full-thickness skin graft with the added advantage that the revascularization is more efficient than that of the full-thickness graft. A particular disadvantage of a full-thickness graft is that the closure of the donor area may be a problem in large grafts. The donor sites of the thick split-thickness skin grafts should be immediately grafted with a thin split-thickness graft in order to obtain primary healing and lessen the discomfort of the patient and the hypertrophic scarring which often follows the healing of donor sites of thick split-thickness grafts.

Full-thickness grafts such as retroauricular or supraclavicular skin are the preferred grafts when available. These full-thickness grafts are relatively thin and become rapidly revascularized. They are excellent substitutes for the skin of the lower eyelids and lips. Full-thickness skin grafts from the inner aspect of the arm have similar qualities, but the color match is often not satisfactory.

SKIN FLAPS: LOCAL, REGIONAL, AND DISTANT. While skin grafts are preferable to skin flaps, particularly in the mobile areas of the face, they do not provide a satisfactory repair in burns with deep tissue destruction extending to the frontal or other cranial bones, the nasal bones, or the mental symphysis. When cranial bone is exposed, the outer table is removed and skin grafts applied over the area after it has become covered by a layer of granulation tissue. A scalp flap or a flap from a distant area may be necessary to provide definitive repair of such skin-grafted scalp defects. Skin flaps may also be necessary to reconstruct the nose and to provide sufficient tissue in patients with deep tissue destruction over the mandible.

In the treatment of burn contractures of the neck (see Chapter 34), flaps have been transferred in stages from the abdominal or scapular regions. Tube flaps have lost favor as a method of repairing neck contractures, because of the long, multiple-stage, drawn-out period of treatment. After they have been placed in the cervical area, they must usually be defatted. In addition, they have the disadvantage that the mandibulocervical angle, normally situated at the level of the hyoid bone, is obliterated.

Distant skin flaps are generally considered to be contraindicated in the mobile portions of the face and particularly around the mouth. The rigidity of the flap, when it is transferred from an area such as the abdomen, prevents it from adapting to the underlying mobile tissues (Aubry and Levignac, 1957). The patient smiles beneath his flap.

Skin flaps are indicated in certain areas. The region of the lower lip and chin is an area particularly suited to flap repair when tissue destruction has extended deeply to the mandible and in cases in which repeated grafting has been attempted and has left a wake of contracted tissues and hypertrophic scars. Regional flaps from the upper chest area, from which most of the underlying fat has been excised, are employed if the donor area is available. A tube flap mobilized from the dorsal area, if this donor area is utilizable, or from the abdomen via the wrist as a carrier adapts itself well to the convex surface of the chin and the mandibular area. This area of solid and relatively nonmobile flap tissue interrupts the continuity of the contracted tissues of the lower lip and neck. The lower lip can then be relieved from its position of ectropion, and a thick split-thickness graft can be utilized to furnish the required skin cover.

Advancement, transposition, and rotation flaps of cervical skin (Fig. 33–14) have also been successfully employed for the replacement of burn scars in the lower portions of the cheeks (Sanvenero-Rosselli, 1964). These local flaps are useful for the replacement of hypertrophic scars of the cheeks, and cervical skin is often available for this purpose (Fig. 33–15). They have the merit of restoring hair-bearing skin to the facial area in male patients. Successful use of the Cronin technique of skin grafting of cervical defects has made it possible for the surgeon to transpose or rotate cervical skin flaps for the repair of a facial defect, knowing that he can repair the cervical defect with impunity by means of a thick split-thickness skin graft (see Chapter 34).

When the face alone is involved in the burn and the skin of the neck is available for transplantation, a particularly useful flap in male patients is the 1–2 flap (see Fig. 33–16 and Chapter 6, Fig. 6–38). This flap permits the transplantation of hair-bearing skin from the cervical area to the chin and lower lip regions. In a first stage, the scarred contracted tissues of the chin are excised, and the cervical skin is advanced over the defect. The patient's neck is maintained in flexion in order to relieve tension. Two weeks later, a submandibular incision detaches the advanced cervical skin,

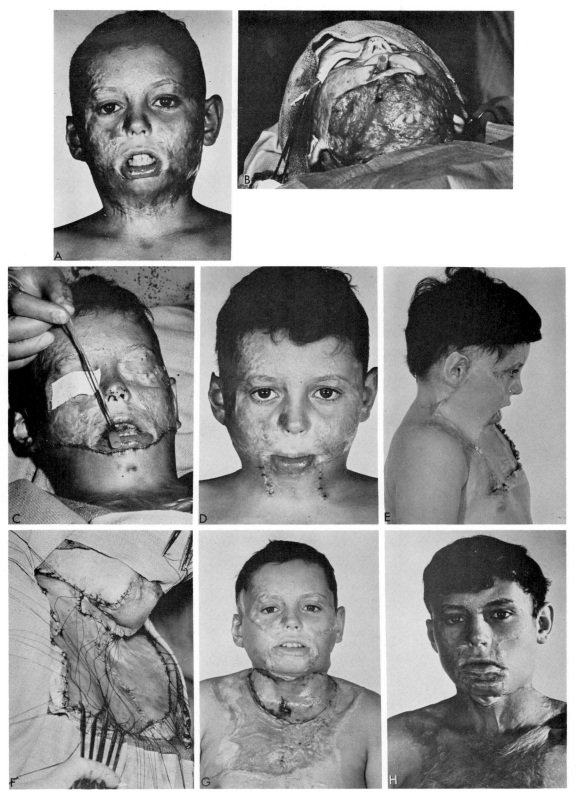

FIGURE 33–14. *A*, Appearance following multiple applications of skin grafts to the cheeks and chin. Note the ectropion of the lower lip. *B*, Following excision of the scar tissue of the cheeks and chin. *C*, Advancement of a large neck flap into the defect. *D*, The intermediate stage following division between the chin and cheek flaps. *E*, Following additional advancement of cheek flaps to the zygomatic area. *F*, *G*, The pedicles have been divided and the defects resurfaced with split-thickness skin grafts. *H*, Final appearance.

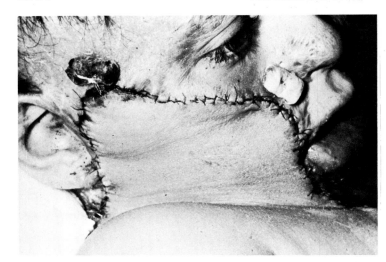

FIGURE 33–15. Advancement flap of cervical skin to resurface the cheek.

which is now an island of skin placed over the chin and lower portion of the face; the neck is extended, and the resulting cervical defect is grafted with a thick split-thickness graft (Converse, 1967). This method has given excellent results for the repair of burn contractures and burn scars in the lower facial area. Because of the discomfort caused by the required flexion of the neck, the 1–2 flap is contraindicated in the older patient. The technique shown in Figure 33–16 eliminates this difficulty when it is combined with the 1–2 advancement flap. In the patient shown in Figure 33–17, two flaps of cervical skin were imbricated, and the resultant defect at the base of the neck was covered by two flaps taken from the chest. The secondary defects on the chest were covered with split-thickness skin grafts.

Forehead flaps are required for the resurfacing of the nose when the scar tissue resulting from the burn extends deeply to the level of the nasal bones and cartilages or when the nose requires elongation to correct the upward contraction of the cartilaginous portion of the nose. Experience with the use of forehead flaps for the repair of cheek defects has shown that they have the same inconvenience as distant flaps in this area—namely, their rigidity interferes with the mobility of the cheeks.

COLOR MATCH IN SKIN REPLACEMENT. When small areas of the face require grafting, the best possible color match should be attempted. Full-thickness skin removed from the retroauricular and supraclavicular areas and from other areas in proximity to the face, such as the cervical and upper thoracic areas, generally fulfills the exigencies of color matching.

In extensive burns of the face, where the texture and color of the healed burned skin differ from those of the nonburned skin of the rest of the body, it is particularly important to avoid using a skin flap or graft which contrasts too greatly in color with the surrounding skin. Scarred forehead skin, healed after superficial burns, may be employed to restore the skin of the nose because its color is similar to that of the surrounding burned tissues. Similarly, superficially scarred cervical skin can be used for the lower portion of the face. A split-thickness skin graft from the cervical area (Edgerton and Hansen, 1960) is the graft of choice in overgrafting of dermal burn scars (see also Chapter 6).

When the facial or cervical areas are extensively burned, thick split-thickness grafts from distant body areas must be employed. The color of the grafted face is often either too dark or too pale. Unfortunately, the surgeon has no choice. While he has relieved the contracture and reconstructed the distorted or missing facial features, the disparity of texture and color marks the individual and sets him apart as a "burned patient."

TREATMENT OF BURN SCARS. One of the most difficult problems during the final stages of rehabilitation is that of the residual burn scars. The contractures have been relieved, and an adequate surface of skin has been restored to permit functional and expressive movements, but scars remain in the wake of the injury and subsequent surgical reconstruction. Scars between the grafts, finely striated and plicated scars of healed areas of superficial burns, and pigmentation of skin grafts are

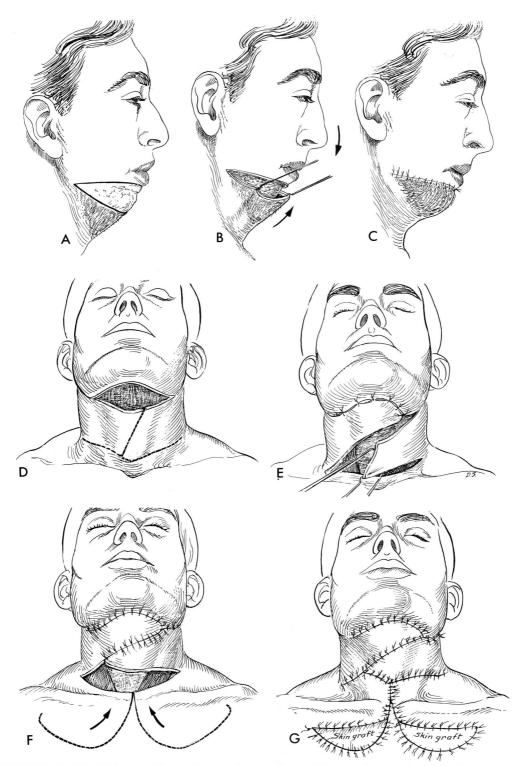

FIGURE 33–16. The l-2 flap combined with secondary cervical and thoracic flaps. *A,* Area of hairless burn scar to be resected. *B,* Cervical skin has been undermined and is advanced over the defect. Hair-bearing cervical skin has replaced hairless scar tissue. *C,* A cervical flap with hair-bearing skin has been advanced. *D,* In a second stage, a horizontal incision is made in the suprahyoid area, thus releasing tension. Cervical flaps are outlined. *E,* The cervical flaps are transposed to cover the suprahyoid defect. *F,* Chest flaps designed to cover the defect at base of the neck. *G,* Chest flaps have been transposed, and skin grafts cover the secondary defects. (Figs. 33–16 and 33–17 from Converse, J. M.: Burn deformities of the face and neck. Surg. Clin. North Am., *47:*323, 1967.)

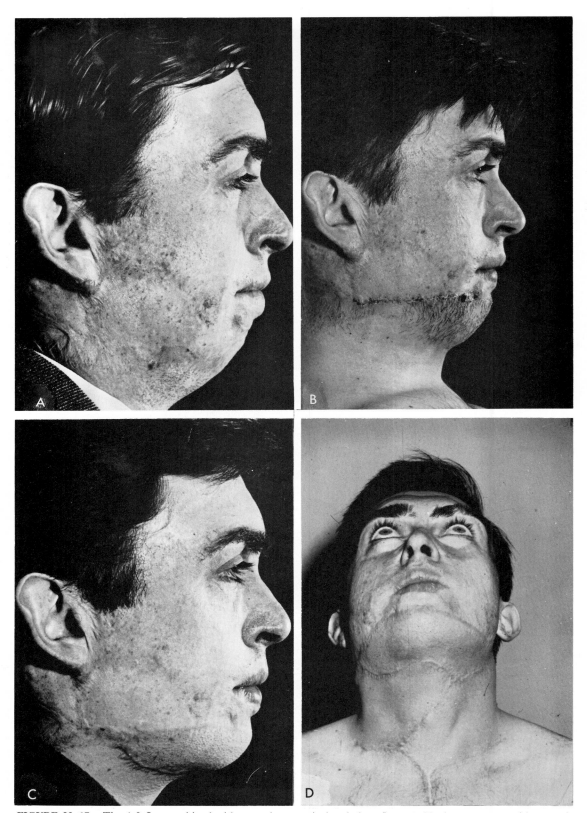

FIGURE 33–17. The 1-2 flap combined with secondary cervical and chest flaps. *A,* Neck contracture with extensive facial burn scars, ectropion of lower lip, and an area of dense, hairless scar tissue over the lower lip and chin. *B,* After advancement of 1-2 flap. *C,* At completion of surgery. Two additional stages have been performed: the procedures illustrated in Figure 33–16, and a final horizontal osteotomy of the mandible with advancement of the lower border of the mandible (see Chapter 30) to increase projection of the chin. *D,* Frontal view showing the cervical and chest flaps.

some of the remaining stigmata of the original accident. Removal or improvement of these scars has a marked psychologic effect on the patient.

In addition to the softening and flattening effect of the passage of time, as stated earlier in the chapter, the release of scar contracture by means of the Z-plasty technique results in an improvement in the quality of the scar tissue, the tissue becoming softer and better-appearing.

Repeated partial (serial) excision is employed in burn scars of moderate size when the surrounding tissue is healthy and elastic. Advancement and rotation flaps are also applicable when sufficient surrounding tissue permits the procedure, particularly when cervical skin is available.

Wide hypertrophic scars require a Z-plasty combined with skin grafting to cover the resultant defect. It can be stated that the thicker the skin graft, the better the result (Skoog, 1963). After an area of hypertrophic scarring has been dissected along the subcicatricial plane of loose connective tissue and resected, only a full-thickness or three-quarter thickness graft will prevent subsequent contraction, wrinkling, and possible recurrence of hypertrophic scarring.

Superficial scars, which are often seen following the spontaneous healing of deep second degree burns, wrinkling, and irregularities are improved by prudent surgical dermabrasion; abrasion may be repeated after a suitable interval of a number of months. Areas of extensive superficial scarring without contracture can be improved by dermabrasion followed by over-

grafting with a relatively thin split-thickness graft (Fig. 33–18) (Hynes, 1957; Rees, and Casson, 1966). These wide areas of scarring following burns are particularly suited to overgrafting, as the scarred skin contains few glandular epithelial elements or hair follicles (see Chapter 6), whereas overgrafting of unscarred skin is followed by a difficult period during which the excretory ducts and hair follicles must make their way through the grafted skin. Overgrafting following surgical abrasion is also useful in the replacement of grafted skin which shows a marked disparity in color. One of our patients complained of his lower eyelids and cheeks, which were skin-grafted and deeply pigmented and detracted from an otherwise satisfactory surgical result. Overgrafting with split-thickness skin grafts removed from the supraclavicular area and the skin at the base of the neck, after ballooning out of the skin of the area with a solution of procaine-epinephrine to facilitate skin graft removal, resulted in a distinct improvement in the patient's appearance.

A recent addition to the armamentarium against hypertrophic scars and keloids is the periodic injection of the scar with triamcinolone acetonide (Kenalog), which has been effective in the resolution of hypertrophic scars (Murray, 1963; Pariser and Murray, 1963; Maguire, 1965; Griffith, 1966; Griffith, Monroe and McKinney, 1970) (see Chapter 16).

ADDITIONAL MEASURES. Among the many procedures which assist in improving facial appearance, mention should be made of the advancement of the lower portion of the body of the mandible by a horizontal osteotomy

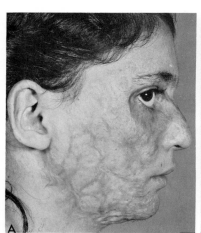 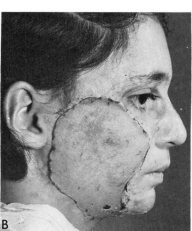 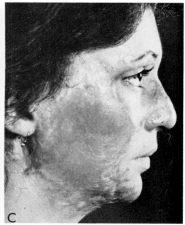

FIGURE 33–18. Dermal overgrafting. *A,* Burn scars of the right cheek. *B,* Immediately following dermabrasion and split-thickness skin grafting. *C,* Final appearance. Cheek is more amenable to the application of cosmetics. (From Kazanjian and Converse.)

through an intraoral approach (see Chapter 30). This procedure corrects the flat chin frequently seen following burns in children. The deformity is the result of soft tissue destruction and continuous pressure exerted during the period of growth over the mandibular symphysis by the scarred soft tissues.

Cosmetics to improve color disparity of the skin grafts, a hairpiece to replace hair-bearing scalp, a prosthetic external ear, and the application of cold permanent wave solution to reconstructed eyebrows in order to direct the hairs outwardly are additional aids in severely burned patients.

Repair of Deformities of Specific Areas

Burn Deformities of the Scalp. The surgical correction of scalp defects has been discussed in Chapter 27.

Burn Deformities of the Forehead. Skin replacement, when necessary, is satisfactorily achieved in most cases by means of a patterned thick split-thickness skin graft which covers the entire forehead from eyebrows to hairline. Lesser deformities respond well to the Z-plasty correction of contractures and other modalities of treatment previously described.

When bone is exposed as a result of deep penetration by a thermal or electric burning agent, a scalp flap will provide satisfactory cover, protect the bone, and prevent its necrosis. After a two- to three-week interval, the flap is raised, and a skin graft can be placed over the regenerated pericranium and subcutaneous tissue supplied by the flap. The hair-bearing portion of the flap can then be returned to the original donor site.

Burn Deformities of the Eyebrows. The surgical technique employed in reconstruction of the eyebrows depends to some extent on the

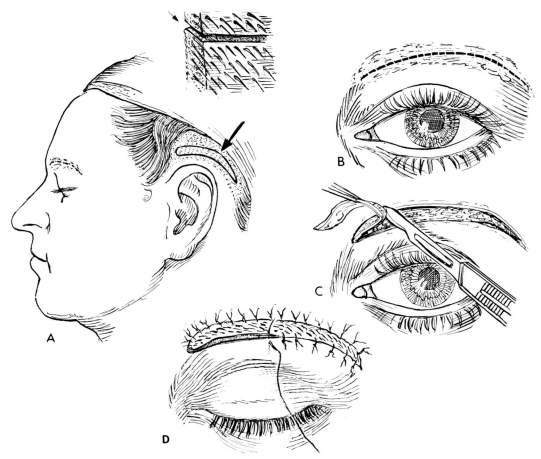

FIGURE 33–19. Reconstruction of eyebrow by a scalp graft. *A*, Removal of strip of scalp from the temporal area. Note the direction of the hair follicles. *B*, Incision made in supraorbital area to receive the scalp transplant. *C*, A strip of skin is removed, providing a bed for the graft. *D*, Scalp graft sutured in position.

desired width of the reconstructed eyebrows (see also Chapter 28). For example, women in our society tend to pluck their eyebrows to a narrow dimension. In such a situation the preferred surgical procedure would be a scalp graft (Figs. 33–19 and 33–20). Excessive defatting of the graft should be avoided to preserve the integrity of the hair follicles. In the reconstruction of the eyebrow in the burned face, one must place a scalp graft into a scarred recipient bed. Consequently, the follicles on the sides of the transplant survive, whereas those in the center of the transplant fail. In the resulting graft there is hair growing along the sides of the transplant with a bare center. When this occurs, the bare central portion can be excised. For this reason the authors feel that in the reconstruction of a burned eyebrow with a scalp graft, the latter should not exceed 3 mm in width. The recipient vascular supply can be increased by making several parallel incisions to receive thin free scalp grafts.

Brent (1975) advocated the insertion of narrow scalp grafts in separate incisions to facilitate vascularization. At a second stage, the intervening area is excised, and the grafts are coupled (see Chapter 28, Fig. 28–96 and p. 958).

On occasion, a satisfactory result can be obtained with a relatively large scalp flap. For a full eyebrow, one must use a scalp flap with its attached superficial temporal artery and vein. The simplest and usually most successful type of scalp flap is one with a cutaneous pedicle (Fig. 33–21). At a second stage, the pedicle is divided and returned to the donor site.

If an island type of scalp flap (Figs. 33–22 and 33–23) is used, care must be exercised not to skeletonize excessively the superficial temporal artery and vein. This often results in additional trauma to the vessels, including possible coagulation or tearing of the vessels. By palpation or with the Doppler flowmeter, one can determine the location of the artery; the incision is made in such a fashion that the artery and vein are not exposed. Care is taken to excise the entire strip, removing the artery and vein with the surrounding subcutaneous tissue. This maneuver provides protection to the vessels and results in fewer postoperative problems.

Another common mistake in eyebrow reconstruction is to place the transplant in such a

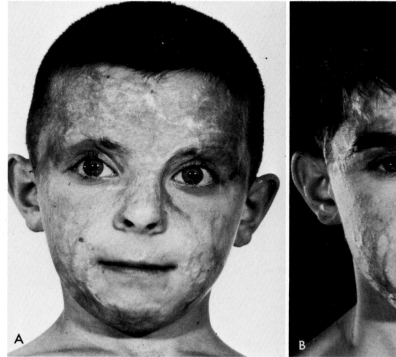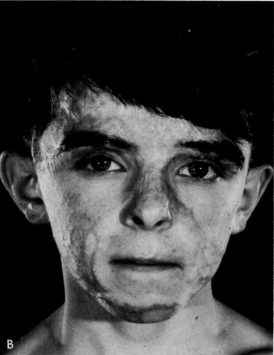

FIGURE 33–20. Reconstruction of eyebrow by free scalp graft. *A*, Preoperative appearance. *B*, Postoperative appearance.

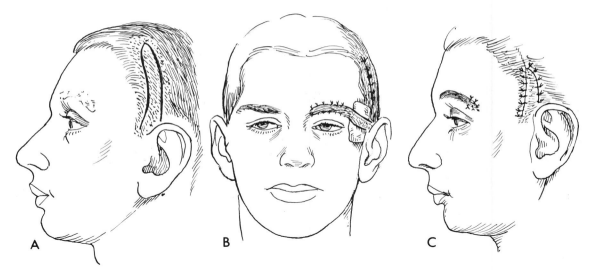

A B C

FIGURE 33–21. Scalp flap with a cutaneous pedicle.

fashion that the hairs do not grow superiorly and laterally. This can be avoided by leaving the donor sites unshaven and by leaving the hair sufficiently long to determine their direction. Therefore, when the transplant is placed in the recipient site, it can be readily determined whether the hairs are growing in the proper direction. A preferred method of immobilization or suturing of the eyebrow has consisted of superficial sutures placed in the epidermis; one should refrain from putting any sutures through the dermis in order to avoid possible trauma to the hair follicles. A light pressure dressing is applied to avoid hematoma formation. It should be emphasized that complete hemostasis must be obtained in the recipient site before applying the scalp transplant.

An alternative and promising method of eyebrow reconstruction is the microvascular free flap of hair-bearing scalp (Harii, Ohmori and Ohmori, 1974). The technique is limited to one stage and assures more precise control of the vascular supply.

Brent (1975) advocated the reconstruction of the sideburns by a high cervico-occipital tube flap as a three-stage procedure. A microvascular free scalp flap can also be employed for this purpose.

Burn Deformities of the Eyelids

INTRINSIC AND EXTRINSIC ECTROPION. Because the eyelid is thin, burns usually cause greater tissue destruction than in the thicker skin of the face. The eyelids consist of loosely attached tissues and are readily submitted to the pull of contracting healed burned tissues over the periphery of the orbital rims. A distinction should therefore be made between *intrinsic* ectropion, in which the cause of ectropion is primarily in the eyelids themselves, and *extrinsic* ectropion caused by loss of skin in the facial area around the eyelids. The pull of the contracting raw area causes ectropion from a distance. This distinction is important clinically, indicating the need for replacement of the eyelid skin proper and also of the adjacent skin.

CHOICE OF SKIN GRAFTS FOR BURN ECTROPION OF THE EYELIDS. A full-thickness graft of eyelid skin provides the most satisfactory skin cover for the eyelids. Such a graft can be taken only from an unburned upper lid. Because the available donor site is limited, the method is not applicable in most cases of burn ectropion.

A thin split-thickness graft from the inner aspect of the upper arm is relatively hairless and is the most suitable type of skin graft for replacing upper eyelid skin (Fig. 33–24), for it remains thin and supple and permits the graft to assume the horizontal folds characteristic of the upper lid (see Fig. 33–27). The color match as a rule improves in time, although some grafts remain white or yellowish white in color. This inconvenience is of lesser importance in the upper than in the lower lid, because most of

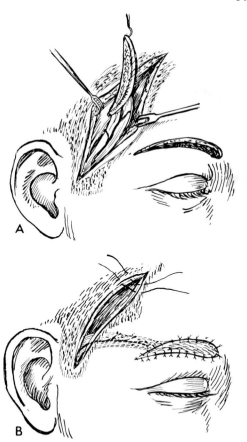

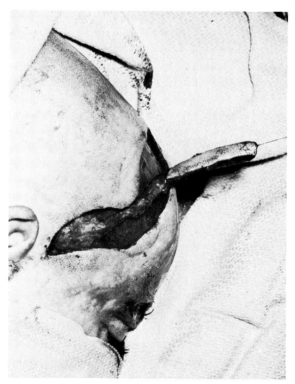

FIGURE 33–23. Island scalp flap prior to insertion in the supraorbital defect.

FIGURE 33–22. Island scalp flap. *A,* Incisions in the temporal and supraorbital areas. An island of scalp is dissected with a pedicle of superficial temporal vessels and surrounding subcutaneous tissue. *B,* The island is sutured in place.

the upper lid is hidden in the normal forward gaze.

One should avoid the use of a thick full-thickness graft in the upper eyelid in most cases, because its thickness and lack of suppleness prevent the formation of the supratarsal fold. In hypertrophic scars of the lateral portion of the lids and periorbital area, full-thickness grafts may be indicated, as they do not contract to the same extent as do thinner grafts. Thin full-thickness grafts from the retroauricular or supraclavicular areas or the inner aspect of the arm are preferable; if these areas are not available, thick split-thickness grafts are an alternative.

A full-thickness graft of skin from the postauricular or supraclavicular regions is the graft of choice for lower lid defects. The lower

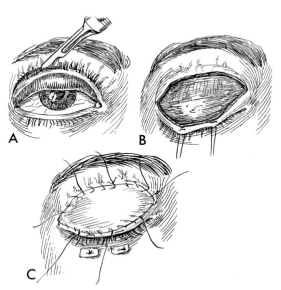

FIGURE 33–24. Corrective surgery of ectropion of the upper eyelid. *A,* Incision made immediately above the lid margin, freeing the lid. *B,* The lid is freed of scar tissue, the margin is brought down into its normal position, and the defect becomes apparent. *C,* Split-thickness skin graft applied to the defect. The graft may be permitted to overlap the edges of the defect when sutured. Two mattress sutures tied over gauze hold the lids together.

eyelid being less mobile than the upper, the relative rigidity of the graft is an asset in maintaining the position of the lid. Although the thin mobile skin of the lower and upper lids is similar in structure, thin grafts are less satisfactory than thicker grafts in the lower lid, for the tendency toward recurrence of ectropion is greater in the lower lid. Full-thickness skin from the retroauricular region (Fig. 33–25) or the supraclavicular area is selected for grafts because of the texture and color match.

TECHNIQUE OF SKIN GRAFTING OF THE UPPER EYELIDS. The eyelid must be freed of scar tissue in order that the margin of the lid may be returned to its normal contact with the lower lid (see Fig. 33–24). Excision should include both the skin scars and most of the fibrotic subcutaneous tissue. Hemostasis is obtained by fine-tipped jeweler's forceps applied to the bleeding points, which are electrocoagulated. A full-thickness graft is removed from the upper lid of the contralateral eye in moderate ectropion, and the graft is sutured to the edges of the defect by carefully placed interrupted sutures. Such a graft may be dressed as early as the third day.

When a split-thickness graft from the inner aspect of the arm is employed, the graft is spread over the defect and is permitted to overlap the wound edges. The margin of the upper lid is temporarily fastened to that of the lower lid by one or two interrupted sutures before the pressure dressing is applied over the skin graft to prevent the opening of the eyelid under the dressing and to avoid corneal abrasion.

Immobilization of the area and pressure over the graft are obtained by a variety of methods, which will be subsequently discussed. A dressing of gauze impregnated with an ointment or mineral oil is placed over the graft. Absorbent cotton (preferably Acrilan cotton) saturated with mineral oil prevents adherence between the dressing and graft. A pressure dressing, retained by a bandage, further immobilizes the region. The cotton is saturated with saline solution to facilitate its removal when the first dressing is changed on the fourth day after the operation.

Outlay technique for burn ectropion of the upper eyelids. This technique (Gillies, 1920) was popularized by McIndoe during the Second World War. Contraction of the skin adjacent to the eyelid can be anticipated in early grafting of extensive burns of the face. The dental compound mold technique is helpful in such grafting, since it permits the introduction of excess skin into the defect and allows for subsequent contraction of the surrounding skin. The ectropic eyelid must be freed of scar tissue by excision of the scar; the excision must often be extended beyond the lateral rim of the orbit. Traction is exerted on a number of special everting vertical mattress sutures to distend the raw area of the lid. The wound edges are slightly undermined above, medially, and laterally for a distance of 0.5 to 1 cm to increase further the size of the defect. Softened dental compound is spread over the defect and introduced beneath the undercut edges of the wound. The compound is chilled and hardened by a stream of sterile ice water and is removed from the wound (Fig. 33–26, *A*). The skin graft, dermal surface outward (Fig. 33–26, *B*), is applied to the compound mold and placed into the defect, and the long ends of the end-on mattress sutures are tied over the mold (Fig. 33–26, *C*). Pledgets of cotton and a pressure dressing are applied over the entire area.

The graft must not be disturbed when the mold is removed at the time of the first dressing on the fifth postoperative day. The excess overlapping skin graft is trimmed with scissors, and the grafted areas are left exposed. Protection by a dressing or an eye shield during sleep may be indicated during the next five days. Figure 33–27 shows photographs of a patient whose severe burn ectropion was successfully repaired by this technique.

The disadvantage of this technique is the resulting ridge at the junction of the skin graft and surrounding skin, a frequent occurrence. To obviate this complication, the following technique is preferred.

The overlapping technique. The overlapping technique (Converse, 1967) is illustrated in Figure 33–28. After an incision is made horizontally across the eyelid along the superior border of the tarsus and extended laterally into the temporal area, the eyelid is freed of scar tissue and, by means of traction sutures, pulled inferiorly, overlapping the lower eyelid. Thus a wide surface of skin graft is assured.

A similar technique is employed in the lower eyelid at a subsequent session. When all four eyelids must be grafted, preference is given to grafting both upper eyelids in the same operating session, covering the eyes, and thus eliminating vision for a few days. There is no inconvenience to doing this when the patient is forewarned. Both upper eyelids are covered with pressure dressings. When one eye is left open, synergistic ocular globe movement on the grafted side may disturb the graft. Howev-

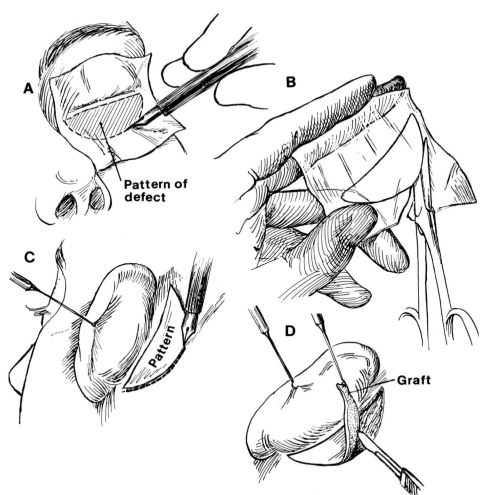

FIGURE 33–25. Full-thickness skin graft for repair of an ectropion of the lower eyelid. *A*, Preparation of a pattern of the defect. *B*, Cutting the pattern. *C*, Tracing the pattern graft in the retroauricular area. *D*, Removal of a full-thickness graft.

er, two of the authors (M.D. and D.L.) prefer to reconstruct the upper and lower lids on one side at the same time. In this way vision is not interrupted. The upper eyelids are grafted with split-thickness skin grafts cut at 0.014 inch; a graft of this thickness preserves the necessary mobility of the upper eyelids. In contrast, the lower eyelids are usually resurfaced with full-thickness retroauricular or supraclavicular skin grafts (see Figs. 33–25, 33–28, and 33–29).

TECHNIQUE OF SKIN GRAFTING OF THE LOWER EYELID. The lower lid is completely freed of all scar tissue until the margin of the lid resumes its normal outline and is reapplied against the globe without tension. Incisions should be extended medially and laterally in order that the graft is applied in a slinglike fashion; it is extended medially to the nose and laterally above the lateral canthus (Fig. 33–30, *A*). This design is essential to maintain the support of the lower eyelid in order to counteract the effect of gravity and prevent a downward pull on the lid. The overlapping technique of fixation maintains the lid margin at the correct level (Fig. 33–30, *B*).

The full-thickness graft, cut to pattern, is anchored in place with fine nonabsorbent suture material. The long ends of a number of sutures are employed to retain a tie-over pressure dressing (Fig. 33–30, *C*). Figure 33–31

Text continued on page 1629.

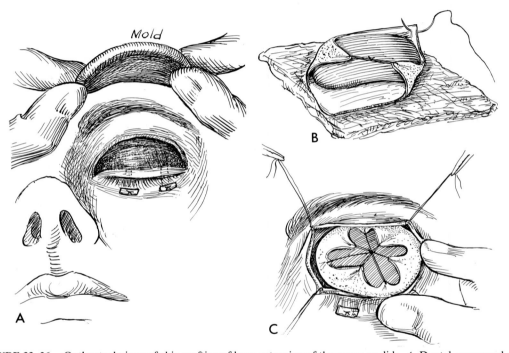

FIGURE 33–26. Outlay technique of skin grafting of burn ectropion of the upper eyelids. *A*, Dental compound molded over the defect. *B*, Compound mold is covered with a skin graft with dermal surface outward. *C*, Compound mold and graft are fitted into the defect and sutured.

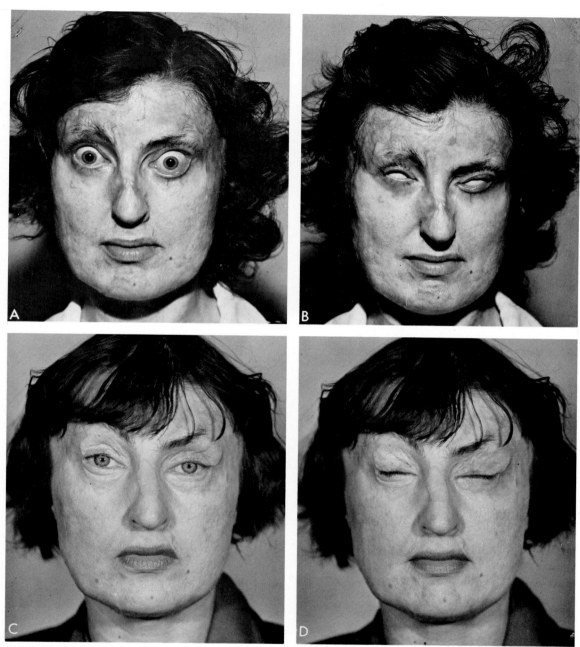

FIGURE 33–27. Skin grafting for burn ectropion of the eyelids. *A*, Ectropion of lids resulting from burns caused by a gasoline explosion. *B*, Exposure of eyeballs due to inability to occlude the lids. *C*, Restoration of eyelid skin by grafting. Upper eyelids were restored by a split-thickness skin graft removed from the inner aspect of the arm and retained by the compound mold technique, as shown in Figure 33–26. Lower eyelids were repaired by full-thickness retroauricular grafts, as shown in Figure 33–30. *D*, After skin grafting, the patient is able to occlude the eyelids. (From Kazanjian and Converse.)

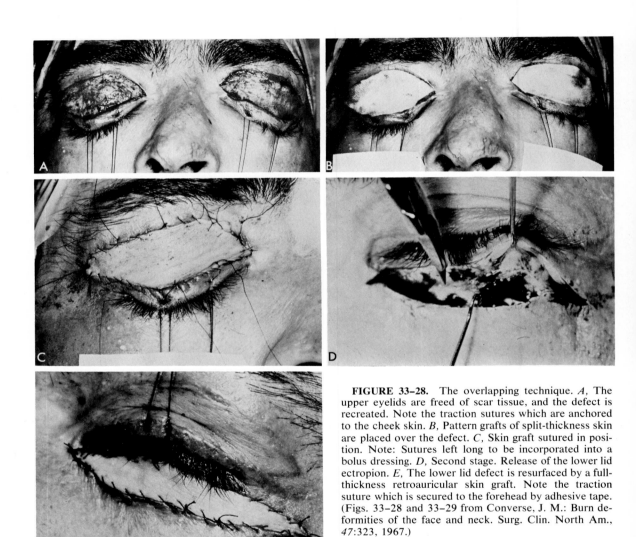

FIGURE 33–28. The overlapping technique. *A,* The upper eyelids are freed of scar tissue, and the defect is recreated. Note the traction sutures which are anchored to the cheek skin. *B,* Pattern grafts of split-thickness skin are placed over the defect. *C,* Skin graft sutured in position. Note: Sutures left long to be incorporated into a bolus dressing. *D,* Second stage. Release of the lower lid ectropion. *E,* The lower lid defect is resurfaced by a full-thickness retroauricular skin graft. Note the traction suture which is secured to the forehead by adhesive tape. (Figs. 33–28 and 33–29 from Converse, J. M.: Burn deformities of the face and neck. Surg. Clin. North Am., 47:323, 1967.)

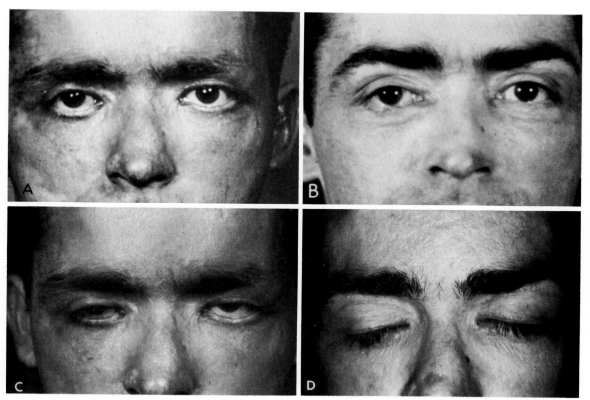

FIGURE 33–29. Repair of moderate burn ectropion by the overlapping technique. *A, C,* Burn ectropion showing inability to occlude the eyelids. *B, D,* Result obtained following repair by technique illustrated in Figure 33–28 in two stages; in a later stage, double-opposing Z-plasties were done in the medial canthal region.

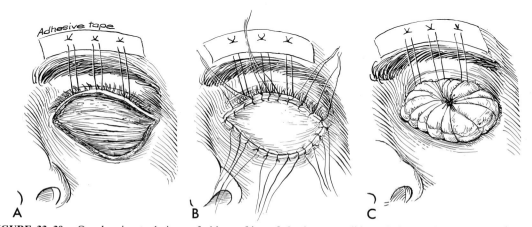

FIGURE 33–30. Overlapping technique of skin grafting of the lower eyelid. *A,* Release of the ectropion. Note the traction sutures suspended to the forehead. *B,* The full-thickness skin graft sutured in place. *C,* Tie-over bolus dressing.

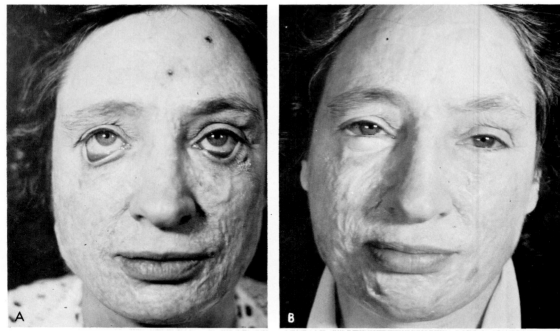

FIGURE 33–31. *A*, Lower eyelid ectropion. *B*, Following reconstruction by technique illustrated in Figure 33–30.

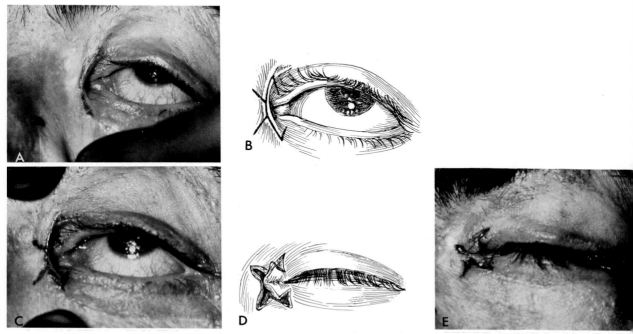

FIGURE 33–32.   Double-opposing Z-plasties. *A*, The epicanthal fold is exaggerated by stretching it. *B, C*, Design of the incisions. *D, E*, Transposition of Z-flaps. (From Converse, J. M.: Burn deformities of the face and neck. Surg. Clin. North Am., *47*:323, 1967.)

shows a patient with burn ectropion of the eyelids before and after surgical correction by scar release and skin grafting.

CONTRACTION OF EYELID SKIN GRAFTS. All healing wounds contract, particularly wounds with total skin loss. Wound contraction is minimized by skin grafting, but a degree of contraction occurs during and after skin grafting. The eyelids, because they are mobile structures and loosely bound, are particularly susceptible to contraction. Such secondary contraction may result in a recurrence of ectropion which, although of a lesser degree, may require additional skin grafting.

Skin grafts applied to burned raw areas contract much more in the early weeks than in the convalescent period later. In cases of moderate burn ectropion without dangerous corneal exposure, postponement permits skin grafting under more favorable conditions with a minimal danger of subsequent contraction. In the interval, release of the extrinsic contracture and skin grafting is completed. It must be emphasized, however, that in extensive skin loss of the eyelids such purposeful postponement of skin grafting may lead to dangerous exposure of the cornea and irrevocable deformity of the lids. In such a

situation, early skin grafting should be done with the realization that there will be subsequent contraction and partial recurrence of the ectropion.

EPICANTHAL FOLDS FOLLOWING SKIN GRAFTING OF THE EYELIDS. Epicanthal folds occur occasionally, especially after grafting of the upper and lower eyelids in the same operative session. After a period of waiting for restoration of eyelid mobility and softening of the skin grafts and scars, the technique of double-opposing Z-plasties (Converse, 1964) has given satisfactory results (Fig. 33–32).

INADVISABILITY OF TARSORRHAPHY AND CONCOMITANT GRAFTING OF THE UPPER AND LOWER EYELIDS IN BURN ECTROPION. The patient shown in Figure 33–33 has the typical appearance seen when a tarsorrhaphy is performed, joining the upper and lower eyelids, and a single graft is placed over the raw areas of both lids. In addition to the destruction of the eyelid margins, the surface area of grafting is inadequate. Repeated additional grafting was required in the upper and lower eyelids as well as in the medial canthal area. In the primary grafting of burned

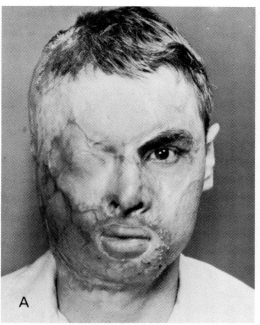 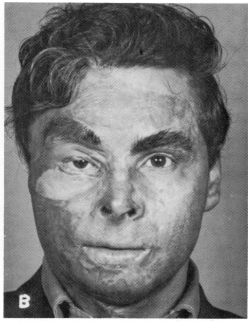

FIGURE 33–33. Extensive burns of the face involving the scalp, eyebrow, eyelids, cheek, and lips. *A,* Preoperative. Note that a complete tarsorrhaphy of his lids was performed and a split-thickness graft placed over the continuous raw area of the upper and lower eyelids. *B,* Tarsorrhaphy was divided and the eyelids separated. The upper eyelid was grafted by means of the overlapping technique. The lower eyelid was also grafted in a later stage by means of the overlapping technique. Note the size of the graft that was required to correct the ectropion. After these two procedures, a skin graft was placed in the medial canthal region, and fixation was obtained by transosseous wiring, as illustrated in Chapter 28, Fig. 28–162. Thus the canthus was successfully replaced in a satisfactory position. Additional reconstructive procedures consisted of transposition of scalp flaps, as illustrated in Chapter 27. A scalp flap was utilized to restore the eyebrow (see Fig. 33–21). A full-thickness skin graft restored adequate length to the upper lip. Ectropion of the lower lip was relieved by Z-plasties and small full-thickness grafts. Additional skin grafts were added to the right cheek. (From Converse, J. M.: Burn deformities of the face and neck. Surg. Clin. North Am., 47:323, 1967.)

eyelids, the plan outlined in this chapter (grafting the upper eyelids in a first stage and the lower lids in a second stage) is usually the preferable technique. An exception is the rare condition in which full-thickness loss of the lid occurs (see Fig. 33–37).

FORWARD DISPLACEMENT OF THE MEDIAL CANTHUS BY CONTRACTURE. The medial canthus can be drawn forward in full-thickness burns of the medial canthal area and side of the nose, thus displacing the lacrimal puncta forward away from the lacrimal lake. The contracture results in a peculiar epicanthal fold, with a forward displacement of the medial portions of both eyelids (Fig. 33–34, *A*). The deformity, resulting in epiphora from the absence of contact of the lacrimal puncta with the ocular globe, must be remedied by resecting the scar tissue, freeing the canthus, and replacing it in its anatomical position. The lacrimal puncta should be located prior to making an incision medial to the medial canthus in order to avoid dividing the canaliculi. A horizontal incision through the medial third of the skin of the upper and lower eyelids is required (Fig. 33–34, *B*), because the skin of the medial aspect of both the upper and lower eyelids is usually deficient. The medial canthus thus resumes a satisfactory position, and the eyelid margins and the lacrimal puncta are once again applied to the globe. The remaining defect is covered with a skin graft (Fig. 33–34, *C*).

Four precautions must be observed to prevent a tendency for recurrence of the deformity: (1) the skin edges of the defect over the nasal area should be widely undermined in order that the skin edges can overlap the graft, which is maintained on a dental compound mold (Fig. 33–34, *C*); (2) the periosteum over the frontal process should be exposed; in some cases it may be necessary to remove the periosteum to ensure adherence of the skin graft to the bone; (3) transnasal wiring may be employed to provide fixation of the graft in the canthal area (see Chapter 28, Fig. 28–162); and (4) a thick skin graft should be employed to minimize subsequent contraction, which is also lessened by the adherence of the skin graft to the denuded bone. Revascularization of skin grafts transplanted over the bare bone occurs satisfactorily in this area despite the removal of the periosteum.

ELONGATION OF THE PALPEBRAL FISSURE. Shortening of the horizontal dimension of the palpebral fissure is a complication in patients with severe burn ectropion of the eyelids, particularly when forward displacement of the medial canthus has occurred. The technique for medial canthoplasty which has consistently given the best results is that suggested by Converse and Smith (1959). After placing an ink dot at the point where the medial canthus should be situated, an oblique incision is made through the outer covering of the scar tissue which joins the eyelids (Fig. 33–35, *A*). A flap of tissue is raised (Fig. 33–35, *B*), exposing the inner lining of the scarred area. An oblique incision in the opposite direction to the preceding one (Fig. 33–35, *C*) outlines a second flap of conjunctiva. Each flap is sutured over the raw surface of the eyelid margin (Fig. 33–35, *D, E*). A new medial canthus is thus formed, exposing the caruncle. The puncta should be located and lacrimal probes placed in the canaliculi prior to incision in order to avoid injury to the lacrimal structures.

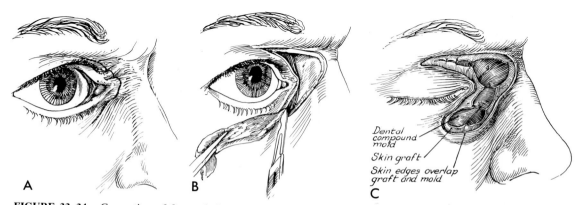

FIGURE 33–34. Correction of forward displacement of the canthus following intrinsic burns. *A,* Typical deformity following burns of the medial canthal area and root of the nose. Canthus is drawn forward, displacing the lacrimal punctum forward. *B,* Excision of scar tissue and freeing of the canthus. *C,* Skin graft maintained on a dental compound mold is placed in the area to cover the defect. (From Converse, J. M., and Smith, B.: Repair of severe burn ectropion of the eyelids. Plast. Reconstr. Surg., *23:*21, 1959.)

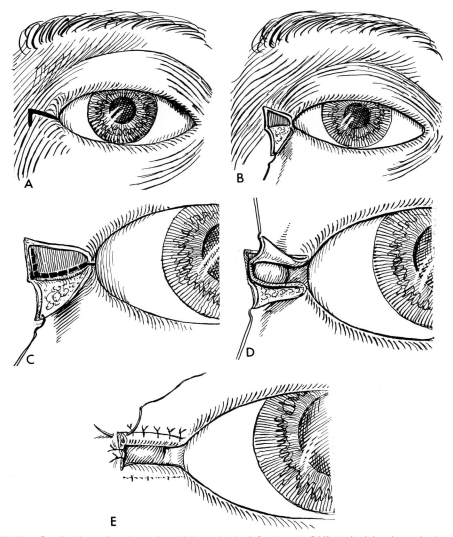

FIGURE 33–35. Canthoplasty for elongation of the palpebral fissure. *A,* Oblique incision is made through the outer covering of scar tissue. *B,* Flap is raised, exposing the inner lining of the scarred area. *C,* Oblique incision is made in an opposite direction to the preceding one, outlining a second flap of conjunctiva. *D, E,* Each flap is sutured over the raw area of the eyelid margin. (Figs. 33–35 to 33–37 from Converse, J. M., and Smith, B.: Repair of severe burn ectropion of the eyelids. Plast. Reconstr. Surg., *23*:21. Copyright 1959, The Williams & Wilkins Company, Baltimore.)

THE TARSOCONJUNCTIVAL FLAP IN SEVERE BURN ECTROPION. Simultaneous skin grafting of both lids is obligatory when a tarsoconjunctival flap is required to reconstruct the lid. This technique (Converse and Smith, 1959) is employed in intractable severe burn ectropion deformity in which a part of the eyelid margins has been destroyed (Fig. 33–36), a condition usually observed in patients with severe burn ectropion who have been unsuccessfully, or only partially successfully, skin grafted in the early stages. The deformity in one case of this type (Fig. 33–36) is characterized by ectropion and short lids of the right eye; a portion of the right lower lid has been destroyed, and there is a forward and lateral displacement of the medial canthus and medial third of the eyelids. The eyelashes of both lids and a considerable amount of the tarsus of the lower lid have been destroyed. The objective of the technique is to remedy the skin deficiency and restore the lower lid by a tarsoconjunctival flap.

Incisions are made at the lid margin of both upper and lower eyelids along the entire length of the margins except for a few millimeters near both the medial and the lateral canthus (Fig.

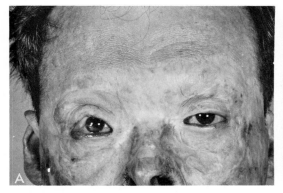

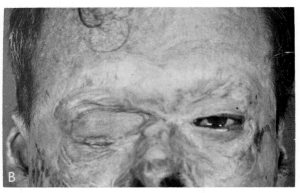

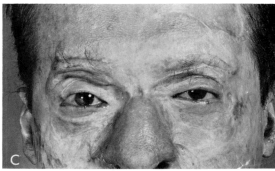

FIGURE 33–36. Extensive facial burns with severe ectropion. *A,* Appearance after multiple unsuccessful attempts at eyelid skin grafting. Note partial full-thickness loss of both lower eyelids and foreshortening of the nose. *B,* Intermediate stage in technique illustrated in Figure 33–37. *C,* Following tarsoconjunctival flap correction of the ectropion of the right eyelids. In addition, the right medial canthal tendon was reattached. The nose has been lengthened and resurfaced by the scalping flap technique.

33–37, *A*). The tarsoconjunctival layer is separated from the superficial soft tissue, which includes orbicularis oculi muscle fibers and skin (Fig. 33–37, *B*). In the lower eyelid the pretarsal fibers of the orbicularis oculi musculature are included in the tarsoconjunctival flap (Fig. 33–37, *C*); these additional muscle fibers are necessary to support the reconstructed lower eyelid. The dissection in the lower lid, therefore, extends along a plane between the skin and the orbicularis oculi muscle fibers. The scar tissue medial to the medial canthus over the frontal process of the maxilla must be resected to permit recession of the medial canthus to its normal position; the procedure is similar to the one previously described (see Fig. 33–34). The margins of the tarsoconjunctival flaps are excised and approximated by a to-and-fro continuous buried 5–0 nylon suture (Fig. 33–37, *D*); the ends of the suture extend out through the skin a short distance from each canthus. The remnants of the scarred lateral layer of the eyelid margins are resected (Fig. 33–37, *D*). The skin edges are widely retracted, exposing a raw area over the tarsoconjunctival layer which is ready to be grafted (Fig. 33–37, *E*); the skin edges retract readily because of the eyelid skin deficiency. The

defect represented by the outer surface of the tarsoconjunctival layer is covered by a split-thickness graft which is maintained on a dental compound mold (Fig. 33–37, *F, G*).

In a later stage, six to eight weeks after the first operation, an incision is made through the tarsoconjunctival layer to separate the upper and lower eyelids (Fig. 33–37, *H*). The incision through the tarsoconjunctival layer is done at a level that allows a sufficient amount of the upper tarsus to be transferred to the lower lid to ensure its stability. The raw surface along the margin of the lids is eliminated by suturing the outer layer of skin to the inner conjunctiva. Figure 33–36 illustrates the result obtained by this technique; the intermediary stage prior to the separation of the lids is shown in Figure 33–36, *B*.

HORIZONTAL MOBILIZATION OF A TARSO-CONJUNCTIVAL FLAP IN FULL-THICKNESS DE-FECTS. In defects causing full-thickness destruction of a portion of the eyelid, such as occurs following chemical burns (Fig. 33–38), the tarsoconjunctival flap is displaced laterally or medially to furnish tissue to fill the gap in the eyelid; skin grafting provides cutaneous coverage (Fig. 33–39).

Text continued on page 1636.

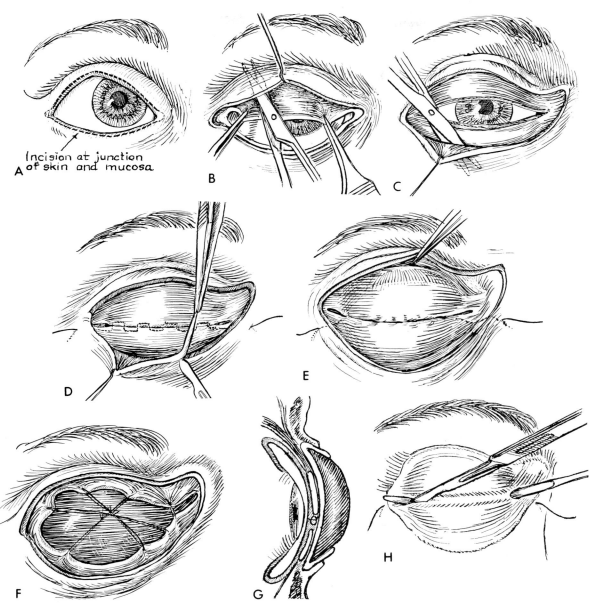

FIGURE 33–37. Tarsoconjunctival flap in severe burn ectropion. *A,* Incision made along the entire margin of both upper and lower eyelids. *B,* Separation of the tarsoconjunctival flap of the upper lid. *C,* Separation of the tarsoconjunctival flap of the lower lid. *D,* Suture of the tarsoconjunctival flaps of the upper and lower eyelids. Excision of the eyelid margin along the edge of the defect. *E,* Skin of eyelids is retracted in every direction to increase the raw surface. Instrument is pointing to the insertion of the levator on the superior tarsus. *F,* Dental compound mold carrying split-thickness skin graft (outlay technique). *G,* Cross section of semiburied mold introducing an excess of skin graft (outlay technique). *H,* In a second stage, the upper and lower eyelids are separated by an incision.

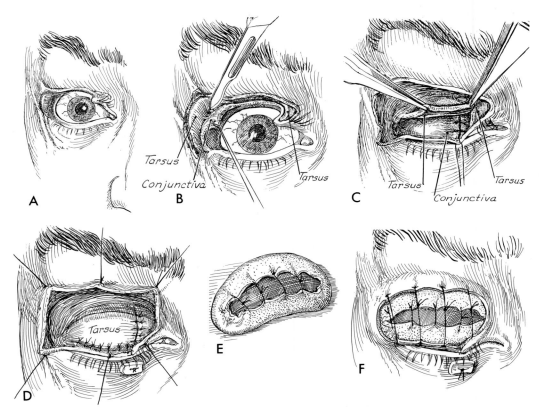

FIGURE 33–38.   Horizontal mobilization of a tarsoconjunctival flap in full-thickness loss of the eyelid resulting from an acid burn. *A*, Burn coloboma of the upper eyelid resulting from full-thickness destruction. *B*, The tarsus and underlying conjunctiva are freed. *C*, The conjunctiva has been dissected from the tarsus and widely undermined; it is mobilized and sutured to the medial conjunctiva with fine catgut sutures. *D*, The tarsus has been mobilized and sutured to the medial component. *E*, Dental compound was softened in warm water and molded into raw area shown in *D*. *F*, The dental compound mold carrying the skin graft is sutured into position; an occlusive suture approximates the lids (see Fig. 33–39). (Figs. 33–38 and 33–39 from Kanzanjian and Converse.)

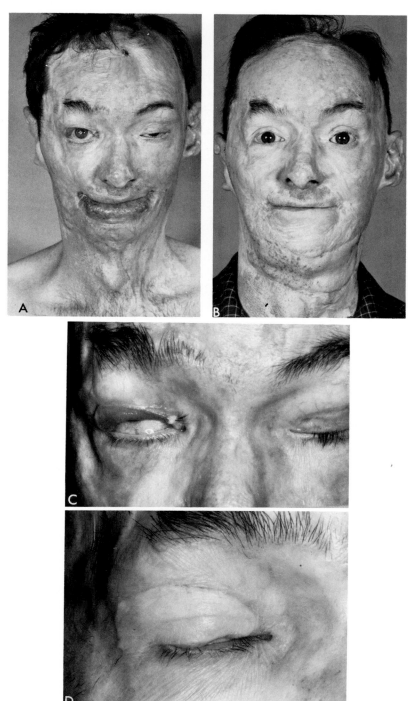

FIGURE 33–39. Multiple burn deformities of the face and neck. Burn coloboma of the right upper eyelid. *A*, Pre-operative appearance. *B*, After reconstruction of the right upper eyelid, as illustrated in Figure 33–38, multiple Z-plasties on the face and neck, skin grafting of the upper and lower lips, and transplantation of a tube skin flap from the thoracic area to the chin. In addition, the oral fissure was diminished in its horizontal dimension by a lateral labiorraphy procedure; at the hospital where he had received initial treatment, the corners of the mouth had been slit to facilitate intratracheal intubation for anesthesia. *C*, Close-up view of the coloboma of the right upper eyelid and the ectropion. *D*, After the operative procedures illustrated in Figure 33–38.

Burn Deformities of the Auricle. The acute management of the burned ear was discussed earlier in the chapter.

Techniques of reconstruction of the auricle in the burned patient are discussed in Chapter 35.

Burn Deformities of the Nose. In Chapter 29, the techniques of skin grafting and flap repair applicable to burn deformities of the nose are discussed. The cartilaginous portion of the nose is retracted upward by the burn contracture of the overlying skin (Fig. 33–40). The nose is foreshortened because of an upward tilt of the nasal tip. The alae are also everted, with exposure of the vibrissae and nasal lining.

When there has been full-thickness destruction of the alar border, the lining may be reconstructed by local tissue. The scarred skin should be excised, the incision above the nasal tip following the contour of the tip and alae (Fig. 33–41). A forehead flap resurfaces the defect as an esthetic unit (see Fig. 33–36, *C*). Nasal vestibular inserts are occasionally required and should be worn for a minimum of six months to avoid vestibular contractures (see Fig. 33–12).

As mentioned earlier in the chapter, skin grafted forehead skin has been used successfully (the scalping flap technique, see Chapter 29).

Burn Deformities of the Cheeks. Cheek scars are excised within the confines of the segmental unit (see Fig. 33–9). Full-thickness grafts of relatively thin skin, such as the supraclavicular or retroauricular skin, are the grafts of choice. Thick split-thickness grafts are the next choice. The dermal onlay technique (Hynes, 1957; Thompson, 1960) is particularly suited for minor to moderate burn cheek scars with surface irregularities (see Fig. 33–18). The technique is discussed in detail in Chapter 6.

Local skin flaps are also indicated in resurfacing burn scars of the cheek. Use of rotation flaps from uninvolved portions of the cheek (Fig. 33–42) and the retroauricular and cervical areas is the preferred technique (see Figs. 33–14 through 33–17).

In the cheek area the surgeon must avoid cutting the peripheral branches of the facial nerve.

Burn Deformities of the Perioral Area and Chin. Following the periorbital and eyelid areas, the perioral region is the next most common site for reconstruction following burn injury. Many patients present a grotesque appearance, with drooling, microstomia, inability to eat, dental caries, and eversion of the lips.

THE UPPER LIP. Burn ectropion of the upper lip is best corrected by a full-thickness retroauricular or supraclavicular skin graft, or by a thick split-thickness skin graft when these sites are not available. The entire esthetic unit, extending between the nasolabial folds, should be resurfaced (Fig. 33–43; see also Fig. 33–33). In excising the scar from the upper lip, it is important to leave some residual scar on the philtrum in the hope of avoiding a flat upper lip and of providing a better profile. Obviously, if the scar in this area remains undisturbed, the potential for contracture in the upper lip is still present. However, the contracture in the upper lip can be released by making an incision at the base of the nose and allowing the upper lip to fall into its anatomical position, leaving the defect in the upper aspect rather than in the lower part of the upper lip. Releasing of the scar should not be done in the lowermost portion of the upper lip, so that bulk can be maintained in this area as much as possible (Fig. 33–43). An

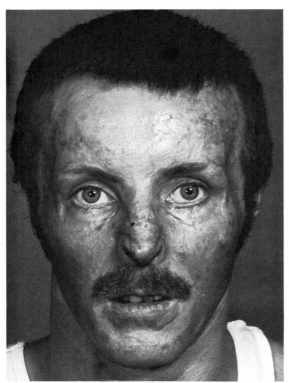

FIGURE 33–40. Burn deformity of the nose. Note the foreshortening of the nose and the retraction of the alar rims with exposure of the vibrissae and nasal lining.

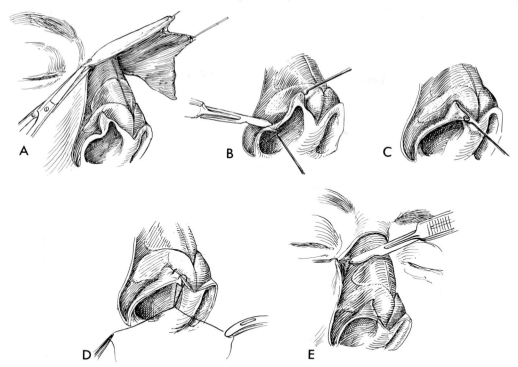

FIGURE 33–41. Preparation of the burned nose prior to the transfer of a forehead flap. *A,* Excision of the scar tissue over the dorsum of the nose. *B,* The alar margins are undermined. *C,* A triangular flap of tissue is turned down as a hinge flap. *D,* The flap is sutured in position. This technique restores the alar margins. *E,* Prior to transfer of the forehead flap, the margins of the wound are undermined to provide further release of the scar contracture.

incision is made in the middle of the philtrum, and the graft is sutured to the resulting defect. The sutures are not removed for 10 to 14 days in an attempt to form as much of the philtrum as possible. In summary, in removing the scar of the upper lip, the incisions are made within the confines of the esthetic unit; all of the scars are removed except for those in the area of the philtrum, where only the epidermis is excised,

leaving the underlying scar. The scar in the upper lip is often advanced into the nasal columella to release the contracted columella. The incision is similar to the forked flap technique

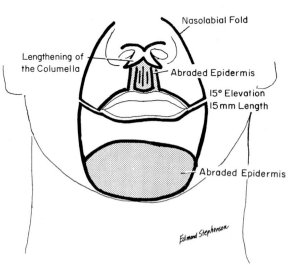

FIGURE 33–43. Esthetic units of the perioral area. In the philtrum, the epidermis should be removed but the underlying scar preserved to give fullness to this region. Note the design of the lip forked flap (Millard, 1958) to lengthen the columella.

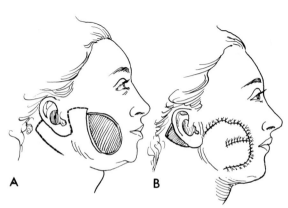

FIGURE 33–42. Local flap coverage of burn scars of the anterior cheek. Retroauricular donor defect can usually be closed primarily.

(Millard, 1958) used to lengthen the columella in cleft lip nose deformities (see Fig. 33–43).

One of the most common technical errors made in reconstructing the upper lip is overcorrection. As a result of gravity, the upper lip does not contract; the resulting elongated upper lip gives the patient a grotesque appearance.

THE LOWER LIP AND THE CHIN. The lines of the incisions in reconstructing the lower lip should also fall within the lines of the esthetic unit. Figure 33–44 illustrates that the incision is extended beyond the corner of the mouth with a slight upward sweep. The thick skin graft will thus suspend the lower lip. In excising the scar of the lower lip, it is important to excise all of the scar, except for an oblong area at the apex of the chin (Fig. 33–44). Because it is difficult to excise uninvolved tissue, the surgeon will frequently defer resecting a small area in the middle aspect of the lower lip. Unfortunately, this area of normal tissue, surrounded by skin graft, always has the appearance of an island and remains obvious. Consequently, it is preferable to excise and sacrifice this area and to place a large graft covering the entire esthetic unit, thus obtaining a more pleasing final appearance (Fig. 33–45).

In the excision of the lower lip and chin, it is important that a circle of scar be left on the apex of the chin (see Fig. 33–44). Too often, excision of all the scar in the lower lip and chin results in a flat chin; retention of the extra tissue at the apex of the chin gives an esthetically more pleasing profile.

The correction of microstomia and deformities of the oral commissure, although frequently done following thermal injury, is discussed in the subsequent section on electrical burns and in Chapter 32.

Skin flaps are useful over the chin area to build up loss of contour due to the loss of the mental fat pad and are acceptable over the parotid-masseteric area. Skin flaps must be employed in deep burns with massive tissue destruction, severe contracture, and hypertrophic scarring (see Figs. 33–14 to 33–16; see also Fig. 33–39).

A rotation or transposed flap from the neck is an excellent technique, as stated earlier in the chapter, to restore hair-bearing skin to the lower portion of the cheek and chin in male patients. The 1–2 advancement flap of Converse not only gives bulk to the mental region but also provides hair-bearing tissue (see Fig. 33–16). It is indicated only in the younger patient who can tolerate the flexed neck position; the technique cannot be employed if the cervical area is skin grafted.

Full-thickness loss of skin following burns usually results in scar contracture of the neck. The looseness of the skin of the cervical area favors wound contraction during healing. The extent of the deformity varies with the amount of skin destruction and the adequacy of early skin replacement by skin grafting. Weblike vertical bands of scar tissue pull the chin downward in some cases, disturbing the normal contour and limiting neck movements. The chin may be bound to the chest by a mass of scar tissue when loss of skin is extensive.

Secondary deformities of the soft tissues due to extensive scar contractures of the neck may include a downward pull of the corners of the mouth, lower lip, cheek tissues, and, in extreme cases, even the lower eyelids. The bony structures may also be affected when contractures, originating during childhood, remain uncorrected for a long period of time; deformity of the mandible may result from the downward pull of the scar. Consequently, reconstruction of the cervical contracture (see Chapter 34) is an integral part of the treatment of lip and cheek deformities in burn patients.

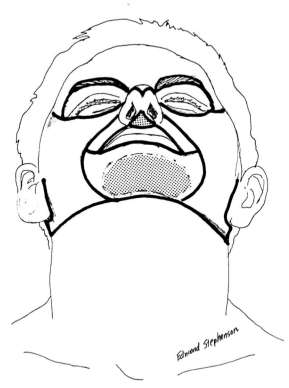

FIGURE 33–44. Incisions for resurfacing the upper and lower lips. At the apex of the mental region, only the epidermis is excised in order to provide chin prominence following skin grafting.

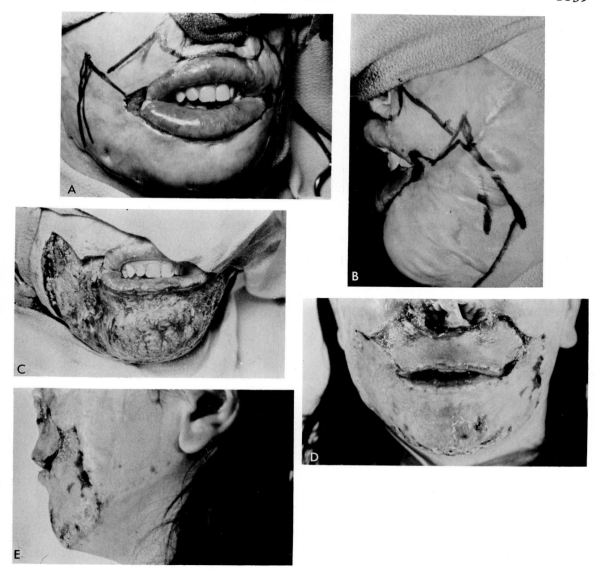

FIGURE 33–45. Resurfacing the perioral area according to designs illustrated in Figures 33–43 and 33–44. *A, B,* Outlines of the incisions. *C,* The scar tissue has been excised. It is preferable to preserve some de-epithelized scar tissue over the mentum to maintain chin projection. *D, E,* Two weeks after thick split-thickness skin grafting.

ELECTRICAL BURNS OF THE PERIORAL REGION

The electrophysical and pathologic aspects of electrical burns were discussed at the beginning of the chapter.

In a review of 43 children with perioral electrical burns, Thompson, Juckes, and Farmer (1965) emphasized that, on occasion, a 110-volt current can be fatal, provided that the contact is large, there is complete grounding, and the current passes through the thorax. The wet lips and mucosa have decreased resistance to electrical current. In their series, 28 of the 43 children were under 2 years of age, and 12 were between the ages of 2 and 4. Thirty-seven of the 43 sucked on or bit the free end of a "live" extension cord; four patients bit directly into the wire; one patient sucked at an electrical outlet, and another bit the coil of an electric fireplace.

Deformities Resulting from Electrical Burns

The lips, alveolar processes, and tongue are involved in live socket burns. Damage to the tongue is not usually severe, although the tip of the tongue may show considerable ulceration in the initial stages. Some impairment occurs when the floor of the mouth is involved, the tongue being bound down by scars which interfere with the normal mobility of the tip.

Burns of the alveolar processes and the teeth are common, with resultant sequestration. Loss of the deciduous incisors may occur, but the development of the permanent teeth is usually not affected. The lip seems to suffer the most extensive damage; the lower lip is usually more severely burned than the upper. The entire thickness of the lip is usually involved, including the mucosa of the inner surface and the alveolar process. The contracting scar causes severe deformities as the wound heals. When the median section of the lip is lost, the remaining lip tissue becomes retracted and adherent to the alveolar process, distorting the lips and interfering with normal function. Part of both upper and lower lips on the injured side becomes adherent when the corner of the mouth is destroyed; scar tissue interferes with the full opening of the mouth and results in microstomia.

In the series reviewed by Thompson, Juckes, and Farmer (1965), only the mucosa was involved in ten patients and the combined red and white lip in 33 patients. There was commissure deformity in ten patients, upper and lower lip involvement in 13, lower lip only in two, upper lip only in six, and tongue and buccal mucosa only without lip involvement in two. There were associated burns of the tongue in 18, of the buccal sulcus in 13, of the alveolus in ten, and of the teeth in four.

Treatment: Early or Late. Electric socket burns are usually full-thickness burns, and the extent of the tissue destruction in the lip can occasionally be determined within a few hours after the accident. Reconstructive procedures can be done early, after excision of the involved tissue. This approach has the advantage of preventing the contracture deformities which are otherwise inevitable and avoids a protracted healing period.

Immediate reconstruction following an electrical burn of the lip is also feasible when the defect is in an anatomically favorable position and is limited in extent. Hyslop (1957) advocated early debridement of the lips and oral commissure with primary reconstruction. He felt that the true line of demarcation was apparent by 12 hours and noted that the involved muscle had a chocolate color.

Unfortunately, many electrical socket burns of the lips and cheeks in children are not seen early and may involve areas less amenable to primary repair. When the burn involves the corner of the mouth, as it frequently does, it is probably preferable to await the spontaneous separation of the eschar and the healing and softening of the wound before undertaking the definitive repair of the resulting defect (Kazanjian and Roopenian, 1954; Thompson and coworkers, 1965; Fogh-Andersen and Sørensen, 1966; Pitts and coworkers, 1969). Early excision also runs the risk of sacrificing valuable uninvolved tissue. Moreover, early assessment of the extent of the burn is often only speculative. It has been our own experience that final reconstruction is best achieved not only after healing of the burn wound but also after a significant period during which the scars are allowed to soften. The waiting period can extend over a year or more. Children have a tendency to develop hypertrophic scarring, and reconstructive procedures done while the scars are hypertrophic may lead to additional hypertrophic scarring. After a period of a year or more, the scars tend to flatten and soften, and the tendency for hypertrophic scarring may have lessened.

Deformities Due to Electrical "Live" Socket Burns

Each case presents its own individual type of deformity, although there appear to be two principal types: (1) those which are limited to the corner of the mouth (commissure), and (2) those involving the loss of a section of the lower lip. When the side of the mouth is involved, the upper and lower lips are adherent for a varying distance from the corner of the mouth.

The reconstruction of lip and commissure defects is discussed in Chapter 32.

TREATMENT OF ESTABLISHED HYPERTROPHIC BURN SCARS

As mentioned earlier in the chapter, treatment is directed at the prevention of hypertrophic scarring by early skin grafting, constant pressure by elasticized face masks, serial splinting (nares, mouth, neck), and exercises of the oral and palpebral sphincters.

If within six months of the burn injury the patient returns with hypertrophic facial scars and the latter are firm and hyperemic, they are still amenable to continuous pressure (face mask) and serial splinting (nose and mouth conformers). Histologic studies have demonstrated that with such therapy there is loosening of the collagen, and individual fibers become apparent (see Fig. 33–6) (Larson and coworkers, 1974).

Injection with triamcinolone acetonide is helpful when dealing with older hypertrophic scars (Griffith, 1966; Griffith and coworkers, 1970). Adjuvant methods include full-thickness replacement with skin grafts or local flaps and dermabrasion with or without overgrafting. Cosmetics, if properly applied, also play a role.

REFERENCES

Abercrombie, M., Flint, M. H., and James, D. W.: Wound contraction in relation to collagen formation in scorbutic guinea-pigs. J. Embryol. Exp. Morphol., 4:67, 1956.

Abercrombie, M., James, D. W., and Newcome, J. F.: Wound contraction in rabbit skin studied by splinting the wound margins. J. Anat., 94:170, 1960.

Apfelberg, D. B., Waisbren, B. S., Masters, F. W., and Robinson, D. W.: Treatment of chondritis in the burned ear by the local instillation of antibiotics. Plast. Reconstr. Surg., 53:179, 1974.

Asch, M. J., Moylan, J. A., Jr., Bruck, H. M., and Pruitt, B. A., Jr.: Ocular complications associated with burns: Review of a five-year experience including 104 patients. J. Trauma, 11:857, 1971.

Aubry, M., and Levignac, J.: Repair of facial defects due to burns. Total reconstruction of the face. Transactions of the First Congress of the International Society of Plastic Surgeons. Baltimore, The Williams & Wilkins Company, 1957, p. 149.

Aufricht, G.: Evaluation of pedicle flaps versus skin grafts in reconstruction of surface defects and scar contractures of chin, cheeks, and neck. Surgery, 15:75, 1944.

Baldridge, R. E.: Electric burns. New Engl. J. Med., 250:46, 1954.

Blocker, T. G.: Free full thickness skin graft for the relief of burn contracture of the neck. South. Surg., 10:849, 1941.

Brent, B.: Reconstruction of ear, eyebrow, and sideburn in the burned patient. Plast. Reconstr. Surg., 55:312, 1975.

Bromberg, B. E., Song, I. C., and Walden, R. H.: Hydrotherapy in chemical burns. Plast. Reconstr. Surg., 35:85, 1965.

Brown, J. B., and Blair, V. P.: Repair of loss of skin from burns. Surg. Gynecol. Obstet., 60:379, 1935.

Brown, J. B., Blair, V. P., and Byars, L. T.: Repair of surface defects from burns and other causes with thick split-skin grafts. South. Med. J., 28:408, 1935.

Bullough, W. S., and Laurence, E. B.: Control of mitotic activity in mouse skin. Dermis and hypodermis. Exp. Cell Res., 21:394, 1960a.

Bullough, W. S., and Laurence, E. B.: Control of epidermal mitotic activity in the mouse. Proc. R. Soc. Lond. [Biol.], 151:517, 1960b.

Constable, J. D., and Carroll, J. M.: The emergency treatment of the exposed cornea in thermal burns. Plast. Reconstr. Surg., 46:309, 1970.

Converse, J. M.: In Converse, J. M. (Ed.): Reconstructive Plastic Surgery. Philadelphia, W. B. Saunders Company, 1964.

Converse, J. M.: Burn deformities of the face and neck. Surg. Clin. North Am., 47:323, 1967.

Converse, J. M.: Skin grafting following full-thickness burns of face. In Kazanjian and Converse's Surgical Treatment of Facial Injuries. 3rd Ed. Baltimore, The Williams & Wilkins Company, 1974, p. 1341.

Converse, J. M., and Robb-Smith, A. H. T.: The healing of surface cutaneous wounds; its analogy with the healing of superficial burns. Ann. Surg., 120:873, 1944.

Converse, J. M., and Smith, B.: Repair of severe burn ectropion of the eyelids. Plast. Reconstr. Surg., 23:21, 1959.

Coughlin, W. T.: Contractures due to burns. Surg. Gynecol. Obstet., 68:352, 1939.

Cronin, T. D.: Successful correction of extensive scar contractures of the neck using split thickness grafts. In Transactions of the First Congress of the International Society of Plastic Surgeons. Baltimore, The Williams & Wilkins Company, 1957, p. 123.

Dale, R. H.: Electrical accidents (a discussion with illustrative cases). Br. J. Plast. Surg., 7:44, 1954.

Davis, J. S.: Relaxation of scar contractures by means of the Z- or reversed Z-type incision; stressing use of scar infiltrated tissues. Ann. Surg., 94:871, 1931.

Di Vincenti, F. C., Pruitt, B. A., and Recklar, J. M.: Inhalation injuries. J. Trauma, 11:109, 1971.

Dowd, C. N.: Some details in the repair of cicatricial contractures of the neck. Surg. Gynecol. Obstet., 44:396, 1927.

Dowling, J. A., Foley, F. D., and Moncrief, J. A.: Chondritis in the burned ear. Plast. Reconstr. Surg., 42:115, 1968.

Edgerton, M. T., and Hansen, F. C.: Matching facial color with split thickness skin grafts from adjacent areas. Plast. Reconstr. Surg., 25:455, 1960.

Feller, I.: Personal communication to D. L. Larson, 1975.

Flagg, S. V., Converse, J. M., and Rapaport, F. T.: Possible deleterious effects of topical agents on the rate of healing of the burn wound. Surg. Forum, 20:501, 1969.

Fogh-Andersen, P., and Sørensen, B: Electric mouth burns in children. Treatment and prevention. Acta Chir. Scand., 131:214, 1966.

Fox, C. L.: Silver sulfadiazine—a new therapy for Pseudomonas infection in burns. Arch. Surg., 96:184, 1968.

Frankelton, W. H.: Neck burns—early and late treatment. In Transactions of the First Congress of the International Society of Plastic Surgeons. Baltimore, The Williams & Wilkins Company, 1957, p. 130.

Furnas, D. W., Bartlett, R. H., and Achauer, B. M.: Burns: Management of the respiratory tract. In Lynch, J. B., and Lewis, S. R. (Eds.): Symposium on the Treatment of Burns. Vol. 5. St. Louis, Mo., C. V. Mosby Company, 1973, p. 49.

Gabbiani, M. G., Ryan, G. B., and Majno, G.: Presence of modified fibroblasts in granulation tissue and their possible role in wound contraction. Experientia, 27:549, 1971.

Gillies, H. D.: Plastic Surgery of the Face. London, Oxford University Press, 1920.

Grant, D. A., Finley, M. D., and Coers, C. R.: Early management of the burned ear. Plast. Reconstr. Surg., *44*:161, 1969.

Greeley, P. W.: Plastic repair of scar contractures. Surgery, *15*:224, 1944.

Griffith, B. H.: The treatment of keloids with triamcinolone acetonide. Plast. Reconstr. Surg., *38*:202, 1966.

Griffith, B. H., Monroe, C. W., and McKinney, P.: A follow-up study on the treatment of keloids with triamcinolone acetonide. Plast. Reconstr. Surg., *46*:145, 1970.

Harii, K., Ohmori, K., and Ohmori, S.: Hair transplantation with free scalp flaps. Plast. Reconstr. Surg., *53*:410, 1974.

Hynes, W.: The treatment of scars by shaving and skin graft. Br. J. Plast. Surg., *10*:1, 1957.

Hyslop, V. B.: Treatment of electric burns of the lips. Plast. Reconstr. Surg., *20*:315, 1957.

Kazanjian, V. H.: The repair of contractures resulting from burns. New Engl. J. Med., *216*:1104, 1936.

Kazanjian, V. H., and Converse, J. M.: The Surgical Treatment of Facial Injuries. Baltimore, The Williams & Wilkins Company, 1949.

Kazanjian, V. H., and Roopenian, A.: The treatment of lip deformities resulting from electric burn. Am. J. Surg., *88*:884, 1954.

Larson, D. L., Abston, S., Evans, E. B., Dobrkovsky, M., and Linares, H. S.: Techniques for decreasing scar formation and contractures in the burned patient. J. Trauma, *11*:807, 1971.

Larson, D. L., Abston, S., Willis, B., Linares, H., Dobrkovsky, M., Evans, E. B., and Lewis, S. R.: Contracture and scar formation in the burn patient. Clinics in Plastic Surgery, *1*:653, 1974.

Larson, D. L.: Personal communication, 1975.

Linares, H. A., Kischer, C. W., Dobrkovsky, M., and Larson, D. L.: On the origin of the hypertrophic scar. J. Trauma, *13*:70, 1973.

Lindberg, R. B., Moncrief, J. A., Switzer, W. E., Order, S. E., and Mills, W.: The successful control of wound sepsis. J. Trauma, *5*:601, 1965.

Longacre, J. J.: Scar Tissue, Its Use and Abuse: The Surgical Correction of Deformation Due to Hypertrophic Scar and the Prevention of its Formation. Springfield, Ill., Charles C Thomas, Publisher, 1972.

MacCollum, D. W.: The early and late treatment of burns in children. Am. J. Surg., *38*:275, 1938.

McIndoe, A.: Total facial reconstruction following burns. Postgrad. Med., *6*:187, 1949.

Maguire, H. C.: Treatment of keloids with triamcinolone acetonide injected intralesionally. J.A.M.A., *192*:325, 1965.

Majno, G., Gabbiani, M. G., Hirschel, B. S., Ryan, G. B., and Statkov, P. R.: Contraction of granulation tissue in vitro: Similarity to smooth muscle. Science, *173*:548, 1971.

Mathews, D.: The late repair of burns. Fortschr. Kiefer. Gesichtschir., *9*:44, 1964.

Millard, D. R., Jr.: Columella lengthening by a forked flap. Plast. Reconstr. Surg., *22*:454, 1958.

Mishima, S., and Maurice, D. M.: The oily layer of the tear film and evaporation from the corneal surface. Exp. Eye Res., *1*:39, 1961.

Mixter, C. G.: Contractions of the neck following burns. New Engl. J. Med., *208*:190, 1933.

Moyer, C. A., Brentano, L., Gravens, D. S., Margraf, H. W., and Monafo, W. W., Jr.: Treatment of large human burns with dressings continuously wet with a 0.5 per cent aqueous solution of silver nitrate. Arch. Surg., *90*:799, 1965.

Murray, R. D.: Kenalog and the treatment of hypertrophic scars and keloids in Negroes and whites. Plast. Reconstr. Surg., *31*:275, 1963.

Padgett, E. C.: The full thickness skin graft in the correction of soft tissue deformities. J.A.M.A., *98*:18, 1932.

Padgett, E. C.: Calibrated intermediate skin grafts. Surg. Gynecol. Obstet., *69*:799, 1939.

Pariser, H., and Murray, P.: Intralesion injections of triamcinolone acetonide. Arch. Dermatol. Syph., *87*:183, 1963.

Phillips, A.: Personal communication, 1975.

Phillips, A. W., and Cope, O.: The revelation of respiratory tract damage as a principal killer of the burned patient. Ann. Surg., *155*:1, 1962.

Pitts, W., Pickrell, K., Quinn, G., and Massengill, R.: Electrical burns of lips and mouth in infants and children. Plast. Reconstr. Surg., *44*:471, 1969.

Pontén, B.: Burns in automobile accidents. Scand. J. Plast. Surg., *2*:104, 1968.

Rees, T. D., and Casson, P. R.: Indications for cutaneous dermal overgrafting. Plast. Reconstr. Surg., *38*:522, 1966.

Roper-Hall, M. J.: Immediate treatment of thermal and chemical burns. *In* Troutman, R. C., Converse, J. M., and Smith, B. (Eds.): Plastic and Reconstructive Surgery of the Eye and Adnexa. Washington, Butterworths, 1962, p. 1991.

Sanvenero-Rosselli, G.: Richlinien für die Narben Korrecture nach Gesichtsverbrennungen. Fortschr. Kiefer. Gesichtschir., *9*:54, 1964.

Scapicchio, A. P., Constable, J. D., and Opitz, B.: Comparative effects of silver nitrate and Sulfamylon acetate on epidermal regeneration. Plast. Reconstr. Surg., *41*:319, 1968.

Sheehan, J. E.: Use of free full thickness skin graft. J.A.M.A., *112*:27, 1939.

Skoog, T.: Surgical Treatment of Burns. A Clinical Report of 789 Cases. Stockholm, Almqvist & Wiksell, 1963.

Smith, F.: Plastic and Reconstructive Surgery. A Manual of Management. Philadelphia, W. B. Saunders Company, 1950.

Spira, M., and Hardy, S. B.: Management of the injured ear. Am. J. Surg., *106*:678, 1963.

Thompson, H. G., Juckes, A. W., and Farmer, A. W.: Electric burns to the mouth in children. Plast. Reconstr. Surg., *35*:466, 1965.

Thompson, N.: Subcutaneous dermis graft. Plast. Reconstr. Surg., *26*:1, 1960.

Tubiana, R.: Thermal burns of the face and eyelids. *In* Smith, B., Converse, J. M., Obear, M., and Wood-Smith, D. (Eds.): The Second International Symposium of the Manhattan Eye, Ear and Throat Hospital on Plastic Surgery of the Eye and Adnexa. St. Louis, Mo., C. V. Mosby Company, 1967, p. 187.

Tumbush, W. T.: Treatment of facial burns. *In* Troutman, R. C., Converse, J. M., and Smith, B. (Eds.): Plastic and Reconstructive Surgery of the Eye and Adnexa. Washington, D.C., Butterworths, 1962, p. 43.

Wallace, A. B.: Treatment of burns; return to basic principles. Br. J. Plast. Surg., *1*:233, 1949.

Watts, G., Grillo, H. C., and Gross, J.: Studies in wound healing. II. Role of granulation tissue in contraction. Ann. Surg., *148*:153, 1958.

Zarem, H. A., and Greer, D. M.: Tongue flap for reconstruction of the lips after electrical burns. Plast. Reconstr. Surg., *53*:310, 1974.

Zikria, B. A., Budd, D. C., Floch, F., and Ferrer, J. M.: What is clinical smoke poisoning? Ann. Surg., *181*:151, 1975.

CHAPTER 34

DEFORMITIES OF THE CERVICAL REGION

THOMAS D. CRONIN, M.D.

SCAR CONTRACTURES OF THE CERVICAL REGION

Scars of the anterior cervical region are particularly troublesome because the area from the chin to the sternum is a concave flexor surface of extreme mobility; an additional complication, as far as skin grafts are concerned, results from movements of the underlying larynx in swallowing. The skin is relatively thin and rather easily destroyed. Vertical incisions in the skin of the anterior cervical area, whether accidental or surgical, are likely to result in contracted scar bands.

Etiology. Most scar contractures of the neck result from thermal burns. Less frequently, neck contractures are caused by electrical, radiation, or chemical burns. Severe infection with gangrene of the skin may also cause scar contractures; surgical or accidental vertical incisions may produce linear scars.

Total Loss of Anterior Neck Skin. The proper treatment of severe and extensive contractures of the anterior neck was at one time a matter of some confusion. Many authorities (Dowd, 1927; Mixter, 1933; MacCollum, 1938a; Coughlin, 1939; Aufricht, 1944; McIndoe, 1949; Smith, 1950) advocated skin flaps, despite the number of operations entailed. Others (Babcock, 1932; Padgett, 1932; Brown and coworkers, 1935; Kazanjian, 1936; Blocker, 1941) recommended full-thickness

skin grafts as a means of avoiding postoperative contracture. Spina (1955) and Pitanguy (1957) have advised coverage with a thick split-thickness skin graft from the chin to the mandibulocervical angle and with a flap to the front of the neck below the mandibulocervical angle. Split-thickness skin grafts have been advocated by Greeley (1944), Padgett and Stephenson (1948), Frackelton (1957), and Brown and McDowell (1958). As ordinarily used, split-thickness skin grafts in these cases have been disappointing because of the high incidence of postoperative contracture and wrinkling of the graft. Preventive measures to avoid contracture were described by the author (Cronin, 1957, 1961, 1973) and make possible the use of split-thickness skin grafts as the treatment of choice, just as in most other locations. In fact, whereas the anterior neck was one of the most unsatisfactory sites for split-thickness skin grafts, successful, wrinkle-free grafts can be reliably obtained with the splinting-pressure technique. Dingman (1961), Mendoza and colleagues (1961), Gottlieb (1963), Cramer (1964), Tanzer (1964), Gibbons (1965), Pitanguy and Bisaggio (1967), Converse (1967), Fujimori and associates (1968), Ousterhout and coworkers (1969), Moore (1970), and Evans and coworkers (1970) have confirmed this principle, although several have suggested modification of the splint.

Burn scar contractures of the neck may involve limited areas, and when these areas are more or less vertical, some type of scar band usually forms. Actually, a complete anterior neck contracture may be simpler to correct than one that involves only a half or a third of the neck. In the former situation all the scar is excised and replaced with a thick split-thickness skin graft, and a uniform result is obtained. However, relief of incomplete contractures with only a split-thickness skin graft may not be ideal, because one part of the neck is covered by normal elastic skin, while the relatively inelastic skin-grafted area stands in marked contrast. Therefore, repair with local flaps or Z-plasties is often preferable, augmented when necessary with split-thickness skin grafts.

Prevention of Contractures. Ideally, scar contractures of the neck should be prevented rather than corrected later. Following a thermal burn the neck should be kept extended and the use of a pillow is avoided. Willis (1970) used isoprene splints molded to the neck early in the healing phase following a thermal burn. To be successful, however, a definitive thick split-thickness skin graft must be applied and splinted within four to six weeks (Fig. 34–1). If the burn wound cannot be prepared for definitive grafting within this time, if the extent of the surrounding burn is so great as to interfere with the proper use of a splint, or if the general condition is such that a definitive graft is not possible, it is preferable to use a thin graft and accept contracture until that time when conditions are favorable for scar excision and application of a thick split-thickness skin graft according to the author's technique.

COMPLETE CONTRACTURES

Anesthesia. The accomplishment of safe anesthesia is perhaps the most important problem to be solved when there is a severe anterior neck contracture. Induction with thiopental (Pentothal), ether, or any of the inhalation gases is likely to result in sudden respiratory obstruction. Introduction of an endotracheal tube under these circumstances may be extremely difficult, if not impossible. The use of a paralyzing agent for intubation would only compound the problem and is, therefore, contraindicated.

According to Wilson and his colleagues (1970), ketamine is the safest anesthetic agent to use in children with severe neck contractures. While producing anesthesia, it also stimulates rather than depresses respiration, and the protective pharyngeal and laryngeal reflexes persist during anesthesia. The authors recommend two alternatives, both involving the use of ketamine. In one method ketamine is used alone. Premedication consists of 0.1 mg scopolamine 1 hour preoperatively; ketamine, 8 mg. per kilogram of body weight, is given intramuscularly in the patient's room. No obstruction occurred with this regimen in the five cases so treated, and the only objection was the accumulation of carbon dioxide if drapes were placed over the airway. Consequently, minimal draping was used in these cases. In a recent personal communication, Wilson (1974) stated that he is administering ketamine alone more frequently and that the following method of endotracheal intubation with halothane is used, mainly when it is necessary to remove the anesthesiologist from the surgical field.

The recommended method is as follows:

1. Premedication is with 0.1 mg. scopolamine 1 hour before surgery.
2. Ketamine, 8 mg./kg., is administered intramuscularly in the patient's room.
3. In the operating room brief administration of halothane is followed by spraying the larynx with 2 per cent to 4 per cent lidocaine, and, after additional inhalation of halothane, nasotracheal intubation is accomplished under direct vision.

Tanzer (1964) and Pitanguy and Bisaggio (1967) have suggested initial incision of the scar contracture under local anesthesia followed in turn by general anesthesia and endotracheal intubation. This is a sound method and should probably be used if there is any question as to the experience of the anesthesiologist with ketamine or if there is a difficult problem with endotracheal intubation.

Excision of the Scar. Complete excision of the scar is indicated to minimize postoperative contracture (Fig. 34–2). If the scar extends over the chin or lower border of the mandible, it is usually advisable to excise this area, because the splint can be made with an extension to press against the grafts (Fig. 34–3). Inferiorly, excision should extend slightly below the clavicles. If a heavy scar is continuous with one over the upper chest, it is advisable to excise as much as possible and to apply split-thickness skin grafts with plans to repeat the procedure at a later date. If this is not done,

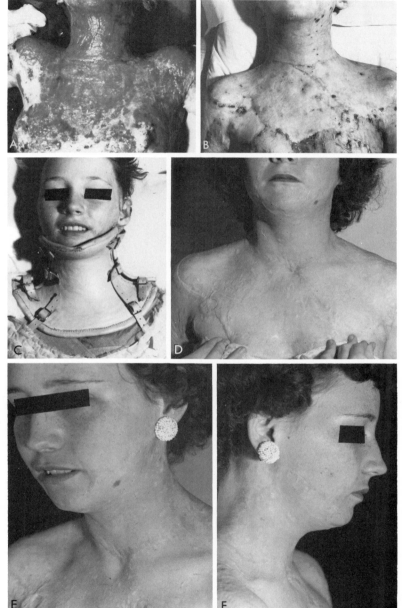

FIGURE 34–1. Patient with thermal burn. *A*, Clean granulating wounds 27 days following thermal burn. *B*, Appearance approximately three weeks after the application of a split-thickness skin graft (0.020 inch) to the neck, shoulders, and upper chest. *C*, Molded splint was worn day and night for six months, and for another three weeks only at night. *D*, Appearance two years later. The circular linear scar on the right side of the chin outlines a small skin graft which was necessary to cover an area of pressure necrosis four months after original grafting. *E*, *F*, Appearance 3½ years after skin grafting. (From Cronin, T. D.: The use of a molded splint to prevent contracture after split-skin grafting on the neck. Plast. Reconstr. Surg., *27*:9. Copyright 1961, The Williams & Wilkins Company, Baltimore.)

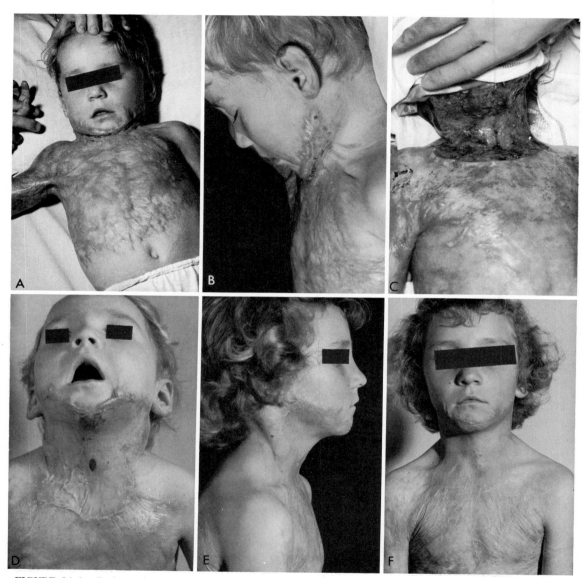

FIGURE 34–2. Patient with thermal burn. *A, B,* Complete contracture of the neck despite skin grafting (applied without splinting). *C,* The neck extended on the operating table after excision of the scar. Note one arm of a Z-plasty on the right margin of the wound. *D,* Loss of skin over the larynx caused by swallowing movements. To avoid this complication, dressings are removed from the neck after the first 24 hours. *E, F,* Appearance almost four years after a single operation to release the scar and apply split-thickness skin grafts. A splint was worn continuously for 6½ months.

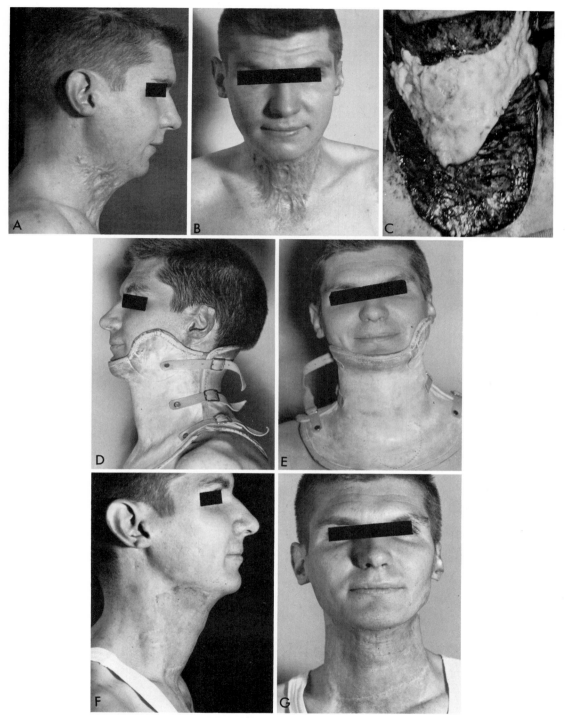

FIGURE 34–3. Patient with neck contracture. *A, B,* Moderate contracture involving most of the anterior aspect of the neck. *C,* After excision the scar has been laid in the center of the wound to show the extent of expansion. Contracted parts of the platysma were excised. A split-thickness skin graft was applied one week later. *D, E,* Splint with extension on one cheek to apply pressure to a graft of this area. The splint was worn continuously for eight months. *F, G,* Appearance eight months after application of the skin graft. Note Z-plasty on the side of the neck at the junction of the graft with the neck skin. (From Cronin, T. D.: The use of a molded splint to prevent contracture after split skin grafting on the neck. Plast. Reconstr. Surg., *27*:11. Copyright 1961, The Williams & Wilkins Company, Baltimore.)

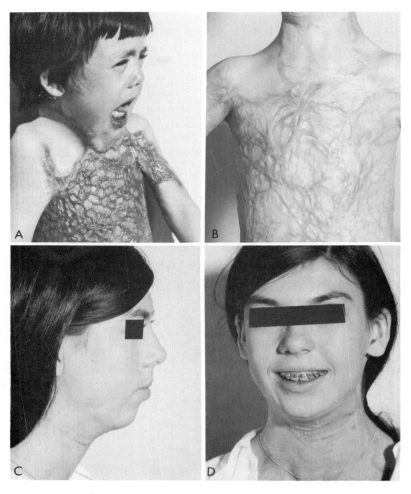

FIGURE 34–4. Patient with contracture of the anterior neck. *A*, Severe contracture of the neck. *B*, Appearance 20 months after grafting. It was later noticed that the extensive chest scar was pulling the neck skin inferiorly. A large area of the chest scar was later excised and a split-thickness skin graft applied. *C, D*, Appearance 12 years later. With growth some vertical tightness developed. A transverse relieving graft can be seen in *D*. (From Cronin, T. D.: Burn scar contractures of the neck. *In* Lynch, J. B., and Lewis, S. R. (Eds.): Symposium on the Treatment of Burns. Vol. 5. St. Louis, Mo., The C. V. Mosby Company, 1973.)

the author has seen continued contracture of the scar pull the newly applied skin graft of the neck toward the chest (Fig. 34–4), thereby impairing its efficiency in relieving the neck contracture.

On each side of the neck, the vertical margins of the wound are interrupted by making one arm of a Z-plasty and transposing it, the other arm to be formed from the skin graft when it is later applied (see Fig. 34–2, *C*). If the chin-neck angle remains obtuse, it may be accentuated by performing a Z-plasty on the platysma muscle and its overlying subcutaneous tissue.

If the neck remains tight after the scar excision, overhead traction can be applied by a hook (made from a Kirschner wire) applied to the symphysis of the mandible for as long as necessary before application of the skin graft (Fig. 34–5). Evans and associates (1970) drilled a wire through the symphysis from side to side for this purpose.

It is never wise to apply the skin grafts at the time of excision, because a 100 per cent take of the graft is extremely important. De-

spite the greatest care, small to large hematomas are prone to occur with loss of the skin graft if it is immediately applied.

The wound may be dressed with fine mesh nitrofurazone (Furacin) gauze and fluffed Kerlix or cotton waste secured by an elastic bandage (see Fig. 34–5, *C*). This dressing, plus padding behind the shoulders, keeps the neck extended and remains unchanged until the skin graft is applied at about five days. Recently the author has been covering the fresh wound with porcine grafts,* which form a perfect dressing, ensuring a sterile wound when removed four or five days later for application of the autogenous skin graft.

Skin Grafting. An interval of five days between scar excision and skin grafting seems to be optimum. By this time, a fine layer of granulation tissue has begun to form. Any areas of fat necrosis can be detected and curetted. With lesser periods, bleeding upon removal of the dressing may still be troublesome.

---

*Obtained from Burn Treatment Skin Bank, Inc., 2430 East Washington Street, Phoenix, Arizona 85034.

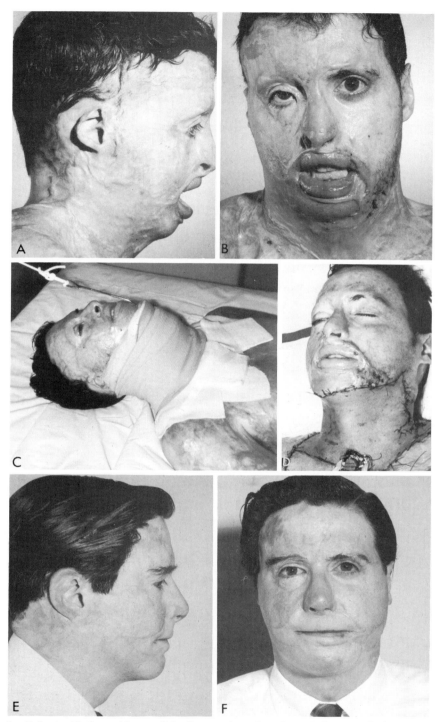

FIGURE 34–5. Patient with thermal burns of the face, neck, and trunk. *A, B,* Proper splinting was not possible after an early skin graft, and a contracture resulted. *C,* Complete extension of the neck was not obtained immediately following scar excision; overhead traction was applied to the symphysis for several days. *D,* Two days after application of a split-thickness skin graft. *E, F,* Appearance two years following thick split-thickness skin grafting and prolonged use of a molded splint. (From Cronin, T. D.: Burn scar contractures of the neck. *In* Lynch, J. B., and Lewis, S. R. (Eds.): Symposium on the Treatment of Burns. Vol. 5. St. Louis, Mo., The C. V. Mosby Company, 1973.)

After five days epithelium begins to grow in from the wound edges and may need to be trimmed, with the possibility of additional bleeding. Further delay would also increase the chance of infection.

The skin graft should be removed in one large piece if possible. The Padgett-Hood or Reese dermatomes are preferred, since a graft 4 × 8 inches (10 × 20 cm) can be obtained, a size usually adequate for a young child. These dermatomes are preferred also because a thick graft (0.020-inch) is desired and can be more accurately obtained than with other dermatomes or knives. If more than one piece is required, the line of junction should be transverse. The grafts should be carefully sutured in a slightly stretched state, completing the second arm of a Z-plasty wherever a first arm has previously been made on the lateral edge of the wound. Scattered interrupted sutures may be left long to tie over a large bolster dressing of fluffed gauze or mechanics waste. The latter is piled on a layer of gauze impregnated with Furacin or an antibiotic ointment. A pressure dressing is preferred initially to ensure that the graft is in contact with the surface depressions and irregularities.

Postoperative Care. On the day after operation, the bolster dressing is removed and the graft is carefully inspected for hematomas and serum collections. Hematomas should be removed with power suction through a small transverse nick in the skin graft. Serum and liquid blood collections may be aspirated with syringe and needle.

The bulky dressing is not reapplied because of the danger of loss of skin over the larynx. The graft tends to stick to the dressing and is therefore prevented from adhering to the moving tissues over the larynx during deglutition (see Fig. 34–2, *D*). The extended position of the neck is, of course, maintained.

If as much as 1 square centimeter of skin is lost, it is advisable to regraft it promptly. If refrigerated skin autograft is available, it can be used. Otherwise, a fresh piece of skin can be procured under local anesthesia. If areas of skin loss are permitted to heal without regrafting, the scars will contract and be unsightly, even though a splint is used.

Daily observation is advisable until it is certain that the splint (see following section) fits well and any pressure points have been detected and corrected by the splint maker. If pressure necrosis of the skin graft develops, the area must be promptly regrafted. The splint should be worn even if there are small unhealed areas, which must be covered with a thin dressing.

Infection is rarely a problem in the clean wound after scar excision but is more likely to occur in primary grafting of granulating burn wounds. It is best, therefore, not to attempt a definitive graft unless the local condition of the wound is ideal.

Moist dressings during the postoperative period lessen the chances of infection when grafting the burn wound.

Preparing the Mold of the Neck. On the first or second day following skin grafting, a plaster mold of the neck is made, preferably with the splint maker present so that he will understand the problem. The graft is covered with strips of Furacin or petrolatum gauze, one or two layers thick. The patient is then allowed to sit up in a comfortable position, with the neck extended slightly. The position must be carefully chosen, because the splint being molded to this exact position and shape determines the contour of the neck when the graft contracts against it. The entire success of this method depends on the accuracy of the mold and the resulting splint.

A strip of malleable metal or cardboard is laid along each side of the neck and shoulders. When removing the cast the line of section through the cast is extended over these strips, which protect the patient's skin from injury. A complete circular cast is applied directly to the neck, the adjacent parts of the shoulders, and the clavicular areas. It extends up to the chin, and if the graft reaches the cheeks, the cast should also cover this area. As the plaster begins to warm, it is cut through on one side and removed. If the plaster has already set, both sides are cut and the two halves of the cast can be separated.

The patient is returned to his bed and to the previous hyperextended position. As mentioned before, the graft is left exposed or it may be covered with a single layer of Furacin or other medicated gauze.

The Splint. The splint is designed to accomplish three goals, all of which are of equal importance:

1. Keep the neck extended
2. Mold the chin-neck angle
3. Apply even pressure to the grafted area

Successful use of the splint presupposes complete surgical correction of the scar contracture and restoration of the cutaneous contour of the neck.

The need for keeping the neck extended is obvious, but the need for applying pressure to the graft and molding the chin-neck line is often overlooked, as it was by Gibbons (1965) and Koepke (1970), who reported the use of only four-post adjustable cervical braces. The four-poster cervical splint fails to achieve two of the three essential goals. Although it may keep the chin elevated, it does not mold the chin-neck angle and it does not apply pressure to all of the graft. The latter is important in preventing the development of a hypertrophic scar and in producing a soft, smooth graft. Koepke and Feller (1971) also described another similar style of brace that applied pressure to the forehead rather than beneath the chin. Martins (1960) tried unsuccessfully to prevent recurrent contracture of the neck after split-thickness skin grafting by placing a child in a plaster head cap and body cast with a metal strut arching from the head to the chest area. Neither of these methods, of course, would prevent the chin from being pulled inferiorly.

In the construction of the splint, a positive model is made from the negative cast by pouring plaster around a heavy wooden post which is inserted in the center and is used as a handle (Fig. 34–6). The negative mold must be kept rigid with no expansion from front to back. After the plaster has set, the negative mold is removed, the rough positive model is smoothed with a coarse file, and a piece of ordinary screen wire, approximately 7 × 35 cm, is used in the manner of a shoeshine cloth. The angle between the chin and neck is deepened, as are the depressions above and below the clavicles and the manubrium sterni. It is necessary, however, to avoid much smoothing of the bony prominences (the clavicles and the inferior border of the mandible), as this would cause undue pressure at these points by the splint.

Lightweight gray horsehide is applied over the area and is worked into all the depressions. A layer of wool felt, 1/8-inch thick (approximately 0.32 cm), is added. In place of the wool felt, 1/4-inch firm foam rubber may be used; it is applied in sections to avoid stretching and consequent thinning in some places.

The main support of the splint is laid on in the form of Celastic, approximately 1/8-inch thick. This material is first soaked in XP 25 solvent for Celastic.* The Celastic is superimposed upon the wool felt and is worked into all the depressions. For adult patients two layers may be advisable to afford additional strength. In order to mold the Celastic firmly to the contours of the model, depressions are accentuated with half-round rubber or felt, and the entire splint is firmly wrapped with heavy elastic tape for 36 to 48 hours. A lightweight horsehide cover completes the build-up. Soft aluminum sheet metal, about 0.05-inch thick, properly molded, may be substituted for the

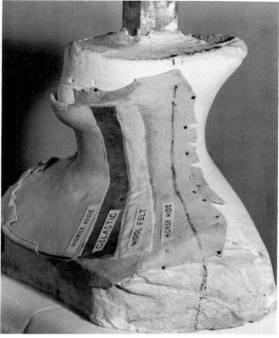

FIGURE 34–6. Plaster (positive) model of the neck, showing the different layers of the splint. (From Cronin, T. D.: The use of a molded splint to prevent contracture after split skin grafting on the neck. Plast. Reconstr. Surg., *27*:14. Copyright 1961, The Williams & Wilkins Company, Baltimore.)

Celastic. It need not be covered with the horsehide on its outer surface.

The splint is made in two parts, front and back, with three buckles on each side and a tapered piece of leather between the two halves. The leather is attached to one half and slides beneath the edge of the other. There should be, between the halves, a distance of 1.5 to 3 cm. If the grafted area extends onto the cheek, the splint is extended to cover it and is reinforced, in this case, by a metal strut.

The splint is usually applied during the second week after grafting. It should be worn continuously day and night for about six months or until the grafted site is soft and pliable and there is no tendency for wrinkling of the graft. This may be determined after five or six months by removing the splint for a few hours or a day at a time, and in turn for longer intervals if there is no wrinkling.

Any splint that will efficiently fulfill the three requirements previously mentioned may be used. Gottlieb (1963), Gibbons (1965), and Converse (1967) have used a ready-made collar, sometimes constructed with the addition of foam rubber. Tanzer (1964) employed a 4-inch block of foam rubber trimmed to fit the neck and secured with an elastic bandage. Frackelton (1957) advised the use of a cervical wrap collar dressing of the Sayre type. Ousterhout

---

*Joseph Jones Company, 186 William Street, New York, N.Y. 10038.

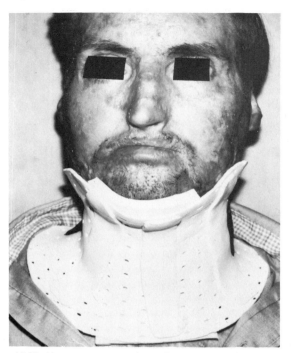

FIGURE 34–7. Orthoplast isoprene splint. (From Cronin, T. D.: Burn scar contractures of the neck. *In* Lynch, J. B., and Lewis, S. R. (Eds.): Symposium on the Treatment of Burns. Vol. 5. St. Louis, Mo., The C. V. Mosby Company, 1973.)

and coworkers (1969) constructed a kidney-shaped inflatable bag with tube and valve to be worn under a ready-made collar. While all of these might produce satisfactory pressure on the skin graft, the cervical wrap and the block of foam rubber might not ensure adequate extension of the neck. None of them would provide sufficient pressure on the skin grafts, either above the mandibular border or below the clavicles. The inflatable bag, moreover, might be difficult to obtain or make.

Willis (1970) has described in detail a splint made of Orthoplast isoprene* (Fig. 34–7). The advantage of this technique is the relative simplicity with which the splint can be made. After softening in hot water, it is molded and shaped to the neck and reinforced with strips of the same material. A Velcro strap is riveted onto the splint and passed around the back of the neck. Moore (1970), a prosthetic dentist, made a splint of cold-curing resin and lined it with a resilent mixture of silicone foam and silicone rubber. When carefully molded, both of these splints would seem to be satisfactory.

---

*Johnson & Johnson, 501 George Street, New Brunswick, N.J. 08903.

Skin Flaps. In the past, skin flaps have been widely used because they undergo little contraction, and if the donor site is carefully selected and the flap is of adequate size, excellent results can be obtained. However, now that postoperative scar contracture can be prevented following the use of thick split-thickness skin grafts on the anterior neck, the need for skin flaps should be greatly reduced. Their use should be limited to repair of severe radiation burns and extremely deep thermal burns with resultant loss of contour, such as that of the chin prominence. Even in such instances, it may be possible to combine a thick split-thickness skin graft applied to most of the neck with a tube flap to augment the chin (Fig. 34–8).

When all or most of the anterior neck skin has been lost, an extremely large flap is required. In an adult this requires a rectangle of at least 15 × 18 cm, entailing the mutilation of some other part of the body, several major operations, and secondary touch-up procedures. Aside from the general risk to the patient of repeated anesthesia, this technique also causes a great economic burden. In the mobilization of large flaps, there is also the risk of partial loss from circulatory embarrassment. Unless expert shaping and thinning of the flap are accomplished, the chin-neck angle can be obscured by the bulky flap.

Sources of Skin Flaps. If adjacent skin is available, its use is generally preferable for convenience and simplicity, although this may result in scarring of an exposed area. When the use of local skin is not possible or desirable, skin flaps should be obtained from parts of the body that are not exposed. Many sources have been used, including the acromiocervical (Fig. 34–9), acromiopectoral (Fig. 34–10), thoracoepigastric (axilloabdominal) (Fig. 34–11), shoulder-back (Fig. 34–12), transabdominal via the forearm (Fig. 34–13), and oblique abdominal via the forearm.

The technique of preparing tube flaps has been described in Chapter 6.

As tube flaps must, of necessity, be prepared in advance, it is important that an accurate estimate be made of the amount of skin that will be needed when the scar is excised and the neck extended. The decision concerning the choice of the donor site may be simple, because in many cases it is determined by finding a large enough skin donor site that is free of burn scar.

Kirschbaum (1958), after treating 31 pa-

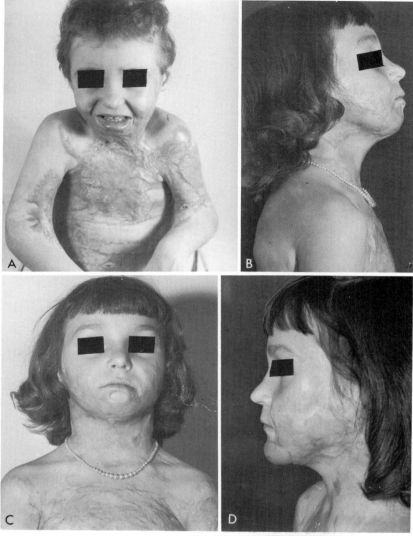

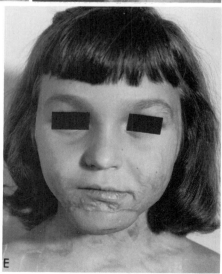

FIGURE 34–8. Patient with scar contracture corrected by skin grafting and skin flap. *A,* Severe contracture of neck. *B, C,* Appearance 19 months after a single operation in which the scar was released and a thick split-thickness skin graft was applied. The splint was worn for seven months. Note the flatness of the chin caused by the depth of the burn. *D, E,* Appearance six weeks after transfer of an oblique abdominal tube flap via the wrist. (From Cronin, T. D.: Burn scar contractures of the neck. *In* Lynch, J. B., and Lewis, S. R. (Eds.): Symposium on the Treatment of Burns. Vol. 5. St. Louis, Mo., The C. V. Mosby Company, 1973.)

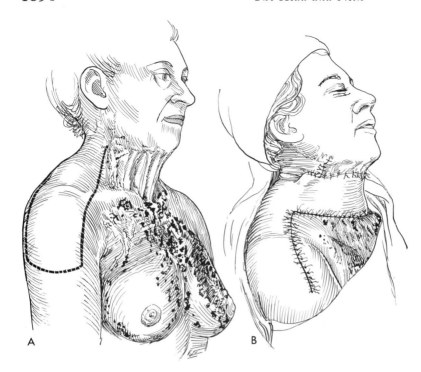

A   B

FIGURE 34–9. Correction by an acromiocervical flap. *A*, A burn scar contracture of the neck. Proposed flap incisions. *B*, Relief of contracture by transposition of a "charretera" (acromiocervical) flap in one stage. (Drawings after photographs from Kirschbaum, 1958.)

tients, advocated the use of the "charretera" flap (acromiocervical) for severe contractures. The flap is raised from the lateral and upper part of the neck and over the entire shoulder to the deltoid area (see Fig. 34–9). It is raised and transferred in one stage at the level of the fascia and can extend beyond the midline of the neck.

Aufricht (1944) has employed a transabdominal flap with transfer via the hand and forearm (see Fig. 34–13). He has also used the axilloabdominal (see Fig. 34–11, *A*) and acromiopectoral flaps (see Fig. 34–10) for chin and neck reconstruction. In regard to securing good cosmetic results with tube flaps, Aufricht (1944) observed:

1. The size of the defect should be carefully considered. There is always a danger of lacking sufficient tissue.

2. Large flaps provide a better cosmetic result than small ones.

3. No old scar should be spared between the transplanted and healthy skin.

4. In extensive reconstruction of the chin, the flap should extend to the vermilion border; even uninvolved skin has to be sacrificed. Small islands of healthy skin spoil the esthetic effect and do not provide functional aid.

5. The flap can be thinned and modeled after transfer has been completed.

Pitanguy and Bisaggio (1967) attached both ends of the transabdominal flap to the forearm, while leaving the middle attached to the abdomen. Along with Spina (1955), they used a split-thickness skin graft from the chin to the mandibulocervical angle and transferred a flap to the anterior aspect of the neck.

Microvascular Surgery. For surgeons trained and experienced in microvascular anastomosis, another method of resurfacing the neck is available. Harii, Ohmori, and Ohmori (1974) transferred groin flaps (Fig. 34–14), ranging in size from 7×14 cm to 18×28 cm, supplied by either the superficial circumflex iliac artery or the superficial epigastric artery and subcutaneous vein. End-to-end anastomosis was made with the facial artery and vein. The donor sites were closed either by primary closure or by split-thickness skin graft.

Eleven patients were corrected by this technique, with an excellent result in nine. There was partial necrosis of one flap and complete necrosis of another. The technique should find wide application in the future because of the elimination of multiple procedures and the shortened period of hospitalization. The subject is discussed in Chapter 14.

Full-Thickness Skin Grafts. A "take" is less certain when full-thickness skin grafts are

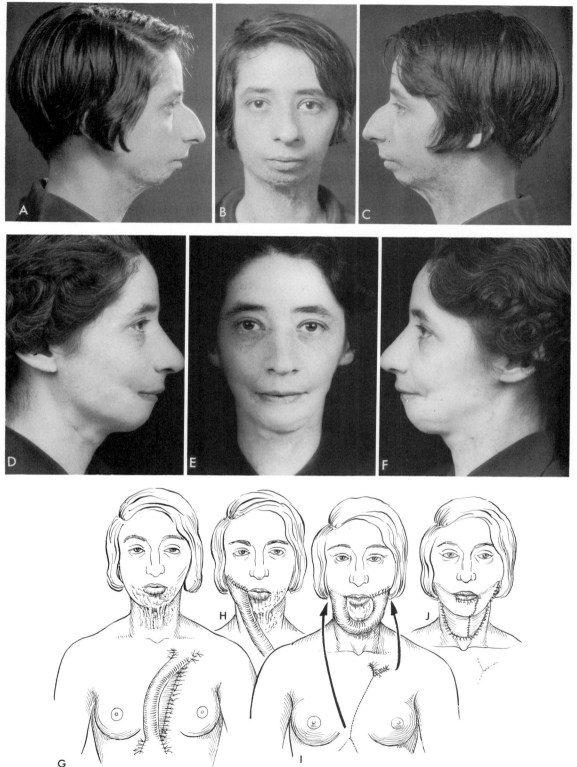

FIGURE 34–10. Correction with an acromiopectoral flap. *A, B, C,* Preoperative photographs of a patient following thermal burn. Hypertrophic scars had been treated with X-ray. Several years later radiation dermatitis and ulceration appeared on the chin despite previous skin grafting procedures. *D, E, F,* Postoperative photographs after reconstruction of the chin and neck with an acromiopectoral tube flap. Patient had also had a corrective rhinoplasty. *G, H, I, J,* Diagrams of the surgical technique. (From Aufricht, G.: Evaluation of pedicle flaps versus skin grafts in reconstruction of surface defects and scar contractures of the chin, cheeks and neck. Surgery, *15:*75, 1944.)

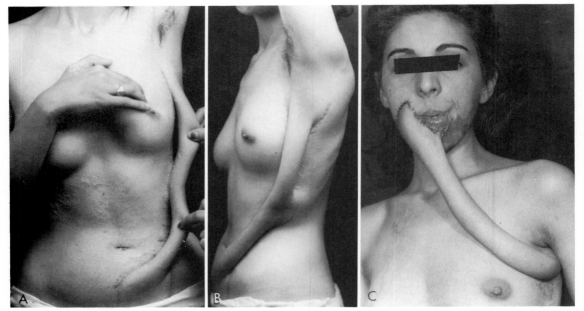

FIGURE 34–11. Correction by a thoracoepigastric (axilloabdominal) tube flap. *A, B,* Frontal and lateral views of axilloabdominal tube flap. *C,* Flap transferred to face.

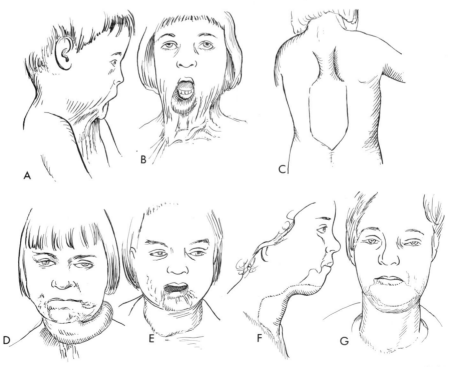

FIGURE 34–12. Correction by a shoulder-back flap. *A, B,* Burn scar contracture. *C,* The only available skin was on the back. Six delaying operations were done before transferring the flap to the neck, as shown in *D, E,* and *F*. After two to three months, the pedicle was divided in stages and spread out on the left side of the neck. *G,* Final result. (Drawings after photographs from Smith, 1950.)

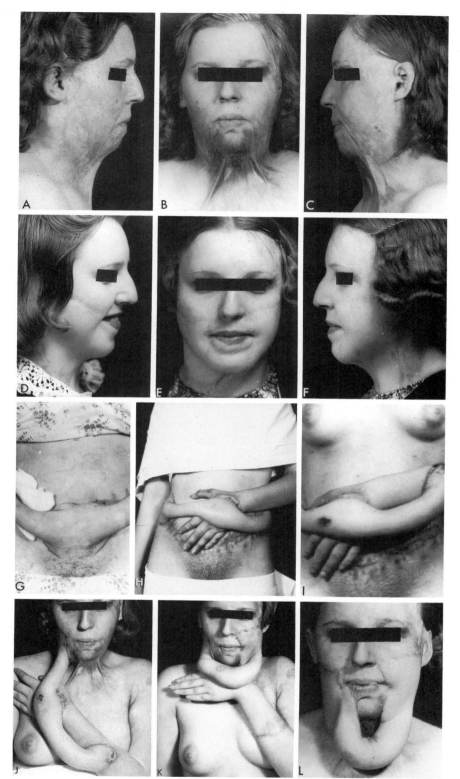

FIGURE 34–13. Correction by a transabdominal flap. *A, B, C,* Preoperative photographs of a patient with a burn scar contracture of the chin, cheeks, and neck. *D, E, F,* Postoperative views after reconstruction with an abdominal tube flap. *G,* Abdominal tube flap, 15 by 45 cm long; the central portion remains attached. *H,* Central portion of abdominal tube flap attached to the dorsum of the hand. *I,* Left end of tube flap attached to the forearm. The dark spot in the center of the tube is a superficial burn caused by hot Negocoll when a moulage was prepared. *J,* Skin tube transferred via hand to face. *K,* Both ends of skin tube attached to the face. The central portion remains attached to the hand. *L,* Skin tube entirely free of intermediary host and vascularized by facial attachments. In a subsequent operation the skin tube was divided and spread over the defect. Note the vertical scar on the left side of the chin in *E* where the flaps were joined. (From Aufricht, G.: Evaluation of pedicle flaps versus skin grafts in reconstruction of surface defects and scar contractures of the chin, cheeks and neck. Surgery, *15:*75, 1944.)

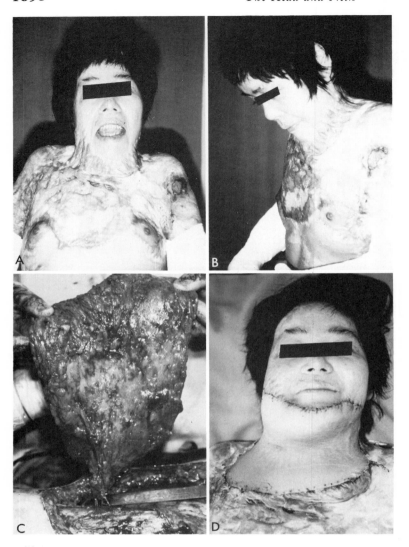

FIGURE 34–14. Correction by a microvascular free groin flap. *A, B,* Scar contracture of the neck three years after a gasoline burn. *C,* Groin flap (28 × 18 cm) based on the superficial epigastric artery and subcutaneous vein. *D,* Appearance of flap two weeks later. Microvascular anastomosis was to the right facial artery and vein. The donor site was covered by a split-thickness skin graft. (Courtesy of K. Harii, J. Ohmori, and S. Ohmori.)

used, because of the difficulty of immobilizing the area and because of the thickness of the grafts. Grafts of this type are less easily obtained than split-thickness skin grafts, and the donor sites must be covered with split-thickness skin grafts. Full-thickness grafts are not recommended in large areas of the neck but may profitably be used in small ones, as there is little postoperative contracture. Brown and McDowell (1958) used full-thickness grafts to restore a chin-neck line after contracture of previously applied split-thickness skin grafts. A transverse incision was made, the defect recreated, and a full-thickness skin graft inserted.

LIMITED CONTRACTURES

In limited contractures, Z-plasties, local flaps, or a combination of local flaps and split-thickness skin grafts may be successfully used.

In using the Z-plasty it should be remembered that one large Z-plasty will give greater length than several small ones in the same area. Mukhin and Mamonov (1970 described a four-flap 90° Z-plasty of the Limberg type with the flaps divided in half.

The use of local transposition flaps combined with split-thickness skin grafts and subsequent prolonged splinting is illustrated in Figure 34–15.

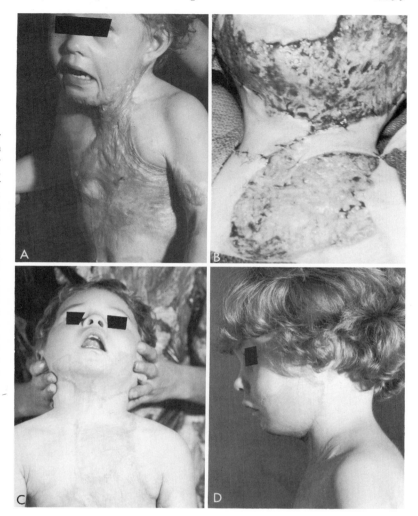

FIGURE 34–15. Correction by transposition flaps combined with skin grafts. *A*, Heavy scar contracture of the left side of the neck, face, and chest. *B*, Excision of scar and transposition of local flaps across the anterior aspect of the neck. *C*, Appearance six months later, showing that the flaps have spread out over the neck; the split-thickness skin grafts above and below the flaps are smooth and soft after wearing a molded splint. *D*, Profile six months following surgery. Note the well-defined chin-neck angle. (From Cronin, T. D.: Burn scar contractures of the neck. *In* Lynch, J. B., and Lewis, S. R. (Eds.): Symposium on the Treatment of Burns. Vol. 5. St. Louis, Mo., The C. V. Mosby Company, 1973.)

CONGENITAL WEBBING OF THE NECK (PTERYGIUM COLLI)

Turner (1938) reported a syndrome in females consisting of webbed neck, infantilism, and cubitus valgus (see Chapter 100). Webbing of the neck was already well known, having been reported by Kobylinski (1883) and named pterygium colli by Funke (1902). Turner (1938) considered these patients to have pituitary insufficiency, but Wilkins and Fleischmann (1944) discovered absence of the ovaries, there being only a streak of rudimentary tissue, and termed the syndrome "ovarian agenesis and dwarfism." Barr, Bertram, and Lindsay (1950) discovered that certain cells of the female contained a peripheral nuclear chromatin mass and that those of males did not.

Polani, Hunter, and Lennox (1954) and Wilkins, Grumbach and Van Wyk (1954) found that the cells of girls with the syndrome described by Turner, for the most part, were chromatin-negative or lacked the typical chromatin mass. In most series about 80 per cent of patients were found to be chromatin-negative. This led investigators to postulate that dysgenesis of the fetal gonad had occurred, resulting in the invariable development of the müllerian structures. Jost (1947) had previously shown that gonadectomy of the fetus in experimental animals resulted in 100 per cent of the offspring being females. In abnormal individuals, however, chromatin negativity or positivity ("nuclear sexing") may not necessarily indicate true chromosomal sex (Polani and coworkers, 1956). Ford and coworkers (1959) suggested "the findings in gonadal dysgenesis might be abnormal sex differentiation following anomalous sex determination in the zygote.''

Tjio and Levan (1956) and Ford and Hamerton (1956) discovered that the human has 46 chromosomes, and with the development of methods by which chromosomes from human cells could be counted, Ford and coworkers (1959) found that girls with the Turner syndrome had only 45 chromosomes, having 44 autosomes and only one sex chromosome—the XO. The absence of the sex chromosome leads not only to aplasia of the gonad but also to the other malformations seen and is now known to be one of a number of chromosomal abnormalities (see Chapter 4). These girls are typically dwarfed, and this may be the only finding, or they may have in addition webbed neck with low, wide hairline, webbed elbows and knees, epicanthal folds, malformation of the mandible, anomalies of the nails, coarctation of the aorta, hypertension of unknown etiology, lymphedema of the hands and feet, and mental retardation.

The diagnosis is made by obtaining a buccal smear and examining the cells for the peripheral chromatin mass. In postpubertal patients the urinary gonadotropins are elevated.

Medical treatment consists of administration of estrogens at the age of puberty. Consultation with the endocrinologist, or interested gynecologist or peditrician, is indicated in the diagnosis and systemic treatment of these patients.

Ulrich-Noonan Syndrome (Turner Phenotype). Other terms for the Ulrich-Noonan syndrome are Bonnevie-Ullrich syndrome and chromatin-positive Turner syndrome. This is one of the most common syndromes transmitted by a mendelian mode. Nora and Sinka (1970) and Levy and coworkers (1970) demonstrated an autosomal dominant mode of inheritance. Nora, Nora and Sinka (1974) stated:

General findings are that the patient with the Ullrich-Noonan syndrome may be male (eliminating XO Turner syndrome) or female and will have normal chromatin and chromosomes for their phenotype sex. Thus, a buccal smear that is chromatin positive with Barr bodies that are normal in size (to differentiate from isochromosome X) and normal in number (to distinguish from XX/XO mosaicism) will represent strong evidence that a female patient with Ullrich-Noonan and Turner stigmata has Ullrich-Noonan syndrome rather than Turner syndrome. The stature is usually, but not invariably small.

Surgical Correction of Cervical Webs. The usual low hairline and its anterior extension on the neck increase the difficulties of designing flaps that will not transpose hair-bearing skin

to the side or front of the neck. If the hair does not encroach on the web, an ordinary large Z-plasty may be done, with the central incision extending from the tip of the mastoid to the acromion, the lateral incisions being directed as seems best in each individual case. The flaps are elevated, and the underlying bands of fibrous tissue are excised; the flaps are transposed and sutured. Either one side or both sides can be corrected at the same time, as in Figure 34–16.

Unfortunately, in the typical Turner's syndrome, the hair extends so far forward on the web and so low on the neck that it is difficult to design a classical Z-plasty with flaps of equal size (Fig. 34–16, C). If the skin of the web is pulled backward, a normal contour is obtained. Some cases may be relieved by excision of a half-moon or ellipse of hair-bearing skin on each side (Fig. 34–17). Foucar (1948) excised an ellipse from the midline of the back of the neck. A combination of excision of hair-bearing skin plus rotation of a flap was described by Schröder (1958). However, his flap, being based below and posteriorly, would in most cases contain hair-bearing skin and would be therefore unsuitable. La Ruffa (1970) described a technique of excision of hair-bearing skin from the upper neck with a Z-plasty below, the posterior arm being based below and the anterior arm above. In this design the posterior flap would ordinarily be hair-bearing and thus unsuitable. It is possible to excise a large amount of hair-bearing skin and rotate an anterior non–hair-bearing flap posteriorly (see Fig. 34–16) (Cronin, 1961).

Mennig (1956) described an operation in which a posterior flap was advanced, and concomitantly the excess hair-bearing skin was excised to improve the hairline.

One male patient, in addition to having club feet and the Robin anomalad with cleft palate and bilateral inguinal hernia, also had a short neck. There was generalized vertical shortening of the skin of the anterior aspect of the neck in addition to lateral webbing (Fig. 34–18). A large Z-plasty on each side of the neck relieved the webbing, but the anterior shortness of skin remained, with resultant limitation of extension. The condition therefore had to be managed as if it were an extensive cicatricial contracture. A transverse incision was made and the skin of the neck retracted widely. A thick split-thickness skin graft was inserted and a molded splint applied. The splint was worn for approximately five months. The use of a split-thickness skin graft in the neck is

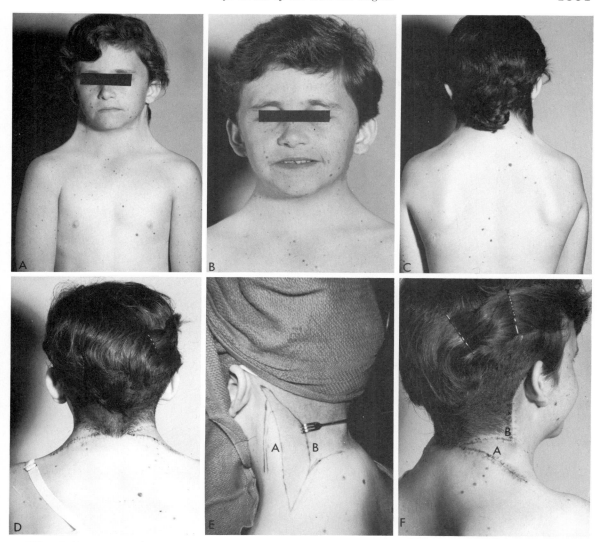

FIGURE 34–16. Pterygium colli in a 15 year old girl with Turner's syndrome (gonadal aplasia). *A*, Note the web from the mastoid to the acromion and the absence of breast development. *B*, Following correction of neck webs. *C*, Note the low, wide hairline on the back of the neck typical of this syndrome. The scar resulted from a thoracotomy to correct coarctation of the aorta. *D*, Ten days after excision of the abnormal hair-bearing skin and correction of the web. *E*, The web is flattened out with a retractor, and the large ellipse of hair-bearing skin to be excised is outlined. Note that the triangular flap (A) of non–hair-bearing skin on the anterior aspect of the web which will be transposed 90 degrees to fill the space created when the horizontal incision is made across the lower part of the neck. *F*, Ten days after excision of the excess hair-bearing skin and transposition of flaps A and B.

unwise unless an accurately molded splint is immediately available.

CONGENITAL MIDLINE CERVICAL CLEFT AND WEB

A congenital midline cervical cleft with webbing is uncommon. Although patients with associated median cleft of the lower lip have been reported, there have been few in whom

cervical webbing existed. Davis (1950) reported such a case, and Wynn-Williams (1952) cited two examples. In the first, a 7 year old child had a midline cleft in the anterior cervical region that extended from the cranial end of the cleft to the symphysis menti. The base of the cleft appeared fibrotic but was not attached to the deeper structures. The floor of the cleft was slightly depressed below the normal skin at its cranial end and gradually increased in depth to end in a blind pit 0.64 cm in depth at the suprasternal notch. The skin in the cleft

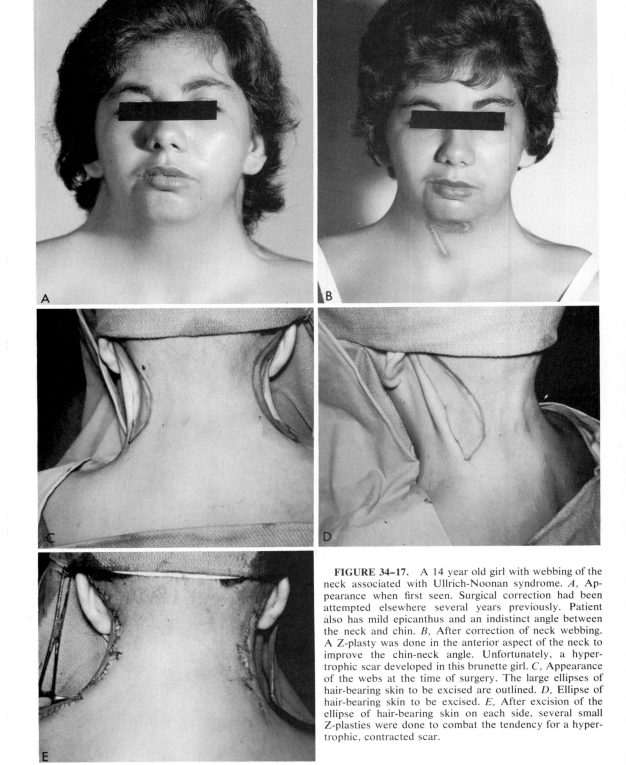

FIGURE 34–17. A 14 year old girl with webbing of the neck associated with Ullrich-Noonan syndrome. *A,* Appearance when first seen. Surgical correction had been attempted elsewhere several years previously. Patient also has mild epicanthus and an indistinct angle between the neck and chin. *B,* After correction of neck webbing. A Z-plasty was done in the anterior aspect of the neck to improve the chin-neck angle. Unfortunately, a hypertrophic scar developed in this brunette girl. *C,* Appearance of the webs at the time of surgery. The large ellipses of hair-bearing skin to be excised are outlined. *D,* Ellipse of hair-bearing skin to be excised. *E,* After excision of the ellipse of hair-bearing skin on each side, several small Z-plasties were done to combat the tendency for a hypertrophic, contracted scar.

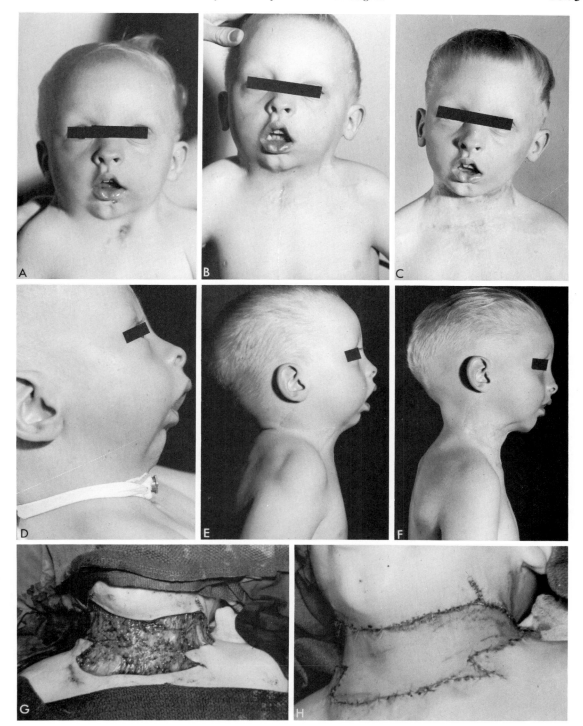

FIGURE 34–18. The Robin anomalad with short neck. *A*, Frontal view. Suturing of the tongue to the lip did not relieve respiratory obstruction, and a tracheotomy had been performed. *B*, Appearance after Z-plasty correction of the lateral webs. *C*, After addition of skin to the neck by the split-thickness skin graft technique. *D*, Lateral view showing generalized vertical shortness of the skin of the neck with lateral webbing. Note tracheostomy tube. *E*, Appearance after Z-plasty on each side of the neck. *F*, Appearance after split-thickness skin grafting of the anterior neck. *G*, Size of the wound after transverse releasing incision of the anterior neck. *H*, Thick (0.017 inch) split-thickness skin graft immediately after application. A special molded collar splint, as shown in Figure 34–3, was worn continuously for five months.

was slightly reddened and had a cracked, desquamating appearance. The cleft was excised and a large Z-plasty done to relieve the web.

The second patient was a 12 year old girl. There was a projecting tag of skin with a small depression in the skin caudal to it in the midline of the neck just below the symphysis menti. The depression was 1.27 cm in length and 0.32 cm wide and was cranial to the hyoid. A subcutaneous fibrous band extended inferiorly from the caudal end of the cleft to the suprasternal notch. The soft tissues of the neck were tight, and the normal chin angle was obliterated. The mandible was underdeveloped. Roentgenograms of the mandible showed a congenital midline cyst. The skin tag and cleft were excised, together with the fibrous band, as far as the suprasternal notch, and a double Z-plasty was done.

There was some hypertrophic scarring of the Z-incision. A similar case is shown in Figure 34–19.

CONGENITAL MUSCULAR TORTICOLLIS

Torticollis (literally "twisted neck") is the term used for both congenital and acquired deformities of both organic and psychogenic origin. The deformity is frequently known as wryneck. Other terms are collum distortum and caput obstipum (Hough, 1934). Scoliosis capitis is descriptive of the skeletal deformity of the head (Middleton, 1930).

The condition results from a shortening of the sternocleidomastoid muscle and is characterized by a tilting of the head to the affected side, while the chin points up and to the opposite side. The shoulder is higher on the affected side, and the external ear may sometimes be more prominent on this side. Either the sternal or the clavicular head may predominate (Figs. 34–20 and 34–21), or both heads may participate equally in the shortness. Attempts to turn the head in the opposite direc-

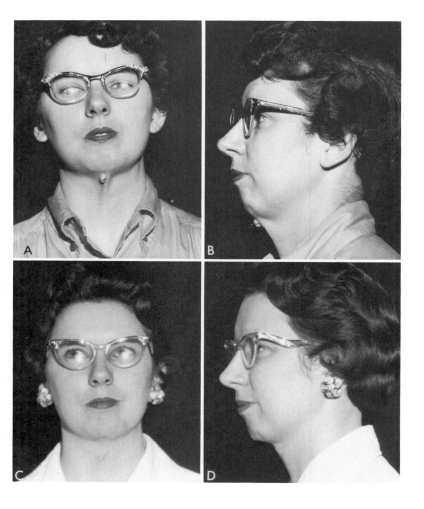

FIGURE 34–19. Congenital midline web of the neck. *A,* Frontal view. *B,* Profile. *C, D,* After excision of the skin tag and Z-plasty correction of the web. (Courtesy of Dr. T. A. Cresswell.)

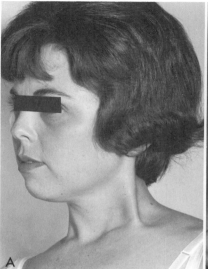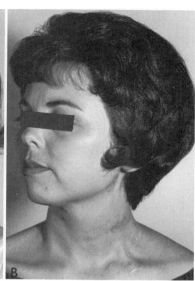

FIGURE 34–20. Thirty year old woman without history of tumor of the sternocleidomastoid muscle. Torticollis was first noted when she was ten years of age. *A*, Shortness predominant in the clavicular head. Note elevation of the shoulder and head tilt. *B*, Appearance following excision of the upper 3.7 cm of the sternocleidomastoid muscle and all of the clavicular head; the sternal head was left intact. Incisions were made just below the tip of the mastoid and another over the middle of the neck. A small stab incision was made over the clavicle, through which a bony exostosis was removed.

tion are limited by the tightness of the shortened sternocleidomastoid muscle. Bilateral torticollis has been reported by Von Muralt (1946).

When the condition persists beyond a few weeks in infancy, an asymmetry develops in which the face and skull on the affected side appear smaller.

The skeletal deformity is reversible if the contracture is released during the period of growth. However, in adults and older teenagers little, if any, change can be expected.

History. Torticollis has been recognized and reported for centuries, and treatment is known to have been attempted long ago. Lidge, Bechtol, and Lambert (1957) stated that Girolama Fabrizio d'Aguapendente (1537–1619) devised an apparatus to correct torticollis. They also credited a Dutch surgeon,

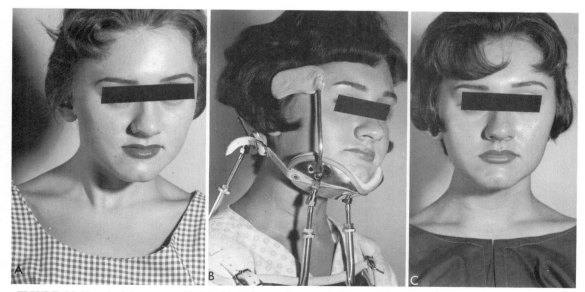

FIGURE 34–21. A sixteen year old girl with a history of sternocleidomastoid "tumor" in infancy. Attempts to correct the head tilt by positioning were not successful. *A*, Frontal view. The sternal head predominates. *B*, Adjustable brace worn for two months following surgery according to the technique of the author. Note extension to the temple to secure additional positive overcorrection of the head tilt. *C*, Appearance two months after surgical correction.

Isacius Minnius, with performance of the first tenotomy. Hulbert (1950), however, stated that tenotomy probably dates at least from the second century. Taylor (1875) was the first to describe the pathology of the sternocleidomastoid muscle.

Classification. Many classifications of the different forms of torticollis have been suggested. The following is a simple classification:

  I. Congenital
     a. Muscular
     b. Vertebral maldevelopment
  II. Acquired
     a. Secondary or acute (cold drafts, infection, or trauma)
     b. Ocular: hypertropia or hypotropia
     c. Spasmodic or neurogenic
     d. Psychogenic

Etiology. The cause of congenital torticollis is unknown. Many explanations have been suggested but none has been fully substantiated.

Stromeyer (1838) suggested that rupture of the sternomastoid and hematoma formation during labor could cause the condition, but the presence of a hematoma has never been demonstrated.

Middleton (1930) offered experimental evidence to support his theory of venous occlusion, and this is perhaps the most reasonable explanation of the pathogenesis which has yet been offered.

Lidge, Bechtol, and Lambert (1957) cited 87 references to the high incidence of breech and other abnormal obstetric presentations, but torticollis has been reported in infants delivered by cesarean section (Roemer, 1954). Chandler (1948) believed that intrauterine malposition causes pressure and ischemia of the muscle, predisposing it to damage by a traumatic or even normal delivery which would not injure a normal muscle. Kiesewetter and others (1955) thought that intrauterine malposition resulting in ischemia and fibrosis of the muscle might be the cause of the abnormal delivery.

Hellstadius (1927) suggested the possibility of a genetic factor, although a positive family history is rarely obtained. Reye (1951) suggested the possibility of a congenital defect in the development of the muscle anlage.

Incidence. Coventry and Harris (1959), in a study of 7835 well infants, found an incidence of 0.4 per cent (35 out of 7835). The "tumor" was first discovered by the physician in half the cases and by the mother in the other half. This could easily explain the lack of a history of "tumor" in some children who subsequently develop torticollis. Hough (1934) cited the following incidence figures: Tubby reported 0.3 per cent of the children in a surgical hospital (8 cases of 2324 admissions at Evelina Hospital for Children), 0.3 per cent of orthopedic cases (15 of 5079 at Royal National Orthopedic Hospital), less than 0.2 per cent of other patients (9 of 5190); Colonna reported 0.5 per cent (269 of 55,000 at the Hospital for the Ruptured and Crippled). Grieve (1946) found only two cases of muscular torticollis among 4500 recruits, as opposed to 16 cases of ocular torticollis in the same group.

No significant differences according to sex or to the side of the neck involved have been noted.

Clinical Course. In the typical case, a firm, cartilaginous-like "tumor" involving the sternocleidomastoid muscle is discovered at about 10 to 14 days after birth, or sooner. The muscle feels short and inelastic. The head may be tilted to the affected side to a variable degree, while the chin points to the opposite side. The cervical vertebrae are normal. Asymmetry of the face and facial skeleton develops. The swelling may increase for two to four weeks and remain stationary for two or three months, gradually regressing and disappearing in four to eight months. In a few cases, residual shortness of the sternocleidomastoid may remain, producing torticollis and asymmetry. In another small group, torticollis may not be apparent until three or four years later, when the neck elongates.

Coventry and Harris (1959) suggested that whether or not torticollis occurs and when it occurs are dependent upon the ratio of normal muscle to fibrous tissue which remains after disappearance of the sternocleidomastoid "tumor" of infancy.

Differential Diagnosis. The history of sternocleidomastoid "tumor," a short sternocleidomastoid muscle in early life with the head tilted to the same side and the face pointing up and to the other side, and normal cervical vertebrae establish the diagnosis of congenital muscular torticollis.

Severe maldevelopment of the cervical vertebrae might rarely be confused with torticollis, but a roentgenogram would clarify the nature of the deformity.

Ocular torticollis is distinguished by a milder degree of head tilt and lack of contracture of the sternocleidomastoid muscle, so that it is possible to straighten the head. The face looks toward the side of tilt and down, whereas in the muscular form the face looks up and away from the side of tilt. Conjugate ocular movements are abnormal, and hypertropia or hypotropia is present.

Secondary torticollis is usually a temporary, acutely painful condition ascribed to exposure to drafts of cold air, pharyngeal or cervical spine infection, or trauma.

Spasmodic torticollis occurs most frequently in adult life and is characterized by recurring attacks of irregular clonic or tonic contractions of neck muscles which cause intermittent rotation and lateral flexion or extension of the head. Grimacing and blepharospasm may also be present. No single etiologic factor has been established.

Pathology. Middleton (1930) described a cut section of the sternocleidomastoid "tumor" as having the appearance of glistening fibrous tissue. Microscopically, young cellular fibrous tissue is seen containing dispersed remnants of muscle fibers. Many of these fibers show absence of nuclei and vacuolation and are undergoing degeneration.

Middleton believed that the microscopic picture in a fully developed case of torticollis could only be interpreted as representing the terminal stage of a sternocleidomastoid tumor. No degenerating muscle or young fibrous tissue is observed; instead, swathes of adult, noncellular fibrous tissue are seen. Scattered throughout it are collections of muscle fibers, which, though smaller than normal and varying in size and outline, are living, healthy fibers and bear no stigmata of degeneration.

No cases of fibrosarcoma of the sternocleidomastoid muscle have been reported (Gruhn and Hurwitt, 1951).

Treatment. In view of the observed tendency for "tumors" of the sternocleidomastoid muscle in infants to disappear spontaneously with no residual shortening, the majority of writers (Hulbert, 1950; Gruhn and Hurwitt, 1951; Horsley and coworkers, 1954; Coventry and Harris, 1959) advised against surgery on the sternocleidomastoid "tumor." They advocate surgery only for those cases in which torticollis persists after a year. The author also recommends this program.

Chandler and Altenberg (1944), Brown and McDowell (1950), and Clader, Sawyer, and McCurdy (1958) advised early complete excision of the fibrous sternocleidomastoid muscle in well-developed cases. Brown performed the resection through a 5-cm collar incision, ligating the external jugular vein but preserving the eleventh cranial nerve, phrenic nerve, internal jugular vein, and carotid artery. If necessary, the deep fascia or scalene muscles or the anterior border of the trapezius are divided. No postoperative splinting is necessary in these infants.

Those who do not operate on the "tumor" usually suggest massage stretching, or the like, but Coventry and Harris (1959) believe no treatment is as effective as the surgical one.

Treatment of a well-established muscular torticollis has included subcutaneous and open tenotomy of the inferior end of the sternocleidomastoid muscle. Lange (Steindler, 1940) divided the muscle at the upper end, and this approach has been combined with an inferior tenotomy. In Foelderl's procedure (Steindler, 1940), the clavicular head is divided at its attachment, and the sternal head is divided near its middle third. The clavicular head is transposed to the distal sternal head and sutured, thereby lengthening the muscle. Ferté (1947) felt that a 4 cm vertical incision between the clavicular and sternal heads, being in the line of traction when the deformity is corrected, may show less tendency to hypertrophy. He also pointed out that the platysma may be shortened, and, if so, it should also be divided; otherwise, failure may result and prolonged overcorrection may be necessary.

In making a decision as to the proper surgical procedure to be chosen, consideration should be given not only to the functional result but also to the cosmetic result, especially in females. Although complete excision of the sternocleidomastoid muscle in infancy does not seem to leave an objectionable hollow in the neck as the child grows, it does so in the teenager or adult. Penn and Kark (1954) performed a dermis-fat graft to correct the unsightly hollow two years after removal of the muscle in a 13 year old girl. Tenotomy at the clavicular end of the muscle may also tend to eliminate the normal prominence of the sternal head.

Recommended Technique. An oblique incision is made about 1.9 cm below the tip of the mastoid down to the muscle. The upper 4 cm of the sternocleidomastoid muscle is exposed, avoiding injury to the greater auricular nerve. The muscle is divided at its bony insertion, great care being taken to identify and preserve the spinal accessory nerve which descends through the muscle. About 2.5 to 4 cm of the muscle is excised. The head is tilted to the opposite side with the chin down and to the affected side, and any other tight fascial or muscle (platysma, anterior scalene, and trapezius) bands are severed. When this has been done, there is usually some tightness remaining in the lower part of the sternocleidomastoid. A short, transverse incision is then made over the muscle about 4 cm above the clavicle. The muscle is completely divided, again with care taken to preserve the spinal accessory nerve. The procedure usually provides freedom of motion of the neck, but the short sternoclavicular heads that remain present an unsightly hollow. If the clavicular head predominates, as in Figure 34–20, the head is completely excised, leaving the sternal head undisturbed.

In all patients who have had torticollis for over a year, it is absolutely essential to hold the head in an overcorrected position for six to eight weeks or longer following the operation; otherwise, the tendency of the patient to hold his head in the former position and the development of scar contracture deep in the wound will result in recurrence of the torticollis.

Soeur (1940) applied a plaster cast from the iliac crest to the top of the head. A ready-made brace* (see Fig. 34–21), which rests on the shoulders and can be adjusted to hold the head in any position, is efficient if properly adjusted. The plaster cast or brace should generally be applied a day or two after operation when the patient has recovered from the effects of the anesthesia.

In severe cases of long-standing torticollis, diplopia may be noted postoperatively, and Soeur (1940) reported that the patient's equilibrium may also be disturbed for a few days.

---

*Hallmark Orthopedic Specialities, 111 N. Santa Anita Blvd., Arcadia, California 91006.

REFERENCES

Aufricht, G.: Evaluation of pedicle flaps versus skin grafts in reconstruction of surface defects and scar contractures of the chin, cheeks and neck. Surgery, *15*:75, 1944.

Babcock, W. W.: Contracted dense scar of the neck despite the use of many Thiersch grafts. Surg. Clin. North Am., *12*:1405, 1932.

Barr, M. L., Bertram, L. F., and Lindsay, H. A.: The morphology of the nerve cell nucleus, according to sex. Anat. Rec., *107*:283, 1950.

Bizzarro, A. H.: Brevicollis. Lancet, *2*:828, 1938.

Blocker, T. G., Jr.: Free full thickness skin grafts for the relief of burn contractures of the neck. South. Surg., *10*:849, 1941.

Brown, J. B., and McDowell, F.: Wry-neck facial distortion prevented by resection of fibrosed sternomastoid muscle in infancy and childhood. Ann. Surg., *131*:721, 1950.

Brown, J. B., and McDowell, F.: Skin grafting. Philadelphia, J. B. Lippincott Company, 1958, p. 234.

Brown, J. B., Byars, L. T., and Blair, V. P.: Repair of surface defects resulting from full thickness loss of skin from burns. South. Med. J., *28*:408, 1935.

Chandler, F. A.: Webbed neck (pterygium colli). Am. J. Dis. Child., *53*:798, 1937.

Chandler, F. A.: Muscular torticollis. J. Bone Joint Surg., *30A*:566, 1948.

Chandler, F. A., and Altenberg, A.: "Congenital" muscular torticollis. J.A.M.A., *125*:476, 1944.

Clader, D. N., Sawyer, K. C., and McCurdy, R. E.: Surgical treatment of congenital torticollis. Am. Surg., *24*:132, 1958.

Converse, J. M.: Burn deformities of the face and neck, reconstructive surgery and rehabilitation. Surg. Clin. North Am., *47*:323, 1967.

Coughlin, W. T.: Contractures due to burns. Surg. Gynecol. Obstet., *68*:352, 1939.

Coventry, M. B., and Harris, I. E.: Congenital muscular torticollis in infancy. J. Bone Joint Surg., *41A*:815, 1959.

Cramer, L. M.: Cervical splinting for burn contracture. Plast. Reconstr. Surg., *34*:293, 1964.

Cronin, T. D.: Successful correction of extensive scar contractures of the neck using split skin grafts. *In* Skoog, T., and Ivy, R. H. (Eds.): Transactions of the International Society of Plastic Surgeons (First Congress, 1955). Baltimore, The Williams & Wilkins Company, 1957, p. 123.

Cronin, T. D.: The use of a molded splint to prevent contracture after split skin grafting on the neck. Plast. Reconstr. Surg., *27*:7, 1961.

Cronin, T. D.: Unpublished method of correcting cervical webs, 1961a.

Cronin, T. D.: Burn scar contractures of the neck. *In* Lynch, J. D., and Lewis, S. R. (Eds.): Symposium on the Treatment of Burns. Vol. 5. St. Louis, Mo., The C. V. Mosby Company, 1973.

Cunningham, G. C., and Harley, J. F.: A case of Turner's syndrome. J. Pediatr., *38*:738, 1951.

Davis, A. D.: Medial cleft of the lower lip and mandible. Plast. Reconstr. Surg., *6*:62, 1950.

Davis, A. D.: Congenital webbing of the neck (pterygium colli). Am. J. Surg., *92*:115, 1956.

Davis, J. S., and Kitlowski, E. A.: The theory and practical use of the Z-incision for the relief of scar contractures. Ann. Surg., *109*:1001, 1939.

Dingman, R. O.: Some applications of Z-plastic procedure. Plast. Reconstr. Surg., *16*:246, 1955.

Dingman, R. O.: The surgical correction of burn scar contractures of the neck. Surg. Clin. North Am., *41*:1169, 1961.

Dowd, C. N.: Some details in the repair of cicatricial contractures of the neck. Surg. Gynecol. Obstet., *44*:396, 1927.

Durham, R. H.: Encyclopedia of Medical Syndromes. New York, Paul B. Hoeber, Inc., 1960.

Evans, E. B., Larson, D. L., Abston, S., and Willis, B.: Prevention and correction of deformity after severe burns. Surg. Clin. North Am., *50*:1361, 1970.

Ferté, A. D.: The role of the platysma muscle in torticollis deformity. Plast. Reconstr. Surg., 2:72, 1947.

Flavell, G.: Webbing of neck with Turner syndrome in the male. Br. J. Surg., 31:150, 1943.

Ford, C. E., and Hamerton, J. L.: Chromosomes of man. Nature, 178:1020, 1956.

Ford, C. E., Jones, K. W., Polani, P. E., de Almeida, J. C., and Briggs, J. H.: A sex-chromosome anomaly in a case of gonadal dysgenesis (Turner's syndrome). Lancet, 1:711, 1959.

Foucar, H. O.: Pterygium colli and allied conditions. Can. Med. Assoc. J., 59:251, 1948.

Frackelton, W. H.: Neck burns—early and late treatment. In Skoog, T., and Ivy, R. H. (Eds.): Transactions of the International Soceity of Plastic Surgeons (First Congress, 1955). Baltimore, The Williams & Wilkins Company, 1957, p. 130.

Fujimori, A., Huramoto, M., and Ofuji, S.: Sponge fixation method of eary scars. Plast. Reconstr. Surg., 42:322, 1968.

Funke: Pterygium colli. Dtsch. Z. Chir., 3:162, 1902.

Furnas, D., and Fischer, G. W.: The Z-plasty: biomechanics and mathematics. Br. J. Plast. Surg., 24:134, 1971.

Gibbons, W. P.: Innovations of skin grafting as applied to chin-chest contractures. Plast. Reconstr. Surg., 35:322, 1965.

Gillies, H.: Experience with tubed pedicle flaps. Surg. Gynecol. Obstet., 60:291, 1935.

Gilmour, J. R.: The essential identity of the Klippel-Feil syndrome and iniencephaly. J. Pathol. Bacteriol., 53:117, 1941.

Ginestet, G., Merville, L., and Dupuis, A.: Le traitement des sequelles de brulures de la face et du cou par lambeaux cylindriques. Ann. Chir. Plast., 4:81, 1959.

Gottlieb, E.: Prolonged postoperative pressure as an adjunct to plastic surgery of the neck. Plast. Reconstr. Surg., 32:600, 606, 1963.

Greeley, P. W.: Plastic repair of scar contractures. Surgery, 15:224, 1944.

Grieve, J.: The relative incidence of sternomastoid and ocular torticollis in air crew recruits. Br. J. Surg., 33:285, 1946.

Gruhn, J., and Hurwitt, E. S.: Fibrous sternomastoid tumor of infancy. Pediatrics, 8:522, 1951.

Harii, K., Ohmori, K., and Ohmori, S.: Personal communication, 1974.

Hellstadius, A.: Torticollis congenita. Acta Chir. Scand., 62:586, 1927.

Horsley, G. E., Pitman, N., and Schuler, J. D.: Fibrous sternocleidomastoid tumor of infancy. J. Tennessee Med. Assoc., 47:20, 1954.

Hough, G. de N., Jr.: Congenital torticollis. Surg. Gynecol. Obstet., 58:972, 1934.

Hulbert, K. F.: Congenital torticollis. J. Bone Joint Surg., 32B:50, 1950.

Jackson, W. P. U., and Sougin-Mibashan, R.: Turner's syndrome in the female. Br. Med. J., 2:368, 1953.

Jones, P. G.: Torticollis in Infancy and Childhood: Sternomastoid Fibrosis and Sternomastoid "Tumor." Springfield, Ill., Charles C Thomas, Publisher, 1968.

Jost, A.: Sur les effets de la castration precoce de l'embryon male de lapin. C. R. Soc. Biol., 141:126, 1947.

Kazanjian, V. H.: The repair of contractures resulting from burns. New Engl. J. Med., 215:1100, 1936.

Kiesewetter, W. B., Nelson, P. K., Palladino, V. S., and Koop, C. E.: Neonatal torticollis. J.A.M.A., 157:1281, 1955.

Kirschbaum, S.: Mento-sternal contracture. Plast. Reconstr. Surg., 21:131, 1958.

Klippel, M., and Feil, A.: Anomalie de la colonne vertébrale par absence des vertébres cervicales-Cage thoracique remontant jusqu'à la base du crane. Bull. Soc. Anat. (Paris), 87:185, 1912.

Kobylinski, O.: Ueber eine flughautahnliche Austreitung am Halse. Arch. Anthropol., 14:343, 1883.

Koepke, G. H.: The role of physical medicine in the treatment of burns. Surg. Clin. North Am., 50:1385, 1970.

Koepke, G. H., and Feller, I.: Physical measures for the prevention and treatment of deformities following burns. J.A.M.A., 199:791, 1971.

La Ruffa, H.: Cirugia de las membranas cervicales alares (Pterygium colli). Boletines y Trabajos Sociedad Argentina de Cirujanos, 31:572, 1970.

Levy, E. P., Pashayan, H., and Fraser, F. C.: XX and XY Turner phenotype in a family. Am. J. Dis. Child., 120:36, 1970.

Lidge, R. T., Bechtol, R. C., and Lambert, C. N.: Congenital muscular torticollis. J. Bone Joint Surg., 39A:1165, 1957.

MacCollum, D. W.: The early and late treatment of burns in children. Am. J. Surg., 39:275, 1938a.

MacCollum, D. W.: Congenital webbing of the neck. New Engl. J. Med., 219:251, 1938b.

McIndoe, A. H.: Total facial reconstruction following burns. Postgrad. Med., 6:187, 1949.

Martins, A. G.: Burn contractures. Br. J. Plast. Surg., 13:152, 1960.

May, H.: The correction of cicatricial deformities. Surg. Clin. North Am., 29:611, 1949.

May, H.: Reconstructive and Reparative Surgery. 2nd Ed. Philadelphia, F. A. Davis Company, 1958.

Mendoza, C. A., Benzecry, A., Hernandez, M. C., Sanchez, C., and DeLima, A.: Prevention of contractures following burns. Bol. Soc. Venez. Cirug., 15:381, 1961.

Mennig, H.: Die plastiche Operation des Pterygium Colli. Z. Laryngol. Rhinol. Otol., 35:153, 1956.

Middleton, D. S.: The pathology of congenital torticollis. Br. J. Surg., 18:188, 1930.

Mixter, C. S.: Contractions of the neck following burns. New Engl. J. Med., 208:190, 1933.

Moore, D. G.: The role of the maxillofacial prosthetist in support of the burn patient. J. Prosthet. Dent., 24:68, 1970.

Mukhin, M. V., and Mamonov, A. F.: Classification of scarred neck contractures and their surgical therapy by methods of local plastic operation. Acta Chir. Plast. (Praha), 12:48, 1970.

Muralt, R. H. von: Bilateral occurrence of congenital muscular torticollis. Helv. Paediatr. Acta, 1:349, 1946.

Nora, J. J., and Sinka, A. K.: Direct male to male transmission of the XX Phenotype. Lancet, 1:250, 1970.

Nora, J. J., Nora, A. H., and Sinka, A. K.: The Ullrich-Noonan syndrome (Turner phenotype). Am. J. Dis. Child., 127:48, 1974.

Ousterhout, D. K., Yeakel, M. H., Lau, B. M., and Tumbush, W. T.: Inflatable splint: an adjunct to prevention and treatment of cervical scar contractures. Br. J. Surg., 22:185, 1969.

Padgett, E. C.: Full thickness skin graft in correction of soft tissue deformities. J.A.M.A., 98:18, 1932.

Padgett, E. C., and Stephenson, K. L.: Plastic and Reconstructive Surgery. Springfield, Ill., Charles C Thomas, Publisher, 1948, p. 627.

Penn, J., and Kark, W.: Surgical treatment of a case of wryneck. S. Afr. Med. J., 28:929, 1954.

Pitanguy, I.: Cervical contractures. *In* Skoog, T., and Ivy, R. H. (Eds.): Transactions of the International Society of Plastic Surgeons (First Congress, 1955). Batlimore, The Williams & Wilkins Company, 1957, p. 147.

Pitanguy, I., and Bisaggio, S.: Retracoes, cicatriciais do pescoco. Rev. Bras. Cirurg., *53*:469, 1967.

Polani, P. E., Hunter, W. F., and Lennox, B.: Chromosomal sex in Turner's syndrome with coarctation of the aorta. Lancet, *2*:120, 1954.

Polani, P. E., Lessof, M. H., and Bishop, P. M. F.: Color blindness in "ovarian agenesis" (gonadal dysplasia). Lancet, *2*:118, 1956.

Reye, R. D. K.: Sternomastoid tumor and congenital muscular torticollis. Med. J. Aust., *1*:867, 1951.

Roemer, F. J.: Relation of torticollis to breech delivery. Am. J. Obstet. Gynecol., *68*:1146, 1954.

Schmid, E., and Romacher, W.: Chirurgie réparatrice du cou et du menton après brulures. Ann. Chir. Plast., *4*:51, 1959.

Schneider, R. W., and McCullagh, E. P.: Infantilism, congenital webbed neck and cubitus valgus (Turner Syndrome). Cleveland Clin. Quart., *10*:112, 1943.

Schröder, F.: Die operative Korrektur des Pterygium Colli. Arch. Klin. Chir., *289*:643, 1958.

Smith, F.: Plastic and Reconstructive Surgery. Philadelphia, W. B. Saunders Company, 1950, p. 666.

Soeur, R.: Treatment of congenital torticollis. J. Bone Joint Surg., *22*:35, 459, 1940.

Sougin-Mibashan, R., and Jackson, W. P. U.: Turner's syndrome in the male. Br. Med. J., *2*:371, 1953.

Spina, V.: Tratamento Cirurgico das Cicatrizes do Pescoco Pos-Queimadura. V. Spina, Sao Paulo, Brazil, 1955.

Steiker, D. D., Mellman, W. J., Bongiovanni, A. M., Eberlain, W. R., and LeBoeuf, G.: Turner's syndrome in the male. J. Pediatr., *58*:321, 1961.

Steindler, A.: Orthopedic Operations. Springfield, Ill., Charles C Thomas, Publisher, 1940.

Stromeyer, G. F. L.: Beitrage zur operativen Orthopädik, Hellwing, Hännover, 1838; cited by Gruhn and Hurwitt (1951).

Tanzer, R. C.: Burn contracture of the neck. Plast. Reconstr. Surg., *33*:207, 1964.

Taylor, F.: Induration of the sternomastoid muscle. Trans. Pathol. Soc. Lond., *26*:224, 1875.

Tjio, J. H., and Levan, A.: The chromosome number of man. Hereditas, *42*:1, 1956.

Turner, H. H.: A syndrome of infantilism, congenital webbed neck, and cubitus valgus. Endocrinology, *23*:566, 1938.

Wilkins, L., and Fleischmann, W.: Ovarian agenesis; pathology, associated clinical symptoms and bearing on theories of sex differentiation. J. Clin. Endocr., *4*:357, 1944.

Wilkins, L., Grumbach, M. M., and Van Wyk, J. J.: Chromosomal sex in ovarian agenesis. J. Clin. Endocr., *14*:1270, 1954.

Willis, B.: The use of orthoplast isoprene splints in the treatment of the acutely burned child. Am. J. Occup. Ther., *24*:187, 1970.

Wilson, R. D.: Personal communication, 1974.

Wilson, R. D., Knapp, C., Traber, D. L., and Evans, B.: Safe management of the child with a contracted neck. South. Med. J., *63*:1420, 1970.

Wynn-Williams, D.: Congenital midline cervical cleft and web. Br. J. Plast. Surg., *5*:87, 1952.

CHAPTER 35

DEFORMITIES OF THE AURICLE

RADFORD C. TANZER, M.D., RICHARD J. BELLUCCI, M.D., JOHN MARQUIS CONVERSE, M.D., AND BURT BRENT, M.D.

Congenital Deformities

RADFORD C. TANZER, M.D.

A radical change in the outlook for the results of ear reconstruction has occurred in recent years. Instead of a feeling of bafflement and frustration, one notes encouraging efforts to construct cosmetically acceptable ears that will relieve the patient's anxiety. Material will be presented in this chapter to help the surgeon choose methods which are least fraught with complications and which will give the greatest insurance of permanence of the reconstructed auricular appendage. Evidence has accumulated that a primary ear reconstruction, using unscarred tissue, has an overriding advantage over a secondary repair and that strict adherence to all of the principles of wound healing is essential to avoid disastrous complications.

HISTORY OF AURICLE RECONSTRUCTION

The first reference to ear reconstruction appeared in the Susruta Samhita (Bhishagratna, 1907), in which a cheek flap was suggested as a substitute for the missing lobule. Tagliacozzi (1597) described the restoration of defects of the upper and lower ear by the use of hairless, retroauricular skin flaps and even suggested the supposedly modern technique of using postauricular wedges to maintain ear position. His contemporary Cortesi (Gnudi and Webster, 1950) emphasized a point that is relevant today—namely that restoration of the upper half of the ear carries the danger of crumpling, whereas the lower half can be much more readily and permanently restored. Dieffenbach (1845) described the restoration of partial defects, and Szymanowski (1870) suggested the complete reconstruction of the auricle by means of bilobular scalp flaps.

Toward the end of the nineteenth century, attention was directed toward the correction of congenital deformities of the ear. Several techniques, many of them revivals of early suggestions, are classified under the section on Prominent Ear.

The surgical correction of microtia received a decided stimulus during the early part of the twentieth century when Gillies (1920) reproduced the auricle by burying carved rib cartilage under the skin of the mastoid region, then lifting it outward and covering the defect with a cervical skin flap. Pierce (1930) refined this method by using a skin graft to cover the new auriculocephalic sulcus and by adding a thin, tubed, cervical skin flap to form the helix. Preserved cartilage allografts and maternal cartilage (Gillies, 1937) were popular for a brief time until both were found to have a high incidence of absorption. Recently, investigative work has centered around the use of autogenous rib or conchal cartilage and of various types of inorganic implants (see section on Complete Hypoplasia).

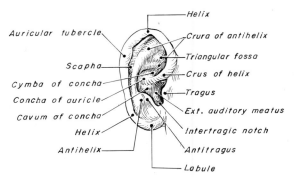

FIGURE 35-1.   Anatomy of the auricle.

The luxuriant blood supply is derived principally from the superficial temporal and posterior auricular arteries. The sensory nerve supply stems mainly from the anterior and posterior branches of the greater auricular nerve, with lesser contributions from the auriculotemporal and lesser occipital nerves (Fig. 35-2, *A, B*). Regional anesthesia of the auricle is readily accomplished by instilling an anesthetic solution along its base anteriorly and posteriorly (Fig. 35-3). At times a supplement may be needed at the posterior wall of the external auditory meatus, an area supplied by the auricular branches of the vagus nerve.

ANATOMY

The auricle (or pinna), diverging from the side of the head at an angle of approximately 30 degrees, consists of a delicate shell of elastic cartilage whose thin integument is more closely adherent laterally than medially. The anatomical landmarks of the auricle are defined in Figure 35-1. The helical border terminates anteriorly in a crus, which lies almost horizontally above the external auditory meatus. The anthelix, crowning the posterior conchal wall, diverges into superior and anterior crura enclosing the triangular fossa. Between the helix and anthelix lies a long, deep furrow, the scapha. The conchal cavity, composed of cymba and cavum, arises from a floor which is at least a centimeter deeper than the overlying tragus and antitragus. Viewed laterally, the denuded cartilage conforms almost exactly to the surface contours, except that the inferior tip of the helical cartilage, the cauda, is separated from the antitragus by a deep fissure and is absent in the fleshy lobule (see Fig. 35-1).

EMBRYOLOGY

The human ear consists of a sound conducting apparatus, which includes both the external and middle ears, and a receptive sense organ, the inner ear. Since the embryologic derivation is quite different, the middle and external ears can undergo anomalous changes in the presence of normal inner ear development, although all components are not infrequently involved.

The Inner Ear. A thickening of the ectoderm, termed the auditory placode, first noted in the three-week embryo dorsal to the future site of the auricle, sinks into the underlying mesenchyme, forming a vesicle called the *otocyst,* which later elongates and divides into a vestibular and cochlear pouch. It attains its final membranous labyrinthine stage before the twelfth week.

The Middle Ear. The middle ear and eustachian tube develop from the first entodermal

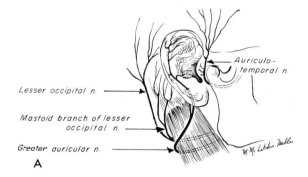

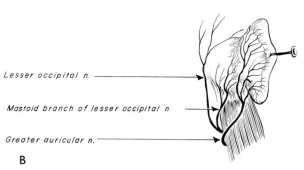

FIGURE 35–2. Sensory nerve supply of the auricle.

pharyngeal pouch, while the otocyst is still connected with the ectoderm. Enlarging rapidly, the pouch comes into temporary contact with the ectoderm, then constricts to form the auditory tube while the blind outer end enlarges to form the tympanic cavity. The ossicles originate in the first and second branchial arches, the incus and malleus arising in the first and the stapes in the second arch (Fig. 35–4).

The External Ear.   The external ear traces development from the first branchial cleft and from portions of the adjacent first (mandibular) and second (hyoid) arches. At the end of the second month the ectoderm sinks inward, forming a funnel-shaped depression, the primary meatus, connected with the expanding tympanic cavity by a solid strand of epithelial cells, the meatal plate, which at the seventh month develops a lumen destined to become the osseous component of the external auditory canal (see Fig. 35–4). The tympanic membrane is represented by a thinned-out diaphragm of mesoderm lying between this canal and the tympanic cavity.

The auricle is formed from six hillocks which first appear in the five-week embryo clustered about the first branchial cleft, three

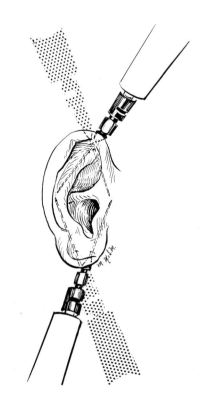

FIGURE 35–3.   Technique of regional anesthesia of the auricle.

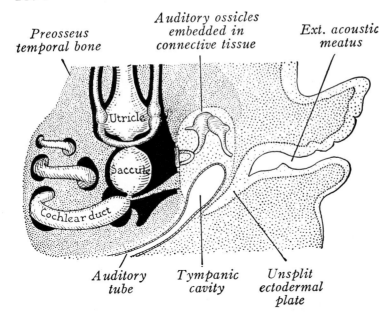

Preosseus temporal bone　*Auditory ossicles embedded in connective tissue*　*Ext. acoustic meatus*

Utricle

Saccule

Cochlear duct

Auditory tube　*Tympanic cavity*　*Unsplit ectodermal plate*

FIGURE 35–4. Partly schematic section of the ear in a three-month embryo. (From Arey, L. B.: Developmental Anatomy. 6th Ed. Philadelphia, W. B. Saunders Company, 1954.)

on the posterior border of the first arch and three on the anterior border of the second arch (Fig. 35–5) (His, 1899; Streeter, 1922; Arey, 1954). Although the relationship of the hillocks to specific pinnal structures is rather obscure, investigations appear to show that the greater contribution comes from the hyoid arch (Streeter, 1922; Wood-Jones and Wen I-Chuan, 1934). The first and sixth hillocks maintain a fairly constant position, marking the sites of development of the tragus and antitragus respectively, whereas the fourth and fifth tubercles expand and rotate across the dorsal end of the cleft, giving rise to the anterior and superior helix and to the adjacent portion of the body of the auricle. Growth of the auricular portion of the mandibular arch is suppressed, contributing to the formation of only the tragus and anterior crus helicis (Streeter, 1922; Wood-Jones and Wen I-Chuan, 1934) (Fig. 35–6).

The auricle and the primary (or cartilaginous) external auditory meatus originally lie quite near the ventral surface of the head, but they migrate in a dorsal and superior direction at the same time that the entire foregut, together with the tympanic cavity, moves ventrally and inferiorly. Eventually, the primary meatus and tympanic cavity reach the same level, and amalgamation begins.

ETIOLOGY

Hereditary Factors. Although no specific chromosomal aberrations have been identified, the hereditary transmission of several types of auricular anomaly has been clearly established. Preauricular pits and sinuses, and a combination of pits, preauricular appendages, cupping deformity, and deafness are all hereditarily dominant (Wildervanck, 1962; Minkowitz and Minkowitz, 1964). Deafness associated with

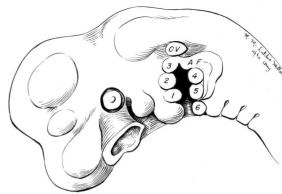

FIGURE 35–5. Development of the auricle in a five-week human embryo: *1* to *6*, elevations (hillocks) on the mandibular and hyoid arches; ov, otic vesicle. (After Arey.)

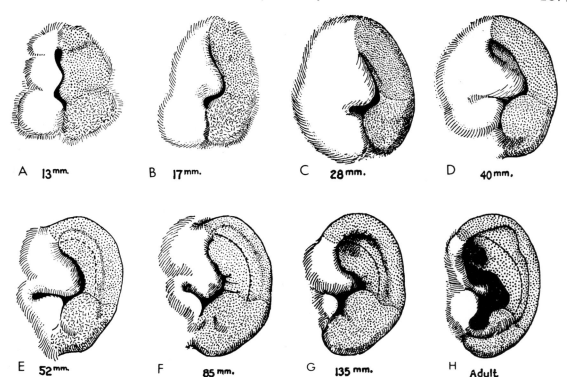

A 13 mm.   B 17 mm.   C 28 mm.   D 40 mm.

E 52 mm.   F 85 mm.   G 135 mm.   H Adult

FIGURE 35–6. Depiction of the retardation of growth of the auricular component of the mandibular arch and the expansion and forward rotation of the component of the hyoid arch. (After Streeter; from Patten, M.: Human Embryology. 3rd Ed. New York, McGraw-Hill Book Company, 1968. Used with permission of McGraw-Hill Book Company.)

several auricular abnormalities has revealed both dominant and recessive characteristics (Königsmark, 1969). The frequent appearance in families of mandibulofacial dysostosis (Rogers, 1964), as well as the cup ear deformity (Potter, 1937; Hanhart, 1949; Erich and Abu-Jamra, 1965; Kessler, 1967), is well known.

Hanhart (1949) found a rather severe form of microtia associated with a cleft or high palate in 10 per cent of family members studied, and Tanzer (1971a), in a study of 43 cases of severe microtia, found ten patients with relatives displaying evidence of the first and second branchial arch syndrome (craniofacial microsomia). Microtia was one of the manifestations in four instances.

Specific Factors. Caronni (1971) is a proponent of McKenzie and Craig's theory (1955) that ear anomalies, together with some other head defects such as cleft palate, are the product of an ischemic factor created by a lag, after the obliteration of the stapedial artery, in the development of an anastomotic circulation to the affected areas through the external carotid and internal maxillary arteries.

The association between rubella appearing during the critical phase of pregnancy and the occurrence of deafness and occasional microtia is well known; other infections may play a less obvious role. Drug ingestion during the first three months of pregnancy should always be investigated, bearing in mind the dramatic teratogenic defects produced by thalidomide. (See also Craniofacial Microsomia, Chapter 54.)

DIAGNOSIS

Classification. Various classifications of congenital auricular deformities have been suggested, none of which is completely satisfactory. Rogers (1968) noted that most types of auricular hypoplasia can be arranged in a descending scale of severity, which corresponds quite closely to the pattern of embryologic development of the auricle as depicted by Streeter (1922). He divides defects into four groups: (1) microtia; (2) lop ear, represented by folding or deficiency of the superior helix and scapha; (3) cup ear, with a deep concha

TABLE 35–1. *Clinical Classification of Auricular Defects (Tanzer)*

I. Anotia
II. Complete hypoplasia (microtia)
   A. With atresia of external auditory canal
   B. Without atresia of external auditory canal
III. Hypoplasia of middle third of the auricle
IV. Hypoplasia of superior third of the auricle
   A. Constricted (cup and lop) ear
   B. Cryptotia
   C. Hypoplasia of entire superior third
V. Prominent ear

and deficiency of the superior helix and anthelical crura; and (4) the common prominent or protruding ear.

Tanzer has used a classification, roughly correlated with embryologic development, which, in addition, conveniently groups according to the surgical approach to reconstruction (Table 35–1).

Associated Deformities. A significant malformation of the auricle occurring as an isolated form is unusual. Sinuses, fistulas, and supernumerary appendages are frequently found along the fusion line between the first and second branchial arch elements, although tracts are occasionally found between the external auditory meatus and the angle of the mandible, presumably associated with abnormal migration of the ear (Fig. 35–7).

One of the commonest associated defects involves the external auditory canal and the contents of the middle ear. The deformity ranges, in the full-blown form of microtia, from atresia of the canal, combined with severely distorted, fused, and hypoplastic ossicles and failure of pneumatization of the mastoid cells, to minor ossicular abnormalities and diminished caliber

of the canal. Hearing impairment is usual. (See Indications, Contraindications, and Timing of Middle Ear Surgery later in chapter.)

The term *first and second branchial arch syndrome* (hemifacial microsomia) has been applied to a condition which, in its fullest genetic expression, includes defects of the external and middle ear, hypoplasia of the mandible, maxilla, and malar and temporal bones, macrostomia, lateral facial clefts, and atrophy of the facial musculature and occasionally of the lingual and palatal muscles and parotid gland (May, 1962; Longacre, DeStefano and Holmstrand, 1963; Grabb, 1965). Characterized initially as a unilateral condition, more careful study has shown a bilateral presence, often only in microform, in almost every instance. Subtle mandibular anomalies are most common (Converse and coworkers, 1973). Gorlin and Pindborg (1964) use the term *hemifacial microsomia* for a unilateral syndrome which is otherwise identical with the foregoing. Converse and coworkers (1974) have popularized the terms *unilateral* and *bilateral facial microsomia*.*

Anomalies of the kidneys and other parts of the urogenital tract have an increased incidence in the presence of microtia (Vincent, Ryan and Longenecker, 1961; Longenecker, Ryan and Vincent, 1965), particularly when accompanied by other evidence of the first and second branchial arch syndrome (Taylor, 1965).

COMPLETE HYPOPLASIA (MICROTIA)

Clinical Characteristics

Microtia, an imprecise term usually applied to severe types of hypoplasia combined with a blind or absent external auditory canal, occurs about once in every 6000 births (Grabb, 1965; Kaseff, 1967). It is twice as frequent in males as in females, and the right-left-bilateral ratio is roughly 5:3:1 (Dupertuis and Musgrave, 1959; Ogino, 1964).

Anotia is extremely rare in Western populations and more frequent in Japan. Almost always one finds at least some semblance of a lobule, lying in a vertical axis, surmounted by a vestige of skin containing a tightly rolled up, two-layered ball of crumpled cartilage, which

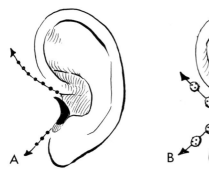

FIGURE 35–7. Line of occurrence of preauricular sinuses (*A*) located slightly posterior to the line of the preauricular appendages (*B*).

*In this text, the term craniofacial microsomia (see Chapter 54) designates the unilateral as well as the bilateral form of the malformation (J.M.C.).

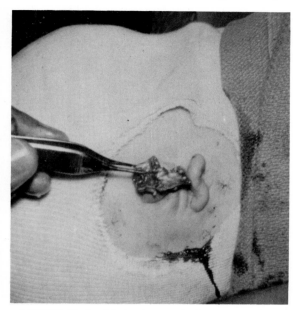

FIGURE 35–8. Diminutive cartilaginous remnant, removed and opened to show the semblance of a tiny auricle.

can be opened to display some rudiments of the auricular structure (Fig. 35–8). Webster (1944) used a flattened sheet of this cartilage as a graft in hopes of obtaining continued growth, but this concept proved to be impractical. The surface of the nubbin usually contains two or three shallow pits, but actual sinus tracts are infrequent. In the most severe forms, atresia of the ear canal is almost invariably present, including absence of the bony canal, but the presence of a diminutive conchal cavity is sometimes combined with a hypoplastic meatus and a canal ending in a blind sac several millimeters below the skin surface. In most instances, the hypoplastic lobule lies superior to the level of the opposite normal lobule, but occasionally an incomplete migration of the ear results in an inferior location.

Preauricular appendages are a frequent concomitant. Approximately half of the cases of microtia are associated with gross forms of hemifacial atrophy, muscle weakness, macrosomia, hypoplasia of the maxilla, mandible, and zygomas, or other evidence of maldevelopment of the first and second branchial arches (Fig. 35–9). Converse and associates (1973, 1974), however, have demonstrated, by tomographic techniques, skeletal evidence of the syndrome in all of their patients with microtia (see Chapter 54).

The Hearing Problem

Pathology. A correlation exists between the severity of the auricular deformity and the middle ear defects. The latter range from isolated deformities of the ossicles, of which fusion or hypoplasia of the malleus and incus are most common, to complete atresia of the tympanic cavity and absence of the ossicles. Although it has been assumed that the inner ear, with its separate embryologic derivation, is unaffected, recent refinements in polytomography have, on the contrary, shown occasional dysplasia and hypoplasia in this area (Nauton and Valvassori, 1968; Reisner, 1969). Aberrant positions of the facial nerve render this structure susceptible to injury during middle ear surgery, particularly in the absence of a pneumatized mastoid (see later in this chapter).

Indications for Operation. The advisability of exploring the middle ear in the presence of microtia is still controversial. The reports by Pattee (1947) and others, using fenestration and later stapes mobilization techniques, stimulated interest in improving hearing in patients with bilateral microtia. The importance of determining, before 1 year of age, whether or not the infant has sufficient auditory acuity to permit the development of communication is obvious. If mechanical aids fail to restore impaired hearing to adequate levels, the otologist

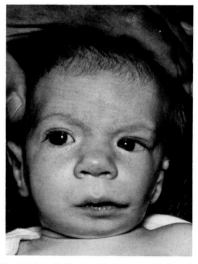

FIGURE 35–9. Patient with hemicraniofacial microsomia (first and second branchial arch syndrome), displaying microtia, macrostomia, hypoplasia of the zygoma, maxilla, and mandible, and soft tissue hypoplasia.

must undertake to correct this surgically. Refinements in technique have encouraged some otologists to expand into the elective field of unilateral deafness (Jahrsdoerfer, 1974; Tanaka, Ishimori and Sekiguchi, 1976), while others question the advisability of operating on microtia if hearing is normal on the opposite side (Bellucci and Converse, 1960; Derlacki, 1968, 1974; Schuknecht, 1971).

Patients with bilateral microtia who can communicate by hearing aids pose another difficult problem. Provided cochlear function is adequate and the mastoid cells are pneumatized, the prospects of establishing binaural hearing at the 20 to 25 decibel range is appealing. Nevertheless, any middle ear surgery makes the auricular reconstruction more complicated. Chronic drainage and infection are frequent postoperative problems, and the gain in auditory acuity is frequently of a temporary nature. Implanting of tympanic membrane allografts with ossicles attached may require a reevaluation of the indications for improving hearing in the presence of congenital auricular deformities (Jahrsdoerfer, 1974).

Unless middle ear surgery becomes urgent in infancy, both otologist and plastic surgeon are well advised to defer any surgery until the age of 5 or 6 and then to plan the complete sequence of events jointly. A pinnal reconstruction can be done after middle ear surgery which has been combined with rotation of the lobule into a transverse position (Nager, 1971; Broadbent and Woolf, 1974). On the other hand, most plastic surgeons prefer to defer the establishment of an external auditory canal and the exploration of the middle ear until the auricular reconstruction has been completed, unless the failure of a hearing aid to restore adequate auditory acuity clearly indicates the otologist's priority. By performing the auricular reconstruction first, valuable retroauricular skin is preserved, and the hazards of working in the presence of scar is avoided.

Edgerton and Nager (1969) suggest completing the auricular reconstruction, turning the whole structure forward on an anteriorly based pedicle in order to permit the otologist complete exposure for the middle ear repair, and then returning the auricle to its former position.

Tanzer (1963, 1971a) has met the objection of the otologist to the restricted exposure imposed by a reconstructed auricle by the use of concurrent procedures. One of the three methods of auricular reconstruction proposed by Tanzer (1959) employs the use of a temporary, skin-lined tunnel beneath the implanted cartilaginous framework, which allows the ear to be easily lifted away from the side of the head, giving wide access to the entire mastoid area (see Fig. 35–24, *B*). At this stage the otologist can correct an aural atresia and explore the tympanic cavity and mastoid without compromising the auricular structure. When he has completed his work (and this can be delayed for years, if necessary, since the auricle at this point has a very presentable appearance), the tunnel can be closed, completing auricular reconstruction (see Fig. 35–24, *C*).

General Considerations

Psychologic Preparation. During the treatment of a child afflicted with microtia, the principal objective is not to produce a commendable ear but to instill in the patient an inner strength which will sustain him through his formative years. An inconspicuous ear contributes significantly to this goal but does not necessarily lead to its fulfillment. This concept should be thoroughly understood by the family before any surgery is started so that the parents and surgeon may unite in minimizing the child's emotional conflicts and in developing within him a realistic acceptance of the surgical result. Every effort should be made to establish a rapport with the youngster, explaining each procedure as it evolves and arousing his interest to the point where he is willing to share this interest with his schoolmates rather than avoid discussion of his abnormality. Complications, which are inevitable, must be carefully explained to the parents and every attempt made to bolster their morale during the periods of ear reconstruction so that their concern will not add to the patient's insecurity.

The study by Adamson, Horton, and Crawford (1965), showing that 40 per cent of children examined in a mental health center were afflicted with congenital ear deformities, suggests some underlying relationship between these abnormalities and character disorders. If a significant character disorder is evident, or if a rapport cannot be established with the parents, discretion calls for delay of the reconstruction and, in some cases, for the use of an artificial prosthesis (Simons, 1974) until prospects for successful surgery are brighter.

Age Factor. The body image concept concerning the face usually manifests itself around the age of 4 or 5 years (Knorr and coworkers, 1974). If possible, the reconstruction should be under way by the time the patient is 6 and entering school, when ridicule and jest by his school mates begin to exact their toll. At age 6 the normal ear has grown to within 6 or 7 mm of its full vertical height (Farkas, 1974), permitting the reconstruction of an ear of matching size with reasonable expectation of symmetry in adult life. Tanzer (1974a) has demonstrated comparable increases in vertical height in both normal and reconstructed ears over 10- to 16-year periods, but the roles played by soft tissues and by cartilage in this growth have not been determined.

The ribs are usually of sufficient size by age 6 to furnish adequate material for the framework. Operation at an earlier age complicates the construction since supplementary blocks of cartilage must be added to give suitable contours and depth. Barinka (1966) deliberately delays the operation until after the age of 10 years when more cartilage is available.

Correlation with the Correction of Associated Deformities. Before any step is taken toward reconstructing the auricle, its timing in relation to the possible surgical correction of soft tissue atrophy, skeletal hypoplasia, or other associated defects should be carefully considered. In general, the sense of psychologic urgency dictates a correction of the ear before other facial asymmetries which are likely to cause less emotional turmoil. The preservation of maximum blood supply to the skin destined to cover the ear calls for the completion of the auricle before the introduction of skin flaps, dermal-fat grafts, injections of liquid silicone for the correction of soft tissue hypoplasia, or bone grafts or inorganic material for the improvement of mandibular hypoplasia. If a mandibular correction is deemed necessary before 7 years of age, every effort should be made to preserve the auricular site intact.

In the presence of skeletal hypoplasia, the proper level of placement of the auricle can usually be determined by locating the superior rim of the reconstructed ear on a plane running across the superior rim of the normal ear, parallel to a line through the inferior corneal margins. Posteriorly, the ear should lie as close to the hairline as possible, actually including some hairy skin if necessary. In dealing with the grosser bony hypoplasia, Converse and coworkers (1973) have noted difficulty in determining the auricular site and have recommended skeletal correction before proceeding

with the ear reconstruction (Chapter 54). When early mandibular surgery is considered essential to the production of facial symmetry and adequate dental occlusion, the ear reconstruction should be delayed.

Avoidance of Scarring. Essential scars on or behind the reconstructed ear are acceptable, but otherwise visible scars should be shunned. The use of cervical tubed skin flaps produces scars which invariably widen, causing an additional source of dissatisfaction. Small preauricular tubes cause inconspicuous scars which are acceptable in augmenting the superior and anterior helix. Larger helical defects can be restored by tubed fascial flaps containing the superficial temporal vessels, which are covered with skin grafts (Dufourmentel, 1958; Cosman and Crikelair, 1966).

Preservation of Auricular Contours. The natural proclivity of skin to tent over depressions may cause a blurring of the concavities of the reconstructed auricle, particularly in the region of the helical sulcus. This unfortunate effect can be effectively counteracted in two ways. First, the depth of the helix can be exaggerated during the construction of the framework, thus compensating for subsequent shrinkage of the helical sulcus. Similarly, the anthelix can be built up by the use of supplementary cartilage strips to delineate more clearly the posterior conchal wall (Spina, Kamakura and Psillakis, 1971). Second, skin tension can be relieved by introducing the auricular framework through a conchal incision (Fig. 35–10). This incision usually corresponds to the vertical scar created by the transposition of the microtic lobule into a transverse position. As the framework slides into its pocket, the covering skin is advanced *centrifugally* and packed into the concavities of the framework, leaving a defect in the conchal floor which can then be covered by a full-thickness skin graft (Tanzer, 1963). This method of inserting the auricular block has the further advantage of preserving the blood supply along the periphery of the ear where maximum vascularization is desired rather than subjecting this region to the vascular damage that accompanies any introduction of a framework through an incision along the hairline.

Skin Cover. The hairline above the site of the proposed reconstruction is usually high enough to avoid interference with adequate positioning of the ear. However, no compro-

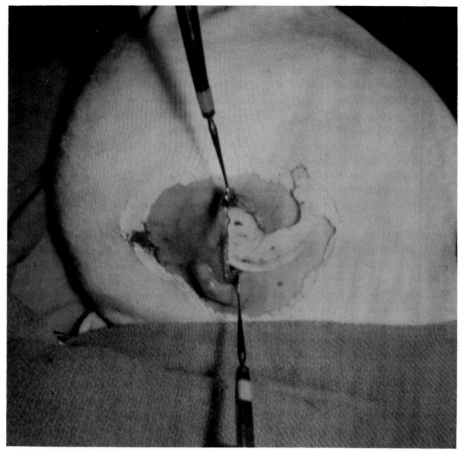

FIGURE 35–10.   The introduction of the cartilage framework through a conchal incision. As skin is advanced centrifugally into the concavities of the framework, the incision spreads open, relieving tension. (See also Fig. 35-18.)

mise should be made in placing the ear at a correct level in relation to the opposite side. A small amount of hairy skin may be permitted to cover the superior helix; in that case, any hair remaining on the ear may be later removed by electrolysis. In the presence of an unusually low hairline, a preliminary resurfacing with hairless skin from the opposite auriculocephalic sulcus or from the supraclavicular region should be done, using a small scalp roll (Letterman and Harding, 1956) (Fig. 35–11). After the framework has been implanted and the ear has been released from the side of the head, the scalp roll should be reopened and returned to its original position. If contraction of the roll prevents its return to the proper level, a correction can be made by undermining and excising a small wedge of redundant scalp (Fig. 35–12).

The Use of Orientation Markings.   During any auricular reconstruction, should it be nec-

essary to mobilize the deformed ear extensively, as for example in relocating a very high lobule, it is easy to lose one's bearings unless guide marks have been established in the first place (Tanzer, 1971b). Two orientation marks are made above and below the vestigial ear, placed well beyond the proposed area of undermining, to avoid any displacement of the marks (Fig. 35–13, *A*). The contour pattern is then held in proper position, with its long axis parallel to the bridge of the nose, while an ink line is drawn across the pattern, in line with the two orientation marks (Fig. 35–13, *B*). The distance between the superior guide mark and the pattern is recorded, and the draping is completed. This reference mechanism, akin to an inertial guidance system, enables the surgeon, at any time during the operation, to place the pattern on its original site, furnishing a guide for the final positioning of the mobilized auricular tissue and the framework.

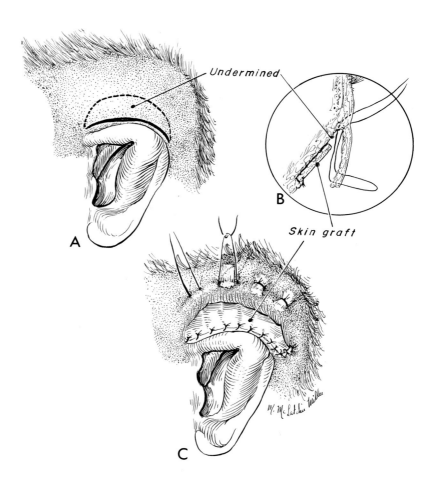

FIGURE 35–11. Use of a scalp roll to furnish additional skin cover. *A*, The incision along the hairline. *B*, Use of a mattress suture to invert the scalp roll. The defect is covered by a full-thickness skin graft. *C*, Sutures are tied over gauze to complete the roll.

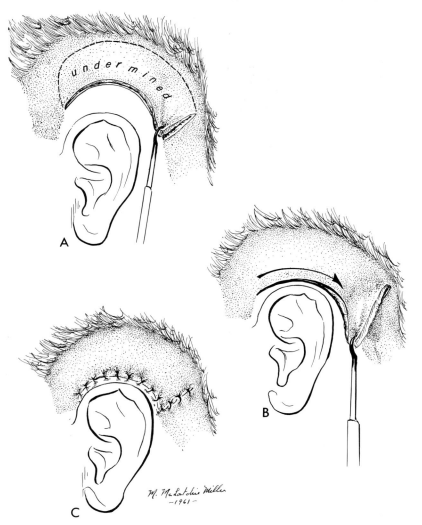

FIGURE 35–12. A method of lowering the hairline after completing a scalp roll (Tanzer).

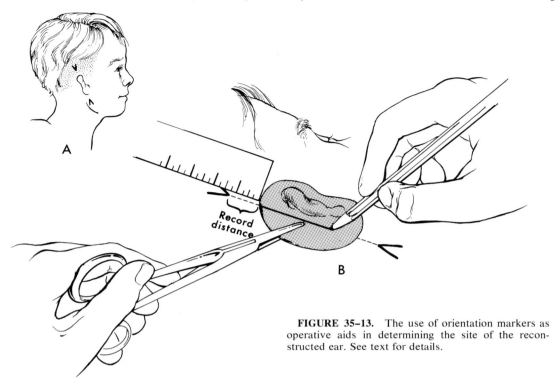

FIGURE 35-13. The use of orientation markers as operative aids in determining the site of the reconstructed ear. See text for details.

Reconstruction with Autogenous Cartilage

Most reconstructive methods follow a general pattern: rotation of the microtic lobule into a transverse position, transplantation of a framework, and elevation of the reconstructed ear from the side of the head, combined with the application of a thick split-thickness or full-thickness graft to the resulting defect. The lobule rotation and implantation of the framework may be combined (Ogino, 1964; Tanzer, 1971a; Fukuda, 1974b) or may be done in the reverse order (Converse, 1955, 1963, 1968; Barinka, 1966).

Once the difficulties of making the framework are overcome, autogenous cartilage offers the best chance of remaining in place without exposure or extrusion. Furthermore, in the unfortunate event that the cartilage becomes exposed during trauma, its viability permits the epithelium to produce a stable, overlying surface by secondary epithelization. Shrinkage and softening occasionally occur, and the innate tendency of cartilage to warp (Gibson and Davis, 1958) must be considered when the structural block is assembled.

Historical Aspects. Interest in the use of autogenous cartilage, which had waned during the early part of World War II, was rekindled by Peer (1943, 1948). Spurred by the demonstration of Young (1941) that diced cartilage would fuse* when laid on a fascial surface. Peer constructed ears with diced rib cartilage which had been allowed to consolidate in the form of an ear within a perforated vitallium mold buried in the abdominal wall. Papers by Webster (1944), Byars and Demere (1950), Dupertuis and Musgrave (1959), Tanzer (1959, 1971a), Converse (1958, 1963, 1968), Converse and Wood-Smith, (1971), Ogino and Yoshikawa (1963), Schmid (1969), Spina (1969), Spina and associates (1971), and Peet (1971) have contributed to current concepts of the use of autogenous costal cartilage in the correction of microtia. Fukuda (1974a) has added many refinements, and Gorney, Murphy and Falces (1971) and Davis (1972) have demonstrated the extended use of conchal cartilage for the same purpose.

Author's Method of Reconstruction. The following method has proved its dependability

---

*Fragments of cartilage are joined by fibrous tissue, in contradistinction to fragments of bone, which join to form a solid block (J. M. C.).

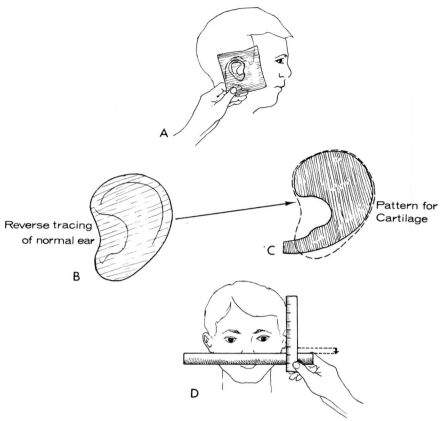

FIGURE 35–14. Tanzer's method of reconstructing the auricle. *A, B,* Tracing the contour of the normal ear. *C,* The contour pattern of the proposed cartilage framework. *D,* Measuring the malalignment of the hypoplastic ear.

in the course of 47 total reconstructions during the past 18 years (Tanzer, 1965, 1971a, 1974a). It is applicable to acquired as well as congenital deformities.

PRELIMINARY STEPS. Prior to operation, a tracing of the normal auricle is made on roentgenographic film (Fig. 35–14, *A*). A second contour pattern of the proposed rib cartilage framework is next made from the reversed original tracing (Fig. 35–14, *B, C*), extending the inferior tip 1 cm beyond the edge of the pattern (this tip will eventually extend into the subcutaneous tissue over the temporomandibular joint, serving to stabilize the framework and to prevent sagging).

The reversed auricular pattern is used to determine the position of the new ear. The long axis should lie roughly parallel to the bridge of the nose, even though this necessitates using some hairy skin (which can be epilated later). The proper vertical adjustment is obtained by placing a straightedge transversely across the inferior tip of the normal lobule, then measuring and recording the distance to the tip of the

microtic lobule (Fig. 30–14, *D*). Most microtic lobules are superior to the transverse line; an occasional low lobule represents incomplete migration. When the deformed ear has a conchal cavity, the pattern should still be placed at the same height as the unaffected ear, and surgical modification of the concha is performed if necessary.

STAGE I: ROTATION OF THE LOBULE. The previously measured level of the tip of the lobule is marked, and the ear contour is traced on the mastoid region, using the gas-sterilized pattern (Fig. 35–15, *B*) with its longitudinal axis parallel to the nasal bridge (Fig. 35–15, *A*). Head draping consists of Stark's doubled length of sterile 6-inch stockinette tied on one end and rolled over the head. (The face on the affected side has been previously covered with sterile cellophane.) An aperture is cut over the ear and cheek, allowing one to watch for facial twitching during the dissection.

The portion of the lobule lying below the cartilaginous remnant is raised; the posterior incision is placed farther from the head than

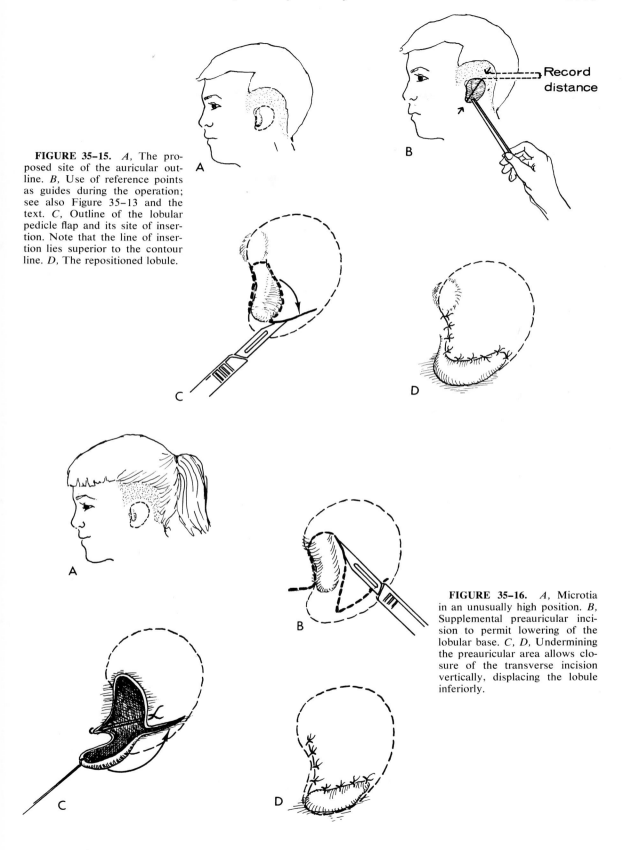

FIGURE 35–15. *A*, The proposed site of the auricular outline. *B*, Use of reference points as guides during the operation; see also Figure 35–13 and the text. *C*, Outline of the lobular pedicle flap and its site of insertion. Note that the line of insertion lies superior to the contour line. *D*, The repositioned lobule.

FIGURE 35–16. *A*, Microtia in an unusually high position. *B*, Supplemental preauricular incision to permit lowering of the lobular base. *C*, *D*, Undermining the preauricular area allows closure of the transverse incision vertically, displacing the lobule inferiorly.

the anterior incision to minimize eversion. When it is rotated into position, the proper line for its insertion will be indicated (Fig. 35–15, C, D). An unusually high lobule may require a supplementary preauricular incision to lower its base to the proper level (Fig. 35–16, A to D).

STAGE II: CONSTRUCTION AND TRANSPLANTATION OF THE FRAMEWORK. Two months later a transverse incision is made over the sixth interspace on the opposite side of the chest (Fig. 35–17, A). The rectus muscle is divided, and the cartilaginous portions of the sixth, seventh, and eighth ribs are exposed and separated from the attached muscles (Fig. 35–17, B). No attempt is made to dissect the ribs from their perichondrial sheaths. After the visi- ble portions of the ribs are freed, the dissection is facilitated by dividing the sixth and seventh ribs at the costochondral junction, lifting them, with the synchondrosis intact, and separating the ribs from the pleura under direct vision. The trunk is flexed and the wound closed in layers.

Working on a carving board, the perichondrium is scraped from the ribs with scalpels, and the outline of the proposed framework is traced across the synchondrosis (Fig. 30–17, C). A moderate defect in the superior scaphal region is acceptable, as it will not be apparent when the framework is embedded. If the seventh rib has insufficient curve to conform to the inferior part of the cartilage pattern, the curve can be accentuated by removing a small wedge from its concave side, leaving a small

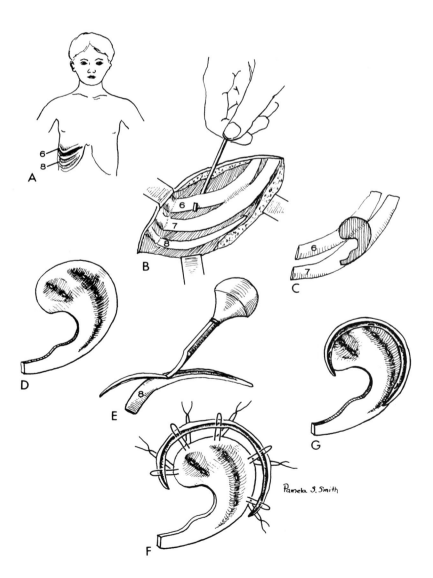

FIGURE 35–17. A, Transverse incision over the contralateral sixth interspace. B, Skeletonizing the sixth, seventh, and eighth rib cartilages. C, The contour pattern superimposed on the cartilaginous base block. D, Completion of the base block, leaving the synchondrosis intact. (Perforations are much larger than shown.) E, Excavation of the visceral side of the eighth rib to form the helix. F, G, Completion of the assembly with wire sutures.

Pamela S. Smith

rim of intact cartilage on the outer edge and closing the wedge with a suture. Using the mold of a random ear as a guide, the concavities are inked in and cut to the proper depth with wood-carving gouges* (Fig. 35–17, *D*). The posterior surface of the eighth rib is thinned out with a U-shaped gouge to create a pliable helix, leaving a platform at its base through which fixation wires may be run (Fig. 35–17, *E*). The medial end of the rib is thinned to form the anterior crus helicis.

*No. 5 and No. 8 wood gouges, approximately 5 mm wide, with palm handles, are available in most craft shops.

The helix is fixed to the flat surface of the base block with mattress sutures of fine stainless steel wire on atraumatic needles (Fig. 35–17, *F, G*). The knots are sunk slightly below the surface in a shallow incision, as described by Converse (1963).

The vertical scar (original site of the lobule) is next excised, the skin within the outline is undermined, staying well below the subdermal plexus, and the ball of native auricular cartilage is removed. When the pocket is dry and completely free of blood clot, the flexible framework is rotated into the cavity (Fig. 35–18, *A*); mattress sutures of 5–0 silk are placed at intervals between the helix and base block

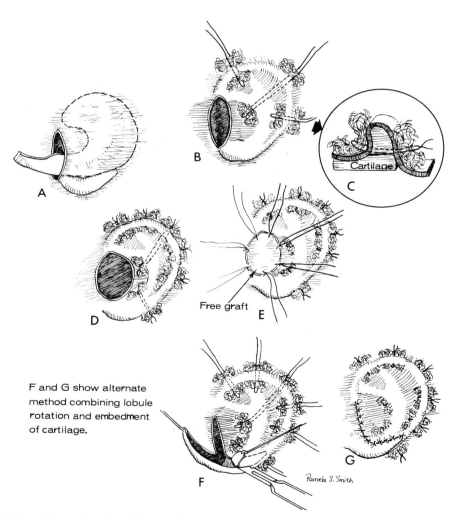

FIGURE 35–18. *A*, Transplantation of the cartilage framework. *B, C*, Placement of compression sutures in the helical and conchal cavities. *D*, A conchal defect is produced by tying compression sutures. *E*, A full-thickness skin graft closes the defect in the conchal floor. *F, G*, An alternative method combining stages I and II. The site of the lobule is only superficially divested of epithelium, to preserve the vascularity of the conchal skin.

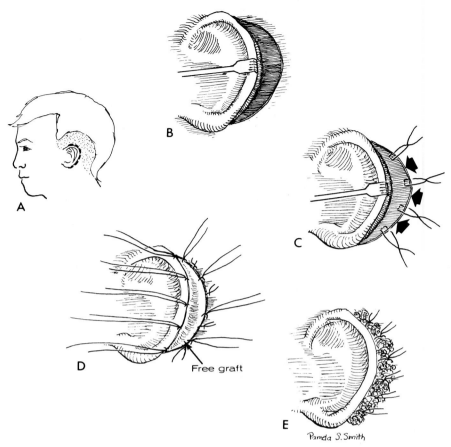

FIGURE 35–19. *A, B,* Creation of an auriculocephalic sulcus. *C,* Advancement of the skin border to minimize the visible skin graft. *D, E,* Tied-in dressing exerts even pressure on the split-thickness skin graft.

and are later tied over gauze pledgets, snugging the skin into the helical sulcus (Fig. 35–18, *B, C*). Occasionally, two or three similar sutures are carried under the entire cartilage block to delineate the posterior and inferior conchal wall (Fig. 35–18, *D*).

As the skin spreads out into the concavities, a defect in the conchal area develops (Fig. 35–18, *D*). The skin margin is tacked down along the edge of this defect, a full-thickness skin graft taken from the opposite auriculocephalic sulcus is anchored (Fig. 35–18, *E*), and tie-over sutures are used to fix a gauze pack. Occasionally, a primary closure of the skin defect can be obtained without tension (Fig. 35–18, *F, G*).

STAGE III: RELEASE OF THE AURICLE FROM THE SIDE OF THE HEAD. Three or four months later, the ear is lifted from the side of the head, the dissection being done most pains-takingly to prevent exposure of cartilage (a small area of exposure may be covered by turning down a flap of contiguous fibrotic, subcutaneous tissue) (Fig. 35–19, *A, B*). The dissection is extended a short distance under the conchal skin to produce an exaggerated auriculocephalic sulcus. The posterior skin edge is advanced and sutured in a forward position (Fig. 35–19, *C*). A thick split-thickness skin graft from the upper thigh is fitted into the defect, and complete hemostasis and absence of blood clot are demonstrated before the final sutures are tied (Fig. 35–19, *D, E*).

STAGE IV: CONSTRUCTION OF THE TRAGUS AND CONCHAL CAVITY. The tragus is formed by carrying a U-shaped incision down almost to the level of the mastoid periosteum (Fig. 35–20, *A*), undermining the flap, and inverting it under itself with three mattress sutures placed into the undermined pocket and onto

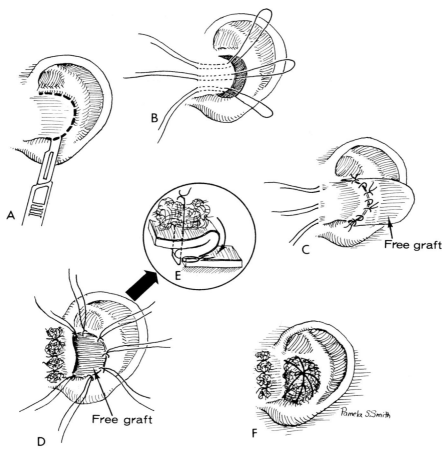

FIGURE 35–20. *A,* Incising a flap to deepen the conchal cavity and form the tragus. *B,* The flap has been undermined, and the inverting sutures are in place. *C,* The addition of a full-thickness skin graft to line the defect. *D, E,* Inversion of the flap by tightening the preauricular sutures. The graft is fixed with tie-over sutures. *F,* Packing of the conchal cavity.

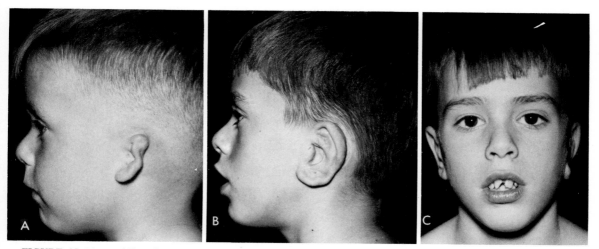

FIGURE 35–21. *A,* Microtia and atresia of the ear canal in a 6 year old boy. *B, C,* Result following four-stage reconstruction and revision of the opposite ear.

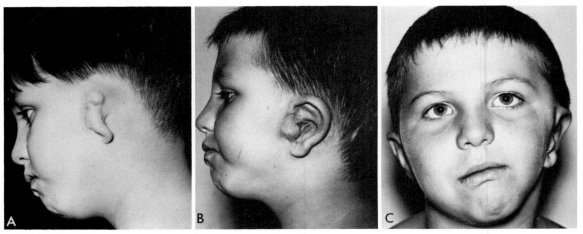

FIGURE 35–22. *A*, Six year old boy with microtia and other evidence of the first and second branchial arch syndrome. *B*, *C*, Result following three-stage reconstruction of the auricle. The preauricular scar marks the site of a row of preauricular pits that were excised in a separate procedure after completion of the reconstruction. Note the associated skeletal deformities.

the preauricular surface (Kirkham, 1940) (Fig. 35–20, *B*). Before the inversion, a full-thickness auriculocephalic graft from the opposite side is sutured with catgut to the flap edge (Fig. 35–20, *C*). As the preauricular sutures are tightened over gauze pledgets, the flap is inverted, pulling the graft into the pseu-

domeatus to line the posterior wall of the pocket and the conchal flap (Fig. 35–20, *D* to *F*).

At the same operation, any minor revisions are completed, and the opposite ear is set closer to the side of the head, if necessary, to obtain symmetry (Fig. 35–21).

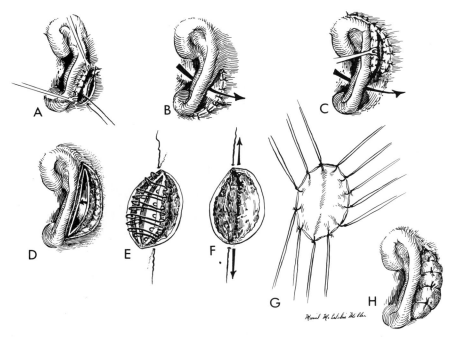

FIGURE 35–23. Use of the temporary tunnel in auricular reconstruction. *A*, *B*, Elevation of the lower half of the ear from the head, closing the raw surfaces with a split-thickness skin graft. The portion of the defect on the side of the head can often be closed primarily. *C*, Completion of the tunnel superiorly. A single skin graft is used to cover the defect. *D* to *H*, Completion of the posterior conchal wall. Narrow flaps based on the margins of the tunnel are closed with an inverting Connell suture of stainless steel wire (*E*, *F*), and the raw surface is covered with a split-thickness skin graft (*G*, *H*).

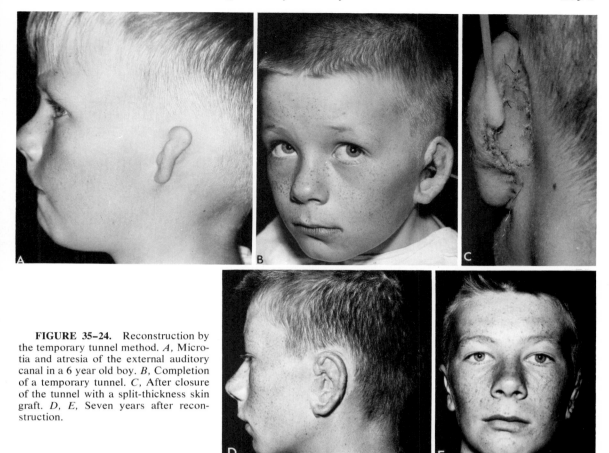

FIGURE 35–24. Reconstruction by the temporary tunnel method. *A*, Microtia and atresia of the external auditory canal in a 6 year old boy. *B*, Completion of a temporary tunnel. *C*, After closure of the tunnel with a split-thickness skin graft. *D*, *E*, Seven years after reconstruction.

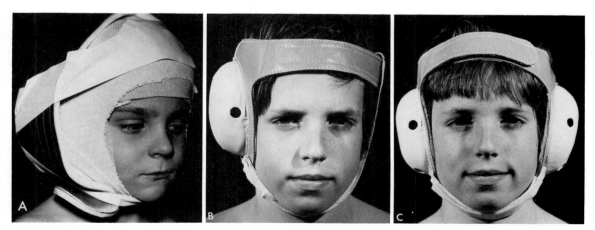

FIGURE 35–25.   Protective devices for postoperative use. *A*, Bulky dressing of fluffed gauze and soft gauze roll, contained in a stockinette head cap and reinforced by a padded aluminum splint. *B*, *C*, Padded leather ear guard, used after removal of the dressing. Right and left models can be made and used unilaterally or bilaterally.

THE THREE-STAGE METHOD. When the lobule is not severely displaced, its rotation and the implantation of the framework can be combined in one procedure. The lobule is raised on its inferiorly based pedicle, and the framework is embedded in the usual manner. The position for the lobule can then be accurately outlined, and a strip of superficial epithelium is excised for the reception of the lobule, leaving a well-vascularized dermal base, which minimizes the hazard of skin necrosis at the inferior conchal angle. This hazard can be significant if the skin is incised completely (see Figs. 35–18, *F, G*, and 35–22).

THE TEMPORARY TUNNEL METHOD. The original, longer method used by the author (Tanzer, 1964) involves the use of a temporary tunnel which is excavated beneath the implanted framework in two stages, serving to bring the ear out at a better angle than the one created by the four-stage method and giving a sharper delineation of the posterior conchal wall (Fig. 35–23, *A* to *C*). The tunnel is closed at the end of the reconstruction to prevent transillumination (Fig. 35–23, *D* to *H*). The superiority of this type of ear over the one produced by the four-stage method is not sufficient to justify its routine use, but it is the method of choice when middle ear exploration is contemplated (Fig. 35–24).

POSTOPERATIVE CARE. A firm, resilient dressing incorporating both ears (Fig. 35–25,

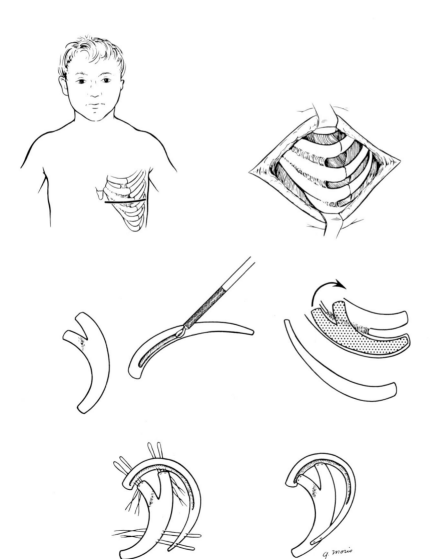

FIGURE 35–26. The Furnas modification of the construction of a framework of autogenous rib cartilage. Wide fenestrations are produced to accentuate the scapha and triangular fossa. (From Furnas, D. W.: Problems in planning reconstruction in microtia. *In* Tanzer, R. C., and Edgerton, M. T. (Eds.): Symposium on Reconstruction of the Auricle. Vol. 10. St. Louis, Mo., C. V. Mosby Company, 1974.)

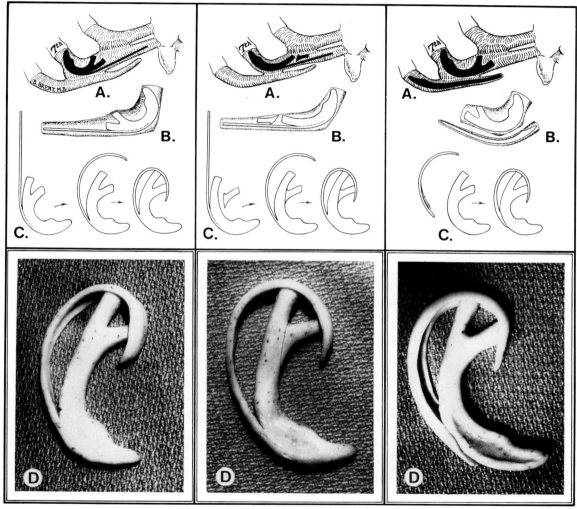

FIGURE 35–27. Fabrication of the expansile framework of Brent in the adult. *A,* The pattern superimposed over the desired ipsilateral rib cartilage. *Left,* One-piece fabrication; *center,* modification for narrow cartilage configuration; *right,* two-piece variation. *B,* The pattern traced on the visceral surface of the rib cartilages. *C,* Assembly of the framework. *D,* The completed framework. (From Brent, B.: Reconstruction of the ear, eyebrow and sideburn in the burned patient. Plast. Reconstr. Surg., *55:*312, 1975. Copyright © 1975, The Williams & Wilkins Company, Baltimore.)

A) is maintained until sutures have been removed and the grafts are healed. A protective helmet, as recommended by Converse (1968), is subsequently worn at night and while the child is at play during intervals between operations and for two months after the last procedure (Tanzer and Chaisson, 1974) (Fig. 35–25, *B, C*). This ensures that the helical rim will not be flattened by pressure during sleep.

RESULTS. In a follow-up of 43 cases extending from six months to 14 years (Tanzer, 1971a), there has been no evidence of softening or shrinkage of cartilage grafts or of exposure of cartilage after completion of the reconstruction. Matthews, Broomhead, and Roxo (1968) have reported six infections in 25 cases, with loss of cartilage in one, and Edgerton (1969) has found absorption in three of his cases.

Alternative Uses of Autogenous Cartilage.*
Barinka (1966) transplants the cartilage framework initially, then rotates the lobule, fillets the native cartilage from the superior remnant, and inverts the skin envelope to form a pocket simulating a pseudomeatus.

Furnas (1974) has modified the construction of the autogenous cartilage framework to provide greater fenestration. The base block, which is made from the sixth and seventh cartilages of the ipsilateral side (Fig. 35–26), is turned over, with the visceral surface outward, and the eighth rib, carved in the form of a

---

*The author's personal experience with these variations has been confined to the methods of Furnas and Brent, both of which have been found to produce satisfactory frameworks.

helix, is wired in three places to the base block.

Brent (1974b) has devised some ingenious methods of carving an "expansile framework" which utilizes the rib cartilage most efficiently and which, like the Furnas technique, results in large fenestrations in the framework. The single rib fabrication (Fig. 35–27) has already been successfully employed in the reconstruction of the adult ear. When using the smaller ribs of a child, he suggests an assembly derived from two ribs (Fig. 35–28).

Converse (1963, 1968; Converse and Wood-Smith, 1971) has utilized a composite graft from the contralateral auricle to form the posterior conchal wall and to hold the ear at the desired angle to the head. The construction and transplantation of the costal cartilage framework in general follow the technique described earlier in the text (see p. 1686), except that the misplaced lobule is left untouched at this time. Later the ear is raised from the side of the head, and the lobule is rotated into a transverse position.

At the third operation, a temporary tunnel is established between the ear framework and the side of the head, and the conchal cavity is excavated in conjunction with a reconstruction of the tragus (Kirkham, 1940). The conchal defect is resurfaced with a full-thickness skin graft (Fig. 35–29).

Finally, the tunnel is closed by means of a composite graft of cartilage from the opposite concha. Originally, a wedge of cartilage, skin-lined on both sides, was employed, but more recently Converse has denuded one side of the composite graft and placed it against a backing

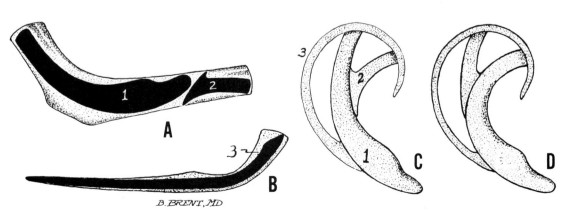

B. BRENT, MD

FIGURE 35–28. Modification of the expansile framework for use in a small child. *A, B,* Film patterns on the visceral surfaces of the contralateral seventh and eighth rib cartilages. *C,* The completed ear framework. *D,* A variation. (From Brent, B.: Ear reconstruction with an expansile framework of autogenous rib cartilage. Plast. Reconstr. Surg., *53*:619. Copyright © 1974. The Williams & Wilkins Company, Baltimore.)

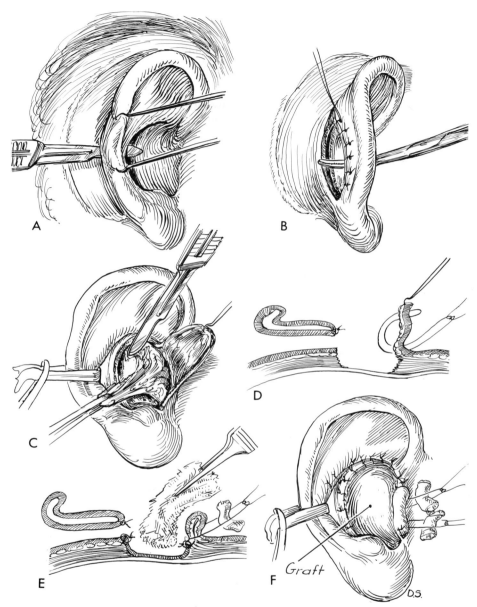

FIGURE 35–29.   The Converse variation of the valise-handle procedure in conjunction with the Kirkham reconstruction of the tragus and deepening of the conchal cavity. *A,* A through-and-through incision is made through the depths of the new retroauricular fold, incising the skin along the anterior border of the cartilaginous implant. *B,* The edge of the skin covering the anteromedial aspect of the cartilaginous framework has been sutured to the edge of the skin covering the posteromedial aspect. *C,* The skin covering the future conchal area is raised as a flap with its pedicle situated anteriorly. The subcutaneous tissue is resected down to the mastoid periosteum. *D,* Resection of the subcutaneous tissue. *E,* Formation of the tragus by the folded flap. *F,* A full-thickness skin graft is placed over the mastoid periosteum and secured by a pressure dressing. (From Converse, J. M.: Construction of the auricle in unilateral microtia. Plast. Reconstr. Surg., *32:*425, 1963.)

of skin turned down from the anterior edge of the reconstructed ear, making sure that the cartilage graft is wedged securely under the lip of the framework to prevent the latter's collapse (Fig. 35–30). The defect in the donor ear is closed primarily to bring the ear closer to the head (Figs. 35–31 and 35–32).

Gorney, Murphy, and Falces (1971) and Gorney (1974) have expanded the use of conchal cartilage for partial defects, as advocated by Adams (1955) and Steffenson (1965), to the treatment of complete microtia. A full conchal graft is lengthened by splicing two segments of the cartilage, and the helix is augmented by a thin cervical tube.

Davis (1972) used a full conchal graft with the expanded ball of native cartilage to form the framework in major reconstructions of

microtia. The rotation of the lobule and the construction of the skeletal structure and the conchal cavity are accomplished in one stage (Fig. 35–33). Although the suitability of conchal cartilage for reconstruction of partial auricular losses has been firmly established, its use in complete reconstruction, particularly in children, is still in a provisional stage.

Alternative Methods of Reconstruction

Inorganic Implants. Materials which have also been used to make the framework include polyethylene, nylon mesh, Marlex, polyester net, and Teflon. Cronin (1966) introduced a silicone elastomer which has had extensive use. Owing to its propensity for extrusion, various modifications of the original design have been

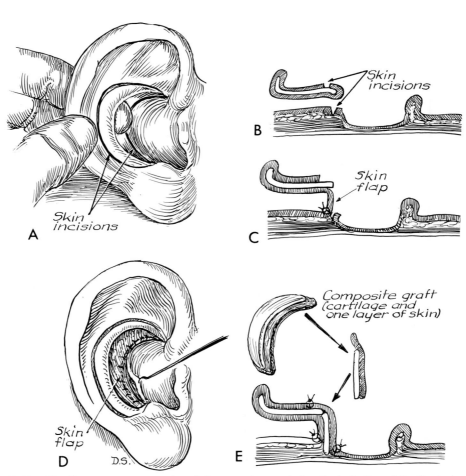

FIGURE 35–30. The Converse reconstruction of the posterior conchal wall. *A,* Outline of the flap to be raised from the skin covering the auricular framework. An outline of the incision to be made through the skin-grafted area is also indicated. *B,* The flap is raised. *C,* The free edge of the flap is sutured into the incision made in the skin-grafted area. *D,* Use of the flap to form the posterior skin of the new concha. *E,* Application of a conchal composite graft.

Illustration continued on the opposite page

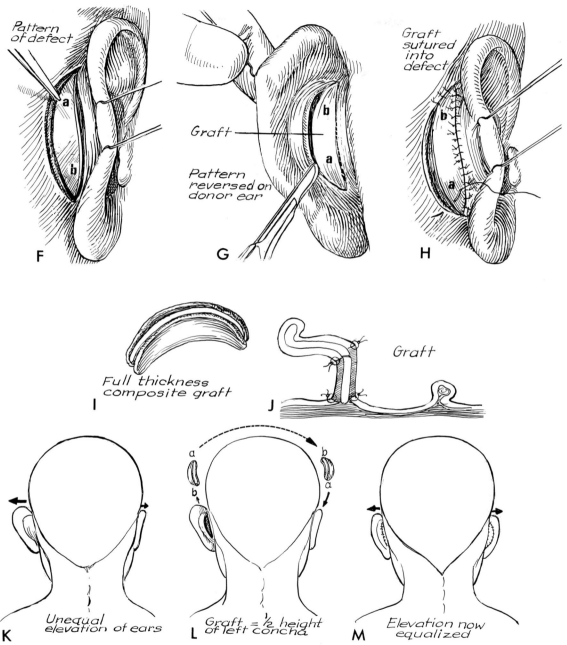

FIGURE 35–30 *Continued. F, G,* A variation: a composite graft of skin and cartilage removed from the contra-lateral concha is employed to form the skeletal framework and anterior cutaneous layer of the new concha. *H* to *J,* The composite graft sutured into position. *K* to *M,* Posterior view of results of composite graft in donor and recipient ears. (From Converse, J. M.: Construction of the auricle in unilateral microtia. Plast. Reconstr. Surg., *32*:425, 1963.)

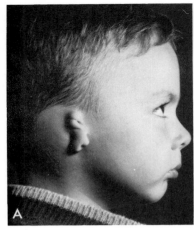

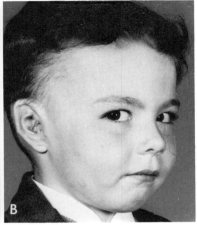

FIGURE 35–31. 2A, Typical microtia in 7 year old boy. B, Result following reconstruction of main framework from costal cartilage and of posterior conchal wall from composite graft taken from the contralateral ear. (From Converse, J. M.: Construction of the auricle in congenital microtia. Plast. Reconstr. Surg., *32*:425. Copyright © 1963, The Williams & Wilkins Company, Baltimore.)

FIGURE 35–32. *A*, Microtia in a 7-year-old boy. *B*, Appearance two years after reconstruction. The concha was reconstructed by the technique illustrated in Figure 35–30, *F* to *M*. *C*, Preoperative lateral view. *D*, Postoperative anterolateral view.

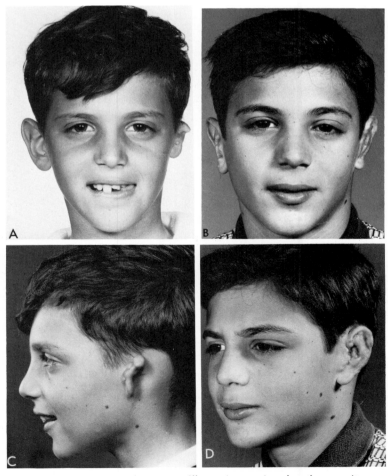

Illustration continued on the opposite page

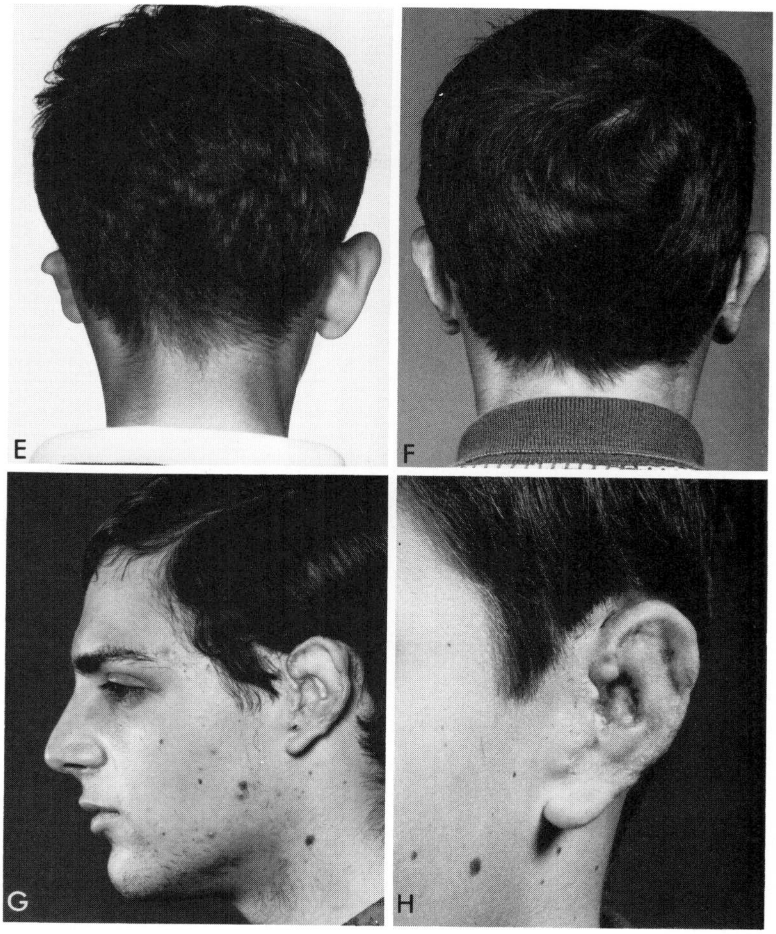

FIGURE 35–32 *Continued. E*, Preoperative rear view. *F*, Postoperative rear view. Note the adequate protrusion of the reconstructed ear obtained by the conchal graft and the symmetry of the two ears. The unaffected auricle was brought closer to the head by a protruding ear operation. *G, H*, Nine years after surgery. (*A* to *D* from Converse, J. M.: Construction of the auricle in congenital microtia. Plast. Reconstr. Surg., *32*:425. Copyright © 1963, The Williams & Wilkins Company, Baltimore.)

made by several surgeons in an attempt to prevent exposure of the frame, including wrapping the rim with Dacron mesh, Dacron velour, and autogenous fascia lata.

SILASTIC TECHNIQUE. In his latest modification, Cronin (1971, 1974) performs a two-stage procedure for correcting microtia (Fig. 35–34, *A*). A preformed, perforated frame of silicone rubber is prepared by suturing a strip of fascia lata around the helix (Fig. 35–34, *B*). This assembly is introduced into a subcutaneous pocket through a central incision paralleling the vertical lobule. Usually the lobule is rotated into a transverse position at the same time (Fig. 30–34, *C*). The use of suction causes the skin to conform to the contours of the framework. At a second operation the reconstructed ear is raised from the side of the head, and the defect is covered with a full-thickness skin graft (Fig. 35–34, *D, E*).

RESULTS. Cronin (1974) reported 13 complete and 8 incomplete reconstructions of primary microtia, of which 6 required removal of the implant. An accumulated total of 131 other cases of microtia treated by Silastic reconstruction reported up to 1973 (Curtin and Bader, 1969; Edgerton and Nager, 1969; Carroll and Peterson, 1971; Davis and Jones, 1971; Lynch and coworkers, 1972; Monroe, 1972; Wray and Hoopes, 1973) has shown a 30 per cent failure rate. More recent reports (Monroe, 1974; Ohmori, 1974; Ohmori and coworkers, 1974) have shown a decreased early failure rate, but their short follow-up periods give no assurance that the continuing danger of extrusion has been avoided. The exposed position of the auricle presents a constant hazard to the thinly covered implant. The failure rate during the operative and early postoperative phases is highest among those surgeons performing only occasional reconstructions and diminishes somewhat as experi-

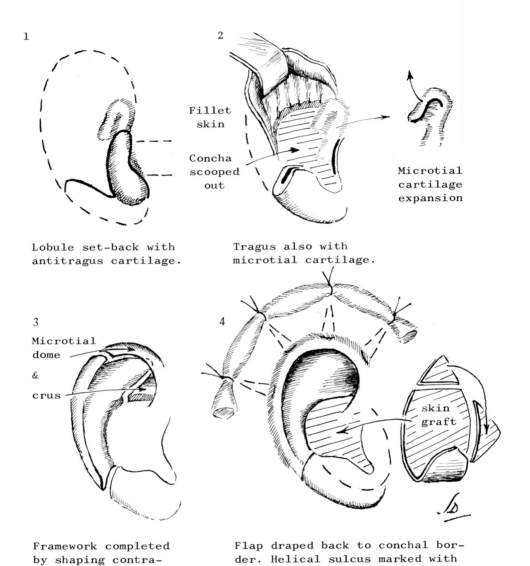

1

Lobule set-back with
antitragus cartilage.

2

Fillet
skin

Concha
scooped
out

Microtial
cartilage
expansion

Tragus also with
microtial cartilage.

3

Microtial
dome
&
crus

Framework completed
by shaping contra-
lateral conchal
cartilage graft.

4

skin
graft

Flap draped back to conchal border. Helical sulcus marked with
bolsters. Full-thickness retro-
aural skin for conchal floor, but
upper triangle used to line tragus.

FIGURE 35–33. Davis technique for constructing the auricular framework from the existing cartilage, to which conchal cartilage from the opposite ear is added.

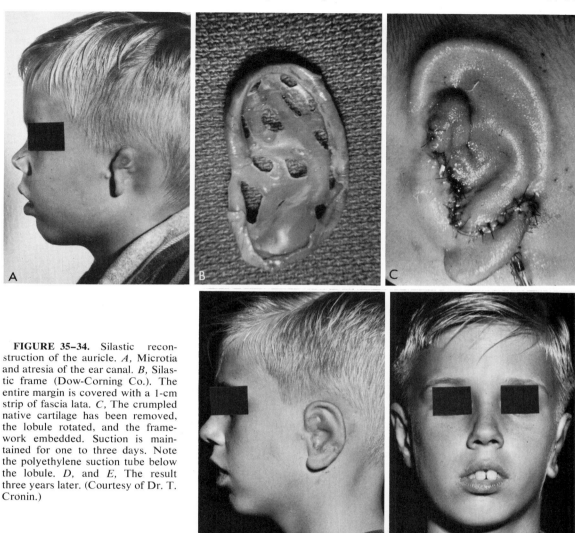

FIGURE 35–34. Silastic reconstruction of the auricle. *A,* Microtia and atresia of the ear canal. *B,* Silastic frame (Dow-Corning Co.). The entire margin is covered with a 1-cm strip of fascia lata. *C,* The crumpled native cartilage has been removed, the lobule rotated, and the framework embedded. Suction is maintained for one to three days. Note the polyethylene suction tube below the lobule. *D,* and *E,* The result three years later. (Courtesy of Dr. T. Cronin.)

ence in coping with complications increases. Edgerton and Bacchetta (1974) have developed salvage techniques for reclaiming ears in which the frameworks have been exposed. These shoring-up procedures are likely to result in bulkier auricles with blurred convolutions. The durability of salvaged reconstructions is precarious because of the presence of scar, which furnishes a locus minoris resistentiae through which the implant pursues its inexorable course to extrusion.

Cartilage Allografts. Gillies (1937) advocated the use of maternal cartilage, contending later that many of these grafts remained unaltered for years. Gibson (1968) and Converse

(1974a) have reported survival of some of these grafts. Because of the deformity at the donor site and in view of other evidence of absorption, the method has been largely abandoned (see footnote on page 308).

Preserved Cartilage. Preserved cartilage allografts were once used extensively (Kirkman, 1940; Brown and coworkers, 1947; Pierce, Klabunde and Brobst, 1952), but the extremely high rate of softening and absorption (Dupertuis and Musgrave, 1959) brought the method into disrepute. During the past ten years, reports by European authors have revived interest in this procedure. Gibson (1968) has presented evidence that quick-frozen allografts survive if they are not exposed to antiseptics and attributes absorption mainly to the presence of clot. Limberg (1962) constructed the auricle in two stages, injecting diced cadaver cartilage through a syringe to build up auricular contours, then bringing the consolidated mass out from the head. Stable results up to five years were reported in 32 cases. Alichniewicz, Bardach, and Kozlowski (1964) and Kruchinsky (1969) have also reported favorable results with cartilage.*

Complications

Exposure of the Framework. This complication has caused more distress to plastic surgeons and their patients during the past 20 years than any other problem, since the use of inorganic implants renders the reconstruction particularly vulnerable to extrusion. Cronin (1971) has enumerated the principal causes: (1) excessive thinning of the skin cover during the preparation of the pocket, (2) the presence of scar, (3) undue tension of the skin investing the implant, (4) trauma, and (5) infection. The danger of exposure can be reduced by strict adherence to basic principles of surgery, namely gentle and painstaking preparation of

---

*These reports should be considered with a certain degree of skepticism (J. M. C.).

the undermined skin and flaps, revision of scars before starting the reconstruction, the addition of skin grafts or flaps when needed to relax tension, the avoidance of undue pressure from dressings or during sleep, and meticulous hemostasis and the elimination of dead space at all times.

Once exposure has occurred, Cronin advises the circulation of an antibiotic solution through the wound, followed by secondary closure. If a reasonable trial fails, the implant should be removed and the skin cover kept expanded until a secondary reconstruction can be done.

CARTILAGE EXPOSURE. Small areas of exposure will heal spontaneously if drying is prevented by the use of an antibiotic ointment and by protection from trauma. Beveling of the exposed cartilage will hasten sluggish healing. Larger areas of skin loss may require the rotation of a skin flap or the advancement of a viable skin border to close the defect without tension. The latter is particularly useful in treating exposure on the rim of the helix, which has been noted shortly after implantation of the framework. Prompt, definitive action minimizes the chance of chronic infection, which can lead to loss of viability and absorption of the cartilage (Fig. 35–35).

Extrusion of Sutures. Fine metal sutures used to wire the cartilage framework may extrude their knots through the skin graft on the medial surface of the ear. Treatment consists

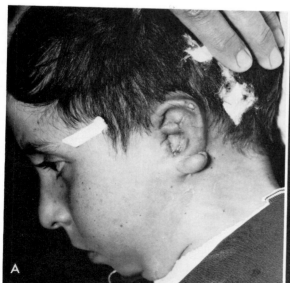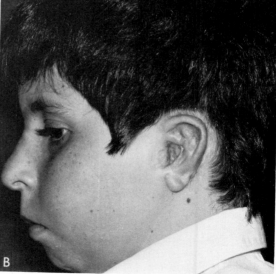

FIGURE 35–35. *A*, Exposure of cartilage near the site of placement of a mattress suture through the helical sulcus during implantation of the framework. *B*, The defect has been closed by advancement of posterior skin. View two years after completion of the reconstruction.

of lifting the knot, clipping one side of the loop, and gently extracting the whole suture.

Pleural Tear. Occasionally, small pleural tears are produced while removing costal cartilage. Positive pressure in the closed anesthesia system keeps the lung expanded until the rent in the pleura is sutured and the chest wall is closed.

Secondary Reconstruction

If the initial result proves unsatisfactory, secondary reconstruction is much more difficult because of the presence of fibrosis. The use of autogenous cartilage is strongly recommended. One crucial decision must be made at the outset: (1) to salvage the existing ear, or (2) to discard the existing structure and to start anew (Tanzer, 1969, 1974b).

Improvement of the Existing Ear. The problem usually results from errors in position, form, or type of skin cover.

ERRORS OF POSITION. A sagging ear requires mobilization and fixation at the proper level by some means such as fascia lata suspension to the temporal bone or periosteum (Edgerton, 1969) or by a cartilage hook (Tanzer, 1972). Failure to align the long axis parallel to the nasal bridge can be corrected by mobilization of the auricle and rotation to the correct angle. An ear that is too close to the side of the head needs a second skin graft to the auriculocephalic sulcus or a retroauricular wedge of cartilage to project the ear at the proper angle (Tanzer, 1963) (Fig. 35–36).

ERRORS OF FORM. A shallow helical sulcus, or a helical rim which has been flattened by pressure during sleep, results in an unpleasant blurring of contour. The sulcus can be restored by removing cartilage with a wood-carving gouge either through broken incisions (Fig. 35–37) or through a single, curved incision which is later closed in the form of an "eave flap" (Tanzer, 1963) (Fig. 35–38). The raw surface can be grafted (Cronin, 1952) or left to granulate (Lewin, 1950).

In the less severe forms of microtia in which

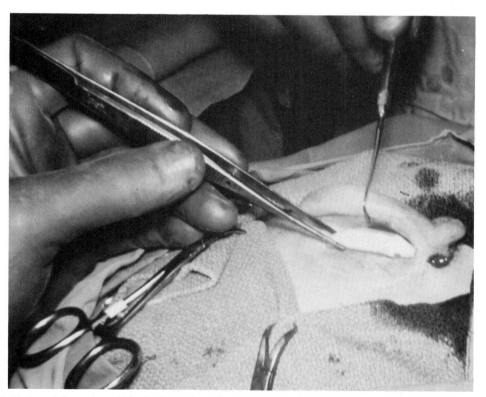

FIGURE 35–36. A boat-shaped block of costal cartilage that will be introduced through an infralobular incision into the retroauricular area in order to project the reconstructed auricle at a proper angle.

some well-vascularized skin is available on the medial wall of the ear, the rolling portion of the helix may be augmented by raising a skin flap from the medial wall, rolling it forward on itself to give a fuller overhang, and covering the medial defect with a skin graft (Matthews, 1943) (Fig. 35–39, *A, B*). A small strip of cartilage may be incorporated within the roll when support is needed (Cronin, 1952) (Fig. 35–39, *C*).

FAULTY SKIN COVER.   Even minor scarring should be revised to give a cleaner appearance; bulky tissue should be thinned; and grafts which are conspicuous because of color should be replaced by the full-thickness type. Electrolysis is the simplest way of removing any residual hair on the auricle.

New Reconstruction. When circumstances dictate a fresh start, any hypertrophic or unsightly scar should be removed, and all previous implants or residual fibrotic, native cartilage should be discarded. Any remaining lobule should be salvaged and rotated into proper position and any usable skin shifted to

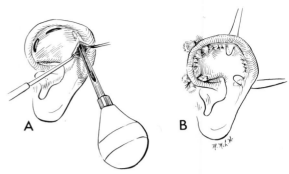

FIGURE 35–37. *A,* Secondary excavation of a shallow helical sulcus through interrupted incisions, using a wood-carving gouge. *B,* The skin is snugged into the deepened sulcus with compression sutures tied over gauze pledgets.

create a single defect, which is then resurfaced with a full-thickness skin graft (Tanzer, 1969). Four months later, a new reconstruction can be undertaken with full recognition of the unlikelihood of producing the finely chiseled out-

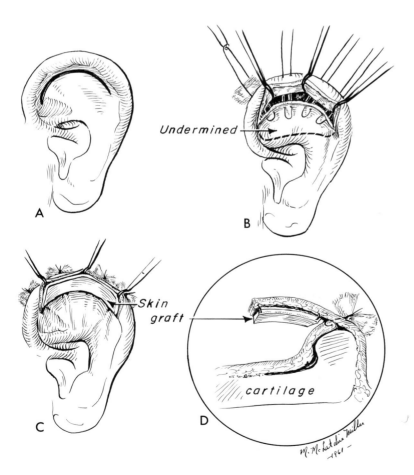

FIGURE 35–38. The eave flap. *A,* The incision for deepening the helical sulcus. *B,* Advancement of scaphal skin into the revised sulcus. *C, D,* The eave flap lined with a skin graft.

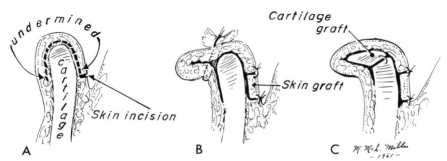

FIGURE 35–39. *A, B,* Method of creating a helical rim by rolling forward the medial auricular skin and covering the defect with a skin graft. *C,* Implantation of a cartilage strip is optional.

lines which are possible when the ear is reconstructed de novo.

HYPOPLASIA OF THE MIDDLE THIRD OF THE AURICLE

One type of diminutive auricle is characterized by a well-developed lobule, together with a helix and scapha of sufficient dimensions to preclude discarding their cartilage, as one would do in preparation for a complete reconstruction. The deformity is essentially an absence of the middle third of the auricle, coupled with a hypoplastic or absent conchal cavity and ear canal. The correction, described by Webster (1944), is started by dividing the superior and inferior components (Fig. 35–40, *A*), spreading them to match the height of the normal ear, and setting each component into a retroauricular incision, so placed as to bring the ear to the same level as its opposite member (Fig. 35–40, *B*). The conchal defect produced by the elevation of the flaps is closed by advancing retroauricular skin (Fig. 35–40, *C*). Later a carved costal or conchal cartilage graft is transplanted to build up the lower helix and posterior conchal wall (Fig. 35–40, *D*). Finally, the ear is released from the head, and a skin graft is applied (Figs. 35–40, *E, F,* and 35–41).

If the constructed helical rim has an inadequate roll, the release of the ear from the head can be combined with the development of a retroauricular skin flap, which is rolled on itself to form the helical fold. The sharpness of the rim is maintained by mattress sutures tied over gauze (see Fig. 35–40, *E, F*). Additional cartilage can be added to the helix at this stage, if needed.

HYPOPLASIA OF THE SUPERIOR THIRD OF THE AURICLE

Anomalies of the upper third of the auricle fall into three general categories: (1) cupping deformities, ranging from minor helical folding to severe hooding; (2) cryptotia; and (3) generalized hypoplasia of the upper part of the ear.

The Constricted Ear

The author has applied the term *constricted ear* to a collection of anomalies, often referred to as *cup* or *lop ear,* in which the helix and scapha are hooded and the body and crura of the anthelix are flattened in varying degrees. One gains the impression that the rim of the helix has been tightened, as if by a purse string. *Group I* includes those lesser deformities, often called lop ear, in which only the helix is involved (Fig. 35–42, *A*). Broadening of the helix may be the only abnormality, but usually the superior rim is squared off, and the cartilage, when exposed, is found to be acutely angulated, even to the point of producing adhesions between the leaf of folded helix and the scapha. *Group II* anomalies include a wide variety of cupping deformities, in which the folding of the anthelix and its superior crus is incomplete or absent and in which the helical rim is pulled over the auricular concavity like a hood (Fig. 35–42, *B*). The more extreme form of cupping *(Group III)* is characterized by a tubular structure, the so-called "cockleshell ear" (Fig. 35–42, *C*) (Tanzer, 1975).

In the severe forms of constriction, the vertical height of the auricle is reduced, and frequently its superior part is pitched forward, causing the anterior helix to lie well in front of

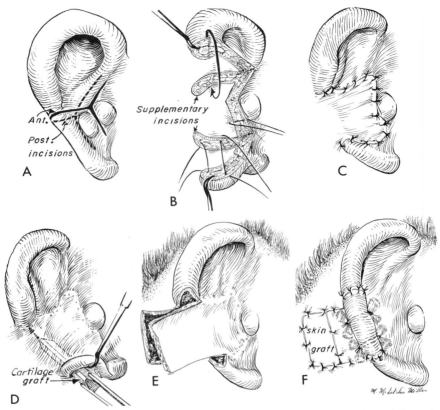

FIGURE 35–40. Reconstruction of the middle third of the auricle. *A, B,* Expansion of the deformed auricle and attachment of the superior and inferior segments to the retroauricular surface. *C,* Advancement of the retroauricular skin to fill the defect. *D,* Introduction of a cartilage block to complete the framework. *E, F,* Release of the ear from the side of the head. The illustrations demonstrate the method of augmenting the helical lip when more definition of the rim is needed.

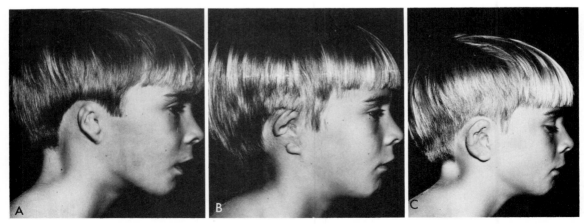

FIGURE 35–41. *A,* Middle third hypoplasia with atresia of the canal. *B,* After expansion of the ear to the proper vertical dimension. *C,* Result following a costal cartilage graft to the helix, a split-thickness skin graft behind the ear, and tragal reconstruction by the method of Kirkham.

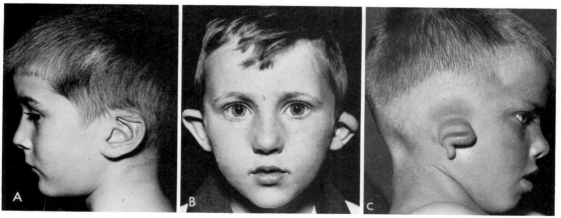

FIGURE 35–42. Varying types of constricted ear. *A,* Involvement of the helix only. *B,* Involvement of the helix and scapha (left auricle). *C,* Severe cupping deformity coupled with incomplete migration of the auricle.

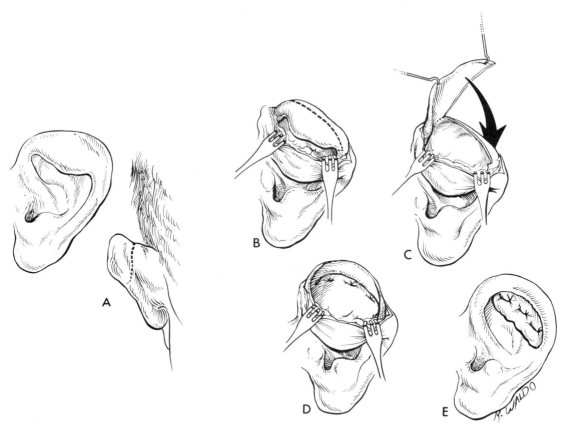

FIGURE 35–43. Correction of group I ear constriction. *A,* The incision for exposure of the skeletal deformity. *B,* The deformed cartilage has been filleted from its soft tissue cover. The line of detachment of the angulated segment is marked. *C,* The deformed cartilage is lifted on a medially based pedicle and rotated into an upright position. *D,* The repositioned cartilage is sutured to the scapha. *E,* The skin is redraped and the helical sulcus is maintained by through-and-through mattress sutures tied over gauze pledgets. (From Tanzer, R. C., *in* Tanzer, R. C., and Edgerton, M. T. (Eds.): Symposium on Reconstruction of the Auricle. St. Louis, Mo., C. V. Mosby Company, 1974, p. 141.)

the vertical plane through the tragus. Due to incomplete migration, the ears are often low-set on the head, causing the ear canals, which are usually present but hypoplastic, to take on an angulated course downward. Ninety per cent of patients have bilateral involvement.

The genetic basis of the deformity has been firmly established as a single, dominant gene, highly variable in expression (see Etiology). Constricted ears comprise approximately 10 per cent of ear anomalies (Cosman, 1974).

Treatment of Group I Constriction. Broadening of the helix is corrected simply by excising an ellipse of helical rim. When the helix is actually flattened against the scapha (Fig. 35–43), the author has used a simple procedure to correct the distortion through a medial incision at least 1 cm from, and parallel to, the superior rim. The entire distorted cartilage is exposed; the angulated helical leaf, which may be tightly bound to the scapha, is dissected free and sutured in proper alignment, as a free graft or as a banner flap, to the medial scaphal surface. The technique raises the height of the ear and restores the helical roll. The roll can be accentuated by scoring. The method is also applicable to lesser forms of the Group II deformity.

Treatment of Group II Constriction. This varied assortment of cupping deformities involving both helix and scapha can be divided, for surgical purposes, into two subgroups, according to the need for supplemental skin to expand the auricular margin. Cartilage revision is required in all instances.

MODERATE DEFORMITY OF HELIX AND SCAPHA. Many of the constricted ear deformities are characterized by insufficient cartilage but adequate skin to cover the framework after its expansion to appropriate height. Lesser degrees of cupping merge with the more exaggerated forms of prominent ear, and the surgical techniques employed for correcting the latter may be enough to restore normal appearance.

HELICAL ADVANCEMENT. Tightness of the helical rim can be relieved by releasing the anterior crus helicis and anterior helix, then sliding this loosened structure superiorly in a V-Y advancement (Holmes, 1949; Becker, 1952; Erich, 1963; Barsky, Kahn and Simon 1964; Kruchinsky, 1966; Stenström, 1974). The incision may have to be extended transversely across the helical sulcus, and the advancement should always be combined with a restoration of the fold of the anthelix and its superior crus.

REMODELING OF CARTILAGE. Ragnell (1951) first introduced the concept of filleting the distorted helix and scapha through an incision on the medial aspect of the auricle, then dividing the exposed cartilage into interdigitating fingers, which are pulled apart to expand the framework. Stephenson (1960) corrected the cupping by radiating incisions in the skeletonized cartilage, permitting a fanlike expansion. Musgrave (1966) has improved the method by adding a strip of conchal cartilage to stabilize the tips of the cartilage fingers and to hold the expanded structure in an upright position (Fig. 35–44). The cartilage fingers can be scored to eliminate some of their curl. Cosman (1974) gained vertical height by dissecting the deformed helical rim as a free-floating "bucket handle," which is sutured in a more superior position.

SEVERE DEFORMITY OF HELIX AND SCAPHA. The more tightly folded forms of constriction not only make the need for supplementary cartilage imperative but also require the rotation of flaps of skin to furnish adequate cover for the expanded rim. The hooded portion can be opened by a vertical incision through all layers, creating a wedge-shaped defect, which is filled by a flap of skin rotated from the medial surface of the auricle (Becker, 1952; Grotting, 1958; Barsky and coworkers, 1964). Kislov (1971) used a lateral wedge

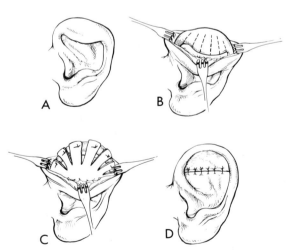

FIGURE 35–44. The Musgrave technique for correction of cup ear. *A*, The deformity. *B*, Folded cartilage is exposed through a lateral incision. *C*, Cartilage fingers are elevated and fixed to a strut of conchal cartilage; the strut is removed through a medial incision when the ear prominence is corrected. *D*, The skin is redraped across the reconstructed framework.

into which a medially based skin flap is rotated, covering a tongue of cartilage which is advanced from the inferior part of the ear. Other methods include the rotation of a cartilage graft on an anteriorly based pedicle to supply the deficiency in the superior third (Davis, 1972, 1974a), and the use of a wedge of composite graft of skin and cartilage from the opposite ear (Becker, 1952; Cardoso and Sperly, 1969).

Treatment of Group III Constriction. In the extreme forms it may be most expedient to split the tubular ear into two segments, setting the raw edge of each component into the retroauricular area, and to proceed with the reconstruction as described under the section on Hypoplasia of the Middle Third of the Auricle.

Cryptotia

Cryptotia or "pocket ear" is a curious anomaly in which the cartilage framework has failed to extrude itself from the side of the head and instead has become buried under the scalp. The auriculocephalic sulcus is obliterated but can be restored by gentle pressure (Fig. 35–45). Usually, the superior antihelical crus is acutely angulated (Ohmori and Matsumoto, 1972), and the cartilaginous helical rim is folded upon itself. Like microtia, it occurs much more frequently in males than in females (Fukuda,

1968, 1974b), but its right-left-bilateral ratio differs (5:3:1 in microtia, 2:1:2 in cryptotia).

Although it is rather rare in the western hemisphere (Sěrcer, 1934), its incidence in Japan has been reported to be as high as 1:400 (Ohmori and Matsumoto, 1972). The cause of the deformity has not been established, although it is presumed to be an aberration in the development of cartilage around the third month of gestation (Sěrcer, 1934; Gosserez and Piers, 1959).

Treatment. Correction of the deformity includes (1) opening and lining the auriculocephalic sulcus, and (2) correcting the malformed cartilage. Deficient skin has been supplemented by the lateral advancement of retroauricular skin (Sěrcer, 1934; Holmes, 1949; Cowan, 1961; Pollock, 1969) and by a vertical V-Y advancement (Kubo, 1938; Fukuda, 1968, 1974b; Ohmori and Matsumoto, 1972). The method requiring the least manipulation of tissue utilizes the skin below the hairline to cover as much of the medial surface of the ear as possible. The hairline is then advanced inferiorly to lessen the raw surface, and the residual defect is closed by a skin graft (Wesser, 1972). Any angulated anthelical cartilage should be straightened before draping the ear with its skin mantle (Fukuda, 1968, 1974b). An angulated helix of the lop type, if present, can be revised to increase vertical height of the ear, as illustrated in Figure 35–43. (See section on Group I ear constriction.)

Hypoplasia of the Entire Superior Third of the Auricle

Infrequently the whole upper third of the auricle is involved in a hypoplastic process which renders the simpler techniques impractical. Effective treatment requires opening up and setting the vestigial parts onto the hairless retroauricular surface and proceeding with a reconstruction of the superior third by one of the methods employed in the correction of post-traumatic defects (see section on Acquired Deformities).

Bilateral Microtia

Bilateral microtia is relatively rare. The reconstructive principles which apply to unilateral microtia also apply to the bilateral deformity. Bilateral microtia is seen in man-

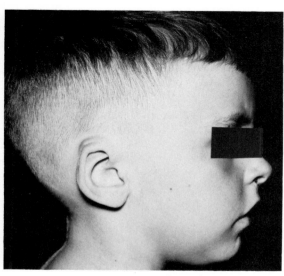

FIGURE 35–45. Cryptotia.

dibulofacial dysostosis (Treacher Collins-Franceschetti-Klein syndrome), in bilateral craniofacial microsomia, and in other rare craniofacial malformations (see Chapters 53, 54, and 55).

PROMINENT EAR

The importance of prominence of the auricle lies not in the fact that it represents a minor embryonic arrest in the final development of convolutions but rather in the fact that Western culture has imposed a stigma on its presence which is not evident in other areas such as Japan, for example, where large ears are considered a sign of good fortune. In view of the psychologic handicap, correction should be accomplished before the child enters school and becomes an object of ridicule and jest.

Pathology

During the third month of gestation, the auricle undergoes increasing protrusion from the side of the head. By the end of the sixth month, the margin of the helix has curled, the body of the antihelix has become definitely folded, and the crura appear (Davis and Kitlowski, 1937). Interference with the normal evolution of this process produces prominent ears.

The usual deformity stems from a failure of folding of the antihelix, which widens the con-

choscaphal angle to as much as 150 degrees or more, producing flattening of the superior crus and, in more severe forms, of the body and inferior crus (Fig. 35–46). In extreme cases one may also note absence of the helical roll, creating a saucerlike structure almost devoid of convolutions, to which the term *shell ear* has been applied. Widening of the conchal wall may occur as an isolated deformity or in conjunction with a lack of antihelical folding. The abnormality is usually bilateral and is frequently noted in parents or siblings.

Clinical Terminology. To avoid confusion, topographic terms are designated as the ear lies in its normal position—for example, *medial* and *lateral* surfaces and *posterior* helical rim. The ambiguous term "postauricular" is avoided.

Treatment

A symmetrical result is important and paradoxically may be more difficult to obtain in unilateral than in bilateral prominence. The most lateral point of the revised ear should lie between 1.7 and 2.0 cm from the head. The convolutions should retain their smooth undulations; the helical contour should be continuously convex; and the rim of the helix, viewed from the front, should be visible behind the body of the antihelix (McDowell, 1968).

To attain these goals, a bewildering array of choices has been suggested, many of which have produced acceptable results, although valid, statistical analysis is meager, making a comparative evaluation virtually impossible. The discerning surgeon will identify the abnormal components that are causing the ear to be conspicuous and will direct corrective surgery to these specific points rather than following stereotyped patterns of correction (Sénéchal and Pech, 1970).

Alteration of Concha. The first attempt at otoplasty, consisting of a simple excision of skin from the auriculocephalic sulcus and suture of the conchal cartilage to the mastoid periosteum, is credited to Dieffenbach (1845), although Rogers (1968) has pointed out that he was actually dealing with post-traumatic deformities. Ely (1881) and others excised a strip of conchal wall, in addition to making a shallower auriculocephalic sulcus, a procedure that is popularly attributed to Morestin (1903). This older method of tacking back the concha to the mastoid periosteum has been revived by

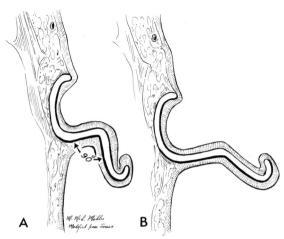

FIGURE 35–46. *A,* Cross section of a normal ear. *B,* Prominent ear resulting from an increased conchoscaphal angle.

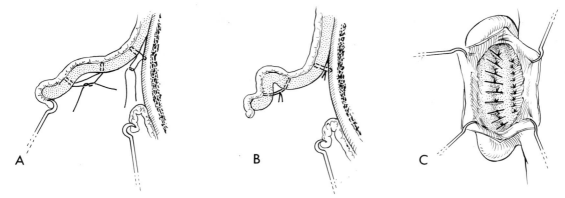

FIGURE 35–47. Technique of reducing prominence by conchomastoid sutures. *A,* Cross section of the auricle, showing placement of the sutures to reduce the conchomastoid angle and to restore the antihelical fold. *B,* Correction of the prominence. *C,* View of the medial surface of the auricular cartilage after correction of the prominence. (From Spira, M., McCrea, P., Gerow, F., and Hardy, B.: Analysis and treatment of the protruding ear. Trans. 4th Internatl. Congr. Plast. Surg. Amsterdam, Excerpta Medica, 1969.)

Owens and Delgado (1955), Stark and Saunders (1962), Paletta, Ship, and Van Norman (1963), Spira, McCrea, Gerow, and Hardy (1969), and Furnas (1968), although it is usually supplemented by a scaphal revision to give a more natural appearance (Fig. 35–47).

REDUCTION OF WIDE CONCHA. An excision of a cartilage ellipse just below the body of the antihelix, extending well into the superior and inferior conchal walls, gives an effective reduction of a prominence due solely to a wide concha. The approach is through a medial incision. Any redundant fold of skin within the conchal cavity should be excised to avoid wrinkling.

Restoration of Antihelical Fold. Luckett (1910) first emphasized the concept that prominence is due to failure of folding of the antihelix and its superior crus and excised a crescent of medial skin and cartilage to restore the fold (Fig. 35–48, *A*). The elimination of the sharp ridge formed by this incision in the cartilage has formed the objective of the majority of subsequent articles.

MODIFICATIONS OF THE LUCKETT INCISION. Erich (1958) made two parallel incisions along the proposed superior crus, creating a narrow strip of cartilage which slides outward, blunting the sharpness of the ridge. Straith (1959) overlapped the edges, Cloutier (1961) beveled the edges, and McDowell (1968) placed the inci-

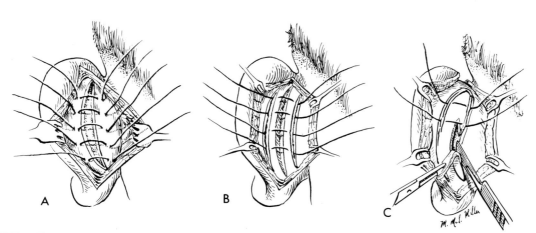

FIGURE 35–48. Evolution of the tubing principle for correction of prominent ears. *A,* Luckett; *B,* Barsky; *C,* Becker.

sion far posteriorly and allowed it to curve into the anterior crus helicis to break the spring.

Alteration of the Medial Cartilaginous Surface. To permit molding, the scaphal cartilage can be weakened by multiple parallel cuts (McEvitt, 1947; Paletta and coworkers, 1963 or by multiple tangential slices in a shingle pattern (Holmes, 1959). Converse, Nigro, Wilson, and Johnson (1955) used abrasion with burrs and wire brushes for the same purpose.

TUBING OF SCAPHAL CARTILAGE. Barsky (1938) suggested incising the anterior and posterior limits of the superior antihelical crus and rolling it into a cornucopia, yet still retaining the central Luckett incision (see Fig. 35–48, *B*). Becker (1949, 1952) and Converse and coworkers (1955) tubed the crus without incising its center (see Fig. 35–48, *C*). In addition to the smooth roll which is formed, tubing has the advantage of encasing a thick scar, which prevents recurrence of the deformity by locking the cartilage into its new position.

Mustardé (1963, 1967), reviving a long-forgotten suggestion of Morestin (1903), restored the roll of the superior crus by inserting a few mattress sutures through the cartilage, without any actual cartilage incisions.

Alteration of the Lateral Cartilaginous Surface. Based on the demonstration by Gibson and Davis (1958) of the propensity of cartilage to curl when one surface is cut, Chongchet (1963) supplemented the Luckett approach by undermining the unfolded surface of the antihelix and scapha anteriorly and making multiple partial thickness vertical incisions to produce folding. Stenström (1963) scored the lateral scaphal surface through a small, medial incision near the cauda helicis, using a short-tined instrument to groove the proposed superior crus. The method does not assure exact control of the amount of roll that will eventually result. Crikelair and Cosman (1964) and Nordzell (1965) described similar methods of producing a permanent curl. The lateral surface has also

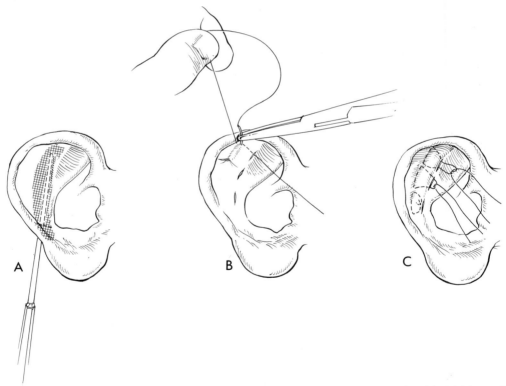

FIGURE 35–49. The Kaye method of correction of the flattening of the antihelix. *A,* A subperichondrial tunnel is made on the lateral surface of the cartilage through a medial incision near the cauda helicis, a sharp-tined instrument produces curling by multiple vertical striations. *B, C,* The proper amount of antihelical roll is maintained by several mattress sutures introduced through tiny incisions along the conchal crest and carried across the antihelical fold through holes in the skin. See text for modification of placement of incisions. (From Kaye, B. L.: A simplified method for correcting the prominent ear. Plast. Reconstr. Surg., *40*:44. Copyright © 1967, The Williams & Wilkins Company, Baltimore.)

been abraded or morselized under direct vision through a lateral incision (Ju, Li and Crikelair, 1963; Courtiss and coworkers, 1973), which permits actual excision of cartilage as well.

Kaye (1967) has advocated a procedure which combines scoring of the superior crus and fixation of the antihelical fold through minimal incisions. A skin tunnel over the lateral antihelix is created through a small incision on the medial auricular surface, either near the cauda helicis or at the tip of the superior crus, and the surface is scored with a sharp-tined instrument (Fig. 35–49, *A*). After a proper curl has been established, several mattress sutures of 5–0 clear nylon are placed through the reconstructed fold of the antihelix to maintain the exact amount of curling desired (Fig. 35–49, *B C*). The knots, which are buried subcutaneously, occasionally erode through the scar some months later. They can be clipped out without losing the curl of the cartilage. Kaye (1973) has found it equally simple to introduce the sutures through small stab incisions on the medial auricular surface, where the thicker soft tissue layer lessens the chance of extrusion of the suture knots.

Author's Preferred Method for Corrective Otoplasty. Long experience with a modification of the techniques advocated by Becker (1952) and Converse and coworkers (1955) has proved it to be dependable and adaptable to almost any combination of the usual abnormalities (Tanzer, 1962). It is particularly valuable in the correction of cases in which all components of the auricle are significantly involved or in which the cartilage is firm and bulky.

TECHNIQUE. Endotreacheal anesthesia is employed when extensive revision is anticipated. The contour of the antihelix and its superior crus, which can be brought into relief by folding the auricle back against the side of the head, is outlined in methylene blue (Fig. 35–50, *A*), and the pattern is transferred to the skin and cartilage of the medial surface of the auricle by a series of punctures with a hypodermic needle which is tipped with dye and then withdrawn (Fig. 35–50, *B*). It is important that the outline should extend well up into the superior scaphal sulcus and that a rim of about 4 mm of cartilage should be left along the base of the helix; otherwise, buckling may occur. A solution of procaine and adrenalin is injected as a hemostatic agent, and the skin is incised

midway between the two rows of dye marks (Fig. 35–50, *C*). After reflecting soft tissues sufficiently to expose the dye marks on the perichondrium (Fig. 35–50, *D*), the latter is incised along the outline, care being taken to preserve small cartilaginous bridges between the horizontal and vertical components (Fig. 35–50, *E*). In fact, the author prefers to omit the short transverse incision at this time, using it later only if necessary to improve contour. In the unusual event that the inferior crus is poorly developed, an incision may be made along this line also.

The pear-shaped antihelical cartilage, with its superior crus, is next rolled into a cornucopia by a series of inverted sutures of 4–0 braided silk, working superiorly until a satisfactory superior crus can be visualized on the lateral surface (Fig. 35–50, *F*). If the cartilage is too thick to bend easily, it may be thinned with an abrasive cylinder or rasp. The lower and narrower part of the pear-shaped cartilage need not be rolled, but any prominence of the tail of the helix should be excised.

The free edge of the concha is next reduced by the removal of successive narrow ellipses until the helix stands about 2 cm from the side of the head (Fig. 35–50, *G*). When cutting down the superior part of the conchal rim, a sharp angle may protrude at the outer edge of the inferior crus. This should be beveled on its lateral surface until the sharpness is relieved.

At this stage one frequently finds that the lower third of the auricle protrudes unduly. This can be improved by continuing the anterior cartilage incision inferiorly and removing a segment of cartilage. If the free edge of the antitragus is too prominent, the cartilaginous ridge can be exposed and trimmed through the original skin incision. Frequently, the reconstructed antihelix tends to slide posteriorly, bringing into sharp relief the cut edge of the concha. Two or three sutures of 4–0 white silk should always be used to hold the free conchal edge loosely to the contiguous edge of the tube, preventing the latter from sliding under the concha.

Having established a satisfactory cartilaginous form, the final positioning of the now mobile auricle can be accomplished by the excision of strips of skin from each side of the incision (Fig. 35–50, *H*). It is well to proceed cautiously, in order to avoid an overcorrection (Fig. 35–51). Rather wide segments of skin must often be excised from the lobule in order to correct eversion. Closure is done in two

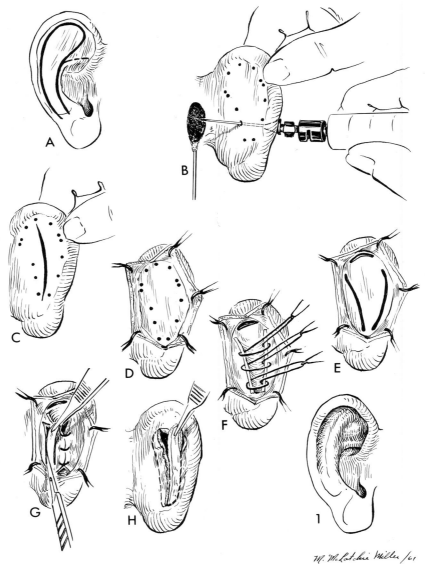

FIGURE 35–50. Complete corrective otoplasty (Tanzer modification of Converse procedure). See text for details.

layers, starting with interrupted, inverted sutures of 5–0 braided silk in the subcutaneous tissue. Plain catgut sutures are used for skin closure to avoid the need for suture removal. When the concha is excessively wide, the removal of a wide segment of conchal cartilage may leave, on the overlying inner conchal wall, an undesirable fold of skin which should be excised. Converse and Wood-Smith (1963, 1971) feel, however, that the redundant skin folds disappear in several months.

After repeating the operation on the oppo-

site side, all concave surfaces are carefully packed with damp cotton; both auricles are packed with fluffed gauze; and a soft gauze roll, elastic bandage, and stockinette head cap are used for fixation. No drains are used, and the dressing is left intact for 12 days. The use of an ear guard at night for another two weeks gives added protection against breaking of the sutures and damage from twisting (see Fig. 35–25).

Converse and Wood-Smith (1963) have more recently modified Converse's original

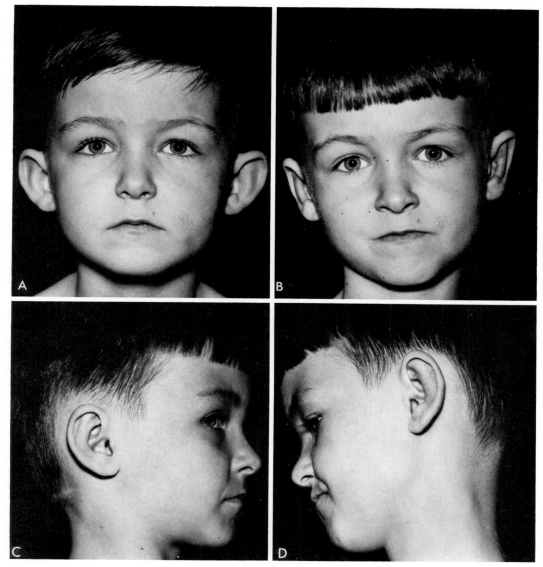

FIGURE 35–51. Correction of prominent ears by cartilage tubing and excision of conchal ellipse. *A,* Heavy, prominent ears, characterized by wide conchae and incomplete folding of the antihelices. *B* to *D,* Result of correction.

procedure, using a separate cartilage incision to reduce the conchal width and confining the anterior tubing incision to the superior crus of the antihelix (Fig. 35–52).

Author's Alternative Technique. A simple procedure combining some of the features of the Stenström, Mustardé, and Converse operations and similar in some respects to the procedure described by Crikelair and Cosman (1964) has proved particularly suitable in the treatment of many of the less severe abnormal-

ities involving failure of folding of the body and superior crus of the antihelix, with or without conchal widening. Proposed contours are dye-marked and the cartilage is exposed, as in the previously described procedure (Fig. 35–53, *A, B*). The cartilage is then incised along the outer mark, and the lateral cartilage surface between the two vertical lines is exposed and scored with a sharp-toothed instrument, such as one tip of a Brown-Adson forceps, to weaken its structure and to produce curling (Fig. 35–53, *C*). Care should be taken to avoid penetrating the full thickness of the

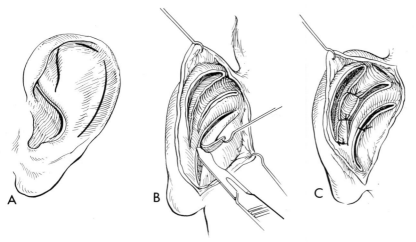

FIGURE 35–52. The Converse revised correction of the prominent ear. *A*, Outline of the cartilage incisions: anterior and posterior limits of the superior crus, the crest of the posterior conchal wall, and the spring-release incision in the superior helical sulcus. *B*, The superior crus has been tubed, and a strip of cartilage is being excised to reduce the width of the conchal wall. *C*, The defect in the conchal cartilage is closed with a single suture. (From Converse, J. M., and Wood-Smith, D.: Technical details in the surgical correction of the lop ear deformity. Plast. Reconstr. Surg., *31*:118. Copyright © 1963, The Williams & Wilkins Company, Baltimore.)

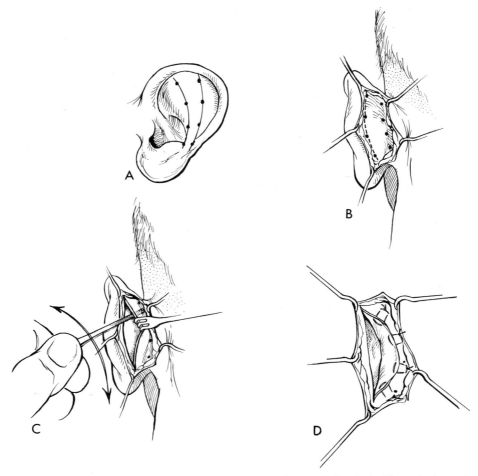

FIGURE 35–53. Correction of prominence due to an isolated superior crus deformity by Tanzer's alternative technique. *A*, Identification of proposed antihelical fold by penetrating dye. *B*, Exposure of dye marks on the medial cartilaginous surface. The broken line indicates the incision through the cartilage. *C*, Scoring of the lateral surface to produce curling. *D*, Final positioning of the rolled cartilage with mattress sutures between the free edge and the medial row of dye marks.

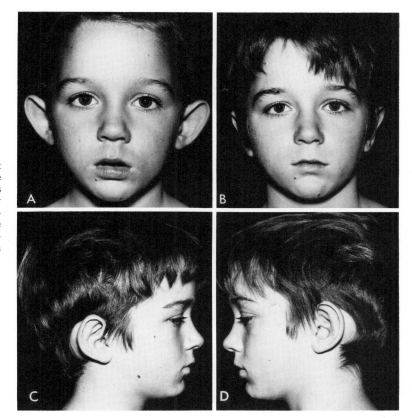

FIGURE 35–54. *A,* Prominent ears characterized by wide conchae and lack of antihelical folds. Previous treatment of the cartilage by mattress sutures resulted only in recurrence. *B* to *D,* Correction by the technique described in Figure 35–53, combined with elliptical excision of the excess conchal cartilage.

cartilage. Moreover, the curling should stop short of the desired roll, as overcorrection is difficult to adjust. The final position of the cartilage roll is established by several mattress sutures of 4–0 braided white silk, which run between the cut edge of the antihelix and the dye mark along the anterior limit of the antihelical fold (Fig. 35–53, *D*). This combination of scoring and suturing offers added security when the need for only a moderate amount of folding reduces the locking effect which scar tissue produces in a fully developed tube (Fig. 35–54).

If a wide conchal wall is playing a role in the prominence, the skin incision may be extended inferiorly and an ellipse of cartilage removed from the posterior conchal wall just below the crest, as previously described. Any prominence of the cauda helicis is reduced, and sufficient skin is excised to afford snug skin closure and to reduce any lobular prominence.

Shell Ear. An absence of the helical fold may occur as an isolated abnormality or in as-

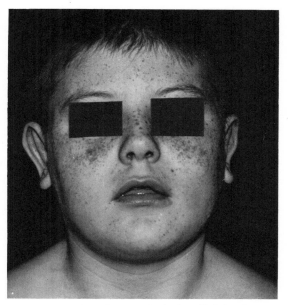

FIGURE 35–55. Concave "telephone" deformity produced by excessive removal of conchal cartilage and medial auricular skin.

sociation with prominent ear. The fold can be restored quite easily by scoring of the medial surface of the helix through small, interrupted skin incisions until an adequate roll has been produced.

Complications

Several pitfalls may beset the operator using the techniques detailed above. Failure to curve the outline of the superior crus well forward into the anterior scapha will give the crus an unnaturally straight, postlike appearance. Failure to remove sufficient cartilage and skin in the su-

perior and inferior thirds or excessive removal of conchal cartilage or skin in the central third may produce unnatural bowing of the entire rim (Fig. 35–55). Lack of attention to proper packing of the convolutions of the auricle or the failure to apply a bulky, well-fitting dressing at the end of the operation may result in the consolidation of the mobilized cartilage in a distorted form or in the ripping out of sutures.

The danger of skin necrosis, hematoma, and infection should be negligible if one adheres to the basic principles of careful handling of skin, meticulous hemostasis, elimination of dead space, and particularly the avoidance of trauma and pressure on the auricles during the first three weeks after operation.

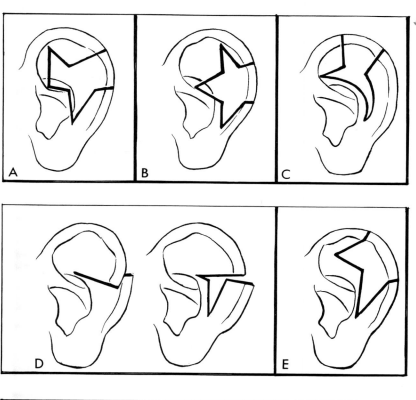

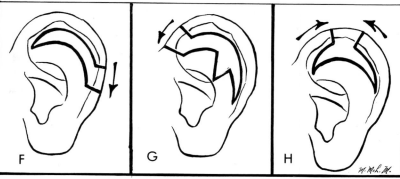

FIGURE 35–56. Correction of macrotia by full-thickness excision of wedges and crescents. *A,* di Martino; *B,* Cocheril; *C,* Cheyne and Burghard; *D,* Binnie; *E,* Day; *F,* Gersuny; *G,* Kölle; *H,* Peer and Walker.

REDUCTION OF THE AURICLE

It is unusual to encounter auricles so large as to require correction. More frequently, one has occasion to perform the reduction of an ear of acceptable proportions to match a reconstructed ear, since this may be simpler than the reconstruction of a large ear.

The earliest operation for the correction of macrotia by di Martino (1856–1857) involved the removal of one central and two subsidiary triangles (Fig. 35–56). Gersuny (1903) introduced the concept of reduction by excision of a long, narrow, scaphal crescent, combined with shortening of the helix, a method which is simple in execution and architecturally sounder than the multiple triangle type of reduction. Peer and Walker (1957) utilized Gersuny's reduction but shortened the superior helix in its center, preserving a more substantial blood supply. Davis (1974) left the medial skin intact, excising a superior scaphal crescent of lateral skin and cartilage, and excised the excess helical rim anteriorly.

A lap joint principle is applicable to the reduction of a hypertrophied lobule, although simple wedge excision rarely produces contracture. Guerrero-Santos (1970) suggested a reduction of the lobule by excising a full thickness wedge whose base lies just inferior to its attachment to the head. The transverse scar falls into a natural indentation of the normal lobule.

Congenital Auricular Malformation: Indications, Contraindications, and Timing of Middle Ear Surgery: An Otologist's Viewpoint

RICHARD J. BELLUCCI, M.D.

With the additional experience gained over a period of 17 years since the initial report of 25 cases of middle ear surgery for congenital auricular malformations (Bellucci and Converse, 1960), only minor changes have been made in the basic surgical technique (Bellucci, 1972a). However, a greater appreciation of the anatomical variations has been obtained, and the indications for middle ear surgery have become more precise. The results of surgery in 23 additional patients have also provided a better understanding of the average hearing improvement possible and have permitted an evaluation of the relative merits of tympanoplastic techniques and fenestration of the horizontal semicircular canal.

INDICATIONS AND CONTRAINDICATIONS

The original group of 25 operations was performed on patients with unilateral as well as bilateral involvement. It was the purpose of the 1960 study to evaluate the effects of the operation on patients with normal hearing in the uninvolved ear, as well as on patients with bilateral atresia of the external auditory canal. It was demonstrated clearly that the construction of the external auditory canal and the repair of the middle ear conductive mechanism did not improve hearing to adequate levels. Usually a hearing level between 20 and 30 decibels was obtained.

PATHOLOGIC FINDINGS

The ossicles were found to be grossly deformed in most cases, and the middle ear could not be exposed sufficiently because of limiting regional anatomy surrounding the aplastic tympanic bone. The facial nerve, which often took a shortened course through the temporal bone, was the most important structure restricting adequate widening of the osseous atresia plate. The tympanic membrane in all cases was absent. The osseous atresia plate, to which the malleus handle was attached by an osseous union, occupied the position of the tympanic membrane (Fig. 35–57). When the osseous atresia plate was removed sufficiently to expose the middle ear in order to perform a tympanoplasty, serious anatomical limitations were often encountered.

In contrast, the horizontal semicircular canal was found to be prominent and accessible in all cases.

The stapes was grossly deformed, rudimentary or fixed, poorly angulated in the oval window, or entirely absent; it was valueless for tympanoplasty in 43 per cent of cases. In some cases normal-appearing crura were entirely separated from the footplate. Fixation of the footplate or continuity between the crura and footplate was sometimes difficult to determine because the oval window was hidden beneath a prominent facial nerve. Consequently, fenestration of the horizontal semicircular canal was often found to be the procedure of choice. When the stapes footplate was normal and mobile and the crura were prominent in position, the autogenous ossicular mass of fused incus and malleus was shaped and repositioned onto the head of the stapes. Under these conditions an allograft incus could also be used. These techniques are adaptable in cases with lesser ossicular malformations in which the stapes is normal and accessible. It is doubtful whether an allograft tympanic membrane could ever be used in these cases. The atresia plate could rarely be widened sufficiently to receive the full-sized allograft tympanic membrane.

Another serious problem encountered has been the inability to widen the osseous atresia plate sufficiently to provide adequate examina-

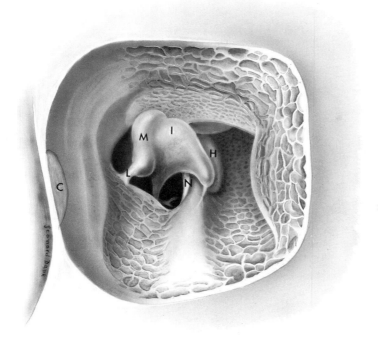

FIGURE 35–57. Typical exposure of the ossicles is demonstrated in a case with adequate cellular development of the mastoid. *C*, Condyle of mandible; *N*, facial nerve; *M*, malleus; *I*, incus; *H*, horizontal semicircular canal; *L*, ligament attaching the malleus to the bone which has formed in place of the eardrum.

tion of the round window. The entire ossicular chain, including the round window, must be examined at surgery. A good exposure of the round window is especially important in cases of severe middle ear malformation. The fenestration operation will not improve hearing unless the round window is well developed and functions normally. When an attempt was made to examine the round window, the facial nerve prevented adequate exposure in 9 of the 48 cases. In the underdeveloped temporal bone, the nerve does not descend directly to the stylomastoid foramen but turns anteriorly at the level of the round window niche to exit from the temporal bone at a level much higher and closer to the temporomandibular joint (Fig. 35–58). If the facial nerve is exposed in the course of widening the atresia plate, it should be decompressed immediately. This procedure ensures against the possibility of having a postoperative facial paresis or paralysis resulting from edema and constriction of the nerve within the bony canal. The additional time and effort involved in the decompression procedure are of little consequence compared with the possibility of an additional facial deformity.

The cavity established by removing mastoid cells in order to form the external auditory canal should not be excessively large. The size of the surgically made external auditory canal will depend on the amount of cellular exentera-tion. If too many cells are removed, a wide, ugly external auditory meatus will result.

On the other hand, surgery is impossible without cellular development of the mastoid. Middle ear surgery is contraindicated in most of these cases. Acellular temporal bones have insufficient space for construction of the external auditory canal between the tegmen antri, sigmoid sinus, and posterior wall of the temporomandibular joint.

Polytomography of the temporal bones is required in the preoperative study of all cases. This technique provides more definitive information than conventional radiography and can assist in determining the distribution and degree of mastoid cell development. The degree of middle ear deformity can be estimated and can be represented by the distance from the horizontal canal to the temporomandibular joint. The course of the facial nerve can also be disclosed by polytomography, and the otologist may be forewarned of an aberrant pathway. Gross errors in development of the inner ear can be observed, and the technique is sometimes useful in estimating the potential of inner ear function.

Although polytomography is of considerable help to the otologist, it does not provide the definitive information required to predict postoperative function. The mobility of the stapes footplate and the development of the round window, which are important factors in middle

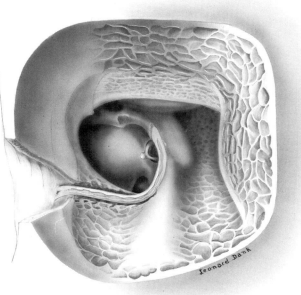

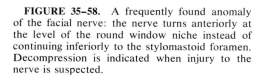

FIGURE 35–58. A frequently found anomaly of the facial nerve: the nerve turns anteriorly at the level of the round window niche instead of continuing inferiorly to the stylomastoid foramen. Decompression is indicated when injury to the nerve is suspected.

ear physiology, can be determined only at the time of surgery.

Thirty-four per cent of the patients developed skin graft problems. The cavities became infected, causing breakdown of the graft which required treatment. In eight cases regrafting of part of the cavity was found to be necessary. In all cases, however, periodic debridement of the postoperative cavity has been necessary.

The open cavity has created some limitations in normal habits of living. Especially in the fenestrated ear, swimming must be avoided if the ear is not protected. Keeping the ear dry is a general requirement in all cases in order to avoid cavity infection.

Gill (1969) reported that a significant percentage of patients with microtia have had infected mastoid cells when explored. This condition has not been observed in our group of patients, as only one patient had middle ear and mastoid secretions resembling those found in chronic secretory otitis media (glue ear). However, the possibility of middle ear and mastoid infection in a congenitally malformed ear should not be overlooked.

POSTOPERATIVE HEARING IMPROVEMENT

The hearing level obtained in cases of ossicular repositioning was slightly better than that obtained with fenestration of the horizontal canal. However, it must be restated that those patients requiring fenestration usually had more serious malformations involving the stapes and the round window. The hearing level in all cases never approached the normal level. The best that could be achieved was a 20 decibel level with the fenestration, and only two patients obtained a 15 decibel level with ossicular repositioning. After fenestration of the horizontal semicircular canal in two patients, there was no change over the preoperative level of hearing. In accounting for these failures, the possibility of cochlear or round window abnormalities exists.

Regression in hearing improvement has been observed following the fenestration operation, especially in children. In 25 per cent of successfully fenestrated patients who had achieved the 30 decibel level, regression in hearing to the 40 decibel level was observed after two years. In the patients having ossicular repositioning, regression in hearing improvement has been found to occur in approximately the same percentage (25 per cent), mostly in ears which have developed infection in the mastoid cavity. The conductive mechanism may have been adversely affected by the infection.

The hearing results obtained with tympanoplasty and fenestration of the horizontal semicircular canal have been tabulated (Table 35-2). In only a few cases were the ossicles found to be adequately shaped to be utilized intact, and the split-thickness skin graft was applied directly over them. The results were not encouraging. Of a total of six patients, only three showed an initial improvement in hearing above the 30 decibel level, and only two maintained the improvement for over two years. Inadequate surgical exposure for examination of the middle ear and graft failure in the postoperative period were considered responsible for these poor results.

TABLE 35-2. *Congenital Auricular Malformation: Hearing Improvement in 48 Cases*

TYPE OF REPAIR	NUMBER OF CASES	AFTER 6 MOS. OVER 30 DECIBELS	AFTER 2 YRS. OVER 30 DECIBELS	NO IMPROVEMENT	IMPROVED BUT NEVER ABOVE 30 DECIBELS
Type II Graft over intact ossicles	6	3	2	0	3
Type III Columella-incus transposition	21	13	10	0	8
Type V Fenestration of horizontal canal	21	16	12	2	2
	48	32 (68%)	24 (51%)	2 (4%)	13 (28%)

Fenestration of the horizontal canal was performed as often as the tympanoplastic procedure. Transposition of the fused malleus and incus over the normal functioning stapes (providing a Type III or columella arrangement) was the most adaptable tympanoplastic technique. When the stapes, for various reasons, was found unsuitable for tympanoplasty, a fenestration of the horizontal canal was performed. The results obtained by these procedures were approximately the same in this group. Although the hearing improved in some cases to a slightly higher level following the tympanoplasty, the fenestration more consistantly improved the hearing to the 30 decibel level. The long-term results, however, in a few cases showed some regression in hearing, probably due to osseous closure of the fenestra.

In general, following middle ear reconstruction approximately 50 per cent of patients maintained the improved hearing above the 30 decibel level for two years. However, 28 per cent of patients studied obtained some improvement in hearing but never attained the 30 decibel level. It must be emphasized that the percentages quoted are based on a small number of patients and may not be statistically significant.

After evaluation of these results it has been considered that the unilateral case does not require middle ear surgery if hearing is within normal limits in the uninvolved ear. Hearing is not improved sufficiently following surgery to compete favorably with the normal ear in providing binaural hearing. Surgery should therefore be limited to patients with bilateral auricular malformation.

TIMING OF MIDDLE EAR SURGERY

The psychologic trauma inflicted on parents of children with malformations often stimulates them to seek early medical advice. It is not uncommon that an infant in the first few weeks of life is brought to the otologist for correction of the hearing defect. There are serious limitations in performing elective surgery at this young age. The otologist, however, must provide a means of communication as soon as possible. In unilateral deformity with normal hearing in the uninvolved ear, no therapy or assistance is required. If poor hearing is present in the uninvolved ear, although external deformity may not be apparent, the patient should receive auditory assistance as soon as possible.

In cases with bilateral malformation of the external ear and absence of an external auditory canal, surgery should be postponed until 4 or 5 years of age. This is the period when pneumatization of the mastoid is complete. In addition, the child also can cooperate in obtaining reliable preoperative hearing tests.

In bilateral involvement, while middle ear surgery must be postponed, it is imperative that the child be provided with a means of communication. Tests should be performed to reveal the presence of bone conduction and of inner ear receptor function. At an early age audiometry is difficult; rotational vestibular tests, however, may offer a clue to the presence of inner ear function. Polytomography may show the presence of gross anatomical abnormalities of the inner ear. A trial of bone conduction hearing aid in the very young child is common practice. A child with bilateral congenital malformation should begin to wear a bone conduction hearing aid by the end of the first year of life. This assistance is essential for hearing as well as for the development of speech and general maturity.

Some controversy exists concerning the time relationship between middle ear surgery and reconstruction of the auricle. As the external canal can be opened only at one precise point, which is governed by the respective anatomical positions of the mastoid and the temporomandibular joint, it is desirable that the middle ear procedure be performed first (refer to p. 1678 for the plastic surgeon's solution). Plastic surgeons have stated that middle ear surgery, when performed as a primary operation, increases the difficulties in the construction of the auricle. As the sculptured cartilage transplant used for the framework of the external ear must be imbedded subcutaneously, the presence of the previously constructed external auditory canal makes this procedure difficult. There is also interference with the blood supply to the transplant when the middle ear surgery has been previously performed. When the cartilage transplant has become well established, it may be elevated and retracted somewhat in order to perform the middle ear surgery. As a secondary procedure, however, the middle ear surgery is more difficult due to limited surgical access and maneuverability. Each case should be discussed by the surgical team before any rehabilitative surgery is begun. In the bilateral congenital auricular defect, hearing should have equal if not prime importance in considering the sequence of the surgical procedures.

A certain number of conclusions can be stated, and they represent the author's opinion concerning this difficult clinical problem:

1. When normal hearing is present in the uninvolved ear, middle ear surgery is not recommended.

2. In cases of bilateral malformation with absence of the external auditory canal, middle ear surgery on both ears is usually required.

3. Middle ear surgery should be coordinated with construction of the auricle whenever possible.

4. In bilateral cases of auricular malformation or in unilateral cases with poor hearing in the unaffected ear, a bone conduction hearing aid should be provided as early as possible. Surgery should be postponed until the child is 4 or 5 years of age.

5. Approximately 60 per cent of the patients have a well-developed and functioning stapes, permitting a tympanoplasty. The fenestration of the horizontal canal is required when the stapes is fixed.

Acquired Deformities

JOHN MARQUIS CONVERSE, M.D., AND BURT BRENT, M.D.

Acquired auricular defects arise from trauma, thermal injury, or tumor excision and result in a wide variety of residual deformities. Because no two acquired auricular defects are exactly identical, the choice of an appropriate reconstructive procedure is limited only by the surgeon's imagination.

DEVELOPMENT OF RECONSTRUCTIVE SURGERY OF THE EAR

The early history of auricular reconstruction centers around the acquired deformity, which was a common result of battle, duel, or intentional punishment. Tagliacozzi (1597) described the preparation of a flap from the arm for repairing a major acquired auricular defect (Gnudi and Webster, 1950) and cited the case of a monk whose ear was "marvelously restored." However, doubts have been cast on the validity of this statement, and according to Bouisson (1870), "The surgeon from Bologna wrote this narrative in an hour of enthusiasm." Ambroise Paré (1575) described the technique of primary suture of the lacerated auricle, although he did not propose an auricular reconstruction.

Roux (1854) stated that his contemporaries considered the reconstruction of the auricle a surgical impossibility: "Where would one obtain all the skin necessary to form a new ear?" He further questioned how one could possibly produce the resilient auricular cartilage and its complicated convoluted shape. He concluded that a prothesis should be used in cases of total destruction of the ear.

Dieffenbach (1845), however, undertook the task of auricular reconstruction on a patient who had been involved in a fight in a public place. A police officer who had been summoned removed the upper portion of the victim's auricle with a single stroke of his saber. The patient was admitted to the Charité Hospital in Berlin, and an auricular reconstruction was begun after the wound was healed. Dieffenbach took a progressive step by performing the reconstruction with a local flap which was doubled upon itself to recreate the two cutaneous layers of an auricle.

Modern advances actually began when Pierce (1930) established the principle of using a cartilage graft to fabricate a framework support when he reconstructed a traumatically amputated auricle.

Attempting to improve the framework contour and to avoid a major operation on the patient, other surgeons turned to fresh and preserved cartilage allografts from unrelated donors, as well as to bovine xenografts (O'Connor and Pierce, 1938; Kirkham, 1940; Converse, 1942; Lamont, 1944; Brown and coworkers, 1947; Gillies and Kristensen, 1951; Steffenson, 1952). However, the cartilage allografts and xenografts became soft and disintegrated over a period of years, the reconstructed auricle lost its upright position and sagged, and sculptural details of the framework were effaced (Gibson and Davis, 1953; Schofield, 1953; Steffenson, 1955; Cannon, 1957).

Young (1944) and Peer (1943, 1944, 1948) emphasized the need for suitably shaped support by developing a technique for the prefabrication of an auricular framework. Chips of autogenous costal cartilage were placed in a two-piece fenestrated mold and then banked in a subcutaneous pocket until the cartilaginous fragments became joined by connective tissue. The unique framework that resulted consistently failed to maintain its contour, but the idea of framework "prefabrication" had been introduced.

In order to fabricate the auricular framework in a leisurely fashion, Converse (1950) advocated resection of the costal cartilage graft and its preservation by refrigeration at 2° C. Sculpturing of the cartilage framework was performed in a separate stage, and its transplantation took place in a third stage, thus avoiding the need for keeping the patient under anesthesia during fabrication of the framework. Brent (1974a) has used a subcutaneous abdominal pocket, as well as overnight refrigeration of the cartilaginous framework, before transplanting it to the auricular region under local anesthesia. This technique of producing a more relaxed "sculpturing atmosphere" is reserved for occasional total ear reconstruction, when prolonged carving time may be required to produce a delicate framework.

The contributions of Tanzer (1959), who introduced the careful sculpturing and assembly of costal cartilage grafts, followed by variations in technique by Converse (1963), made acceptable results in ear reconstruction possible. New designs for more efficient cartilage utilization have been introduced (Brent, 1974a; Furnas, 1974), and the use of auricular cartilage has been revived by Gorney, Murphy, and Falces (1971), Davis (1972), and Gorney (1974). Other techniques will evolve in an attempt to master the difficult task of auricular reconstruction, a problem which has long challenged the plastic surgeon.

SPECIAL CONSIDERATIONS IN ACQUIRED DEFECTS

Although the basic principles of reconstruction are similar to those described in the earlier part of this chapter, unique problems arise which require special consideration.

Except in patients with severe cases of facial microsomia and mandibulofacial dysostosis, in whom the periauricular skin is thin and atrophic, most patients with congenital microtia have an adequate amount of cutaneous tissue to provide skin coverage of good quality. On the other hand, cutaneous resurfacing is often necessary in acquired auricular deformities, since injury to the adjacent skin is common. In cases of thermal injury, the quality of the skin is in reverse proportion to the depth of the burn. Likewise, following tumor therapy, reconstructive attempts are influenced by the nature of the excisional defect and the presence or absence of an irradiated field.

Whereas a central incision is usually made for the introduction of the cartilage framework in congenital microtia (Tanzer, 1959; Converse, 1963), a variety of incisions are utilized in acquired partial losses, depending on the reconstructive technique chosen to reconstruct each individual defect.

Partial defects of the auricle can be repaired by various techniques and are often more easily remedied than congenital microtia. However, successful reconstruction of acquired defects may be extremely difficult or impossible — for example, in patients who have suffered total traumatic loss of the auricle in which the local soft tissues are destroyed or deeply scarred.

REPLANTATION OF THE AMPUTATED AURICLE

Replantation of amputated segments of the auricle was practiced in the seventeenth century. Cocheril (1894) cited the memoirs of Strafford written during the reign of the English King Charles I. Among the punishments inflicted to reduce Puritan and colonist opposition to the regime was the frequent process of nailing the victim's ears to a wooden post prior to amputating them. Among the many victims who endured this punishment, three have been specifically documented; a minister in the government, Burton; a lawyer, Prynne; and a physician, Bartwick. Prynne had had his ears cut off earlier for publishing a book which was considered offensive to the Queen. When he appeared before the Tribunal a second time, the presiding judge was surprised to see Prynne with two normal-appearing ears. Prynne's ears were exposed but showed the signs of mutilation. Prynne was condemned to have his ears amputated a second time, and immediately after the punishment was executed he retrieved the amputated parts, hoping to have them sutured back to their original site as had been done previously. No information is available about the fate of Burton's ears. Concerning the fate of our fellow physician, Bartwick, we know that his wife collected the amputated parts, placing them carefully into a handkerchief, hoping to have them replanted. All this took place between 1630 and 1640, long before any author had reported replanting an amputated ear.

Cocheril cited many examples of successful replantations during the nineteenth century and stated, "It is difficult to doubt the good faith of these authors: the prestige attached to their names; the clarity of their reports; the official approval given to their reports should suffice to consider them as veracious. The vascularity of the auricle, the rapid healing of wounds of this structure..., the fact that the vessels remain gaping, ready to receive nourishing fluid—all militate in favor of the veracity of the reports." The only information missing in all of these reports is the size of the amputated parts.

To the modern plastic surgeon, the choice of a salvage procedure is influenced by the size of the amputated portion and the condition of the tissues of the amputated segment, of the stump, and of the surrounding tissues, particularly in the retroauricular area. A clean-cut amputation gives the surgeon a better chance for success; a mangled and avulsed auricle and surrounding tissues with exposed bone render the task of reconstruction difficult or impossible. Small amputated segments are replaced as composite grafts with good assurance of suc-

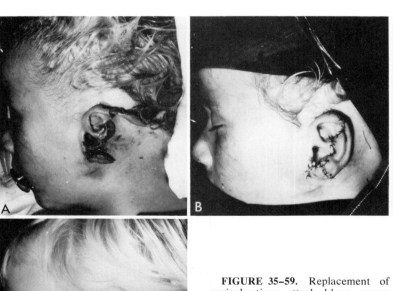

FIGURE 35–59. Replacement of auricular tissue attached by a narrow pedicle. *A,* Near avulsion of the auricle as a result of a dog bite. *B,* Appearance after repair of the auricular segment which is nourished by a narrow superior pedicle. *C,* Appearance of the ear one year after the injury. (Patient of Dr. Andries Molenaar.)

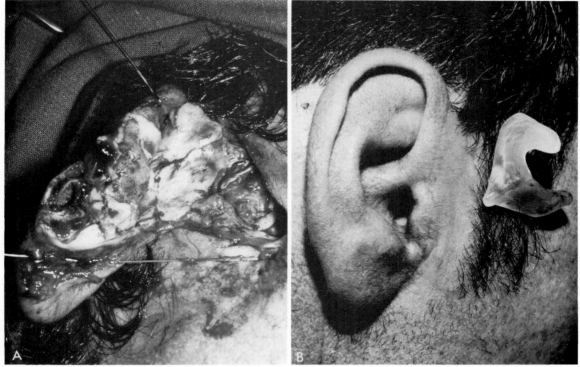

FIGURE 35–60. Repair of a major auricular avulsion. *A*, Avulsed ear remains attached by a narrow pedicle which maintains its viability; the canal is transected. *B*, Result following repair of the canal and maintenance of an acrylic mold for four months.

cess. Larger amputated segments and subtotal amputation require further consideration.

Replacement of Auricular Tissue Attached by a Narrow Pedicle. The rich vascularization of the ear and the fact that major vessels extend through the periphery of the auricle make it possible to replace successfully the partly avulsed auricular tissue, even though the remaining attachment is tenuous (Figs. 35–59 and 35–60).

Replantation of Auricular Tissue as a Composite Graft. The completely detached auricular tissue, even when the piece of auricle is quite large, may survive successfully when replaced as a composite graft, provided that the host bed is able to revascularize the graft (Fig. 35–61).

Replantation of Auricular Cartilage. The most difficult structure to reproduce in auricular reconstruction is the cartilaginous framework, and the salvage and use of denuded auricular cartilage were recommended by Greeley (1944), Suraci (1944), Conway, Neumann, Gelb, Leveridge, and Joseph (1948),

and Musgrave and Garrett (1967). Various techniques have been employed to preserve the cartilage from an avulsed ear. The skin may be removed and the cartilage buried either under the retroauricular skin (Sexton, 1955) or in a cervical pocket (Conroy, 1972). When the cartilage is placed under the skin of the retroauricular area (Bonanno and Converse, 1974), this latter orthotopic replantation of the cartilage obviously can be employed only if the regional cutaneous tissues are in good condition (Figs. 35–62 and 35–63).

An advantage of the tunnel procedure (Converse, 1958) illustrated in Figure 35–62 is the preservation of the retroauricular fold. Split-thickness skin grafts cover the two raw areas when the auricle is raised in a second stage six to eight weeks after subcutaneous placement of the cartilage of the amputated auricular tissue (Fig. 35–62, *G*).

Replantation of the Dermabraded Amputated Auricle. Mladick, Horton, Adamson, and Cohen (1971) and Mladick and Carraway (1973) have advocated a technique of enhancing revascularization of the replanted auricle by dermabrasion. The amputated ear is first dermabraded and then reattached to its stump; the reattached ear is buried in a subcutaneous postauricular pocket, thus allowing revascularization through the exposed dermis of the dermabraded auricle (Fig. 35–64). Two weeks later, the ear is exteriorized by blunt dissection from its covering flap, which is allowed to slide behind the helical rim; the subcutaneous attachments of the posteromedial auricular surface are left intact at this time; the exposed raw auricular surface is dressed, and epithelization begins within several days. One week later, the medial auricular attachments are separated by blunt dissection, which permits the flap to slide forward to the sulcus region. The ear continues to epithelize and becomes healed with routine wound care. The success of this technique in both cited cases is an incentive for further employment of this technique, provided local tissue conditions are favorable.

Replantation of the Amputated Auricle upon Removal of Medial Auricular Skin and Fenestration of Cartilage. Baudet, Tramond, and Goumain (1972) removed the skin from the posteromedial portion of the amputated part, fenestrated the cartilage (Fig. 35–65, A to D), and placed the auricular segment into a raw area established by raising a flap of retroauricular-mastoid skin (Fig. 35–65, E). The carti-

laginous windows (Fig. 35–65, D) allowed direct contact of the auricular skin with the recipient site, thus facilitating its revascularization. Although some distortion of the superior helical border occurred (Fig. 35–66), the result was satisfactory. The helical deformity could be readily improved by the inclusion of a carved cartilage strut. Brent suggested circumventing residual deformity by fenestrating the amputated auricular portion in such a manner as to create a basic "expansile design" cartilaginous framework support prior to replantation (see Fig. 35–65, F).

Replantation of the Amputated Auricle as a Composite Graft. McDowell (1971) reported the replantation of a major portion (50 per cent) of an auricle by Winter. After debridement, skin sutures alone were employed to reattach the auricular segment. Careful postoperative care was administered by McDowell; blisters were opened and dead epithelium trimmed; the ear was dressed with fine mesh Xeroform gauze, which was changed every three days. The transplant was successful despite some crumpling of the upper helical borders, which was corrected 15 months after replantation by means of a small curved strut of cartilage from the contralateral auricle. Gifford (1972) reported an excellent result following replantation of a smaller amputated segment of the upper half of the ear.

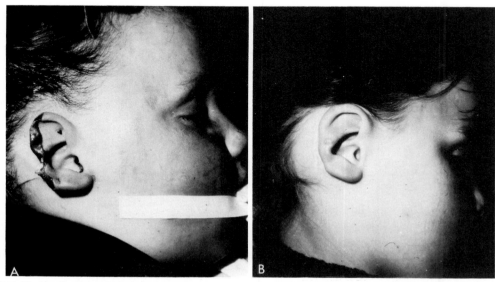

FIGURE 35–61. Replantation of auricular tissue as a composite graft. *A,* Loss of a portion of the scapha and helix resulting from a dog bite. *B,* The amputated segment was retrieved and sutured in position as a composite graft, with this result two years after the operation. (Patient of Dr. Andries Molenaar.)

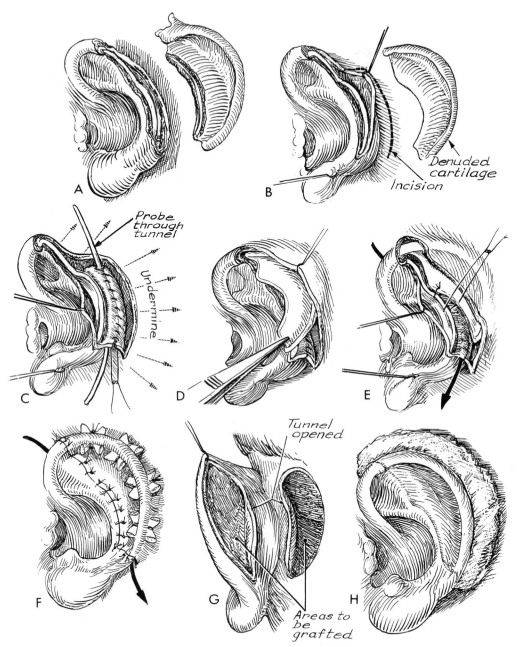

FIGURE 35–62. Replantation of the cartilage of the amputated auricle. *A*, The segment of the auricle amputated (see also Fig. 35–63). *B*, The denuded auricular cartilage, with an outline of the incision for the tunnel procedure (see Figs. 35–103 and 35–104). *C*, The incision is made, the cutaneous tissues are undermined, and the anterior skin edge of the incision is sutured to the medial skin edge of the stump (tunnel procedure). *D*, The cartilage is placed subcutaneously. *E*, The posterior skin edge of the incision is sutured to the lateral skin edge of the stump (the arrow indicates the tunnel). *F*, The suture is completed. End-on mattress sutures are tied over cotton bolsters to snug the skin to the cartilage (the arrow indicates the tunnel). *G*, Second stage: the auricle is raised. Note the preservation of the retroauricular fold. The two raw areas are skin grafted. *H*, A pressure dressing is placed over the skin grafts. (Figs. 35–62 and 35–63 are from Bonanno, P. C., and Converse, J. M.: The orthotopic replantation of the auricular cartilage in the amputated ear: Use of the tunnel procedure. *In* Kazanjian and Converse.)

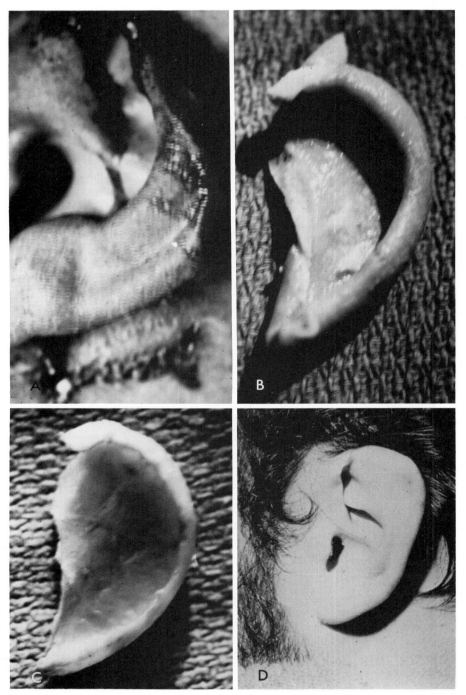

FIGURE 35–63. Replantation of the cartilage of the amputated auricle. *A*, The major portion of the scapha was amputated by a dog bite. *B*, The amputated segment. *C*, The cartilage denuded of soft tissue. *D*, The final appearance of the ear reconstructed according to the technique shown in Figure 35–62.

A surprisingly successful replantation of an amputated ear was reported by Clemons and Connelly (1973). The major portion of the pinna, the earlobe, and a portion of the concha were amputated (Fig. 35–67, *A, B*). Reattachment following debridement was accomplished 5½ hours after amputation. The patient was treated with vasodilators, heparinization, and antibiotics, and 24 hours after its replantation, multiple small incisions were made over the reattached ear's entire surface to relieve venous congestion by promoting capillary bleed-ing. On the fifth postoperative day, the heparin was discontinued and the patient was given two units of whole blood. The edema and venous congestion had been appreciably reduced at that time. Desquamation of the epidermis occurred, but the cutaneous surface re-epithelized with the exception of a small area of full-thickness loss in the posterior auricular area. The final result was excellent (Fig. 35–67, *C, D*).

The success of auricular replantation, as in all replantation procedures, depends on the cir-

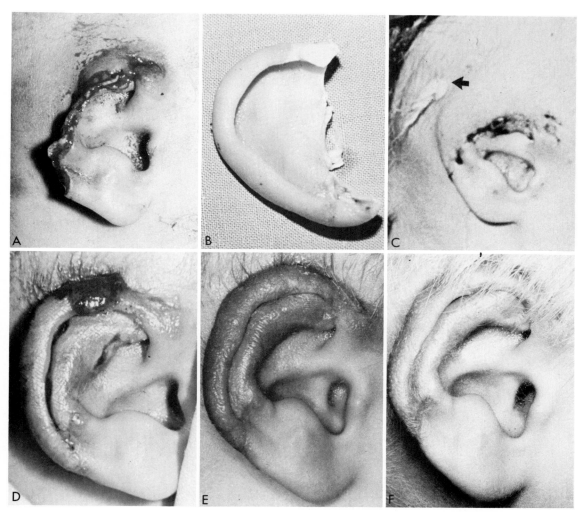

FIGURE 35–64. Reattachment of the severed auricle by dermabrasion and subcutaneous "pocketing." *A,* The amputated stump. *B,* The severed part. *C,* The dermabraded reattached part is buried in a postauricular pocket; a traction suture (arrow) from the helix flattens out the auricle to gain better apposition of the tissues. *D,* The ear has been exteriorized and is almost completely epithelized (see text for details); one granulating area is seen at the superior margin. *E,* One month after injury, the ear has a red flush over the reattached segment. *F,* Appearance at five months. (From Mladick, R., and Carraway, J.: Ear reattachment by the modified pocket principle. Plast. Reconstr. Surg., *51*:584. Copyright © 1973, The Williams & Wilkins Company, Baltimore.)

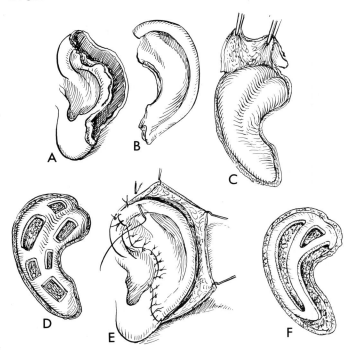

FIGURE 35–65. Replantation of the amputated auricle after removal of the postero-medial auricular skin and fenestration of the cartilage (after Baudet and associates, 1972). *A, B,* The extent of the amputation. *C,* Skin removed from the medial aspect of the amputated part. *D,* Windows cut through the cartilage. *E,* Reattachment of the amputated part; the denuded portion of the auricle is applied against the raw surface in the auriculomastoid area. *F,* Technique of fenestration suggested by Brent to prevent the deformity seen in Figure 35–66, *D.*

cumstances of the accident, the availability of specialized professional talent, the recuperation of the severed part, and the time interval between amputation and reattachment. A simple but valuable measure is to preserve the amputated part in an ordinary refrigerator at a temperature above 0° C or in a container filled with ice until surgical talent is available.

The Future: Microsurgery. The anatomical arrangement of the auricular vessels is particularly favorable for a microsurgical anastomosis of the amputated auricle's vessels to those of the host bed. At this writing, this procedure has not been reported.

DEFORMITIES WITHOUT LOSS OF AURICULAR TISSUE

Irregularities in Contour

The most common traumatic auricular deformities without actual tissue loss are due to faulty approximation of full thickness lacerations, usually resulting in distortion and notching of the helical border.

Meticulous approximation by carefully placed sutures is essential in the primary suturing of lacerations or in the secondary repair of maladjusted tissues. The techniques of Z-plasty, stepping, halving, or dovetailing the edges of the cartilage and soft tissue wound are important measures in preventing recurrence of contour irregularities. The sutures may be left in position for a long period, if necessary, without fear of suture marks or epithelization along the suture tract, the auricle being a privileged area in this regard.

Otohematoma: "Cauliflower Ear." A condition frequently observed in pugilists, this type of deformity is caused by hemorrhage resulting from a direct blow or excessive traction on the auricle. Blood collects between the perichondrium and cartilage, and the clot becomes fibrosed, causing a thickening which obliterates the convolutions of the auricle. This process is similar to that which produces thickening of the septal cartilage, another frequent deformity in boxers.

Early preventive treatment, after hematoma has occurred, requires incision and drainage of the blood clots and serum. The incision through the skin and perichondrium should be long enough to permit retraction, inspection, and the application of a large suction tip for the aspiration of blood clots. Compression sutures, preferably, or continuous suction are

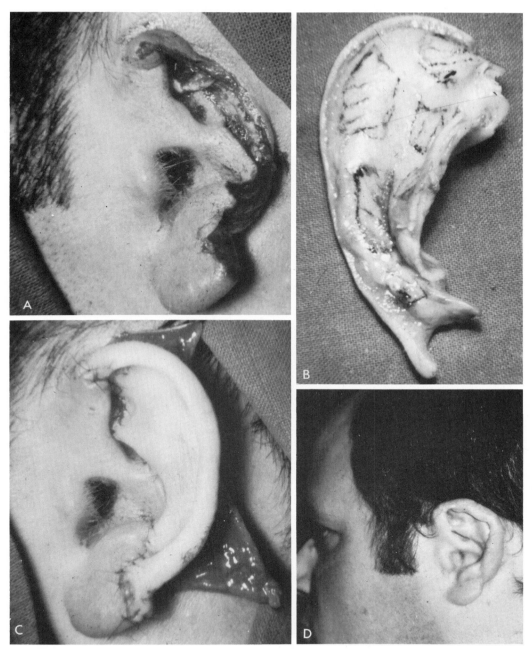

FIGURE 35–66. Replantation of the amputated auricle after removal of the posteromedial auricular skin and fenestration of the cartilage. *A*, Appearance of the stump of the amputated auricle. *B*, The denuded medial aspect of the cartilage; the outlines of the windows to be cut through the cartilage are indicated. *C*, The auricle immediately after reattachment. *D*, Final appearance. (Courtesy of D. F. J. Baudet.)

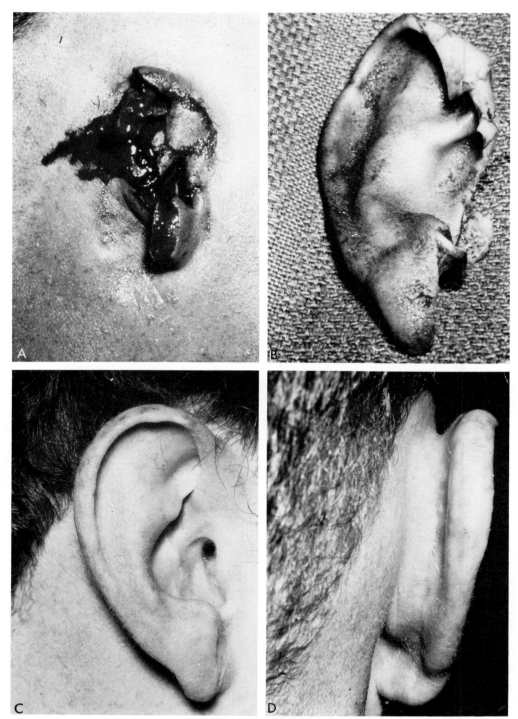

FIGURE 35–67. Replantation of a totally amputated auricle as a composite graft. *A,* The stump of the amputated auricle 5½ hours after the accident. *B,* The amputated part includes the pinna, the earlobe, and part of the concha. *C, D,* The final result after reattachment. See text for details. (Courtesy of Doctors Clemons and Connelly, 1973.)

required to prevent recurrence of the hematoma (Tanzer, 1951; Kelleher, Sullivan, Baibak and Dean, 1967).

The technique for late treatment of the cauliflower ear deformity consists in carving out the thickened tissue in order to improve the auricular contour. The thickened tissue consists not only of fibrous tissue but also of new cartilage which has formed in the blood-filled space between the perichondrium and the cartilage. The carving of the thickened tissue includes both the fibrous tissue and the newly formed cartilage (Skoog and coworkers, 1975). Exposure is obtained by raising a skin flap through carefully placed incisions; after the carving process, it is important to apply a pressure dressing to assure coaptation of the soft tissues to the cartilaginous framework and to prevent hematoma. Dental compound is an excellent pressure material which can be molded into the convolutions of the auricle, but it should be employed only by those familiar with its use.

Stenosis of the External Auditory Canal. The concha is prolonged inward by the external auditory canal through an opening, the meatus, through which lacerations may extend and ultimately produce stenosis.

Circular lacerations involving the canal should be carefully sutured whenever possible, and the canal should be kept packed tightly during the healing period (see Fig. 35–60). A small prosthetic appliance should be prepared to keep the canal open by taking an impression with dental compound, from which a perforated mold of acrylic resin is made. The tendency for stenosis disappears after three or four months, and the wearing of such a prosthetic support during this period minimizes the danger of stenosis (Fig. 35–68). When the concha has been destroyed by traumatic avulsion or thermal injury and only the proximal end of the external auditory canal remains, there is a tendency for the peripheral scar to obliterate the auditory meatus.

Cicatricial stenosis of the external auditory meatus and canal is remedied by Z-plasties of the cicatricial bands (Steffenson, 1946). In severe stenosis, when the meatus is closed and the canal is filled with scar tissue, the cicatricial tissue must be excised; the skin defect is repaired by means of the skin graft inlay technique. A full-thickness retroauricular graft, carefully thinned with sharp scissors, is one of the best skin grafts for this purpose. Two impressions of the canal are taken with dental compound. One impression serves to apply the graft firmly within the canal until the skin graft has taken; the other impression is duplicated in clear acrylic and should be worn by the patient for a period of three or four months to counteract the tendency for secondary contraction of the graft and subsequent stenosis. A detail worth noting is that the mold should be prepared in such a manner that the distal portion

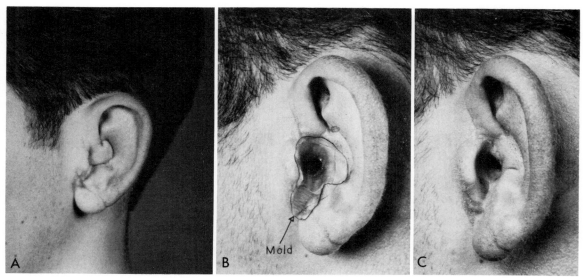

FIGURE 35–68. Traumatic stenosis of the external auditory canal. *A,* Stenosis of the external auditory canal resulting from laceration. *B,* Acrylic mold worn after skin grafting. *C,* Result obtained: the canal remains patent. (From Converse, J. M.: Reconstruction of the auricle. Plast. Reconstr. Surg., *22*:150. Copyright © 1958, The Williams & Wilkins Company, Baltimore.)

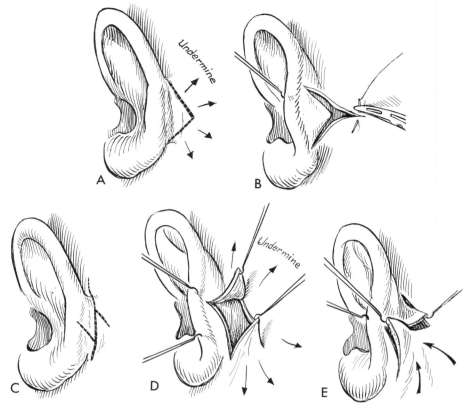

FIGURE 35–69. Freeing an auricular adhesion. *A, B,* The V-Y advancement technique. *C* to *E,* The Z-plasty technique.

of the mold itself fills the concha; this precaution ensures the stability of the prosthesis (Fig. 35–68).

DEFORMITIES WITH LOSS OF AURICULAR TISSUE

These deformities may result from loss of skin or cartilage or full thickness loss of auricular tissue.

Loss of Auricular Skin. Auricular trauma which results only in skin loss is usually secondary to burns. Loss of retroauricular skin results in adhesions between the ear and the mastoid region, whereas skin loss from the anterolateral surface may cause forward folding of the ear. The former condition is corrected by either release and skin grafting or V-Y advancement and Z-plasty (Fig. 35–69). The latter condition may require division and re-expansion of the auricle with interposition of a local flap (Fig. 35–70).

When a burn destroys the skin, the cartilage becomes involved also, and the result is a full thickness defect of the auricle (see Chapter 33 for early treatment of the burned ear). However, partial thickness burns which are adequately treated may heal with only varying degrees of contraction and thinning of the helical border.

Loss of the Helical Rim. In this type of deformity, the posteromedial aspect of the auricle fortunately is usually spared, and the skin is available for reconstructive purposes. The auricle appears thinned, although with little or no loss of cartilage (Fig. 35–71). Restoration is achieved by advancing the skin from the posteromedial area. An incision is made behind the retroauricular fold over the skin covering the mastoid process, and the skin over the posteromedial aspect of the auricle is dissected from the cartilage; the dissection is extended

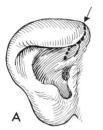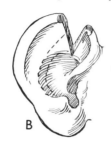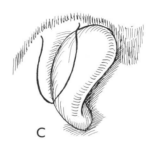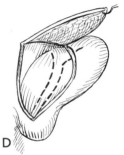

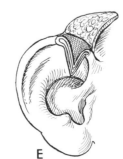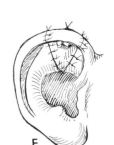

FIGURE 35–70. Correction of an ear deformity due to the loss of tissue at the anterosuperior portion of the auricle. *A,* The deformity caused by the loss of tissue. *B,* After incision through the full thickness of the auricle and restoration of the remaining structures to their anatomical position. *C,* A posterior auricular flap is outlined. *D,* The flap has been raised. *E,* A cartilage graft can be placed in the triangular defect; the flap is ready for coverage. *F,* The operation completed. This type of defect can also be satisfactorily corrected by a composite graft from the contralateral auricle.

to the helical border and over a portion of the anterolateral aspect of the auricle (Fig. 35–72). The skin on the medial aspect of the auricle is advanced to its lateral surface, and vertical mattress sutures anchor the advanced skin to the cartilage. If the deformity is unilateral, the retroauricular defect is covered by a full-thickness skin graft from behind the unaffected ear; if bilateral, a full-thickness supraclavicular graft in male patients, or a thick split-thickness graft from another donor site is used. This technique, which Converse has used for many years, has proved to be most successful.

Still other techniques can be employed for

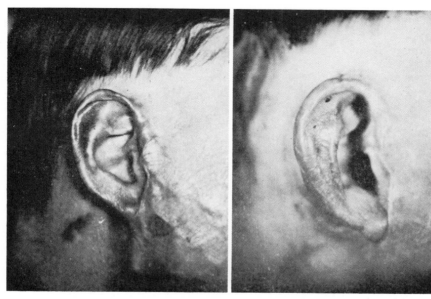

FIGURE 35–71. Thinned helical border secondary to a thermal burn. *A,* Thinning of the helix as a result of a gasoline explosion burn. *B,* The result obtained by mobilization of the auricular skin as illustrated in Figure 35–72.

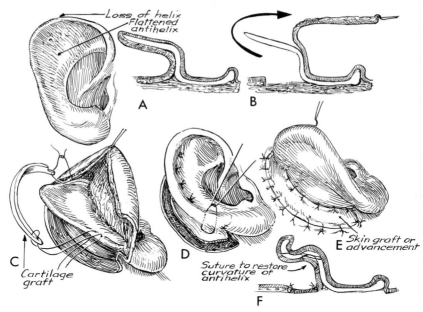

FIGURE 35–72. Advancement of the retroauricular skin for a cutaneous deficiency of the helix. This technique can be employed in combination with a cartilage transplant to restore the missing framework. *A,* The line of incision behind the retroauricular fold. *B,* The retroauricular skin raised. *C,* The cartilaginous ear framework exposed. *D,* The retroauricular skin has been advanced, forming a new helical border, and immobilized with vertical mattress sutures. *E,* The resulting retroauricular defect. *F,* The donor defect covered with a skin graft.

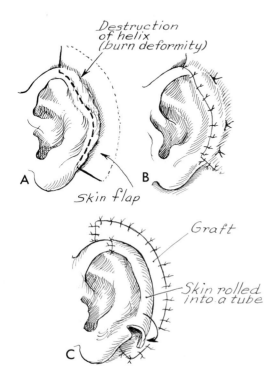

FIGURE 35–73. Technique for restoring the helical margin. *A,* Outline of the incisions for an advancement flap from the retroauricular area. *B,* The advancement flap sutured in position. *C,* In a second stage, the pedicle of the advancement flap has been sectioned, the flap rolled into a tube, and the resulting defect covered by a split-thickness skin graft. (After Padgett and Stephenson, 1948.)

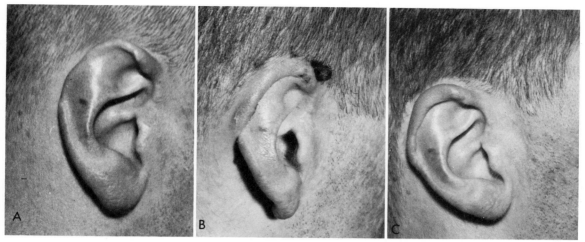

FIGURE 35–74. Helical reconstruction with a postauricular flap. *A*, Acquired loss of the helical rim. *B*, The postauricular flap in position over the auricular margin. *C*, The completed reconstruction, following division of the flap. (From Lewin, M.: Formation of the helix with a post-auricular flap. Plast. Reconstr. Surg., *5*:452. Copyright © 1950, The Williams & Wilkins Company, Baltimore.)

restoration of the helical rim when healthy retroauricular skin is available (Fig. 35–73). Lewin (1950) advanced a rectangular flap from this region, fixing it to the helical margin with some overlap. The overhanging advancement flap was lined with a skin graft or allowed to granulate and curl to produce a lipped rim; a secondary procedure is necessary to divide the tunnel, and satisfactory results have been obtained with this technique (Fig. 35–74).

Although skin tubes are generally to be avoided in total ear reconstruction, they can be valuable in acquired partial auricular defects; thin caliber tubes are useful in helical reconstruction when appropriately employed. When meticulous technique is utilized in conjunction with careful case selection, a fine helical rim can be reconstructed. The presence of good skin in the auriculocephalic fold minimizes tube migration and secondary deformity, and when local conditions permit, a preauricular tube can be useful (Figs. 35–75 and 35–76).

Tube flaps can also be constructed from the supraclavicular area (most suitably in male patients), and occasionally a thin caliber tube cervical flap constructed parallel to the lines of minimal tension of the skin may be desirable (see Fig. 35–76, *C*). In the latter, a horizontal tube is preferable to a vertical one, in order to avoid hypertrophic scarring in the donor

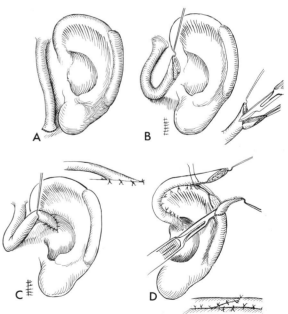

FIGURE 35–75. Stages in the transfer of a preauricular tube to the auricle. *A*, The dotted line indicates the level of the incision through the lower attachment of the tube. *B*, The lower end of the tube is beveled prior to transplantation. *C*, Attachment along a beveled plane (see inset) in the concha. *D*, Attachment of the remainder of the tube to the helical margin. The end of the tube is sutured to a previously inserted retroauricular tube by a beveled line of junction to prevent notching. (From Converse, J. M.: Reconstruction of the auricle. Plast. Reconstr. Surg., *22*:150. Copyright © 1958, The Williams & Wilkins Company, Baltimore.)

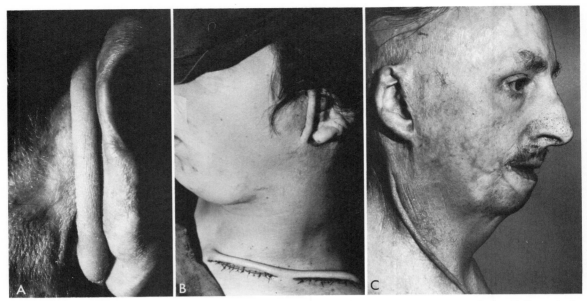

FIGURE 35–76.   Donor sites for construction of fine caliber tubes in helical repair. *A*, Retroauricular. B, Preauricular and supraclavicular; note the bridge in the latter tube. *C*, Cervical; the bridge has been divided previously.

region. Finally, tube flaps may also be constructed from the medial aspect of the arm, usually in children, since they are better candidates for tolerating the acrobatic position required during the tube's transfer.

Migration of fine caliber tubes must be accomplished carefully, following adequate tissue maturation, and unless the tube flap is opened and fully inserted over the helical margin, it will tend to droop over the scapha during subsequent months (Fig. 35–77). The addition of cartilage is often necessary and preferable to tubed helical rim reconstruction, but meticulous technique in employing the latter will provide pleasing results (Fig. 35–78).

A variety of other techniques are available to increase helical definition. When perichondritis or hematoma have resulted in the accumulation of fibrous tissue and newly formed cartilage in the prehelical region, the sulcus can be recreated by an incision through the posteromedial skin and cartilage; this segment is then advanced laterally, and the resultant medial defect is filled with a skin graft (Fig. 35–79). The "eave flap" technique (Cronin, 1952) has been described in the first section of this chapter (see Fig. 35–38) and is another effective method to gain helical sharpness (Figs. 35–80 and 35–81).

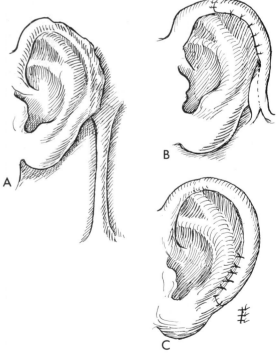

FIGURE 35–77.   The use of a fine caliber tube flap for reconstructing the helical border. *A*, A cervical tube flap prepared; one end of the flap has been moved to the tip of the mastoid process. *B*, The tube flap is inserted onto the helical rim. *C*, The operation completed. This procedure is preferable in female patients, who can hide the usually conspicuous scar along the hairline.

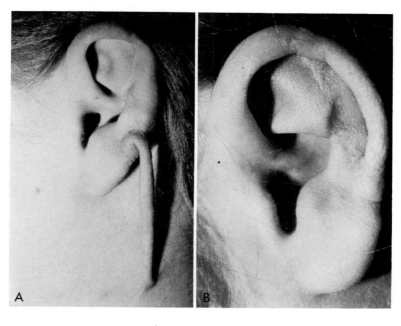

FIGURE 35-78. Helical restoration with a fine caliber tube. *A*, Migration of the supraclavicular tube to the ear with traumatic helical loss. *B*, Completion of the helical reconstruction; note the splice of the superior junction by a Z-plasty.

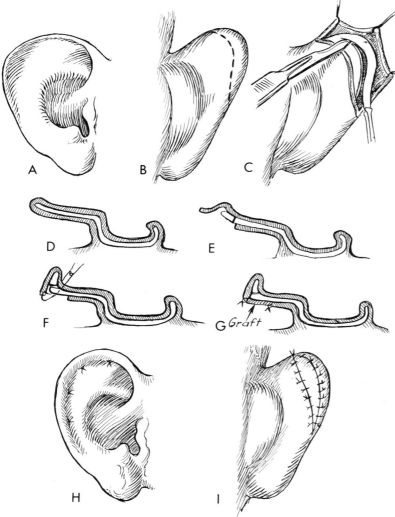

FIGURE 35-79. Reconstruction of the helical rim by an advancement flap containing scaphal cartilage. *A*, The typical shape of the auricle with a thinned helical rim following a burn. *B*, The outline of the incision. *C*, A segment of cartilage is incised along the rim. *D*, A sectional view showing the absent protruding cartilage forming the helical rim. *E*, The line indicates the incision through the auricular cartilage. *F*, The suture rotates the cartilage to form the protrusion of the helical rim. *G*, The skin has been advanced, and a full-thickness retroauricular graft from the contralateral ear (or from another part of the same ear) is in position. *H*, Mattress sutures maintain the rotated cartilage and advanced skin. *I*, A skin graft has been sutured into position over the resulting raw area. (After Cronin, 1952.)

1741

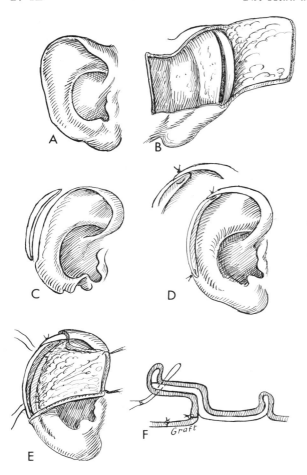

FIGURE 35–80. Reconstruction of the helical rim after partial loss. *A*, The appearance of the auricle with partial loss of the cartilage of the helical rim. *B*, An anteriorly based flap has been raised, and a segment of cartilage removed from the posterior aspect of the helix of the contralateral auricle has been turned upside down and is ready to be sutured into position. *C*, The auricular cartilage and graft. *D*, Technique of anchoring the graft to the adjacent cartilage by mattress sutures. *E*, The flap is ready to be replaced. *F*, Sectional view showing the cartilage graft in position. The skin flap has been advanced, and the resulting raw area is covered with a skin graft.

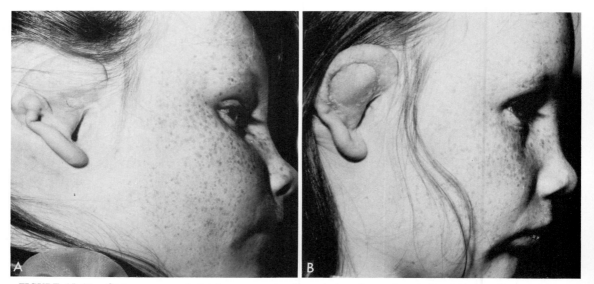

FIGURE 35–81. Common errors in total ear reconstruction. *A*, A patient referred after initial cartilage grafting and lobule rotation. Note the improper forward tilt of the ear, poor positioning of the ear lobe, and lack of helical definition. *B*, "Touch-up" procedures consist of lobule repositioning and the Cronin "eave flap" procedure (see Fig. 35–38) to improve definition.

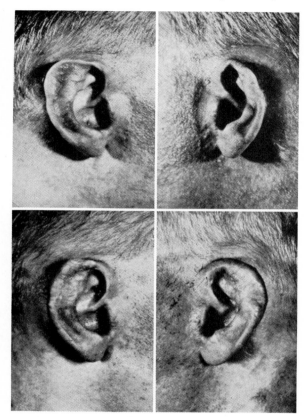

Loss of Auricular Cartilage. Loss of auricular cartilage alone is usually due to exposure of the cartilage by the destruction of the covering skin, as occurs following a burn. When auricular cartilage has become exposed by destruction of an area of overlying skin in a full thickness burn, spreading perichondritis may result in the crumpling of the major portion of the auricular cartilage. The ear loses its upright position, thus becoming a mass of retracted and crumpled soft tissue. Replacement of a cartilaginous framework between the cutaneous layers of the ear is possible only after adequate re-expansion of the soft tissue. A technique to achieve this goal is illustrated later in the text (see Fig. 35–106). Occasionally, the cartilaginous support may be lost secondary to other types of acute trauma (see Fig. 35–107).

Loss of auricular skin may be accompanied by helical cartilage destruction in thermal injury (see Fig. 35–82), and the correction of this deformity can be accomplished by skin advancement as previously described. The cartilage deficiency is simultaneously corrected with a strip of cartilage from the scaphal region of the contralateral auricle or with a small costal cartilage graft which has been carved to shape (Fig. 35–82).

Various techniques are available for providing replacement of cartilage deficiencies not limited to the helical rim. A cartilage graft from the conchal or scaphal region of the deformed or contralateral ear serves well for small defects, whereas costal cartilage may be required for larger deficiencies (Fig. 35–83). These techniques are described later in the chapter.

FIGURE 35–82. Helical losses secondary to a steam burn from the exploding boiler of a derailed locomotive. *A,* Thinning of the helical border of the right ear. *B,* Helicoscaphal loss of the left ear. *C, D,* Reconstruction by retroauricular skin advancement as shown in Figure 35–72. The framework deficiencies were restored with carved autogenous rib cartilage. (From Converse, J. M.: Reconstruction of the auricle. Plast. Reconstr. Surg., 22:150. Copyright © 1958, The Williams & Wilkins Company, Baltimore.)

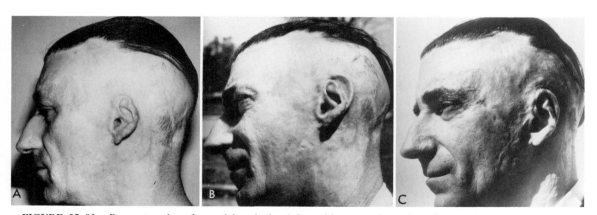

FIGURE 35–83. Reconstruction of a partial auricular defect with a carved costal cartilage graft. *A,* Thermal burn deformity in which the helix and the entire scapha were destroyed. *B,* Six weeks after implantation of a carved cartilage graft. *C,* Final appearance following routine elevation and skin grafting. (From Brent, B.: Ear reconstruction with an expansile framework of autogenous rib cartilage. Plast. Reconstr. Surg., 53:619. Copyright © 1974, The Williams & Wilkins Company, Baltimore.)

FULL THICKNESS DEFECTS OF THE AURICLE

For purposes of classification, full thickness defects of the ear may be divided into six groups: defects of the upper third, middle third, and lower third; partial and total loss; and loss of the lobule of the ear.

Major Auricular Loss Following Trauma

Loss of a major portion of the auricle or the entire ear itself may result from a razor slash, flying glass, a gunshot wound, flame or radiation burns, human or dog bites, or a shearing injury in an automobile accident. Complete traumatic loss of the auricle is an unusual occurrence, for a portion of the concha and the external auditory canal are usually preserved even in cases of severe injury.

When a large portion of the auricle or the entire ear has been destroyed, a number of requirements must be met in successive stages: (1) a suitable skin covering devoid of hair follicles, (2) a framework of cartilage to maintain the upright position of the reconstructed auricle and to represent its characteristic convolutions, and (3) a covering of skin for the posteromedial aspect of the auricular framework after it is raised from the mastoid area. A number of additional ''retouching'' procedures are often necessary in order to achieve satisfactory contour of the reconstructed auricle.

The Skin Covering. The presence of supple and well-vascularized skin is a sine qua non for success in auricular reconstruction. The qual- ity of the residual local soft tissues varies in traumatic defects. When amputation of the auricle is by means of a clean-cut laceration, the local residual skin remains relatively unscarred and thus may be utilized. Likewise, minimally scarred skin following healed partial thickness burns may be of sufficiently good quality to avoid skin grafting. However, if the auricle has been avulsed, destroyed by a burn, or injured by a gunshot, the area may show multiple linear or surface scars, thus necessitating excision and replacement with a skin graft before the auricular reconstruction begins. Should this be necessary, a full-thickness graft from the contralateral retroauricular region or supraclavicular area is most suitable for this purpose, although a thick split-thickness graft will suffice if the former is not available (see Fig. 35–86, *C*). It is essential that the skin overlying a cartilage graft have an adequate blood supply and is sufficiently loose to avoid pressure which might contribute to ultimate cartilage absorption. Therefore, the skin graft must be allowed to mature for a number of months before proceeding to cartilage transplantation.

In conjunction with assessment of the local tissues, one must give consideration to the hairline postion, since its natural location often leaves the surgeon with no choice but to place the cartilage framework beneath it (see the first section of this chapter). The presence of hair on the reconstructed ear represents a major problem which is most difficult to remedy. When the density of the hair follicles is such that it cannot be eradicated by electrolysis, late excision of the hair-bearing tissue and replacement with a skin graft may be required.

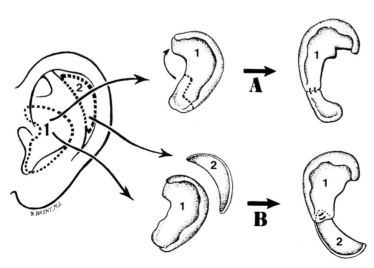

FIGURE 35–84. The use of auricular cartilage for framework fabrication in major auricular reconstruction. *A,* Sectioning and splicing of conchal cartilage; concha is rotated 90 degrees (technique of Gorney, Murphy, and Falces). *B,* The combination of conchal and scaphal cartilage; the conchal piece is rotated 90 degrees (technique of Brent.)

The Auricular Framework. An adequate cartilaginous framework is the key to satisfactory reconstruction in a traumatic auricular loss. The delicate form and elastic properties of the natural auricular support cannot be duplicated with costal cartilage; hence, the avulsed auricular cartilage should be utilized whenever feasible (see Figs. 35–62 and 35–63).

Use of conchal cartilage from the contralateral unaffected ear has been advocated by Kazanjian (1949), Adams (1955), Steffenson (1965), Gorney, Murphy, and Falces (1971), and Davis (1972) and is particularly useful for reconstructing partial auricular defects. The cartilage graft is removed through an incision on the medial auricular surface following precise marking and needle tattooing over the anterolateral surface; careful application of a contoured dressing of cotton or sponge rubber, which is maintained for several weeks, is an important measure in preventing donor ear deformity.

By sectioning and splicing the conchal cartilage graft, a somewhat larger framework can be fabricated for reconstructing larger defects, as demonstrated by Gorney, Murphy, and Falces (1971) (Figs. 35–84 and 35–85). They have stressed the preservation of the basic auricular framework, i.e., the helical and antihelical struts, to prevent donor ear distortion. Complying with this principle, the scaphal cartilage can be utilized in combination with a conchal cartilage to obtain a slightly larger framework (Brent, 1975) (see Fig. 35–84).

For larger defects, costal cartilage is often required. The technique for removing and sculpturing a costal cartilage graft has been described in the first section of this chapter. When adequate skin coverage has been provided, the technique for framework fabrication is similar to that employed in congenital microtia (Figs. 35–86 and 35–87). Likewise, Brent has employed his expansile framework variation (Fig. 35–27) with effective results in the total reconstruction of burned ears (Figs. 35–88 and 35–89).

Planning and Positioning of the Proposed Auricular Reconstruction. Meticulous attention to details is imperative in auricular reconstruction, and careful planning is essential long before the actual surgery takes place. A radiographic film pattern made preoperatively from the patient's opposite normal ear, then reversed, is an invaluable reference for framework fabrication during surgery (Fig. 35–90).

As emphasized previously in this chapter, proper orientation of the reconstructed ear is absolutely essential, as improper positioning will spoil an otherwise well-reconstructed ear (see Fig. 35–81). Topographical relationships between the ear and its adjacent facial features have been described by Broadbent and

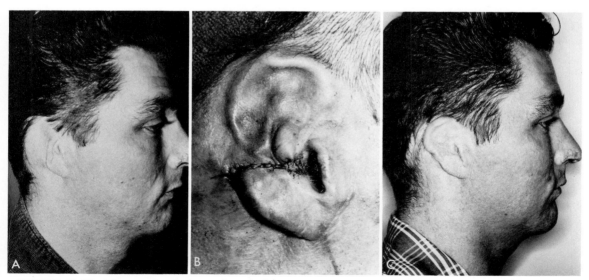

FIGURE 35–85. The use of auricular cartilage for framework support in the reconstruction of the burned ear. *A*, Burn deformity of the ear. *B*, Appearance after the first stage of reconstruction. *C*, The final result. (From Gorney, M., Murphy, S., and Falces, E.: Spliced autogenous conchal cartilage in secondary ear reconstruction. Plast. Reconstr. Surg., 47:432. Copyright © 1971, The Williams & Wilkins Company, Baltimore.)

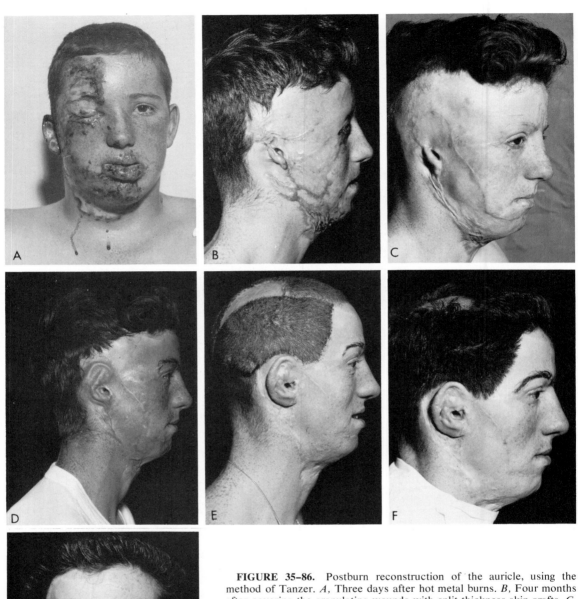

FIGURE 35–86. Postburn reconstruction of the auricle, using the method of Tanzer. *A*, Three days after hot metal burns. *B*, Four months after covering the granulating wounds with split-thickness skin grafts. *C*, After substitution of a thicker skin graft in preparation for ear reconstruction. Full-thickness grafts to the lids and a parietal scalp graft to the right eyebrow have been completed. *D*, Twelve months after embedding the costal cartilage framework. The long axis of the new ear is tilted forward; it should lie parallel to the nasal bridge. *E*, After restoration of the auriculocephalic sulcus. The hairline has been restored by a rotation scalp flap, *F*, *G*, Final views. The conspicuousness of the auditory canal could be partially concealed by a cartilage graft to the tragus. (From Tanzer, R. C.: The reconstruction of acquired defects of the ear. Plast. Reconstr. Surg., *35*:355, Copyright © 1965. The Williams & Wilkins Company, Baltimore.)

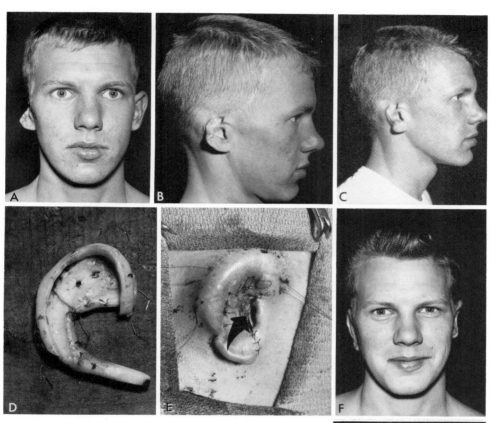

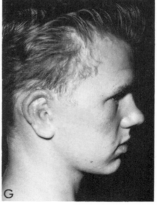

FIGURE 35–87. Avulsion of the auricle associated with a compound fracture of the temporal bone, reconstructed by the method of Tanzer. *A, B,* After initial debridement and repair. *C,* After scar revision and excision of a cartilage wedge to permit setting-in of the lobule. *D,* The completed costal cartilage graft, with wire sutures still untrimmed. Knotted rather than twisted sutures are now used, and the framework is constructed more thinly with larger perforations. *E,* Embedment of the cartilage graft. Compression sutures will be tied over pledgets of gauze to snug the skin cover into the helical sulcus. The arrow indicates the skin defect resulting from the advancement of skin posteriorly and superiorly to fill the helical sulcus. *F, G,* After completion of the reconstruction and revision of the left auricle. (From Tanzer, R. C.: The reconstruction of acquired defects of the ear. Plast. Reconstr. Surg., *35*:355. Copyright © 1965, The Williams & Wilkins Company, Baltimore.)

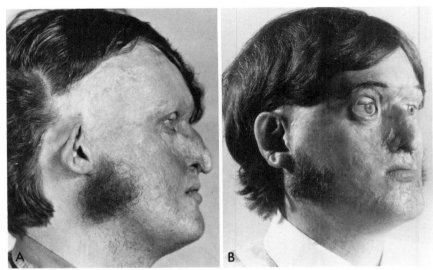

FIGURE 35–88.   Reconstruction of the ear with an expansile framework of autogenous rib cartilage. *A,* The appearance of a Vietnam war veteran following a white phosphorus burn. *B,* Ear reconstruction with an expansile framework (see Fig. 35–27) transplanted following overnight refrigeration; eyebrows reconstructed with scalp grafts; and nasal contouring accomplished with a cartilage graft and a nasolabial flap. The eyes are prosthetic. (From Brent, B.: Ear reconstruction with an expansile framework of autogenous rib cartilage. Plast. Reconstr. Surg., *53*:619. Copyright © 1974, The Williams & Wilkins Company, Baltimore.)

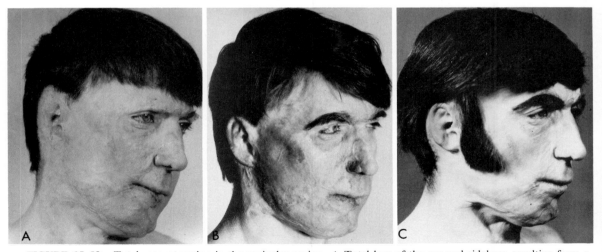

FIGURE 35–89.   Total reconstruction in the auricular region. *A,* Total loss of the ear and sideburn resulting from a burn. *B,* The result obtained with an autogenous costal cartilage framework. The eyebrow has also been reconstructed using scalp grafts. *C,* Restoration of the sideburn completes the reconstruction and complements the reconstituted auricle; the sideburn reconstruction was accomplished with a rectangular scalp flap transposed onto a cervicooccipital tube. (From Brent, B.: Reconstruction of the ear, eyebrow and sideburn in the burned patient. Plast. Reconstr. Surg., *55*:312. Copyright © 1975, The Williams & Wilkins Company, Baltimore.)

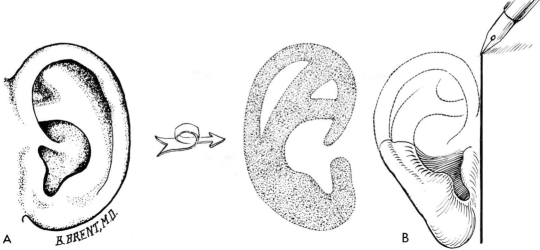

FIGURE 35–90. Preoperative planning for auricular reconstruction. *A,* From the contralateral ear, a radiographic film pattern is traced and used in reverse as a reference during surgery. *B,* The lobe, tragus, and forward helical curve should be behind a straight line. (*A,* from Brent, B.: Reconstruction of the ear, eyebrow and sideburn in the burned patient. Plast. Reconstr. Surg., *55*:312, 1975; *B* from Converse, J. M.: Reconstruction of the auricle. Plast. Reconstr. Surg., *22*:150. Copyright © 1958, The Williams & Wilkins Company, Baltimore.)

Mathews (1957) and further stressed by Gorney, Murphy, and Falces (1971). A simple guideline is the parallelogram used by Brent (1975a) (Fig. 35–91); however, owing to some variance in each individual ear's axis, it is necessary to compare the position of the patient's unaffected ear with its adjacent facial features during the planning stage. A photograph of the patient's contralateral profile is a helpful aid while planning the reconstruction and when embedding the framework (see also Figs. 35–13 to 35–15).

Maintaining an adequate auriculocephalic angle in the reconstructed ear is a difficult problem. The techniques employed by Tanzer and Converse have been discussed in the first section of this chapter. An additional method, endorsed by Gorney (1974) and Edgerton and Bacchetta (1974), is the "sling flap," devised by Steffenson (1952). By this technique, a narrow, inferiorly based triangular flap is transposed into the auriculocephalic sulcus, and a skin graft is placed on each side of the flap (Fig. 35–92). Brent has found it expedient to suture a one-piece graft into place, with the center portion of the graft overlying the triangular flap. At the first dressing change, this overlying portion, which often may become

FIGURE 35–91. Determination of the location of the ear by the parallelogram method (the contralateral unburned side of the patient in Fig. 35–89). The axis of the ear is parallel to the profile of the nose, and the vertical dimension is defined by the glabella and the subnasale. (From Brent, B.: Reconstruction of the ear, eyebrow and sideburn in the burned patient. Plast. Reconstr. Surg., *55*:312. Copyright © 1975, The Williams & Wilkins Company, Baltimore.)

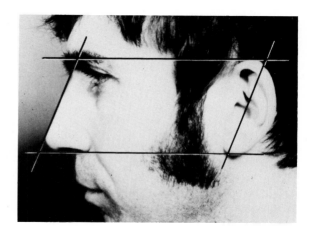

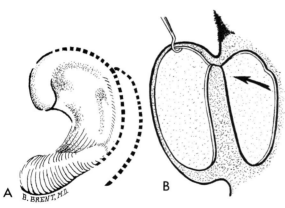

FIGURE 35–92. Maintaining the projection of the constructed auricle with a transposition flap. *A,* Incisions outlined for elevation of the auricle and creation of a narrow, inferiorly based flap. *B,* The flap is transposed to the posteromedial auricular surface at its junction with the new sulcus; the raw surfaces are covered by skin grafts. Interposition of the flap reduces the tendency toward obliteration of the auriculocephalic sulcus. (After Steffenson.)

revascularized by the bridging phenomenon, is merely snipped away, leaving healthy skin grafts on either side of the now exposed triangular flap.

Inorganic Implants. The vicissitudes of surgeons who employ inorganic implants to replace the cartilaginous auricle have been recounted in the earlier part of this chapter. It must be emphasized that, after failure due to extrusion of an inorganic implant, not only is the surgeon "back to zero," having imposed a series of operations upon the patient, but also the reconstructed auricle has become a crumpled mass of scarred soft tissue, which is often an insurmountable handicap.

Recent reports indicating high percentages of rejection of inorganic implants at the International Conference on the Diagnosis and Treatment of Craniofacial Anomalies (1971) and the Symposium on Reconstruction of the Auricle of the Education Foundation of the American Society of Plastic and Reconstructive Surgery (1973) have suggested that the bell tolls, in fact the knell has already sounded, for the inorganic implant as a framework for the auricle.

The Auricular Prosthesis. Because of the multiplicity of operations, the frequent complications, and the poor esthetic results often obtained, many surgeons are prone to suggest the use of a prosthetic ear rather than to submit a patient to surgery. An auricular prosthesis,

however, is not a panacea. Although the immediate result is usually good, the prosthesis often causes skin irritation and requires periodic replacement because of changes in color and texture. The patient in some cases dislikes an "artificial part" and fears it will embarrass him by falling off at inappropriate times. One of the most difficult problems associated with an auricular prosthesis is the seasonal change in each patient's skin color, a phenomenon which dictates his using different-colored auricles in summer and winter. Auricular prostheses in children are not practical. Artificial ears should be reserved for use in inoperable cases and in older individuals, when they are practical if not invaluable items. The attachment by means of a surgically created subcutaneous tunnel (Ombrédanne 1956) has not proved successful.

In conclusion, it is generally agreed that total reconstruction of the ear remains a difficult surgical problem and is not a procedure to be attempted in a hurried manner. Careful, deliberate, and precise planning and technique are essential. As Converse has stated (1958), to construct a structurally thin, well-shaped auricle which protrudes from the side of the head with an adequate retroauricular fold, the surgeon must walk a tightrope, balancing between beauty and blood supply.

Partial Auricular Loss

Partial acquired auricular defects constitute the greatest number of ear deformities confronting the plastic surgeon. The choice of the reconstructive procedure is influenced by the nature of the defect, and it behooves the surgeon to familiarize himself with a variety of techniques.

Composite Grafts. Small to moderate sized defects may be repaired with composite grafts from the unaffected ear, particularly if the latter is large and protruding (Day, 1921; Adams, 1955; Pegram and Peterson, 1956; Nagel, 1972). The wedge-shaped composite graft, preferably less than 1.5 cm in width, is resected from the scapha and helix of the unaffected ear and transplanted into a clean-cut defect on the contralateral ear (Fig. 35–93). The success rate of composite grafts can be enhanced by removing a portion of the skin and cartilage, thus converting part of the "wedge" to a full-thickness skin graft, which is readily vascularized by a recipient advancement flap mobil-

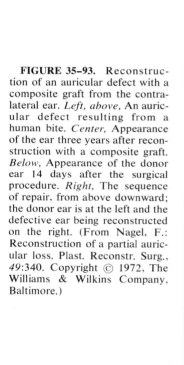

FIGURE 35–93. Reconstruction of an auricular defect with a composite graft from the contralateral ear. *Left, above,* An auricular defect resulting from a human bite. *Center,* Appearance of the ear three years after reconstruction with a composite graft. *Below,* Appearance of the donor ear 14 days after the surgical procedure. *Right,* The sequence of repair, from above downward; the donor ear is at the left and the defective ear being reconstructed on the right. (From Nagel, F.: Reconstruction of a partial auricular loss. Plast. Reconstr. Surg., *49*:340. Copyright © 1972, The Williams & Wilkins Company, Baltimore.)

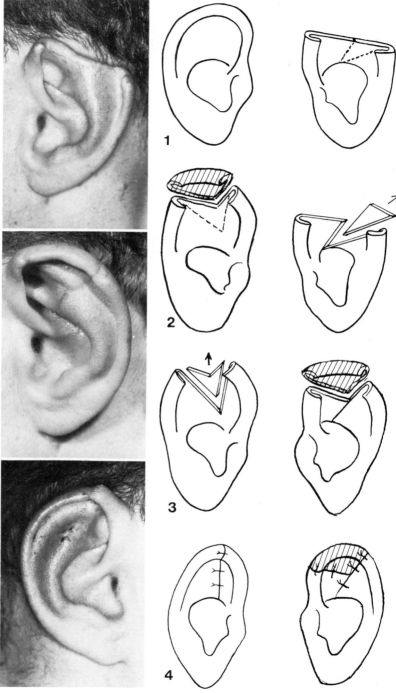

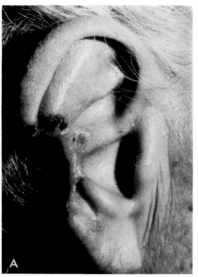
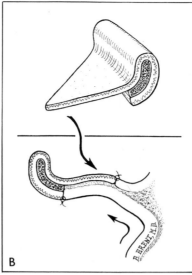
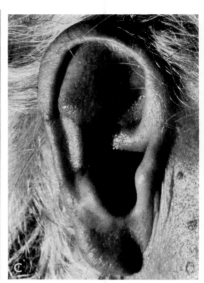

FIGURE 35–94. Enhancement of composite graft revascularization by decreasing "composite bulk." *A,* Auricular defect with residual chondrodermatitis. *B,* The bulkiness of the composite graft is decreased by removing the posteromedial auricular skin and cartilage while preserving a cartilage strut in the helical rim. A retroauricular flap is advanced to serve as a recipient bed for the remaining anterolateral cutaneous portion of the wedge-shaped graft. *C,* The final result.

ized from the loose retroauricular skin (Brent, 1975a). A strut of the helical cartilage is preserved within the graft for contour and support (Fig. 35–94).

Despite a slight tendency toward shrinkage after transplantation, the composite graft offers a simple and expeditious reconstructive technique for partial auricular defects.

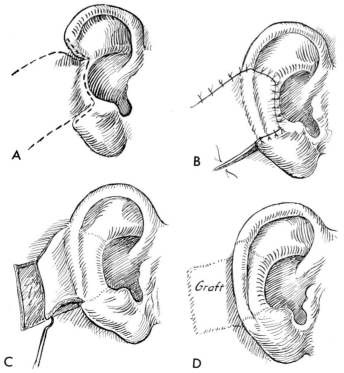

FIGURE 35–95. Dieffenbach's technique for reconstruction of the middle third of the auricle, drawn from his description (1829–1834). *A,* The defect and the outline of the flap. *B,* The flap advanced over the defect. *C, D,* In a second stage, the base of the flap is divided and the flap is folded around the posteromedial aspect of the auricle.

Auricular Cartilage. Auricular cartilage is particularly useful in the reconstruction of partial auricular defects, and its use as a graft has been described earlier in this chapter (see Figs. 35–84 and 35–85). Auricular cartilage may be included within a reconstructive flap either as a graft or as a "composite component" of the repair. Dieffenbach's early description (1829–1834) of a flap employed to repair a middle-third auricular defect indicates that he did not use a cartilage graft for support (Fig. 35–95). Navabi (1964) used Dieffenbach's flap and added a cartilage graft removed from the contralateral scapha (Fig. 35–96). Millard's chondrocutaneous flap (1966) is an interesting alternative to the latter.

Several other "composite flaps" containing auricular cartilage have been described. Upper

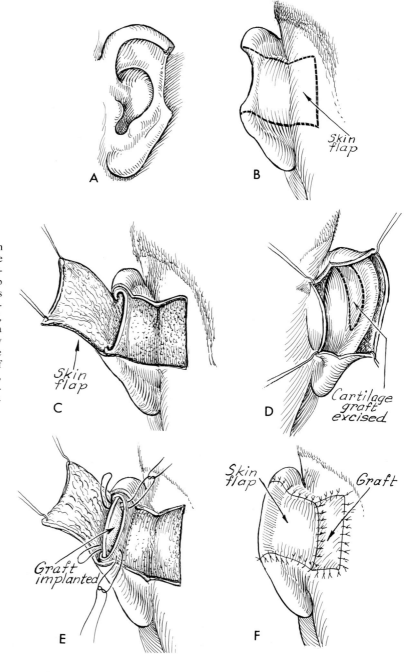

FIGURE 35–96. Reconstruction of a defect in the middle third of the auricle. *A*, The defect. *B*, The outline of the skin flap. *C*, The skin flap is raised. *D*, An ellipse of cartilage is excised from the contralateral auricle. *E*, The graft is in position. *F*, The flap has been advanced, and a skin graft covers the resulting raw area. (After Navabi, A.: One-stage reconstruction of partial defect of the auricle. Plast. Reconstr. Surg., *233*:77. Copyright © 1964, The Williams & Wilkins Company, Baltimore.)

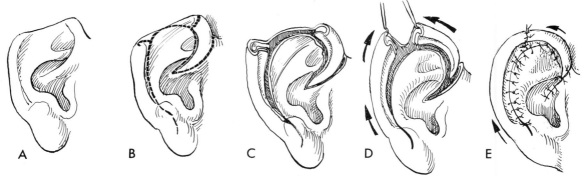

FIGURE 35–97. Helical defect repaired by advancement of auricular skin and cartilage. *A,* Defect of the upper portion of the auricle. *B,* Lines of full thickness incisions through skin and cartilage. *C,* The incisions completed; note the downward extension into the ear lobe. *D,* The skin-cartilage flaps mobilized. *E,* The repair completed. (After Antia, N. H., and Buch, V. I.: Chondrocutaneous advancement of flap for the marginal defect of the ear. Plast. Reconstr. Surg., *39:*472. Copyright © 1967, The Williams & Wilkins Company, Baltimore.)

FIGURE 35–98. *A,* Traumatic defect of the superior helical region. *B,* Repair by helical advancement as illustrated in Figure 35–97. (From Antia, N. H., and Buch, V. I.: Chondrocutaneous advancement of flap for the margical defect of the ear. Plast. Reconstr. Surg., *39:*472. Copyright © 1967, The Williams & Wilkins Company, Baltimore.)

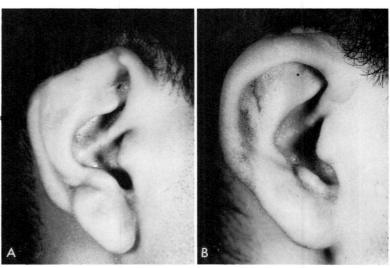

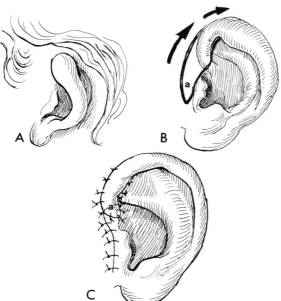

FIGURE 35–99. A technique for release of circumferential tension caused by loss of tissue. *A,* The upper portion of the scapha and the helix have been constricted downward by loss of tissue in the anterosuperior portion of the auricle. *B,* The outline of a flap is indicated, and the flap has been displaced upward, reconstituting the anterior portion of the helix and allowing the auricle to resume its upright position. *C,* The preauricular donor site of the flap is closed by V-Y advancement. In longstanding deformities of this type, an operation similar to that employed for correction of protruding ears is often necessary in the same stage.

helicoscaphal defects are repaired by advancing the entire helix based on the mobilized medial auricular skin (Antia and Buch, 1967). The gain in length of the crus helicis is accomplished by V-Y advancement, similar to the technique illustrated in Figure 35–99. This is an expeditious technique which gives excellent results in moderate defects (Fig. 35–97), and although the size of the auricle is diminished, this is proportional to the size of the original defect (Figs. 35–98 and 35–99).

The use of a composite flap of conchal cartilage and skin rotated upward on a narrow anterior soft tissue pedicle (Fig. 35–100) has been employed successfully by Davis (1974c). The conchal donor area is covered with a full-thickness retroauricular graft from the unaffected ear; the raw medial surface of the mobilized concha is skin-grafted also.

Costal Cartilage. In larger defects, costal cartilage can be used to furnish the required framework in the reconstruction of acquired auricular deformities (Converse, 1958, 1963; Converse and Wood-Smith, 1971; Alexandrov, 1964; Tanzer, 1965; Barinka, 1966; Brent, 1974a, b, 1975a).

Following healing of traumatic auricular defects, the adjacent portions of the ear are often contracted toward the defect; thus the apparent defect appears to be smaller in size than the true defect; the remaining portions of the

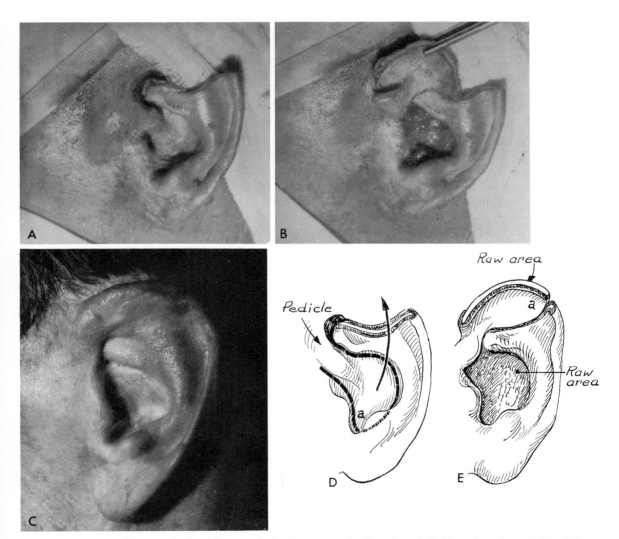

FIGURE 35–100. Upper auricular defect repaired with a composite flap of conchal skin and cartilage. *A*, The defect. *B*, The composite conchal flap elevated. *C*, The final appearance. *D, E,* Diagram of the procedure, indicating the incisions and the raw surfaces to be grafted. The anterior cutaneous pedicle (crus helix) maintains the blood supply. (After Davis, 1974.)

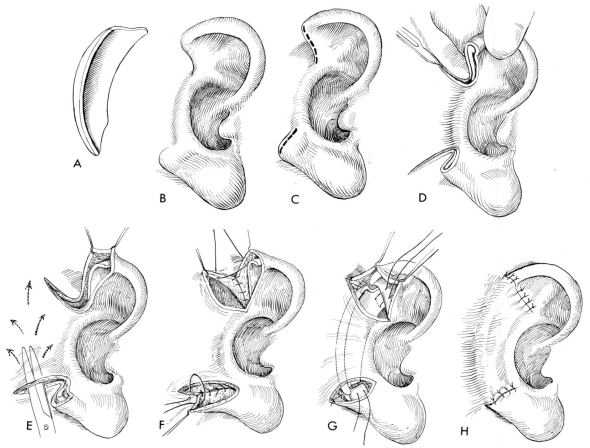

FIGURE 35–101. Repair of a defect of the middle third of the auricle. *A,* Carved costal cartilage graft. *B,* The defect. *C,* Incisions through the margins of the defect. *D,* Incisions through the edge of the defect are extended backward through the skin of the mastoid area. *E,* The skin of the mastoid area is undermined between the two incisions. *F,* The medial edge of the incision at the border of the auricular defect is sutured to the upper edge of the postauricular incision. A similar type of suture is placed at the lower edge of the defect. *G,* The cartilage graft is placed under the skin of the mastoid area and anchored to the auricular cartilage by means of catgut sutures. *H,* Suture of the skin incision (Figures 35–101 to 35–108 are from Converse, J. M.: Reconstruction of the auricle. Plast. Reconstr. Surg., *22*:150; 230. Copyright © 1958, The Williams & Wilkins Company, Baltimore.)

auricle are displaced as a result of the contracture. It is essential to replace the remaining portions of the auricle in correct anatomical position to obtain the size of the actual defect. The scar tissue is resected, and the portions of the auricle on each side of the defect are replaced in their anatomical positons. Occasionally, curling of the cartilage as a result of contraction may require additional correction by one of the techniques used for the repair of protruding ear deformities.

Two oblique incisions delineate the upper and lower limits of the defect on the retroauricular skin. The edges of the cut sections of the remaining portions of the auricle are then sutured to the margins of these oblique incisions (Fig. 35–101, *A* to *F*). A carved cartilage transplant is placed beneath the skin which is situated between the two oblique incisions (Fig. 35–101, *G, H*) and is joined to the adjacent auricular cartilage.

After an interval of three months, a curved

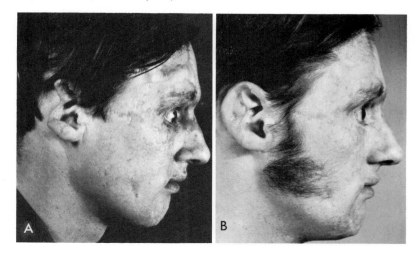

FIGURE 35–102. Repair of a middle third auricular defect with a carved costal cartilage graft. *A*, Traumatic loss of the middle third of the auricle in a Vietnam war veteran. *B*, Repair by the technique of Converse illustrated in Figure 35–101.

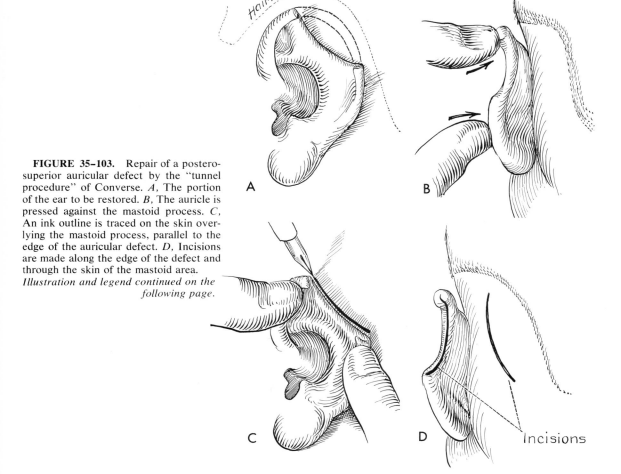

FIGURE 35–103. Repair of a postero-superior auricular defect by the "tunnel procedure" of Converse. *A*, The portion of the ear to be restored. *B*, The auricle is pressed against the mastoid process. *C*, An ink outline is traced on the skin overlying the mastoid process, parallel to the edge of the auricular defect. *D*, Incisions are made along the edge of the defect and through the skin of the mastoid area. *Illustration and legend continued on the following page.*

The Head and Neck

incision is made at a distance from the posterior edge of the cartilage transplant, which is then raised from the subjacent retroauricular tissues. Care is taken to include a layer of subcutaneous tissue over the cartilage; this precaution is necessary, as skin will not survive over denuded cartilage. A split-thickness skin graft covers the defect behind the cartilage

transplant and over the mastoid area. An example of reconstruction by this technique is seen in Figure 35–102.

The Tunnel Procedure. The tunnel procedure (Converse, 1958) is an effective technique for moderate sized defects of the auricle, and in major defects it has the advantage of pre-

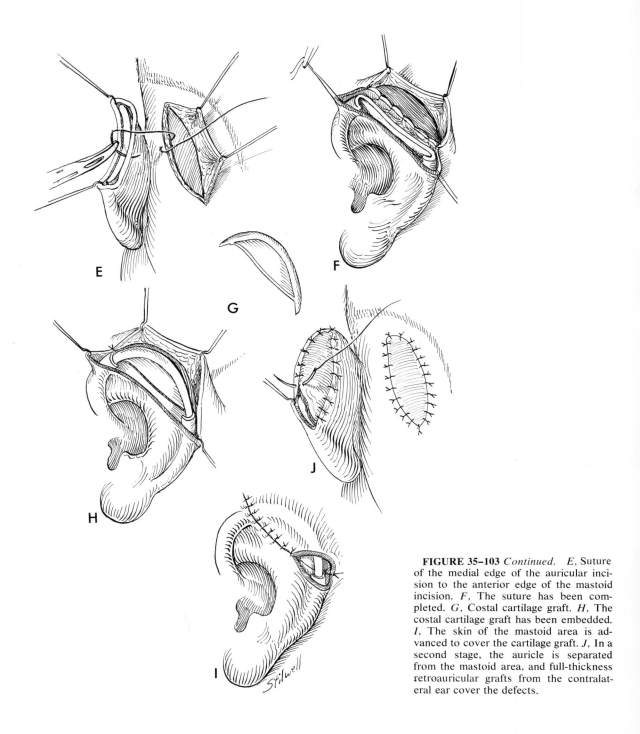

FIGURE 35–103 *Continued. E*, Suture of the medial edge of the auricular incision to the anterior edge of the mastoid incision. *F*, The suture has been completed. *G*, Costal cartilage graft. *H*, The costal cartilage graft has been embedded. *I*, The skin of the mastoid area is advanced to cover the cartilage graft. *J*, In a second stage, the auricle is separated from the mastoid area, and full-thickness retroauricular grafts from the contralateral ear cover the defects.

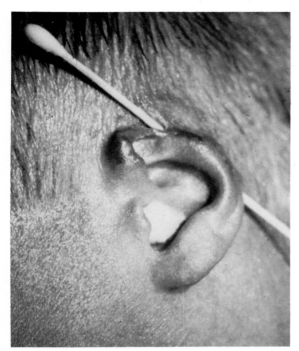

FIGURE 35–104. The tunnel being cleansed by a cotton-tipped applicator. The advantage of the "tunnel procedure" is that it preserves the auriculocephalic sulcus.

serving the retroauricular fold. Figure 35–103 illustrates the repair of a moderate sized defect. The auricle is pressed against the mastoid area, and an ink line is drawn on the skin in this area, the line being parallel and adjacent to the edge of the auricular defect (Fig. 35–103, *B, C*). Incisions are made through the skin along the ink line and also through the edge of the auricular defect (Fig. 35–103, *D*). The medial edge of the auricular incision is sutured to the anterior edge of the mastoid skin incision (Fig. 35–103, *E, F*). A carved costal cartilage transplant is then placed in the soft tissue bed and is joined to the edges of the auricular cartilage defect (Fig. 35–103, *G, H*). The mastoid skin, which has been undermined, is advanced to cover the cartilage transplant, and the edge of this skin flap is sutured to the lateral edge of the auricular skin (Fig. 35–103, *H, I*). A healing and vascularization period of two or three months is permitted; during this period the cutaneous tunnel behind the auricle must be cleansed with cotton-tipped applicators (Fig. 35–104). The auricle is detached in a second stage, and the resulting elliptical raw areas are grafted with full-thickness retroauricular skin from the opposite ear, one on the

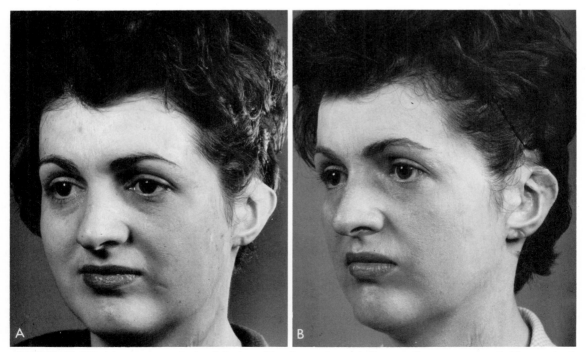

FIGURE 35–105. A superior auricular defect resulting from a burn. *A,* Preoperative appearance. *B,* The result obtained by the "tunnel procedure" of Converse shown in Figure 35–103.

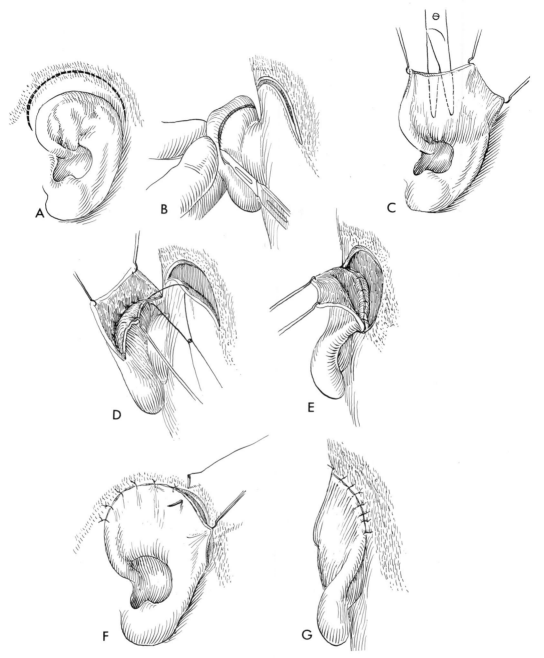

FIGURE 35–106. Use of the tunnel procedure for auricular collapse resulting from loss of cartilage due to peri-chondritis as a result of a burn and exposure of the cartilage. *A*, The collapsed scapha and the outline of the incision in the scalp. *B*, The line of incision along the medial aspect of the helix. *C*, The skin of the ear is widely undermined, and the remaining fibrotic tissue and cartilage is excised. *D*, The first stage of the tunnel procedure. *E*, The medial flaps have been sutured. *F*, The lateral auricular skin is sutured to the scalp incision. *G*, The operation is completed. In a second stage, a carved costal cartilage graft will be placed between the flaps. In a later stage, the auricle will be separated from the side of the head, as illustrated in Figure 35–103, *J*.

auricle and the other on the mastoid area (Fig. 35–103, *J*). Figure 35–105 illustrates a patient with an auricular defect repaired by this technique.

The tunnel procedure may also be employed to re-expand the soft tissues of a contracted auricle resulting from loss of the cartilaginous framework. A curved incision is made near the hairline, and an additional incision is made near the border of the helix, but on the medial aspect of the auricle (Fig. 35–106). A cleavage plane is sought, and the lateral and medial cutaneous layers are separated (Fig. 35–106, *C*). The lower margin of the medial auricular incision is sutured to the lower edge of the hairline incision (Fig. 35–106, *D*, *E*), and the remaining edge of auricular skin is sutured to the upper edge of the hairline incision (Fig. 35–106, *F*, *G*). Before an attempt is made to place a cartilage framework between the cutaneous layers, a sufficient maturation period is required to permit softening of the scar tissue and revascularization of the area. A further maturation is allowed before separating the cartilage-supported auricle from the mastoid area and skin grafting the retroauricular defect (Fig. 35–107).

A modification of the tunnel procedure can be used when the helical rim is intact in an otherwise scarred, contracted ear (Fig. 35–108). The helix is freed of scar tissue and retracted (Fig. 35–108, *A*). The scarred skin and cartilage are resected through the full thickness of the auricle (Fig. 35–108, *B*), and corresponding mastoid skin is outlined and incised; the edges of the skin are undermined over a short distance (Fig. 35–108, *C*, *D*, *E*). The undermined edge of the mastoid skin is then sutured to the auricular skin along the posterior edge of the excised area, leaving a tunnel which preserves the postauricular fold (Fig. 35–108, *F*). The helix is sutured (Fig. 35–108, *G*), and in a second stage, a costal cartilage graft is transplanted to provide support for the auricle (Fig. 35–108, *H*).

Reconstruction of the Earlobe

The most common earlobe deformity is a traumatic cleft, which is caused by traction on an earring in the pierced earlobe. The repair is made by simply excising the cleft margins and suturing the fresh edges together; incorporation of a Z-plasty will help to prevent notching. Pardue (1973) has suggested rolling in a small adjacent flap to line the repair so that an earring can once again be worn without resting against the suture line (Fig. 35–109).

Construction of an earlobe is rarely required in congenital microtia, as the lobe is formed by

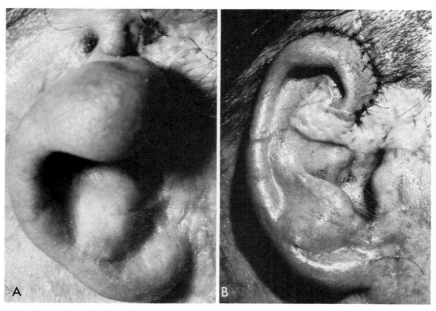

FIGURE 35–107. Expansion of the soft tissues of the auricle. *A*, Loss of cartilaginous support of the upper third of the ear secondary to abrasive trauma. *B*, Expansion of the soft tissues according to the technique illustrated in Figure 35–106.

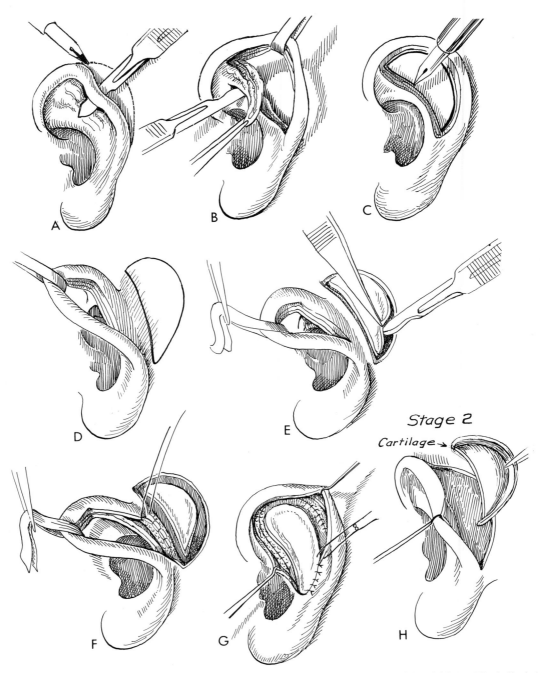

FIGURE 35–108. Another technique for repair of the collapsed auricle following perichondritis. *A*, The helical rim is freed from the remainder of the auricle. It will be sutured into the incision outlined in ink. *B*, The full thickness of fibrotic auricular tissue is resected. *C*, An area of retroauricular skin is outlined. *D*, The auricular defect and the outlined retroauricular skin. *E*, The edges of the retroauricular skin are undermined. *F*, Suturing for the tunnel procedure. *G*, Suture of the retroauricular skin to the edges of the auricular defect. *H*, In a later stage, a carved costal cartilage graft is inserted to replace the missing cartilage. In a final stage, the auricle will be raised and the raw areas covered with skin grafts.

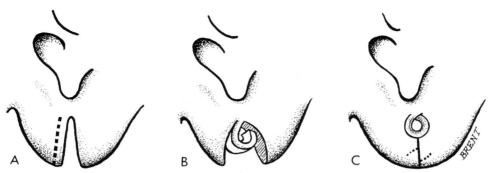

FIGURE 35–109. Repair of a traumatic earlobe cleft with preservation of the perforation for an earring. *A*, A flap is prepared by a parallel incision on one side of the cleft; the other side is freshened by excision of the margin. *B*, The flap is rolled in to provide a lining for preservation of the earring tract. *C*, Closure is completed; a small Z-plasty may be incorporated. (After Pardue, 1973.)

the repositioning of auricular remnants. However, a portion of the lobe or the entire lobe may be missing in traumatic deformities of the ear, and a variety of techniques for its reconstruction have been proposed.

One procedure, described by Gavello (quoted by Nélaton and Ombrédanne, 1907), consists of preparing a bilobed flap; the posterior lobe is folded under the anterior one, thus serving as the inner lining of the new ear lobule (Fig. 35–110).

Another simpler technique (Converse, 1958) is begun by first inking an outline of the new earlobe's shape, allowing an increase in size of approximately one third (Fig. 35–111). Then the superiorly based flap is raised from its bed, and a full-thickness graft of retroauricular or supraclavicular skin is used to cover the entire donor defect produced (Fig. 35–111, *B*). At the uppermost portion of the defect, where the

flap is attached at the base of its pedicle, the skin graft is reflected downward, covering the raw undersurface of the flap (Fig. 35–111, *B*). As the flap heals, the tendency for its edges to curl toward the skin-grafted surface is accentuated, thus simulating the shape of a lobe (Fig. 35–111, *C, D*).

Nélaton and Ombrédanne (1907) advocated a technique which requires two stages. In this method, a long, inferiorly based mastoid flap is raised and attached to the inferior margin of the ear; it is subsequently divided and folded upon itself to form a lobe (Fig. 35–112). A refinement of this technique, advocated by Davis (1974c), consists of turning down a hinge flap from the lateral auricular surface to serve as a lining (Fig. 35–113). Subba Rao (1968) also employs a hinge flap, but this is reflected from the medial auricular surface and is used to create the lobe rather than the lining; it is lined with a

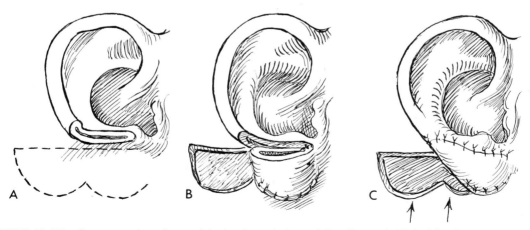

FIGURE 35–110. Reconstruction of an earlobe by the technique of Gavello. *A*, A bilobed flap is prepared. *B*, The posterior flap is folded under the anterior one. *C*, The resulting defect is closed by direct approximation. (After Nélaton and Ombrédanne, 1907.)

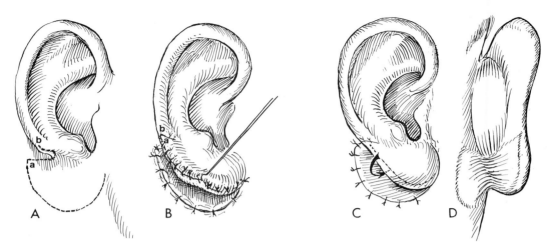

FIGURE 35–111. Reconstruction of an earlobe (Converse). *A*, The design of the flap. *B*, The posterosuperior angle of the flap has been inserted into the lower portion of the helical border. The raw surfaces are covered by full-thickness skin grafts. *C*, As healing takes place, the edge of the flap tends to roll on itself. *D*, The postoperative appearance of the new lobe. (From Converse, J. M.: Reconstruction of the auricle. Plast. Reconstr. Surg., *22*:150, 1958.)

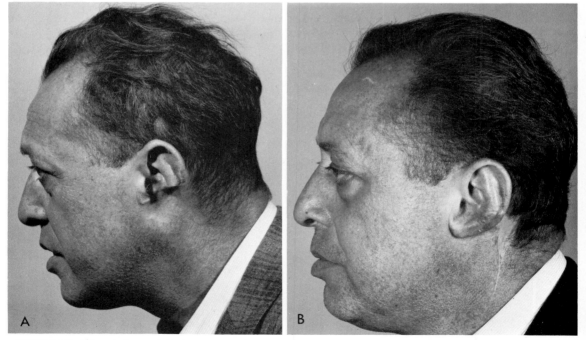

FIGURE 35–112. *A*, Loss of the lower part of the auricle. *B*, The result obtained with a flap based on the mastoid process and folded upon itself. Note the scar of the approximated edges of the flap's donor site. (Patient of Dr. Cary L. Guy.)

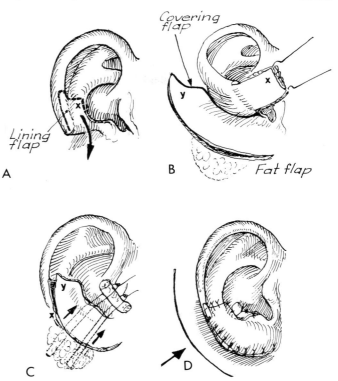

FIGURE 35–113. Reconstruction of the lower portion of the auricle and the earlobe. *A*, The defect and the outline of the lining flap. *B*, The outline of the cover flap and of the fat flap used for fill. *C*, The lining flap is covered by the cover flap and the fat flap is introduced between them. *D*, The secondary defect is closed by direct approximation. (Courtesy of Dr. J. Davis.)

full-thickness skin graft (Fig. 35–114). Zenteno Alanis (1970) folded a preoperatively designed vertical flap (Fig. 35–115), a modification of the technique employed by Paletta (1967).

There is an advantage in reconstructing the earlobe with auricular tissue whenever possible, as a good color and texture match is obtained and a potential hypertrophic scar in the infra-auricular area is avoided. Converse (1974b) employed two flaps to accomplish this objective; one is raised from the medial auricular surface and turned down as a hinge flap, and the other is taken from the retroauricular sulcus area to line the hinge flap (Fig. 35–116).

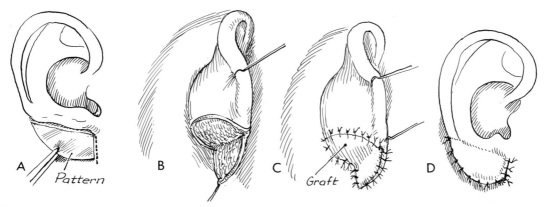

FIGURE 35–114. Reconstruction of the earlobe. *A*, Pattern of the proposed earlobe in position. The pattern is then turned upside down on the posteromedial aspect of the auricle, and a flap is outlined. *B*, The outlined flap is turned down as a hinge flap. *C*, The flap is sutured into the vertical incision made on a line drawn inferiorly from the tragus. A full-thickness skin graft covers the raw area of the flap and auricle. *D*, The operation completed. (Modified after Subba Rao, 1968.)

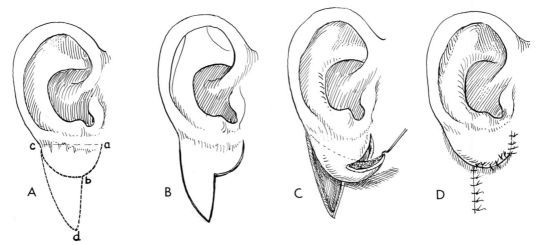

FIGURE 35–115. Reconstruction of the earlobe. *A*, The curved line *abc* outlines the proposed earlobe as measured on the unaffected contralateral auricle. A vertical flap is then outlined; line *bd* is equal in length to line *ab*, and *cd* is equal to *ca*. *B*, Incisions are made through the outlined skin and subcutaneous tissue. *C*, The vertical flap is raised from the underlying tissue as far upward as the horizontal line *ac*, and the tip of the flap is sutured to point *a*. *D*, The operation completed. (After Zenteno Alanis, 1970.)

Brent (1976) utilized a fleur-de-lis–shaped auriculomastoid flap for this purpose (Figs. 35–117 and 35–118). The upper portion of this single flap, which is folded upon itself, comes from the medial auricular surface, whereas its "reverse-contour" portion is raised from the mastoid region; the mastoid defect is closed by direct approximation, and the auricular donor region is covered with a skin graft (see Fig. 35–117).

Benign Tumors

Sebaceous cysts of the auricle are common tumors which are often treated improperly or neglected. They are most often found on the medial aspect of the ear, particularly in the lobe, and should be removed in toto during the quiescent period. Excision should be performed through the medial surface of the lobule to minimize deformity.

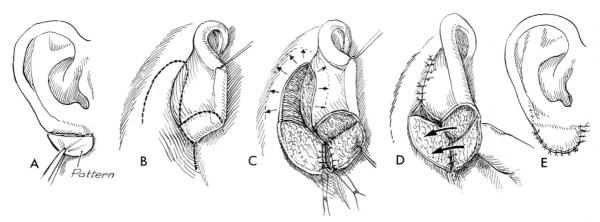

FIGURE 35–116. Reconstruction of the earlobe by a two-flap technique (Converse). *A*, The pattern of the planned earlobe. *B*, The pattern has been placed on the posteromedial aspect of the auricle and an outline made. The outline of the second flap from the retroauricular area is also shown; note the line of the vertical incision for insertion of the lobe. *C*, Each of the flaps is sutured to an edge of the vertical incision, thus anchoring the new earlobe. *D*, The two flaps are sutured to each other. *E*, The operation completed. (From Kazanjian and Converse.)

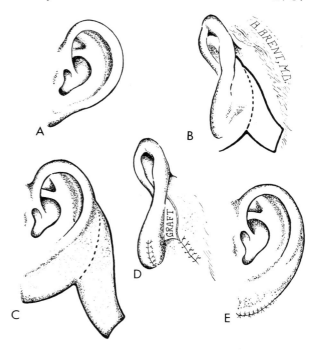

FIGURE 35–117. Construction of an earlobe with a reverse contoured flap. *A*, The earlobe deficiency. *B*, An auriculomastoid flap outlined. *C*, The elevated flap hanging as a curtain from the inferior auricular border. *D*, The flap folded under and sutured and the mastoid defect closed. A small graft is placed over the auricular donor defect. *E*, The completed earlobe, exaggerated by one-third to allow for shrinkage. (Figures 35–117 and 35–118 are from Brent, B.: Earlobe reconstruction with an auriculo-mastoid flap. Plast. Reconstr. Surg., *57*:389. Copyright ©1976, The Williams and Wilkins Company, Baltimore.)

The most common auricular lesion is actinic keratosis; it occurs most frequently in outdoor workers with fair complexions. Other benign auricular lesions are granuloma pyogenicum, beryllium granuloma, verruca contagiosa, verruca senilis, cylindroma, nevus, papilloma, lipoma, lymphangioma, leiomyoma, and chondroma. The treatment of these tumors is surgical excision. Keloid of the earlobe is common; the treatment of this lesion is discussed in Chapter 16.

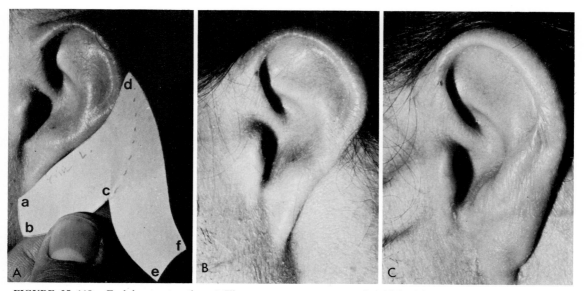

FIGURE 35–118. Earlobe construction. *A*, The reverse contour pattern, in which *ab* is equal to *ef*, *bc* to *ce*, and *ad* to *df*. *B*, Congenital deficiency of lobular tissue. *C*, Completed construction by the technique illustrated in Figure 35–117.

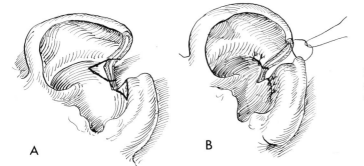

FIGURE 35–119. Wedge resection of a helical tumor. *A,* The tumor has been excised, and secondary wedges are outlined to facilitate closure of the defect. *B,* Details of the closure.

Malignant Tumors

Over 5 per cent of skin cancers involve the auricle (Arons and Sadin, 1971), usually basal cell or squamous cell carcinomas. A lesser percentage are malignant melanomas. The first report concerning malignant tumors of the auricle was that of Kretschman (1886–87). Broders (1921) provided a sizable early review, and Fredericks (1956) and Conway (1959) followed suit. More recently, Hoopes (1974) has updated the literature and recorded considerable information on the various methods of treating malignant auricular tumors.

When first seen, the cartilage is involved by direct extension in about one-third of the cutaneous carcinomas of the auricle. For this reason and because cartilage is an excellent barrier to the spread of tumor, the cartilage must be included in the surgical excision of the lesion (Hoopes, 1974).

Involvement of the cervical lymph nodes is extremely rare in basal cell carcinoma of the auricle but is present in about one-third of all squamous cell carcinomas and malignant melanomas.

The treatment of choice is wide excision. The majority of malignant lesions are located on the helical rim and can be eradicated with a wedge excision (Fig. 35–119) and primary closure or a helical advancement, as previously described. Many of the tumors located on the lateral and medial auricular surfaces can be treated adequately by excision and subsequent skin grafting or by local flap coverage; others will require a definitive reconstructive procedure by an appropriate method chosen from those previously described in this chapter. Radiation therapy is poorly tolerated by auricular cartilage and is of no value in the management of recurrences and metastases.

When the cancer is large and includes cartilaginous invasion, total ablation of the auricle with surrounding soft tissue is essential. Radical resection of the cervical lymph nodes in continuity with resection of the involved auricle should be performed in patients with lymph node metastases; melanomas demand early radical intervention. At times, radical resection in continuity with the temporal bone is the only hope of effecting a cure in auricular cancer (Parsons and Lewis, 1954; Lewis, 1960; Mladick and coworkers, 1974).

Patients requiring total auricular ablation usually are in an older age group and generally are not candidates for total auricular reconstruction. A prosthetic replacement of the auricle is often preferred, but if total reconstruction of the auricle is indicated, it is advisable to postpone reconstruction until the threat of recurrence is well past.

REFERENCES

Adams, W. M.: Construction of the upper half of the auricle utilizing a composite concha cartilage graft with perichondrium attached on both sides. Plast. Reconstr. Surg., *16*:88, 1955.

Adamson, J. E., Horton, C. E., and Crawford, H. H.: The growth pattern of the external ear. Plast. Reconstr. Surg., *36*:466, 1965.

Alexandrov, N. M.: Traumatic defects of the auricle and methods of their repair. Acta Chir. Plast. (Praha), *6*:302, 1964.

Alichniewicz, A., Bardach, J., and Kozlowski, H.: Research on grafted conserved homogenous cartilage. Acta Chir. Plast. (Praha), *6*:229, 1964.

Antia, N. H., and Buch, V. I.: Chondrocutaneous advancement of flap for the marginal defect of the ear. Plast. Reconstr. Surg., *39*:472, 1967.

Arey, L. B.: Developmental Anatomy. 6th Ed. Philadelphia, W. B. Saunders Company, 1954.

Arons, M. D., and Sadin, R. C.: Auricular cancer. Am. J. Surg., *122*:770, 1971.

Barinka, L.: Congenital malformations of the auricle and their reconstruction by a new method. Acta Chir. Plast., *8*:53, 1966.

Barsky, A. J.: Plastic Surgery. Philadelphia, W. B. Saunders Company, 1938.

Barsky, A. J., Kahn, S., and Simon, B. E.: Principles and Practice of Plastic Surgery. New York, McGraw-Hill Book Company, 1964, p. 303.

Baudet, J., Tramond, P., and Goumain, A.: A propos d'un procédé original de réimplantation d'un pavillon de l'oreille totalement séparé. Ann. Chir. Plast., *17*:67, 1972.

Becker, O. J.: Surgical correction of the abnormally protruding ear. Arch. Otolaryngol., *50*:541, 1949.

Becker, O. J.: Correction of the protruding deformed ear. Br. J. Plast. Surg., *5*:187, 1952.

Bellucci, R. J.: Discussion. *In* International Conference on Craniofacial Anomalies, New York, 1971.

Bellucci, R. J.: Congenital auricular malformations: Indications, contraindications and timing of middle ear surgery. Ann. Otol., Rhinol. Laryngol., *81*:659, 1972a.

Bellucci, R. J.: Split thickness grafts in surgery of the ear. *In* Conley, J., and Dickinson, J. (Eds.): Proc. First Internatl. Symposium on Plastic and Reconstructive Surgery of the Face and Neck. Vol. 2, Rehabilitative Surgery. New York, Grune & Stratton, 1972b.

Bellucci, R. J., and Converse, J. M.: The problem of congenital auricular malformation. I. Construction of the external auditory canal. II. Construction of the auricle in congenital microtia. Trans. Am. Acad. Ophthalmol. Otolaryngol., *64*:840, 1960.

Bhishagratna, K. K. L.: An English Translation of the Susruta Samhita. Calcutta, Wilkins Press, 1907.

Bonanno, P. C., and Converse, J. M.: *In* Kazanjian, V. H., and Converse, J. M.: Surgical Treatment of Facial Injuries. 3rd ed. Baltimore, The Williams & Wilkins Company, 1974, p. 1292.

Bouisson, M.: De l'amputation du pavillon de l'oreille; étude chirurgical. Gaz. Méd. Paris, *25*:320, 1870.

Brent, B.: Problems associated with total auricular reconstruction (discussion). *In* Tanzer, R. C., and Edgerton, M. T. (eds.): Symposium on Reconstruction of the Auricle. St. Louis, Mo., C. V. Mosby Company, 1974a.

Brent, B.: Ear reconstruction with an expansile framework of autogenous rib cartilage. Plast. Reconstr. Surg., *53*:619, 1974b.

Brent, B.: Reconstruction of ear, eyebrow and sideburn in the burned patient. Plast. Reconstr. Surg., *55*:312, 1975.

Brent, B.: Earlobe construction with an auriculomastoid flap. Plast. Reconstr. Surg., *57*:389, 1976.

Broadbent, T. R., and Mathews, V. I.: Artistic relationships in surface anatomy of the face. Plast. Reconstr. Surg., *20*:1, 1957.

Broadbent, T. R., and Woolf, R. M.: A bilateral approach to the middle ear. *In* Tanzer, R. C., and Edgerton, M. T. (Eds.): Symposium on Reconstruction of the Auricle. St. Louis, Mo., C. V. Mosby Company, 1974, p. 168.

Broders, A. C.: Epithelioma of the ear: A study of 63 cases. Surg. Clin. North Am., *1*:1401, 1921.

Brown, J. B., Cannon, B., Lischer, C. E., Davis, W. B., and Moore, A.: Surgical substitution for losses of the external ear: Simplified local flap method of reconstruction. Surg. Gynecol. Obstet., *84*:192, 1947.

Byars, L. T., and DeMere, M.: Restoration of missing ear. Plast. Reconstr. Surg., *5*:66, 1950.

Cannon, B.: Personal communication, 1957.

Cardoso, A. D., and Sperly, A. E.: The use of composite grafts to correct the cup ear and to repair small losses of the auricle. Trans. Fourth Internatl. Congr. Plast. Surg. Amsterdam, Excerpta Medica, 1969, p. 667.

Caronni, E.: Embryogenesis and classification of branchial auricular dysplasia. Trans. Fifth Internatl. Congr. Plast. Surg. Melbourne, Australia, Butterworth, 1971, p. 435.

Carroll, D. B., and Peterson, R. A.: Variations of the Tanzer theme. Proc. 40th Annual Meeting Am. Soc. Plast. Reconstr. Surg., Montreal, 1971.

Chongchet, V.: A method of anthelix reconstruction. Br. J. Plast. Surg., *16*:268, 1963.

Clemons, J. E., and Connelly, M. V.: Reattachment of a totally amputated auricle. Arch. Otolaryngol., *97*:269, 1973.

Cloutier, A. M.: Correction of outstanding ears. Plast. Reconstr. Surg., *28*:412, 1961.

Cocheril, R. C.: Essai sur la restauration du pavillon de l'oreille. Thèse pour le Doctorat en Médecine. Lille, L. Danel, 1894.

Conroy, C. C.: Salvage of an amputated ear. Plast. Reconstr. Surg., *49*:564, 1972.

Converse, J. M., quoted by Gillies, H.: Technic in the construction of an auricle. Trans. Am. Acad. Ophthalmol. Otolaryngol., *46*:119, 1942.

Converse, J. M.: Reconstruction of the external ear by prefabricated framework of refrigerated bone and cartilage. Plast. Reconstr. Surg., *5*:148, 1950.

Converse, J. M.: Reconstruction of the auricle. Plast. Reconstr. Surg., *22*:150, 230, 1958.

Converse, J. M.: Construction of the auricle in congenital microtia. Plast. Reconstr. Surg., *32*:425, 1963.

Converse, J. M.: Construction of the auricle in unilateral microtia. Trans. Am. Acad. Ophthalmol. Otolaryngol., *72*:995, 1968.

Converse, J. M.: Construction of the auricle in unilateral congenital microtia. Trans. Fourth Internatl. Congr. Plast. Surg. Amsterdam, Excerpta Medica, 1969, p. 619.

Converse, J. M.: Personal communication, 1974a.

Converse, J. M.: Traumatic deformities of the auricle. *In* Kazanjian, V. H., and Converse, J. M.: Surgical Treatment of Facial Injuries. 3rd ed. Baltimore, The Williams & Wilkins Company, 1974b, Chapter 28.

Converse, J. M., and Wood-Smith, D.: Technical details in the surgical correction of the lop ear deformity. Plast. Reconstr. Surg., *31*:118, 1963.

Converse, J. M., and Wood-Smith, D.: Corrective and reconstructive surgery in deformities of the auricle in children. *In* Mustardé, J. C. (Ed.): Plastic Surgery in Infancy and Childhood. Edinburgh, Churchill-Livingstone, 1971.

Converse, J. M., Nigro, A., Wilson, F. A., and Johnson, N.: A technique for surgical correction of lop ears. Plast. Reconstr. Surg., *15*:411, 1955.

Converse, J. M., Coccaro, P. J., Becker, M., and Wood-Smith, D.: On hemifacial microsomia. Plast. Reconstr. Surg., *51*:268, 1973.

Converse, J. M., Wood-Smith, D., McCarthy, J. G., Coccaro, P. J., and Becker, M. H.: Bilateral facial microsomia. Plast. Reconstr. Surg., *54*:413, 1974.

Conway, H.: The surgical treatment of tumors of the external ear, auditory canal and mastoid. *In* Pack, G. T., and Ariel, I. M. (Eds.): Treatment of Cancer and Allied Diseases. Vol. 3, Tumors of the Head and Neck. New York, Paul B. Hoeber, Inc., 1959.

Conway, H., Neumann, C. G., Golb, J., Leveridge, L. L., and Joseph, J. M.: Reconstruction of the external ear. Ann. Surg., *128*:226, 1948.

Cosman, B.: Repair of moderate cup ear deformities. *In* Tanzer, R. C., and Edgerton, M. T. (eds.): Symposium on Reconstruction of the Auricle. St. Louis, Mo., C. V. Mosby Company, 1974, p. 118.

Cosman, B., and Crikelair, G. F.: The composed tube pedicle in ear helix reconstruction. Plast. Reconstr. Surg., *37*:517, 1966.

Courtiss, E. H., Webster, R. C., and White, M. F.: Otoplasty: Direct surgical approach. *In* Masters, F. W., and Lewis, J. R. (Eds.): Symposium on Aesthetic Surgery of the Nose, Ears and Chin. St. Louis, Mo., C. V. Mosby Company, 1973, p. 128.

Cowan, R. J.: Cryptotia. Plast. Reconstr. Surg., 27:209, 1961.

Crikelair, G. F., and Cosman, B.: Another solution for the problem of the prominent ear. Ann. Surg., 160:324, 1964.

Cronin, T. D.: One stage reconstruction of the helix: Two improved methods. Plast. Reconstr. Surg., 9:547, 1952.

Cronin. T. D.: Use of a Silastic frame for total and subtotal reconstruction of the external ear: Preliminary report. Plast. Reconstr. Surg., 37:399, 1966.

Cronin, T. D.: Reconstruction of the external ear with a Silastic frame. Trans. Fifth Internatl. Congr. Plast. Surg. Melbourne, Australia, Butterworth, 1971, p. 452.

Cronin, T. D.: Use of a Silastic frame for reconstruction of the auricle. *In* Tanzer, R. C., and Edgerton, M. T. (Eds.): Symposium on Reconstruction of the Auricle. St. Louis, Mo., C. V. Mosby Company, 1974, p. 33.

Curtin, J. W., and Bader, K. F.: Improved techniques for the successful silicone reconstruction of the external ear. Plast. Reconstr. Surg., 44:372, 1969.

Davis, J. E.: On auricular reconstruction. Internatl. Microform J. Aesthetic Plast. Surg., Otoplasty, 1972-C.

Davis, J. E.: Repair of severe cup ear deformities. *In* Tanzer, R. C., and Edgerton, M. T. (Edts.): Symposium on Reconstruction of the Auricle. St. Louis, Mo., C. V. Mosby Company, 1974a.

Davis, J. E.: Discussion of reduction of the auricle. *In* Tanzer, R. C., and Edgerton, M. T. (Eds.): Symposium on Reconstruction of the Auricle. St. Louis, Mo., C. V. Mosby Company, 1974b, p. 105.

Davis, J. E.: Repair of traumatic defects of the auricle. *In* Tanzer, R. C., and Edgerton, M. T. (Eds.): Symposium on Reconstruction of the Auricle. St. Louis, Mo., C. V. Mosby Company, 1947c, p. 247.

Davis, J. S., and Kitlowski, E. A.: Abnormal prominence of the ears: A method of readjustment. Surgery, 2:835, 1937.

Davis, P. R. B., and Jones, S. M.: The complications of Silastic implants. Br. J. Plast. Surg., 24:405, 1971.

Day, H. F.: Reconstruction of the ears. Boston Med. Surg. J., 185:146, 1921.

Derlacki, E. L.: The role of the otologist in the management of microtia and related malformation of the hearing apparatus. Trans. Am. Acad. Ophthalmol. Otolaryngol., 72:980, 1968.

Derlacki, E. L.: Preoperative evaluation of congenital malformations of the conductive hearing mechanism. *In* Tanzer, R. C., and Edgerton, M. T. (Eds.): Symposium on Reconstruction of the Auricle. St. Louis, Mo., C. V. Mosby Company, 1974, p. 161.

Dieffenbach, J. F.: Die operative Chirurgie. Leipzig, F. A. Brockhaus, 1845.

diMartino, G.: Anomalie du pavillon de l'oreille et procédé d'otomiose. Bull. Acad. Med. (Paris), 22:17, 1856–57.

Dufourmentel, C.: La greffe libre tubulée: Nouvel artifice pour la réflection de l'hélix au cours de la reconstruction du pavillon de l'oreille. Ann. Chir. Plast., 3:311, 1958.

Dupertuis, S. M., and Musgrave, R. M.: Experiences with the reconstruction of the congenitally deformed ear. Plast. Reconstr. Surg., 23:361, 1959.

Edgerton, M. T.: Ear reconstruction in children with congenital atresia and stenosis. Plast. Reconstr. Surg., 43:373, 1969.

Edgerton, M. T., and Bacchetta, C.: Principles in the use and salvage of implants in ear reconstruction. *In* Tanzer, R. C., and Edgerton, M. T. (Eds.): Symposium on Reconstruction of the Auricle. St. Louis, Mo., C. V. Mosby Company, 1974, p. 58.

Edgerton, M. T., and Nager, G. T.: Surgical reconstruction of the ear for congenital absence. Trans. Fourth Internatl. Congr. Plast. Surg. Amsterdam, Excerpta Medica, 1969, p. 687.

Ely, E. T.: An operation for prominence of the auricles. Arch. Otolaryngol., 10:97, 1881.

Erich, J. B.: Surgical treatment of protruding ears. Eye, Ear, Nose Throat Monthly, 37:390, 1958.

Erich, J. B.: Plastic correction of the lop ear. Proc. Staff Meet. Mayo Clin., 38:96, 1963.

Erich, J. B., and Abu-Jamra, F. N.: Congenital cup-shaped deformity of the ears: Transmitted through four generations. Mayo Clin. Proc., 40:597, 1965.

Farkas, L. G.: Growth of normal and reconstructed auricles. *In* Tanzer, R. C., and Edgerton, M. T. (Eds.): Symposium on Reconstruction of the Auricle. St. Louis, Mo., C. V. Mosby Company, 1974, p. 24.

Fredericks, S.: External ear malignancy. Br. J. Plast. Surg., 9:136, 1956.

Fukuda, O.: Otoplasty of cryptotia. Jap. J. Plast. Surg., 11:117, 1968.

Fukuda, O.: The microtic ear: Survey of 180 cases in 10 years. Plast. Reconstr. Surg., 53:458, 1974a.

Fukuda, O.: Discussion of cryptotia. *In* Tanzer, R. C., and Edgerton, M. T. (Eds.): Symposium on Reconstruction of the Auricle. St. Louis, Mo., C. V. Mosby Company, 1974b, p. 146.

Furnas, D. W.: Correction of prominent ears by conchomastoid sutures. Plast. Reconstr. Surg., 42:189, 1968.

Furnas, D. W.: Problems in planning reconstruction in microtia. *In* Tanzer, R. C., and Edgerton, M. T. (Eds.): Symposium on Reconstruction of the Auricle. St. Louis, Mo., C. V. Mosby Company, 1974, p. 93.

Gavello, P.: Quoted by Nélaton, C., and Ombrédanne, L.: Les Autoplasties. Paris, G. Steinheil, 1907.

Gersuny, R.: Ueber einige kosmetische Operationen. Wien. Med. Wochenschr., 53:2253, 1903.

Gibson, T.: Bone and cartilage transplantation. *In* Rapaport, T., and Dausset, J. (Eds.): Human Transplantation. New York, Grune & Stratton, 1968.

Gibson, T., and Davis, W. B.: Fate of preserved bovine cartilage implants in man. Br. J. Plast. Surg., 6:4, 1953.

Gibson, T., and Davis, W.: The distortion of autogenous cartilage grafts: Its cause and prevention. Br. J. Plast. Surg., 10:257, 1958.

Gifford, G. H.: Replantation of severed part of an ear. Plast. Reconstr. Surg., 49:202, 1972.

Gill, N. W.: Congenital atresia of the ear: A review of the surgical findings in 83 cases. J. Laryngol., 83:551, 1969.

Gillies, H.: Plastic Surgery of the Face. London, H. Frowde, Hodder & Stoughton, 1920.

Gillies, H.: Reconstruction of the external ear with special reference to the use of maternal ear cartilages as the supporting structure. Rev. Chir. Structive, 7:169, 1937.

Gillies, H. D., and Kristensen, H. K.: Ox cartilage in plastic surgery. Br. J. Plast. Surg., 4:63, 1951.

Gnudi, M. T., and Webster, J. P.: The Life and Times of Gaspar Tagliacozzi. New York, Reichner, 1950.

Gorlin, R. J., and Pindborg, J. J.: Syndromes of the Head and Neck. New York, McGraw-Hill Book Company, 1964.

Gorney, M.: The ear as a donor site: Anatomic and technical guidelines. *In* Tanzer, R. C., and Edgerton, M. T. (Eds.): Symposium on Reconstruction of the Auricle. St. Louis, Mo., C. V. Mosby Company, 1974, p. 106.

Gorney, M., Murphy, S., and Falces, E.: Spliced autogenous conchal cartilage in secondary ear reconstruction. Plast. Reconstr. Surg., 47:432, 1971.

Gosserez, M., and Piers, J. H.: Invagination congénitale du pavillon de l'oreille. Ann. Chir. Plast., 4:143, 1959.

Grabb, W. C.: The first and second branchial arch syndrome. Plast. Reconstr. Surg., 36:485, 1965.

Greeley, P. W.: Reconstruction of the external ear. U.S. Naval Med. Bull., 42:1323, 1944.

Grotting, J. K.: Otoplasty for congenital cupped and prominent ears using a postauricular flap. Plast. Reconstr. Surg., 22:164, 1958.

Guerrero-Santos, J.: Correction of hypertrophied earlobes in leprosy. Plast. Reconstr. Surg., 46:381, 1970.

Hanhart, E.: Nachweis einer einfach-dominanten, unkomplizierten sowie einer unregelmässig-dominanten, mit Atresia auris, Palatoschisis und anderen Deformationen verbundenen Anlage zu Ohrmuschel-verkümmerung (Mikrotie). Arch. der Julius Klaus-Stift, 24:374, 1949.

His, W.: Zur Entwickelung des Acusticofacialisgebiets beim Menschen. Arch. Anat. Phys. Anat., Suppl., 1899.

Holmes, E. M.: The microtic ear. Arch. Otolaryngol., 49:243, 1949.

Holmes, E. M.: A new procedure for correcting outstanding ears. Arch. Otolaryngol., 69:409, 1959.

Hoopes, J. E.: Reconstruction of the auricle after tumor resection. *In* Tanzer, R. C., and Edgerton, M. T. (Eds.): Symposium on Reconstruction of the Auricle. St. Louis, Mo., C. V. Mosby Company, 1974.

Jahrsdoerfer, R. A.: Congenital ear atresia. *In* Tanzer, R. C., and Edgerton, M. T. (Eds.): Symposium on Reconstruction of the Auricle. St. Louis, Mo., C. V. Mosby Company, 1974, p. 150.

Ju, D. M. C., Li, C., and Crikelair, G. F.: The surgical correction of protruding ears. Plast. Reconstr. Surg., 32:283, 1963.

Kaseff, L. G.: Investigation of congenital malformations of the ears with tomography. Plast. Reconstr. Surg., 39:283, 1967.

Kaye, B. L.: A simplified method for correcting the prominent ear. Plast. Reconstr. Surg., 40:44, 1967.

Kaye, B. L.: Follow-up clinic: Current comment on 1967 article. Plast. Reconstr. Surg., 52:184, 1973.

Kazanjian, V. H.: Deformities of the external ear. *In* Kazanjian, V. H., and Converse, J. M.: The Surgical Treatment of Facial Injuries. Baltimore, Williams & Wilkins Co., 1949, Chapter 28.

Kelleher, J., Sullivan, K., Baibak, G., and Dean, R.: The wrestler's ear. Plast. Reconstr. Surg., 40:540, 1967.

Kessler, L.: Beobachtung einer über 6 Generationen einfach-dominant vererbten Mikrotie 1. Grades. HNO, 15:113, 1967.

Kirkham, H. J. D.: The use of preserved cartilage in ear reconstruction. Ann. Surg., 11:896, 1940.

Kislov, R.: Surgical correction of the cupped ear. Plast. Reconstr. Surg., 48:121, 1971.

Knorr, N. J., Edgerton, M. T., and Barbarie, M.: Psychologic factors in the reconstruction of the ear. *In* Tanzer, R. C., and Edgerton, M. T. (Eds.): Symposium on Reconstruction of the Auricle. St. Louis, Mo., C. V. Mosby Company, 1974, p. 187.

Königsmark, B. W.: Hereditary deafness in man. New Engl. J. Med., 281:713, 1969.

Kretschman, F.: Ueber Carcinome des Schläfenbeines. Arch. Ohrenheilk., 24:231, 1886–87.

Kruchinsky, G. V.: A new method of correction of flattened ear. Stomatologia, 4:37, 1966.

Kruchinsky, G. V.: Reinforcement of auricular cartilage for total otoplasty. Stomatologia, 6:51, 1969.

Kubo, I.: Über das Taschenohr (Kubo) und die plastische Operation dieser Missbildung. Jap. J. Med. Sci., XII, Oto-rhino-laryngol. Internatl. 2, Abstract 55, 1938.

Lamont, E. S.: Reconstruction plastic surgery of absent ear with necrocartilage, original method. Arch. Surg. (Chicago), 48:53, 1944.

Letterman, G. S., and Harding, R. L.: The management of the hairline in ear reconstruction. Plast. Reconstr. Surg., 18:199, 1956.

Lewin, M.: Formation of the helix with a post-auricular flap. Plast. Reconstr. Surg., 5:432, 1950.

Lewis, J. S.: Cancer of the ear. Laryngoscope, 70:551, 1960.

Limberg, H. A.: Late results of homotransplantation with chopped cartilage. Acta Chir. Plast. (Praha), 4:59, 1962.

Longacre, J. J., de Stefano, G. A., and Holmstrand, K. E.: The surgical management of first and second branchial arch syndromes. Plast. Reconstr. Surg., 31:507, 1963.

Longenecker, C. G., Ryan, R. F., and Vincent, R. W.: Malformations of the ear as a clue to urogenital anomalies: Report of six additional cases. Plast. Reconstr. Surg., 35:303, 1965.

Luckett, W. H.: A new operation for prominent ears based on the anatomy of the deformity. Surg. Gynecol. Obstet., 10:635, 1910.

Lynch, J. B., Pousti, A., Doyle, J., and Lewis, S.: Our experiences with Silastic ear implants. Plast. Reconstr. Surg., 49:283, 1972.

McDowell, A. J.: Goals in otoplasty for protruding ears. Plast. Reconstr. Surg., 41:17, 1968.

McDowell, F.: Successful replantation of severed half of ear. Plast. Reconstr. Surg., 48:281, 1971.

McEvitt, W. G.: The problem of the protruding ear. Plast. Reconstr. Surg., 2:481, 1947.

McKenzie, J., and Craig, J.: Mandibulo-facial dysostosis (Treacher Collins syndrome). Arch Dis. Child., 30:391, 1955.

Matthews, D. N.: The Surgery of Repair, Injuries and Burns. Oxford, Blackwell Scientific Publications, 1943.

Matthews, D., Broomhead, I., and Roxo, C.: Preliminary report on twenty-five cases of external ear construction in children. Br. J. Plast. Surg., 21:45, 1968.

May, H.: Transverse facial clefts and their repair. Plast. Reconstr. Surg., 29:240, 1962.

Millard, D. R.: Chondrocutaneous flap in partial auricular repair. Plast. Reconstr. Surg., 37:523, 1966.

Minkowitz, S., and Minkowitz, F.: Congenital aural sinuses. Surg. Gynecol. Obstet., 118:4, 1964.

Mladick, R. A., and Carraway, J. H.: Ear reattachment by modified pocket principle. Plast. Reconstr. Surg., 51:584, 1973.

Mladick, R. A., Horton, C. E., Adamson, J. E., and Cohen, B. I.: Pocket principle: A new technique for reattachment of a severed ear part. Plast. Reconstr. Surg., 48:219, 1971.

Mladick, R. A., Horton, C. E., Adamson, J. E., and Carraway, J. H.: The core resection for malignant tumors of the auricular area and subjacent bones. Plast. Reconstr. Surg., 53:281, 1974.

Monroe, C. W.: Our experiences with the silicone ear framework: A report of 17 cases in 15 patients. Plast. Reconstr. Surg., 49:428, 1972.

Monroe, C. W.: Discussion of panel on microtia. *In* Tanzer, R. C., and Edgerton, M. T. (Eds.): Symposium on Reconstruction of the Auricle. St. Louis, Mo., C. V. Mosby Company, 1974, p. 77.

Morestin, H.: De la reposition et du plissement cosmétiques du pavillon de l'oreille. Rev. Orthopédie, 14:289, 1903.

Musgrave, R. H.: A variation on the correction of the congenital lop ear. Plast. Reconstr. Surg., 37:394, 1966.

Musgrave, R. H., and Garrett, W. S.: Management of avulsion injuries of the external ear. Plast. Reconstr. Surg., 40:534, 1967.

Mustardé, J. C.: The correction of prominent ears using simple mattress sutures. Br. J. Plast. Surg., 16:170, 1963.

Mustardé, J. C.: The treatment of prominent ears by

buried mattress sutures: A ten-year survey. Plast. Reconstr. Surg., *39*:382, 1967.

Mustardé, J. C.: Plastic Surgery in Infancy and Childhood. Edinburgh, Churchill-Livingstone, 1971.

Nagel, F.: Reconstruction of a partial auricular loss. Plast. Reconstr. Surg., *49*:340, 1972.

Nager, G. T.: Congenital aural atresia: Anatomy and surgical management. Birth Defects: Orig. Art. Ser., Vol. 7, 1971.

Nauton, R., and Valvassori, G.: Inner ear anomalies: Their association with atresia. Laryngoscope, *78*:1041, 1968.

Navabi, A.: One-stage reconstruction of partial defect of the auricle. Plast. Reconstr. Surg., *33*:77, 1964.

Nélaton, C., and Ombrédanne, L.: Les Autoplasties. Paris, G. Steinheil, 1907.

Nordzell, B.: A new method for correction of protruding ears. Acta Chir. Scand., *129*:317, 1965.

O'Connor, G. B., and Pierce, G. W.: Refrigerated cartilage isografts. Surg. Gynecol. Obstet., *67*:796, 1938.

Ogino, Y.: Reconstruction of the external ear. Trans. Third Internatl. Congr. Plast. Surg. Amsterdam, Excerpta Medica, 1964, p. 461.

Ogino, Y., and Yoshikawa, Y.: Plastic surgery for the congenital anomaly of the ear. Keisei Geka, *6*:79, 1963.

Ohmori, S.: Congenital deformities of the auricle. Clinics in Plastic Surgery, *1*:3, 1974.

Ohmori, S., and Matsumoto, K.: Treatment of cryptotia, using Teflon string. Plast. Reconstr. Surg., *49*:33, 1972.

Ohmori, S., Matsumoto, K., and Nakai, H.: Follow-up study on reconstruction of microtia with a silicone framework. Plast. Reconstr. Surg., *53*:555, 1974.

Ombrédanne, L.: Technique de la fixation des oreilles artificielles. Ann. Otolaryngol., *73*:951, 1956.

Owens, N., and Delgado, D. D.: The management of outstanding ears. South. Med. J., *58*:32, 1955.

Padgett, E. C., and Stephenson, K. L.: Plastic and Reconstructive Surgery. Springfield, Ill., Charles C Thomas, Publisher, 1948.

Paletta, F. X.: Pediatric Plastic Surgery. Vol. 1, Trauma. St. Louis, Mo., C. V. Mosby Company, 1967, pp. 205–209.

Paletta, F., Ship, A., and Van Norman, R.: Double spring release in otoplasty for prominent ears. Am. J. Surg., *106*:506, 1963.

Pardue, A. M.: Repair of torn earlobe with preservation of the perforation for an earring. Plast. Reconstr. Surg., *51*:472, 1973.

Paré, A.: Les oeuvres de M. Ambroise Paré conseiller et premier chirurgien du roy. Paris, G. Buone, 1575.

Parsons, H., and Lewis, J. S.: Subtotal resection of the temporal bone for cancer of the ear. Cancer, *7*:995, 1954.

Pattee, G. L.: An operation to improve hearing in cases of congenital atresia of the external auditory meatus. Arch. Otolaryngol., *45*:568, 1947.

Peer, L. A.: Diced cartilage grafts: New method for repair of skull defects, mastoid fistula and other deformities. Arch. Otolaryngol., *38*:156, 1943.

Peer, L. A.: Cartilage grafting. Surg. Clin. North Am., *24*:404, 1944.

Peer, L. A.: Reconstruction of the auricle with diced cartilage grafts in a vitallium ear mold. Plast. Reconstr. Surg., *3*:653, 1948.

Peer, L. A., and Walker, J. C.: Total reconstruction of the ear. J. Int. Coll. Surg., *27*:290, 1957.

Peet, E.: Congenital Absence of the Ear. Edinburgh, E. & S. Livingstone, 1971.

Pegram, M., and Peterson, R.: Repair of partial defect of ear. Plast. Reconstr. Surg., *18*:305, 1956.

Pierce, G. W.: Reconstruction of the external ear. Surg. Gynecol. Obstet., *50*:601, 1930.

Pierce, G. W., Klabunde, E. H., and Brobst, H. T.: Further observations on reconstruction of the external ear. Plast. Reconstr. Surg., *10*:395, 1952.

Pollock, W. J.: Technique for correction of cryptotia. Plast. Reconstr. Surg., *44*:501, 1969.

Potter, E. L.: A hereditary ear malformation transmitted through five generations. J. Heredity, *28*:255, 1937.

Ragnell, A.: A new method of shaping deformed ears. Br. J. Plast. Surg., *4*:202, 1951.

Reisner, K.: Tomography in inner and middle ear malformations: Value, limits, results. Radiology, *92*:11, 1969.

Rogers, B.: Berry-Treacher Collins syndrome: A review of 200 cases. Br. J. Plast. Surg., *17*:109, 1964.

Rogers, B.: Microtia, lop, cup and protruding ears: Four directly inherited deformities? Plast. Reconstr. Surg., *41*:208, 1968.

Roux, P. J.: Chirurgie réparatrice. Quarante Années de Pratique Chirurgicale, *1*:91, 1854.

Schmid, E.: Methods for reconstruction of the ear. Trans. Fourth Internatl. Congr. Plast. Surg. Amsterdam, Excerpta Medica, 1969, p. 635.

Schofield, A. L.: Preliminary report on use of preserved homogenous cartilage implants. Br. J. Plast. Surg., *6*:26, 1953.

Schuknecht, H.: Anatomical variants and anomalies of surgical significance. (Gavin Livingstone Memorial Lecture.) J. Laryngol. Otol., *85*:1238, 1971.

Sénéchal, G., and Pech, A.: Chirurgie du pavillon de l'oreille. Paris, Librairie Arnette, 1970.

Sĕrcer, A.: Beitrag zur Kenntnis der Formanomalien des aüsseren Ohres. Acta Otolaryngol., *20*:59, 1934.

Sexton, R. P.: Utilization of the amputated ear cartilage. Plast. Reconstr. Surg., *15*:419, 1955.

Simons, J. N.: The role of the prosthesis in the correction of ear deformities. *In* Tanzer, R. C., and Edgerton, M. T. (Eds.): Symposium on Reconstruction of the Auricle. St. Louis, Mo., C. V. Mosby Company, 1974, p. 178.

Skoog, T., Ohlson, L., and Sohn, S. A.: The chondrogenic potential of the perichondrium. Chir. Plast., *3*:84, 1975.

Spina, V.: Microtia: A simplified three-stage technique. Trans. Fourth Internatl. Congr. Plast. Surg. Amsterdam, Excerpta Medica, 1969, p. 672.

Spina, V., Kamakura, L., and Psillakis, J. M.: Total reconstruction of the ear in congenital microtia. Plast. Reconstr. Surg., *48*:349, 1971.

Spira, M., McCrea, R., Gerow, F. J., and Hardy, S. B.: Analysis and treatment of the protruding ear. Trans. Fourth Internatl. Congr. Plast. Surg. Amsterdam, Excerpta Medica, 1969, p. 1090.

Stark, R. B., and Saunders, D. E.: Natural appearance restored to the unduly prominent ear. Br. J. Plast. Surg., *15*:385, 1962.

Steffensen, W. H.: Method of correcting atresia of ear canal. Plast. Reconstr. Surg., *1*:329, 1946.

Steffensen, W. H.: Comments on total reconstruction of the external ear. Plast. Reconstr. Surg., *10*:186, 1952.

Steffensen, W. H.: Comments on reconstruction of the external ear. Plast. Reconstr. Surg., *16*:194, 1955.

Steffensen, W. H.: A method of total ear reconstruction. Plast. Reconstr. Surg., *36*:97, 1965.

Stenström, S. J.: A "natural" technique for correction of congenitally prominent ears. Plast. Reconstr. Surg., *32*:509, 1963.

Stenström, S. J.: Cosmetic deformities of the ears. *In* Grabb, W. C., and Smith, J. W.: Plastic Surgery: A Concise Guide to Clinical Practice. 2nd ed. Boston, Little, Brown and Company, 1974, p. 595.

Stephenson, K. L.: Correction of a lop ear deformity. Plast. Reconstr. Surg., 26:540, 1960.

Straith, R. E.: Correction of the protruding ear. Plast. Reconstr. Surg., 24:277, 1959.

Streeter, G. L.: Development of the auricle in the human embryo. Carnegie Contrib. Embryol., 14:111, 1922.

Subba Rao, Y. V., and Venkateswara Rao, P.: A quick technique for earlobe reconstruction. Plast. Reconstr. Surg., 41:13, 1968.

Suraci, A. J.: Plastic reconstruction of acquired defects of the ear. Am. J. Surg., 66:196, 1944.

Szymanowski, J. von: Handbuch der operativen Chirurgie. Braunschwig, F. Ziewig und Sohn, 1870.

Tagliacozzi, G.: De Curtorum Chirurgia per Insitionem. Bindoni, 1597.

Tanaka, F., Ishimori, Y., and Sekiguchi, J.: An attempt to perform simultaneously plastic surgery for microtia and creation of the external auditory canal. Trans. Sixth Internatl. Congr. Plast. Surg. Amsterdam, Excerpta Medica, 1976.

Tanzer, R. C.: Prevention of postoperative hematoma, with a note on the use of the compression suture. Surg. Forum, 2:210, 1951.

Tanzer, R. C.: Total reconstruction of the external ear. Plast. Reconstr. Surg., 23:1, 1959.

Tanzer, R. C.: The correction of prominent ears. Plast. Reconstr. Surg., 30:236, 1962.

Tanzer, R. C.: An analysis of ear reconstruction. Plast. Reconstr. Surg., 31:16, 1963.

Tanzer, R. C.: Congenital deformities of the auricle. *In* Converse, J. M. (Ed.): Reconstructive Plastic Surgery. Philadelphia, W. B. Saunders Company, 1964, p. 1073.

Tanzer, R. C.: The reconstruction of acquired defects of the ear. Plast. Reconstr. Surg., 35:355, 1965.

Tanzer, R. C.: Secondary reconstruction of microtia. Plast. Reconstr. Surg., 43:345, 1969.

Tanzer, R. C.: Total reconstruction of the auricle. The evolution of a plan of treatment. Plast. Reconstr. Surg., 47:523, 1971a.

Tanzer, R. C.: Reconstruction of the auricle in four stages. Trans. Fifth Internatl. Congr. Plast. Surg. Melbourne, Australia, Butterworth, 1971b, p. 445.

Tanzer, R. C.: Reconstruction of the auricle. *In* Goldwyn, R. M.: The Unfavorable Result in Plastic Surgery. Boston, Little, Brown and Company, 1972, p. 147.

Tanzer, R. C.: Correction of microtia with autogenous costal cartilage. *In* Tanzer, R. C., and Edgerton, M. T. (Eds.): Symposium on Reconstruction of the Auricle. St. Louis, Mo., C. V. Mosby Company, 1974a, p. 47.

Tanzer, R. C.: Secondary reconstruction of the auricle. *In* Tanzer, R. C., and Edgerton, M. T. (Eds.): Symposium on Reconstruction of the Auricle. St. Louis, Mo., C. V. Mosby Company, 1974b, p. 238.

Tanzer, R. C., and Chaisson, R.: A protective guard for use during reconstruction of the auricle. Plast. Reconstr. Surg., 53:236, 1974.

Tanzer, R. C.: The constricted (cup and lop) ear. Plast. Reconstr. Surg., 55:406, 1975.

Taylor, W. C.: Deformity of ears and kidneys. Can. Med. Assoc. J., 93:107, 1965.

Vincent, R. W., Ryan, R. F., and Longenecker, C. G.: Malformation of ear associated with urogenital anomalies. Plast. Reconstr. Surg., 28:214, 1961.

Webster, J. P.: Some procedures for the correction of ear deformities. Trans. Am. Soc. Plast. Reconstr. Surg., 13th annual meeting, 1944, p. 123.

Wesser, D. R.: Repair of a cryptotic ear with a trefoil flap. Case report. Plast. Reconstr. Surg., 50:192, 1972.

Wildervanck, L. S.: Hereditary malformations of the ear in three generations: Marginal pits, preauricular appendages, malformations of the auricle and conductive deafness. Acta Otolaryngol., 54:553, 1962.

Wood-Jones, F., and Wen I-Chuan: The development of the external ear. J. Anat. (Lond.), 68:525, 1934.

Wray, R. C., and Hoopes, J. E.: Silastic frameworks in total reconstruction of the auricle. Br. J. Plast. Surg., 26:296, 1973.

Young, F.: Autogenous cartilage grafts: An experimental study. Surgery, 10:7, 1941.

Young, F.: Cast and precast cartilage grafts. Surgery, 15:735, 1944.

Zenteno Alanis, S.: A new method for earlobe reconstruction. Plast. Reconstr. Surg., 45:254, 1970.

CHAPTER 36

FACIAL PALSY

BROMLEY S. FREEMAN, M.D.

Autogenous Muscle Grafts
Noel Thompson, F.R.C.S.

Cross-Face Nerve Grafts
Hans Anderl, M.D.

A patient with complete unilateral peripheral facial palsy presents an appalling picture. At rest, there is sagging of the affected side of the face—drooping of the eyebrow, the cheek, the angle of the mouth, and the lip. Upon voluntary action of the superficial muscles of facial expression, the deformity becomes more severe. Under emotional stress, the patient is a caricature of physical affliction, distressing not only to himself and his close friends but also to the casual observer.

Unilateral paralysis permits the unopposed muscles of the unaffected side of the face to exert an abnormal pull on the palsied side. Prolonged absence of antagonists leads to chronic spasticity of the uninvolved mimetic muscles, even in the ipsilateral levator palpebrae, and a typical appearance of deformity. The voluntary or emotional elevation or wrinkling of the forehead, the contraction of the lids and nasal muscles, and the elevation of the active side of the mouth in a smile or grimace contrast with the flaccid paralyzed side, the wide staring palpebral fissure with exposed sclera, and the twist of the nose to the unaffected side, following the distorted oral fissure. Drooling and ballooning of the cheek while eating, persistent epiphora and muffled or garbled speech are merely outward signs of the mental distress which the patient is suffering.

Although the facial nerve (or seventh cranial nerve) has varied functions, both motor and sensory, in facial palsy it is not the associated disturbances of taste, touch, salivation, or hearing that call for treatment, but the deformity caused by the paralysis of the muscles of expression and the loss of facial sphincteric control. Bell (1821) thought of the facial nerve or the "portio dura" of the seventh cranial nerve as the "respiratory" nerve of the face; it is unquestionably part of the communication system.

Restoration of the conduction of the facial nerve is not always possible, but many small operative procedures can be performed to lift these patients from a state of despondency to one of relative happiness. Simple techniques rapidly performed under local anesthesia can aid even the very young and the aged in bearing their affliction with equanimity. The victims of strokes, cerebral trauma, or operative intervention can be helped emotionally and physically as much by facial operative procedures as by the hypnotic and relaxation techniques used in physical rehabilitation for the release of spastic, antagonistic muscles in the trunk and extremities.

All functions of the facial nerve except those concerned with musculature control of the face can be disregarded except for diagnostic purposes. The primary aims of therapy in facial palsy are to restore (1) an acceptable appearance of the face at rest, (2) symmetry with voluntary motion, and (3) if at all possible, normal facial appearance by combining muscular balance and control while expressing emotion. Another important aim is restoration of sphincteric control of the orbital, nasal, oral, and buccopharyngeal apertures.

HISTORY

In 1814 Charles Bell sectioned the facial nerve of a monkey, noted that a facial paralysis on the same side resulted, and thus proved that the nerve was responsible for facial expression.

"On cutting of the respiratory nerve on the face of a monkey, the very peculiar activity of his features on that side ceased altogether. The timid motions of his eyelids and eyebrows were lost, and he could not wink on that side; and his lips were drawn to the other side, like a paralytic drunkard, whenever he showed his teeth in rage. I suspect that the influence of passion, as this of smiling or laughing, is lost in consequence of affections that do not destroy the entire power of the nerve."

Although Herbert Mayo in 1822 offered the first clear description of the function of the facial nerve, Bellinghieri in 1818 anticipated Bell's demonstration of 1821 which conclusively proved that the trigeminal was sensory and that the facial nerve was the motor nerve of the superficial muscles of facial expression.

Scientific neurology started with Bell. His classic clinical description of facial paralysis in humans is as follows:

"The muscles of the cheek on the left side are wasted and there appears to remain nothing but the thin integument, which hangs upon the side of the face, as if dead, without having any action in them or wrinkles, as in the right cheek; and when he speaks, this cheek is alternately puffed out and then collapsed. The air first distending it as if it were a bag and then escaping at the angles of the mouth. His whole mouth is drawn to the right side, thus producing most remarkable distortion of the face. Whatever action there is in the mouth is altogether owing to the contraction of the muscles on the right side of it; and left angle hangs loose and it is quite passive; and the saliva is allowed to flow constantly out of the lower lip on this side."

ANATOMY

The Intratemporal Facial Nerve. The supranuclear and infranuclear pathways form the trunk of the facial nerve, which leaves the pons, crosses the subarachnoid space to the internal auditory meatus, and enters the facial canal of the temporal bone. The *greater superficial petrosal nerve* (the most proximal branch of the facial nerve) arises at the level of the geniculate ganglion. It supplies secretomotor fibers to the lacrimal gland and conveys taste from the soft palate and probably the deep pressure sense and pain from the skin, muscles, and bones of the face. The *nerve to the stapedius* arises above the chorda tympani in the vertical portion of the facial nerve. It exerts a protec-

FIGURE 36–1. The extratemporal portion of the facial nerve showing the multiple anastomoses between the facial and trigeminal nerves in and around the muscles of expression (modified from Shapiro).

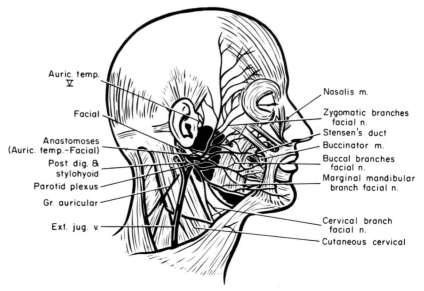

Auric. temp. V

Facial

Anastomoses (Auric. temp.–Facial)

Post dig. & stylohyoid

Parotid plexus

Gr. auricular

Ext. jug. v.

Nasalis m.

Zygomatic branches facial n.

Stensen's duct

Buccinator m.

Buccal branches facial n.

Marginal mandibular branch facial n.

Cervical branch facial n.

Cutaneous cervical

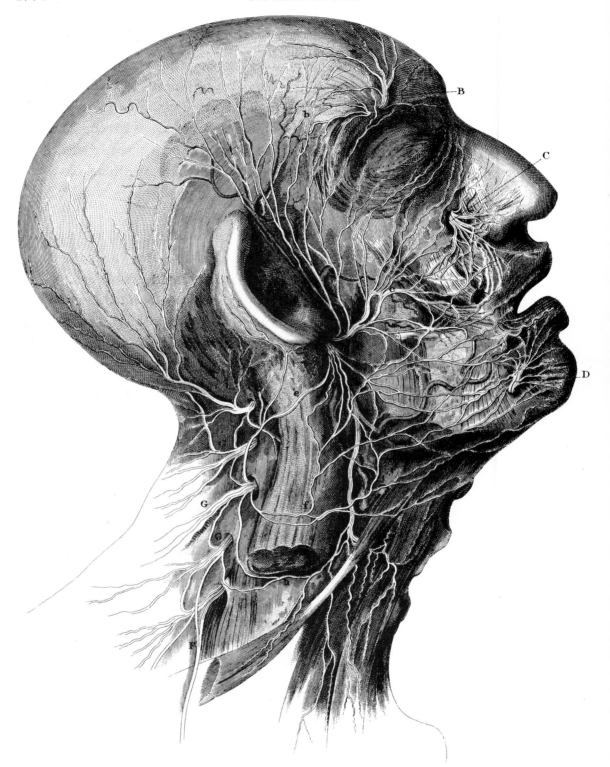

FIGURE 36–2.   The facial nerve (Bell, 1821).

tive dampening effect upon sound vibrations reaching the inner ear and is activated reflexly by sounds of fairly high intensity. Of the three branches of the nerve within the temporal bones, the *chorda tympani* is the most peripheral. It arises 4 to 6 mm above the stylomastoid foramen and contains secretomotor fibers to the submaxillary and sublingual glands, as well as taste fibers from the anterior two-thirds of the upper lateral half of the tongue (Kettel, 1959).

The Extratemporal Nerve. A simplified outline of the extratemporal facial nerve is shown in Figure 36–1 (Shapiro, 1954) and can be contrasted with the drawing of Charles Bell (Fig. 36–2). In the infant, the facial nerve lies superficially. It is almost subcutaneous as it emerges from the stylomastoid foramen, since it lacks the protection of the mastoid process, as yet not developed, and also because the increase in the depth of the nerve is related to the progressive increase of the overlying soft tissue as the child grows older (Sammarco, Ryan and Longenecker, 1966).

The first branch of the facial nerve as it leaves the stylomastoid foramen is the *posterior auricular,* which extends upward between the parotid gland and the anterior border of the sternocleidomastoid muscle and is seen in the notch between the external auditory meatus and the mastoid process. The occipitalis, the posterior auricular, part of the superior auricular muscles, and the intrinsic muscles of the auricle are supplied by this nerve, which also carries a part of the sensory fibers running to the ear. Slightly distally, the facial nerve sends a branch to the posterior belly of the digastric muscle and to the stylohyoid muscle before entering the parotid gland.

A significant study of the surgical anatomy of the facial nerve and the parotid gland is that of Davis and coworkers (1956). Recognition of the bilaminar structure of the parotid gland and of the positions of the posterior and anterior facial veins, the transverse facial artery, and the external carotid artery is emphasized. The so-called "capsule" of the parotid gland beneath the panniculus adiposus, which may contain a considerable amount of fat, is a membranous portion of the fascia of the face; it is not a capsule in the usual sense, as it merely passes over the area and is bounded by the sternocleidomastoid, the zygomaticus, the platysma and the triangularis muscles, which are enclosed. The external part of the nonfatty stratum contains the muscles of facial expression; the internal lamina covers the muscles of mastication. The laminae join at the periphery of the parotid gland to form an envelope which is perforated by the branches of the facial·nerve.

A review of the dissection and sketches by the anatomists of the past century, particularly those of Charles Bell (Fig. 36–2), demonstrates the intricacy of the plexiform arrangement of the branches of the facial nerve. The branches are arbitrarily simplified into two main divisions of *temporofacial* and *cervicofacial,* from which divide the temporal, zygomatic, buccal, marginal mandibular, and cervical rami. McCormack, Cauldwell, and Anson (1945) classified facial nerves from a hundred dissections and divided them into eight major types, with many variants according to the type of branching and major anastomoses.

The multiple connections between the branches of the facial nerve shown in the original plates of Fyfe (1814) and Bell (1821) are confirmed by the dissections of Rhoton and Lineweaver (1976) using the operating microscope (Fig. 36–3). A rich parotid nerve plexus was a consistent finding, with multiple and unpredictable connections between the major branches (Fig. 36–3, *A*). McCormack, Cauldwell and Anson (1945) and Davis and associates (1956) described the anatomy and pattern of distribution of the facial nerve. They did not note, however, that the facial nerve does not lie in a single plane. Rhoton and Lineweaver found that in five of 18 dissected specimens, nerve branches were situated lateral to the main branches (Fig. 36–3, *B* and *C*). These extraplanar branches arose from proximal portions of the buccal branches and descended into the area of distribution of the mandibular marginal branches. Rhoton and Lineweaver propose that a microsurgical approach might be the safest approach to facial nerve dissection during operative procedures.

Conley (1976), in the course of over 1000 parotidectomies, failed to observe a consistent pattern of distribution of the facial nerve. One hundred photographs were taken during the operations after dissection of the facial nerve branches; no two patterns of distribution were identical. Conley (1973) observed that the buccal and zygomatic branches have connections in 80 per cent of the cases, whereas the marginal mandibular and buccal branches are connected in only 5 to 12 per cent of the dissections performed. Dingman and Grabb (1962) found connections between the marginal mandibular and buccal branches in only 5 per cent of their dissected specimens.

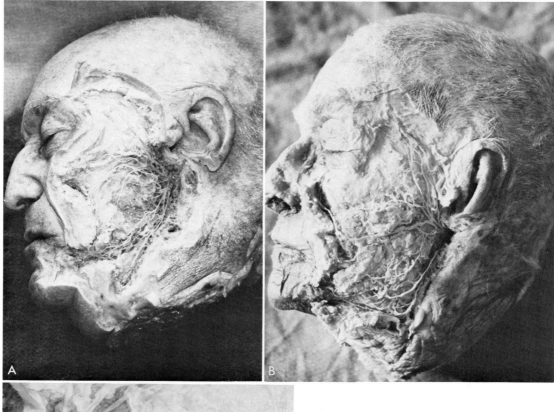

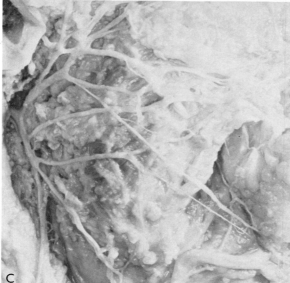

FIGURE 36–3. Anatomy of the facial nerve (dissected with the operating microscope). *A*, A complex specimen showing multiple connections between the major branches. *B*, Specimen showing a simpler pattern of distribution with two extraplanar branches arising from the main buccal trunk and descending into the lower portion of the face. *C*, Dissection of the right facial nerve. Note the single extraplanar branch arising from a buccal nerve, crossing over two other large branches and finally intermingling with some of the upturning offshoots of the marginal mandibular nerve. (Courtesy of Dr. A. L. Rhoton and Mr. W. Lineweaver.)

The *temporal branches* innervate the anterior auricular and part of the superior auricular muscles, and the muscles of the forehead, including the major portion of the orbicularis oculi muscle. The *zygomatic branches* also supply the orbicularis oculi muscle, the muscles around the nares, and the elevators of the upper lip; the *buccal branches* supply most of the musculature around the lip. The lower branches of the buccal and of the *marginalis mandibularis* supply the musculature of the lower lip, and the *cervical branches* innervate the platysma.

Surgical Exposure of the Facial Nerve. The surgeon exploring this field should be familiar with the various techniques of exposing the nerve: (1) locating the major trunk at the stylomastoid foramen and progressing peripherally; (2) exposing and following the marginal mandibular branch proximally to the major branching; or (3) exposing the terminal zygomatic, temporal, or buccal branches distal, or anterior, to the parotid gland and tracing them proximally. The anastomoses are delicate and multiple and can be confusing unless the field is bloodless and the lighting and exposure adequate (Fig. 36–3). In children, the surgeon must be even more cautious, for the facial nerve is superficial in its posterior portion, and the peripheral branches are of gossamer weight and easily damaged.

Knowledge of the variants of the marginal mandibular and the lower buccal branches can prevent unrecognized severance of the facial nerve, with residual and embarrassing palsy. This is the area often transgressed by surgeons in simple operative procedures and one of the most frequent sites of partial facial paralysis. Paralysis of the buccal and marginal mandibular branches produces the most severe facial deformity, since these branches serve the most mobile portion of the face. Variants of the marginal mandibular branch are frequent and must be looked for in all operative procedures near the angle of the mandible in an area extending from the anterior border of the sternocleidomastoid muscle forward for a width of 2.5 cm from the upper margin of the mandible to about 1.5 cm below the lower margin.

Dingman and Grabb (1962) studied the relations of the marginal mandibular branch of the facial nerve to the mandible, and its relation to the external maxillary artery. Posterior to the artery the mandibular branch extended above the inferior border of the mandible in 81 per cent of the specimens. In the other 19 per cent the trunk, or one or more of its branches, extended in an arc, the lowest point 1 cm or less below the inferior border of the mandible; anterior to the external maxillary artery all of the subdivisions of the marginal mandibular nerve were above the inferior border of the mandible.

In a number of specimens peripheral anastomoses of the lowest branch of the mandibular branch with the cervical rami were found. Branches anterior to the external maxillary artery and below the border of the mandible innervate the platysma muscle and not the other depressor muscles of the lip. In 98 per cent of the specimens, the mandibular branch was intimately related to the superficial surface of the posterior facial vein as the nerve made its way from the region of the stylomastoid foramen to the muscles of the lower lip. Multiple major branches of the mandibular branch were present, with a single branch in one-fifth of the specimens. Continuity of the anterior portion of the platysma and quadratus labii inferioris muscle across the inferior border of the mandible was corroborated and was felt to be a factor in some immediate postoperative alterations in the position of the angle of the mouth.

Influence of Other Factors on the Position of the Branches of the Facial Nerve. The relation of the head to the neck, its rotation, flexion, and extension at the time of injury or surgery, as well as the gross physical condition of the tissues, obesity, relaxed aging skin, or the turgor of puberty, all influence the position of the mandibular branch in the *living* patient as compared to a *fixed* specimen. In the living patient past middle age, the mandibular branch drops well below the angle of the mandible; in a child it is considerably higher. Often the facial nerve lies between a large superficial lobe and a variably sized deep lobe of the parotid gland. This finding leads the experienced surgeon to search out the filaments of the facial nerve anterior to the parotid gland, enter the cleavage plane between the superficial and deep nerves, and, by gently retracting the anterior lobe, extend the dissection from anterior to posterior, until the isthmus is reached (Byars, 1952). Laxity of the subcutaneous tissue in the cachectic patient and the variability of position of the submaxillary gland in the aged keep the branches at different levels. Knowledge of the various types of branching encountered in the dissection of the faciocervical halves (Fig. 36–4) is helpful, especially when the facial nerve branches must be dissected out of scar tissue prior to an anastomosis or graft.

The Vascular Supply. The blood supply of the extratemporal segment of the facial nerve at the stylomastoid foramen is furnished by a branch from the *stylomastoid artery* (from the posterior auricular artery). The facial nerve also receives twigs from the *occipital artery* and in the parotid from the *superficial temporal* and the *transverse facial arteries*. Fine and delicate arteriae comitantes accompany and enter the terminal branches that leave the parotid gland. The facial nerve is enclosed in the fallopian canal and the stylomastoid artery exits from the fallopian canal and the stylomastoid foramen. The nerve and the vessel cannot expand or avoid compression in this rigid bony enclosure, hence the multiple irregular and bizarre syndromes that occur secondary to intratemporal vascular changes. As in all nerves, the blood supply of the facial nerve travels along the sheath and dissection must of neces-

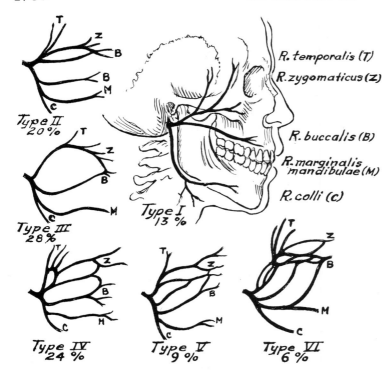

R. temporalis (T)
R. zygomaticus (Z)
R. buccalis (B)
R. marginalis mandibulae (M)
R. colli (c)

Type II 20%
Type III 28%
Type I 13%
Type IV 24%
Type V 9%
Type VI 6%

FIGURE 36–4. Various types of branching of the facial nerve. (Redrawn from Davis, R. A., Anson, B. J., Budinger, J. M., and Kurth, L. E.: Surgical anatomy of the facial nerve and parotid gland based upon a study of 350 cervico-facial halves. Surg. Gynecol. Obstet., *102*:385, 1956.)

sity disturb the delicate branches (Blunt, 1954).

The Facial Muscles. The facial musculature of expression owes its origin to a wide, thin band of muscle found in reptiles, the sphincter colli, innervated by a branch of the seventh cranial nerve. This muscle has grown forward over the face in mammals, and its one nerve, which innervated the muscular matrix, now supplies the 30-odd derivative mimetic muscles (Huber, 1931; Kent, 1969).

The superficial facial muscles control the movements of the soft tissues of the face and do not act upon the bones. The muscular fibers divide into a series of bundles, which penetrate the dermis to terminate in a fanlike manner immediately below the basal epidermal layer. The fibers can contract independently to produce fine shades of expression; the muscles interweave, usually in one plane, but some—the caninus, corrugator, and buccinator muscles—located at a deeper level, interweave in two planes.

All of the mimetic muscles derive their nerve supply from the facial nerve, whose branches enter the muscles in their deeper and more lateral or posterior portions. Facial wrinkles are produced by repeated contraction of the underlying muscles of facial expression.

The shortening of the muscles, without shortening the skin, causes the skin to adapt itself by forming folds at right angles to the line of contraction of the underlying muscle. In general, the muscles act in unison; for example, the nasolabial fold, formed by the attachment of the zygomaticus, quadratus labii superioris, caninus, and risorius, is made more prominent by the junction of the tightly knit orbicularis oris and the loosely bound muscles over the buccal fat pads of the cheek.

The conjoint areas of insertion are the sphincters of the orbicularis oculi and the orbicularis oris muscles (and to a lesser extent, the nares). Areas of antagonism are found in the midline of the face, giving rise to the vertical lines of flexion or expression.

The muscles that are most important in facial palsy are shown in Figure 36–5. In the cervical region, the platysma, innervated by the lowest cervical branches of the facial nerve, augments the depressor action of the lower group of circumoral muscles. The deeply lying stylohyoid, the posterior belly of the digastric, and the tiny stapedius muscle in the middle ear, also innervated by the facial nerve, are of relative academic interest in facial paralysis.

The lower group of circumoral muscles consists of the *triangularis,* the *quadratus labii in-*

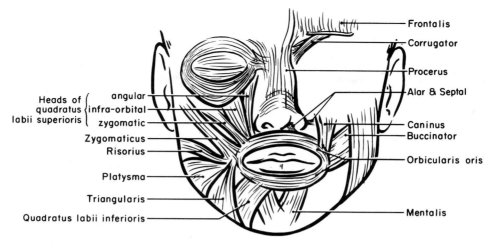

Heads of { angular
quadratus { infra-orbital
labii superioris { zygomatic
Zygomaticus
Risorius
Platysma
Triangularis
Quadratus labii inferioris

Frontalis
Corrugator
Procerus
Alar & Septal
Caninus
Buccinator
Orbicularis oris
Mentalis

FIGURE 36–5. The muscles of facial expression: the deeper mimetic muscles on the right side, the more superficial on the left. (This drawing does not show the interweaving fibers of the various muscles to form the orbicularis oris, but regards them as individual muscles seemingly attached to a central raphé. Close examination at the time of surgery shows that the muscles interweave to form the orbicularis oris, which is really a composite muscle.)

ferioris, and the *platysma,* which depress the corner of the mouth and the lower lip, and the deep lying *mentalis,* which draws the skin down, forcing the lower lip against the gum. The upper group of muscles, the *zygomaticus,* the *risorius,* the *quadratus labii superioris,* with its three heads, and the *caninus* elevate the upper lip, pull the angle of the mouth, and widen the external nares. The *orbicularis oris* is in reality a group of muscles arranged in a sphincteric fashion about the mouth, interwoven and in direct continuation with the adjacent muscles which blend to form it, and inserted partially into the skin and partially into the mucosa of the lips. Through its action, the orbicularis oris puckers the lips, draws them inward at the corners, protrudes them, or presses them against the teeth. The *buccinator,* a deep and powerful muscle, passes through the orbicularis oris to the mucosa, and it is responsible for flattening the cheek against the teeth and maintaining its shape against internal pressure. This must be regarded as part of the pharyngo-bucco-orbicularis oris sphincter, which consists of the orbicularis oris muscle complex, the buccinator muscle, and the buccopharyngeal segment of the superior constrictor muscle which joins the buccinator at the pterygomandibular raphé. The junction of the corresponding muscles of both sides is at the pharyngeal raphé (Fig. 36–6).

The nasal muscles, the *nasalis,* the *depressor septi nasi,* and the *dilator* muscles, act as nares sphincters. Of the orbital group, the chief muscle is the *orbicularis oculi,* which is divided into a superficial orbital portion, extending out to join with the adjacent facial muscles, and a deep, or palpebral, portion. The latter

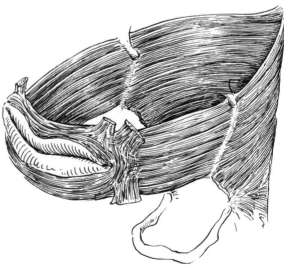

FIGURE 36–6. The pharyngobucco-orbicularis sphincter consists of the orbicularis oris muscle complex, the buccinator muscle, and the buccopharyngeal segment of the superior constrictor muscle, which joins the buccinator at the pterygomandibular raphé. The junction of the corresponding muscles of both sides of the pharyngeal raphé completes the sphincter. (From Freeman, B. S.: Late reconstruction of the lax oral sphincter in facial paralysis. Plast. Reconstr. Surg., *51*:144, 1973. Copyright ©1973, The Williams & Wilkins Company, Baltimore.)

alone can occlude the eyelids; contraction of the orbital portion brings the skin of the forehead and eyelids downward and shades the eyes. The *procerus* and the *corrugator supercilii* muscles produce transverse wrinkles at the root of the nose and draw the eyebrows medially to form vertical wrinkles, respectively. The extrinsic muscles of the ear consist of the *anterior auricular* muscle, the *posterior auricular* muscle, and the *superior auricular* muscle, which are of relatively minor importance. The major muscles of the scalp are the *occipitalis* and *frontalis;* the latter, a thin muscle covering the forehead, wrinkles the forehead and tends to act with the procerus, the corrugator supercilii, and the orbicularis oculi muscles. The frontalis muscles are innervated by the temporal branches of the facial nerve, the occipital by the postauricular branches. Like most anatomical drawings of the facial or mimetic muscles, Figure 36–5 exaggerates the thickness and size of these relatively delicate muscles.

The Muscles of Mastication. The masseter, temporalis, and anterior digastric muscles are innervated by branches of the mandibular division of the trigeminal nerve and are used in reconstruction (Fig. 36–7). The masseter muscles consist of two sets of fibers, the superficial and the deep. The outer or superficial portion, which is the larger, has its origin on the anterior two-thirds of the inferior border of the zygomatic bone. The deep fibers arise from the posterior third of the zygoma and zygomatic arch and the inner surface. The deep part of the muscle extends inferiorly to insert along the posterior and upper portion of the ramus. The superficial portion extends down and backward, intermingling with the deep fibers, and inserts into the outer surface of the lower portion of the mandible and the mandibular angle. Innervation is by the masseteric branch, which passes through the mandibular notch and enters the muscle deeply. The posterior deep temporal nerve passes with the masseteric nerve above the superior head of the external pterygoid muscle and enters the muscle in two main divisions.

The fan-shaped temporalis muscle originates from the temporal bone and the temporal fascia. The converging fibers pass under the zygomatic arch to insert into the anterior border and apex of the coronoid process of the mandible. A few fibers attach to the anterior border of the mandibular ramus. The muscle is innervated by the temporal branch of the mandibular motor nerve (fifth cranial nerve), which emerges from the foramen ovale and passes into the infratemporal fossa. One branch goes to the masseter muscle and another to the temporalis. The nerve to the temporalis muscle splits into posterior and anterior branches. The anterior branch runs with the buccinator nerve superior to the buccinator muscle, supplies the buccinator superiorly, and enters the anterior deep portion of the temporalis muscle at about the level of the zygomatic arch. These three major divisions of the nerve should theoretically permit the splitting of this large, fleshy

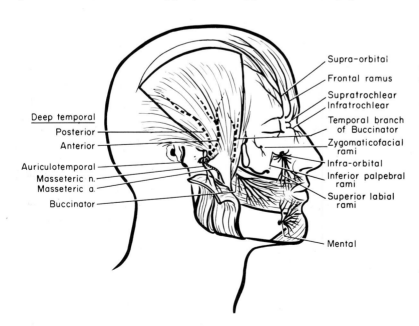

Deep temporal
— Posterior
— Anterior
Auriculotemporal
Masseteric n.
Masseteric a.
Buccinator

Supra-orbital
Frontal ramus
Supratrochlear
Infratrochlear
Temporal branch of Buccinator
Zygomaticofacial rami
Infra-orbital
Inferior palpebral rami
Superior labial rami

Mental

FIGURE 36–7. Ramifications of the trigeminal nerve showing the muscular branches to the masseter and temporal muscles. Note the direction of the masseteric and the deep temporal nerves. Section of the masseter muscle as indicated extends somewhat posteriorly and preserves the nerve. (Frequently blunt dissection may stimulate the nerve and cause contraction of the muscle, thus warning the surgeon to go no higher.) When the fan-shaped major portion of the temporalis muscle is freed, muscle splitting must be done bluntly to prevent direct nerve injury. This is also necessary when the masseter muscle is being split, to avoid tearing the nerve to the deep portion of the masseter, which passes inferiorly and anteriorly.

muscle into three separate but unequal segments, each supplied by an individual branch. However, the pattern is not quite that unvarying.

ANTERIOR BELLY OF THE DIGASTRIC. The anterior belly of the digastric, covered by the external layer of deep cervical fascia, originates on the inner surface of the mandible and is attached by the conjoint digastric tendon to the hyoid bone by an aponeurotic attachment. Innervated by the mylohyoid branch of the inferior alveolar nerve (fifth cranial nerve), the anterior belly is not involved in facial nerve paralysis.

PATHOLOGY

The Effects of Nerve Injury. Nerve injuries can be subdivided into various types: simple block of the axon with no histologically detectable changes, destruction of the axon, discontinuity of the sheath, funicular disorganization, and severance of the nerve trunk. Various lesions can be present, depending upon the etiologic factors, whether infection, thrombosis, pressure, direct trauma, or impact (Fig. 36–8).

The effects of these injuries are degeneration both distally and proximally and the formation and subsequent shrinkage of Schwann cell tubes (Gutmann and Young, 1944). Regenerating axons have varying chances of being confined to their original endoneural tubes and directed to the exact original end organs without cross-shunting. Interfunicular fibrosis and scar tissue may block the regenerating axons, and these are no longer confined to endoneural tubes within the original funiculi. Functional recovery, with or without surgery, is depend-

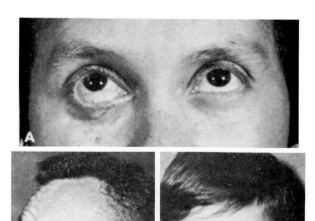

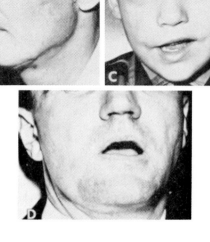

FIGURE 36–8. Partial facial nerve palsies. Severance of *(A)* the branches to the right lower lid by a rock; *(B)* the temporal branch to the frontalis by a broken bottle; *(C)* the buccal branch to the upper lip by a broken stick; and *(D)* the marginal mandibular branch by a retractor.

ent on a high incidence of axonal sprouting, axonal loss, retrograde neuronal degeneration, severe fibrosis and erroneous irregular cross-shunting. Hence the importance of early and accurate diagnosis and treatment. Sunderland (1952) stated, "the distal stump retains the capacity of transmitting axones to the periphery for at least twelve months and muscle function can be fully restored following reinnervation even at that time." Recent studies have shown that even several years after the onset of total facial paralysis reinervation can be restored (Conley, 1973). This is in accord with clinical results.

Even mild stretching can cause damage to epineural vessels with resulting patchy ischemia; severe stretching can cause perineural rupture and herniation, followed by endoneural fibrosis and impairment of regeneration of a grossly intact nerve trunk (Denny-Brown and Brenner, 1944). Although slender nerves may be stretched and stripped for mobilization prior to approximation, the longitudinal vascular chain must be carefully preserved or further damage will be added to the initial trauma.

The review of the microscopic study of nerve vascularity illustrates this point (Smith, 1966). Studies of the mesoneurium of peripheral nerves and the author's clinical experience support the presence of a similar structure in the facial nerve.

Traumatic nerve paralysis can be divided into three types:

1. *Neurapraxia*, in which only the myelin sheath is affected. It occurs some days after trauma and disappears spontaneously and completely.

2. *Axonotmesis*, in which the neural element is separated and damaged but the neurilemmal sheath is not interrupted, and the patient may make a spontaneous, if incomplete, recovery.

3. *Neurotmesis*, in which the neural elements as well as the nerve sheaths are completely interrupted, by either operative intervention or external trauma. Wallerian degeneration occurs with axonotmesis and neurotmesis but not with neurapraxia.

If facial nerve paralysis is noted immediately after a laceration, exploration to determine the exact type of injury is indicated. The longer exploration is delayed, the poorer will be the results of repair. Some fibrosis of paralyzed facial muscles occurs in a year; after this period the degenerative muscular changes are more progressive, often militating against a satisfactory functional result from any type of nerve repair (Seddon, 1954).

DENERVATED MUSCLE ATROPHIES. Upon reinnervation, the characteristics of normal muscle begin to return, but recovery is never complete. In the latest stages of regeneration studied, there still remains an increase in connective tissue, an increase in the numbers of nuclei, and a persistence of small fibers. When neural fasciculi are misdirected in the course of reinnervation, the missed muscle fibers continue to degenerate (Slaughter, 1935).

ETIOLOGY

The etiology of facial paralysis is varied. The literature of "Bell's palsy" from the early nineteenth century to the present is replete with many causes and a multitude of treatments. It is not within the scope of this chapter to discuss the treatment of Bell's palsy, but a brief note on the etiology is of interest. The simplest chill, cold, or ague or the most complicated sequence of allergic and immunologic phenomena may herald its onset. Infections — viral, bacterial, or spirochetal — cerebritis, facial nuclear and endotemporal irritation, meningitis, osteomyelitis, and parotitis have been considered to be causes. The lesions may be due to degenerative changes in the arteries (aneurysms, thromboses), in the nerves, as in alcoholic neuritis and polyneuritis, and in the muscles (myasthenia gravis). Developmental anomalies such as central nuclear agenesis, ischemic changes in the pons or fallopian canal, and tumors — intracerebral, intratemporal, and parotid — have caused paralysis. Trauma, surgical and accidental, due to blasts or electricity, to scalpel, retractor, or a blunt object, has been implicated. For many years surgical incisions and neoplastic changes predominated as causal factors. Automobile accidents and cerebral arteriosclerotic disease currently appear to predominate. In a review by the Central Registry, Joint Study of Extracranial Arterial Occlusions of 2,574 Patients with Limb Paralysis Secondary to Stroke, approximately 70 per cent of patients had an accompanying facial paralysis, and an additional 350 patients (5.4 per cent) had facial paralysis without involvement of the limbs (Field, 1971).

Acute lesions of the facial nerve usually involve the extratemporal portion. Any operative procedure distal to the stylomastoid foramen presents the risk of severance of the nerve. Inflammatory swelling, abscess, lymphadenopathy, and benign and malignant tumors can distort the architecture and confuse the surgeon; anomalies both of position and number of branches can lead to unintentional severance of the nerve. Other handicaps are improper operative position, the hanging jowls of the aged, and the turgid subcutaneous fat layer of the infant. Simple stab incisions for drainage, retroauricular in children or pre-auricular in adults, may damage the nerve. An incision to explore the frontozygomatic junction in a maxillofacial fracture can sever the zygomatic branches. The application of obstetrical forceps can crush the nerve during delivery.

Whenever possible, the nerve should be repaired as soon as the injury is recognized. When segments of the nerve must be removed in the course of an ablative operation, immediate grafting should be practiced to reestablish the continuity.

Postponement of repair seems to have been unduly influenced by the report of Martin and Helsper (1957) showing spontaneous recovery of function following segmental operative defects of facial nerves in adults. These workers have proposed the hypothesis that spontaneous return of movements of the face after resection of the seventh cranial nerve is due to "re-establishment of motor pathways to facial musculature by way of the fifth cranial nerve." As only 28.5 per cent of those afflicted had some *minor* return of motion, the value of delay is questioned. James, Karlan, Kensey and Meagher (1960) suggested that the reinnervation (in dogs) is via the regenerating facial or seventh nerve and its anastomoses. Conley (1961) has shown responses in the seventh cranial nerve, or some segment, to electrical nerve testing in as high as 71 per cent of the patients receiving autogenous nerve grafts. Of the 27 patients reported by Conley, 13 or 46 per cent of the patients with autogenous nerve grafts were classified as having a good result. In a personal series of 30 patients, 95 per cent had evidence of reinnervation of muscle, and in 90 per cent the results were classified as "good" (Freeman, 1972a). If a direct channel is offered, why chance the open sea? The spontaneous recoveries seen have been inadequate to maintain emotional or involuntary response in the facial muscles. The brilliant results published by Bunnell (1952), Maxwell (1954), and Beahrs, Judd, and Woodington (1961) show that it is unnecessary to take the statistically long odds offered by those who look for spontaneous recovery.

DIAGNOSIS

Clinical Examination. Bell's description of a patient with unilateral facial paralysis cannot be improved upon.

The patient should be examined in action. The motor function is tested by having the patient wrinkle his forehead, close his eyes, show his teeth, purse his lips, and dilate and contract his nares. As a matter of routine, the face can be subdivided into six examining areas and the response to attempted volitional control noted—forehead furrowing, eyebrows corrugating, squeezing the eyelids tightly, nose wrinkling, teeth showing, lips puckering, and in the neck, platysma tightening. Ballooning or puffing out the cheeks, chewing, swallowing, spitting, and speech should also be checked. Subjective sensory disturbances of taste (ageusia) and hearing (dysacusis), as well as any unusual history of twitching or facial pain, should be noted. All patients with facial and head injuries or tumors should be routinely checked for possible weakness of the facial muscles.

Muscular tone and symmetry are noted at rest and in motion, when the patient smiles or cries spontaneously or talks with great emotion. These maneuvers may point to "thalamic" facial weakness of the supranuclear type, in which voluntary action may be normal but muscular weakness is present during emotional episodes. Suspicious areas are then checked, not according to the electrical method of Duchenne, but more simply, by the clinician running the gamut of facial contortions and the patient copying the examiner's grimaces. A knowledge of the various mimetic muscles and a perusal of the section on facial motions in the classic work of Duchenne of Boulogne (1862) or Duval's textbook on *Artistic Anatomy* (1905) will prepare one for the task. A modern "beautifying" exercise tome, which is excellent for the anatomical and photographic delineation of expressions, is that of Craig (1970). It is especially helpful for instructing patients in exercises.

With the patient's face at rest, changes of the "irritative" type, twitches or even spasms, are sought as evidence of partially returning, or even misdirected, nerve fibrils (see section on Residuals of Facial Paralysis). The lines of expression usually have disappeared, including the nasolabial fold. As a result of paralysis of the buccinator and the orbicularis oris muscles, whistling or puffing up the cheeks causes air to escape at the angle of the mouth on the affected side. Similarly, the patient drools food and saliva during mastication. There is usually a slight speech defect, and the articulation of labials is interfered with. Paralysis of the platysma can be checked when the patient depresses his chin against finger resistance. Late physical signs include nasal and septal deviation to the contralateral side and, not infrequently, nasal obstruction. Buccal and mucosal protrusion and erosion are prominent in neglected cases.

OCULAR SIGNS.   In complete unilateral facial palsy the *palpebral fissure cannot be closed* on the affected side. Although passive closure may occur during sleep because of relaxation of the levator palpebrae superioris muscle, an attempt at closing the eye results in a movement of the eyeball upward and inward, until the cornea passes under the upper lid. The paralyzed lower lid exposes the sclera. Eversion of the lid margin prevents contact of the lacrimal punctum against the eyeball, interfering with the tear drainage. Palsy of the orbicularis oculi muscle hampers collection of the tears by the lacrimal sac. The punctum becomes stenosed and the exposed caruncle hypertrophies. Increased conjunctival exposure leads to increased lacrimal secretion, and the sagging lid collects the tears in the midportion of the lacrimal lake away from the canthi, thus interfering with normal drainage.

LOCATION OF THE LESION.   A number of tests can be employed to assist in determining where the continuity of the facial nerve is interrupted. *Bilateral facial paralysis* is rare. It results in expressionless features, with the inability to smile, to close the eyes, to elevate the eyebrows, to wrinkle the forehead, or to show the teeth. There is profuse tearing and the acts of mastication and speech are considerably interfered with. Bilateral congenital facial paralysis associated with bilateral abducens cranial nerve palsy (Möbius syndrome), although uncommon, is striking and variable in extent and degree and may involve all of the cranial nerves (Rogers, 1964). A distinguishing feature of *supranuclear paralysis* is the preservation of the action of the orbicularis oculi and frontalis muscles associated with paralysis of the lower facial muscles on the side opposite the cerebral lesion. The eye can be closed, the eyebrow elevated, and the forehead wrinkled, but the muscles of the lower two-thirds of the face are flaccid. An unusual facial weakness of the supranuclear type is sometimes detected only when the patient smiles spontaneously and a "thalamic" facial weakness is present. Associated lesions, such as abducens palsy,

may accompany facial nuclear lesions secondary to poliomyelitis. Associated nerve palsies and anesthesia of the other cranial nerves must be searched for and noted, especially after trauma and after removal of intracranial tumors. Unilateral facial weakness, partial or complete, in the newborn (*neonatal facial asymmetry*) can be studied only by electrodiagnostic studies under general anesthesia. Diagnostic biopsies have indicated that the palsy is due to agenesis of the affected muscle rather than to a neural lesion (McHugh and co-workers, 1969).

Diagnosis of the site of intratemporal interruption of the nerve.   To determine the level of nerve block, the function of the three major branches of the nerve which arise within the temporal bone may be tested. The *chorda tympani* contains secretomotor fibers to the submaxillary and sublingual glands, as well as taste fibers from the anterior two-thirds of the upper lateral half of the tongue. The gustatory function is tested either by galvanic current, noting the difference between the metallic taste on the sound side of the tongue and the sensation of the electric shock on the affected side, or by an applicator moistened with a bitter solution.

Patients questioned about their reaction to loud sound may give a clear-cut history that the sound of high-pitched children's voices and of the clashing of dishes is almost intolerable in the early stages of paralysis involving the *nerve to the stapedius muscle.*

The greater superficial petrosal nerve (the most proximal branch) arises at the level of the geniculate ganglion. It supplies secretomotor fibers to the lacrimal gland and conveys taste from the soft palate and deep proprioceptive fibers. The rate of secretion of the lacrimal gland is studied by Cawthorne's (1956) modification of Schirmer's test: a strip of filter paper hooked over the lower lid acts as a wick; the patient is given a whiff of ammonia, and the rate of flow along it is compared with that of a similar strip applied to the opposite eye. Taste sensitivity of the soft palate may be investigated as described for the tongue.

Diagnosis in Acute Trauma.   Facial lacerations producing injury to the facial nerve are more frequent than is generally supposed. Segmental divisions of the facial nerve, anastomoses between the branches of the nerve, and the power of regeneration of the facial nerve (with the exception of the frontalis and marginal mandibular branches) have minimized the number of paralyses after severance. The current increase in the number of maxillofacial injuries, particularly in automobile accidents, has led to an increasing incidence of facial nerve severance. Facial paralysis may be easily missed in an unconscious patient or in a patient with a bandaged head; unless the paralysis has been specifically looked for initially and the state of facial movements reported in the notes, a history of onset one or two days later cannot be relied upon. Later swelling of the face may further delay diagnosis.

ELECTRODIAGNOSTIC TESTS

Electrodiagnostic tests are extremely helpful to the clinician. Standardized testing procedures in nerve and muscle diseases assist in making a differential diagnosis but are not always readily available. Electrodiagnostic testing consists of stimulating tests, recording tests, and combined stimulating and recording tests (Rosenthal, 1961).

Stimulating Tests

GALVANIC TONGUE STIMULATION. Anodal galvanic stimulation of the tongue (electrogustometry) has been developed and consists of measuring the threshold of the anterolateral tongue region to acid taste with the application of a low galvanic current up to 100 microamps from a battery generator (Krarup, 1958). The test is considered normal if the unilateral threshold is less than 10 microamps or there is a difference of 5 microamps between the two sides (Taverner and coworkers, 1967). The patients with abnormal galvanic thresholds do not always develop denervation. In addition, some patients with normal results have shown later denervation, but if there is a difference of approximately 100 microamps after five days of paralysis, denervation can be expected. This technique, however, has limitations, depending upon patient cooperation, and can be abnormal in heavy smokers. Consequently, it is not a definitive answer but may be of value earlier than nerve conduction tests.

CHRONAXIE. Measuring *chronaxie* is the easiest of the stimulating tests. A chronaximeter is a muscle stimulator so constructed that the strength of the electrical stimulus and its duration may be varied through wide limits, and these parameters are read directly from the recording dials on the machine. There are two major types of chronaximeters: the *con-stant current* type in which the voltage is the variable, and the *constant voltage* type in which the current flow is the variable.

In order to determine the chronaxie of a given muscle, one must first obtain the *rheobase*. The rheobase is defined as that strength of electrical stimulus acting over an infinite period of time which results in a mechanical muscle twitch. Bipolar electrodes are placed over the motor point of a given muscle. The chronaximeter is set at a given strength of stimulus, long enough to be considered infinite in time. If the strength is sufficient to be threshold for that particular muscle, a resulting muscle twitch is seen. If the strength is not of sufficient intensity, no response occurs and the intensity must be increased until threshold is reached.

The next step is to determine the *chronaxie,* the duration of stimulus twice the rheobase in strength which is necessary to produce a muscle twitch similar to that obtained in determining the rheobase. Having determined the rheobase, one keeps the stimulating electrode in situ and doubles the strength of the stimulus. Its duration, however, is calibrated in tenths of a millisecond; and in order to determine the chronaxie, which is a measure of the stimulus duration, one needs to move to longer duration positions until one observes the same muscle twitch as that determined for the rheobase. This is repeated for every muscle which is to be tested.

Essentially, the test is performed to determine whether the nerve pathway to the muscle is intact. If the nerve-muscle pathway is intact, the chronaxie is one millisecond or less. If, however, the nerve is injured, it will be necessary to *increase* the duration of stimulus at the motor point to a much longer period, so that the muscle fiber is stimulated. Since muscle is not nearly as sensitive to electrical stimuli as intact nerve tissue, it will take a much longer duration of stimulus to fire the muscle and produce a muscle twitch. In other words, the chronaxie in denervation will be prolonged above one millisecond, and one probably can then make a diagnosis of lower motor neuron disease and suggest other tests. Any pathologic process which impairs the ability of the lower motor neuron to conduct an impulse will produce an abnormal chronaxie.

It should be emphasized that this is a gross test and that there has to be a substantial amount of nerve damage before the test shows any abnormality. If only a few axons in a nerve are diseased, there may be a sufficient number of normal axons present to mask the effects of the diseased units. Therefore a normal chronaxie, in itself, is insufficient evidence that no abnormality exists. Consideration of the more sensitive recording tests may help to clear up any doubts when the chronaxie does not offer the information anticipated from the clinical picture. On the other hand, chronaxie significantly elevated above one millisecond is unequivocal evidence of denervation. Prognostically, the chronaxie can be useful in determining whether reinnervation will occur. If, for example, in a facial (Bell's) palsy, the first chronaxie determination is elevated and a subsequent test shows that it is returning to normal, this may indicate a favorable prognosis for recovery. On the other hand, if the chronaxie remains elevated after a significant period of time, the prognosis for reinnervation may be poor.

After injury, approximately two weeks elapse before nerve deterioration develops to the point where the chronaxie is elevated. This means that for about two weeks after injury or disease the chronaxie will be normal and, therefore, a normal finding during this period has little significance.

STRENGTH-DURATION CURVES. These are graphic measurements of excitability of nerve and muscle. An electrical impulse of long duration (100 milliseconds or more) is passed through the tested muscle, and the amount of current (in milliamperes or volts) required to cause a minimal perceptible contraction is measured. Similarly, the threshold of the contraction at progressively shorter durations, up to 0.01 millisecond, is measured, and a *curve* relating the *strength* of current to the *duration* of impulse is drawn. When the muscle is normally innervated, the current stimulates the fine intramuscular nerve fibers. In a totally denervated muscle the current stimulates the muscle fibers directly and the *response of the muscle* is obtained, as compared with the typical excitability response of nerve. During reinnervation a kinked or broken curve is obtained, which shows elements of both curves, the upper lefthand portion representing a decrease of innervated muscle fibers, similar to the normal nerve response, and the lower righthand portion being that of muscle and similar to the muscle response. This curve shows the ratio of reinnervated to denervated fibers and allows a roughly quantitative determination of the degree of reinnervation.

The earliest sign of reinnervation on the strength-duration curve precedes a clinical contraction by about six to eight weeks. As reinnervation proceeds, changes in the curve are noted. The strength-duration curve shows whether there is any sign of innervation and, if so, roughly how much. The changes in the curve associated with the progress of reinnervation are so reliable that failure to find them indicates a failure of regeneration (Collier, 1953).

It is important to know whether the lesion is in the process of degeneration or is a partial lesion which has ceased to degenerate, hence the value of checking by a strength-duration curve. Absolute evidence of complete denervation cannot be expected for fourteen days after a lesion. However, if there is nerve conduction present and the muscles react strongly seven days after the lesion, it is not likely that the lesion is a severe one. It is wiser to postpone electrical testing of peripheral nerve lesions for 14 days after the injury. Nerve conduction may also be absent when there is gross edema or ischemia.

NERVE CONDUCTION TEST. An indifferent electrode plus an active electrode, which is moved about, stimulates the nerve trunks. After the facial nerve is tested on the normal side and the threshold for conduction measured, the injured nerve is tested. If normal response is obtained only with a current of at least double the normal threshold, nerve conduction is said to be absent. This test can be used to study or detect abnormalities of innervation. In distinguishing partial from complete losses of nerve conduction with clinical paralysis present, the test may indicate that the lesion is complete or there may be a partial lesion and no nerve conduction obtainable.

The facial nerve is maximally stimulated at the angle of the jaw with surface or concentric needle electrodes in the frontalis or orbicularis oris muscles. The evoked muscle potential is displayed on an oscilloscope, and the distal latency is measured from the onset of stimulus. A latency of less than 3.8 msec is considered normal. Studies of normal and abnormal latencies have been done in Bell's palsy (Langworth and Taverner, 1963). After seven days, lack of conductibility is indicative of complete denervation and delay of latency compatible with partial denervation. It has been demonstrated that conductibility may continue up to five to seven days after a complete nerve section before the nerve becomes unexcitable (Gilliatt and Taylor, 1959). Therefore, conduction latencies at this point in time can provide valuable information in terms of prognosis and treatment. The value of nerve conduction latencies in traumatic facial nerve lesions has not been well established. The same general principles would apply during the early stages following injury, but serial studies may be of more value than a single determination.

When conduction of the nerve is blocked there will be clinical paralysis, but in early stages there may be no signs, such as wasting or circulatory disturbance, to distinguish a neurapraxia from an axonotmesis.

EVOKED NERVE ACTION POTENTIALS (NAP). Kline and DeJonge (1968) have stimulated the nerve proximal to the lesion and recorded *evoked nerve action potentials* (NAP) directly from the nerve distal to the level of the lesion. Bipolar stimulating and recording electrodes are used, and a ground electrode may be placed on the neuroma or in adjacent soft tissue to reduce artifact from the muscle contraction. A Grass S-44 stimulator provides a stimulus of variable voltage, duration, and frequency. Stimulus is increased until an evoked potential or muscle contraction or both are obtained. The evoked nerve action potential (NAP) is recorded by an oscilloscope with amplifier and permanently recorded by a Polaroid camera.

Experimental studies with crushed nerves and severed and sutured nerves in primates have shown that one can relate the presence and, in general, the form of such in vivo evoked potentials to the degree of axon population and maturity in regenerating nerves (Kline and DeJonge, 1968). With regenerating primate nerves, evoked potentials could be recorded four to six weeks earlier in severely crushed nerves than in severed and sutured nerves. In vivo evoked potentials can also be recorded weeks to months before electromyographic evidence of reinnervation is present.

NAP recordings have been made on patients with neuromas in continuity. On the basis of the evoked NAP correlated with clinical data, decisions can be made either to resect the neuroma or to leave it intact. If a good potential was obtained, the lesion was left alone, and if one was not, the lesion was resected. To date, there have been no facial nerves with neuromas, but this promises to be a technique of great value, as late lesions in continuity represent a number of puzzling nerve injuries.

Recording Tests

ELECTROMYOGRAPHY. Electromyography is a technique of recording electrical muscle potentials without stimulation. The usual method is to insert a needle electrode into the muscle to be tested, amplify the electropotentials generated by the muscle, visualize these by means of a cathode ray oscilloscope, and make them audible through a speaker. The procedure for electromyography is fairly simple. The needle electrode, which can be monopolar, bipolar, or multipolar, is thrust into the muscle. The muscle is tested at rest and on slight voluntary contraction. Amplification of about one million times is achieved as the amplitudes of these small potentials are in the millivolt range.

The cathode ray oscilloscope indicates potentials by means of a beam of electrons, and the horizontal sweep of the electron beam across the oscilloscope is calibrated to give the duration of the potentials generated. The vertical plates after suitable amplification show, by their deflection of the beam, the amplitude and the shape of the potentials generated. The impulses from the cathode ray tube may be photographed with either a still or movie camera (Fig. 36–9 and accompanying data).

What are we looking for in electromyography? We are seeking to determine: (1) Is the muscle denervated? (2) Is intrinsic muscle disease present? With electromyography changes can be detected before there is clinical evidence of denervation. In addition, electromyography can also demonstrate evidence of reinnervation before it is clinically evident.

When normal muscle is tested at rest, there is electrical silence, since a striated muscle does not generate electrical potentials in the resting state. Spontaneous electrical activity present in the muscle at rest is a definite sign of disease. When the patient is asked to contract the muscle *partially,* motor unit potentials of 500 to 1000 microvolts in amplitude and 4 to 8 milliseconds in duration are generated. The patient is then asked to contract the muscle *maximally.* Maximal contraction activates many motor units which fire asynchronously, and the electrical pattern recorded is known as an *interference pattern* because the activity of individual units can no longer be distinguished. The three-step analysis is made of each muscle to be tested, with notation regarding the size, shape, and duration of the potentials generated.

When a nerve has been *transected completely,* fibrillation potentials are found in the muscle while it is at rest, after a two-week period during which the distal segment degenerates completely. When deprived of the nerve supply, the individual muscle fibers become hyperirritable and may fire spontaneously. The

MUSCLES	FIBRILLATION	FASCICULATION	VOLUNTARY MOTOR UNIT POTENTIALS
Rt. frontalis Lateral portion	2 Plus	0	From 25 to 50% of the total normal number are seen during attempted voluntary contraction by the patient; most of these potentials are "nascent" polyphasic potentials of the type seen during earliest reinnervation (see graph).
Medial portion	Trace to 1 Plus	0	Only one or two giant, rapid-firing polyphasic potentials present during attempted maximal voluntary contraction.
Rt. orbicularis oculi (Corrugator portion)	0	0	Normal
Lt. frontalis	0	0	Normal

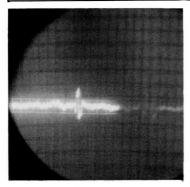

FIGURE 36–9. Electromyographic study of reinnervation of the right frontalis muscle. The inset shows polyphasic voluntary motor unit potentials.

potential thus generated has a very brief duration, is of low voltage, and will be recorded as a *fibrillation potential.* With complete denervation, attempts at voluntary contraction do not result in the appearance of motor unit discharge; the fibrillation potentials continue unchanged.

Partial denervation. The characteristic electromyographic picture of partial denervation is that of fibrillation or fasciculation potentials at rest, normal motor unit potentials on slight voluntary contraction, and an inability to recruit additional motor units on maximal contraction, with poor interference pattern development. In addition, on slight voluntary contraction, one may see an increase in polyphasic potentials or observe the presence of giant potentials (increased amplitude). These usually mean that reinnervation has occurred. Since the nerve fibers may grow sporadically and may innervate fibers which they did not originally innervate, *asynchrony* may develop, producing polyphasic potentials. If more muscle fibers are now innervated by growth of the nerve fiber, the innervation ratio will be increased, producing giant potentials. *No matter what the cause of the damage, electromyographic findings reflect only the damage and not the cause.*

Myopathic pattern. The findings in intrinsic muscle disease, such as muscular dystrophy, are fairly characteristic and may be differentiated from those of lower motor neuron disease. The classic electromyographic findings in myopathic disease are silence at rest; low voltage motor unit potentials on slight voluntary contraction; and a low voltage, short duration interference pattern on maximal voluntary contraction. In myasthenia gravis, with the patient contracting maximally, there is a progressive decrease in amplitude of the potentials as fatigue increases (Rosenthal, 1961).

Electromyographic values are important not only to note the progression of nerve changes in traumatic paralysis but also to note the comparative percentile weaknesses of various groups of muscles in well-established partial central paralysis. Two typical examples follow:

1. Two weeks after a temporomandibular arthroplasty, the immediately paralyzed fron-

ELECTROMYOGRAPHY			
MUSCLES	FIBRILLATION	FASCICULATION	VOLUNTARY MOTOR UNIT POTENTIALS
Rt. Frontalis	0 (gritty sensation on needle electrode insertion)	0	None seen
Lt. Frontalis	"	0	None seen
Rt. Zygomaticus	0	0	Essentially normal in form and in total numbers.
Lt. Zygomaticus	0	0	About 25% of the expected normal number were seen during what appeared to be maximal voluntary contractions; these potentials were relatively normal in form.
Rt. Orbicularis Oris	0	0	Essentially normal in form and in total numbers.
Lt. Orbicularis Oris	0	0	Same as left zygomaticus (above).
Rt. Depressor Anguli Oris	0	0	Essentially normal in form and in total numbers.
Lt. Depressor Anguli Oris	0	0	Same as left zygomaticus (above), except about 50% of the expected normal number were present.

COMMENT: This examination confirms the clinical impression of total paresis of the frontalis muscles bilaterally. Further, the gritty sensation on electrode insertion suggests fibrous replacement of muscle has occurred.

FIGURE 36–10. Electromyographic report on a child with facial paralysis prior to masseter muscle transposition.

talis showed changes indicative of a regenerating nerve; hence, there was no need for surgical exploration for possible anastomosis of the temporal branch (see Fig. 36–9).

2. A study of the muscles of a child of 6 with bilateral facial paralysis, having more marked weakness of one-half of the lower face than of the other, showed that during voluntary maximal contraction the muscles of the lower face had less than 25 per cent of the average number of motor unit potentials. It was felt that the difference was sufficient to warrant a muscle transposition. The charts in Figures 36–10 and 36–11 show the typical report.

There are two critical periods in the course of facial paralysis when exact information on the pathologic state of the nerve is especially necessary to serve as a control: the first seven days after onset, and the period between two and three months later, when reinnervation may be progressing, even though there is no clinical sign of returning movement. During the first two or three days, the problem is to determine whether there is severance of the nerve or an interference with conduction. At this time *quantitative conduction tests are made*. To avoid the possibility of impeding reinnervation by surgical intervention, the presence of polyphasic multiunit action potentials and the progressive diminution of fibrillation action potentials can be searched for and detected with electromyography, many weeks before facial movements can be seen.

Only by testing for nerve conduction by quantitative stimuli, in the first few days after onset, can the surgeon learn whether a nerve is degenerating. After the fifteenth day, *intensity duration curves* give more exact information as to the degree of denervation. The only available method for detecting reinnervation before clinical recovery has taken place is by electromyography. Precise methods of electrodiagnosis are as necessary in the management of facial paralysis as any accurate laboratory examination.

Mention should be made of the Nessel succinyl test (Miehlke, 1973), which involves administration of one tenth the normal dose of succinylcholine intravenously and causes a sustained (about 10 second) contraction of the paralyzed side of the face only, due to hypersensitivity of the denervated muscle. This is considered to be the definitive test for judging the possibilities of *muscle* function.

Miehlke stated that degeneration or interruption of more than 80 per cent of the nerve fibers is necessary to cause severe asymmetry of facial expression.

THE METHODIST HOSPITAL
TEXAS MEDICAL CENTER
HOUSTON, TEXAS

FORM PM-10 12/63

DATE *February 6, 1974*

REPORT OF ELECTROMYOGRAPHY/ELECTRODIAGNOSTIC STUDIES:

Batchelor, Gayle   Referred by:
Inpatient 239A Annex   Dr. B. S. Freeman
21-31-49

RIGHT FACIAL NERVE:

Threshold of excitation - 5.0 milliamps
Latency - 3.0 milliseconds
Evoked potential - duration 16 milliseconds
orbicularis oris - amplitude 2.5 millivolts

EMG - interference pattern slightly decreased.

LEFT FACIAL NERVE:

Threshold of excitation - no response
Latency - over frontalis - 10.5 milliseconds
         over orbicularis oculi - 3.3 milliseconds
         over orbicularis oris - 7.5 milliseconds
Evoked potential - frontalis muscle - amplitude 1.5 millivolts
                                      duration 2.5 milliseconds
              orbicularis oculi - amplitude 0.7 millivolts
                                  duration 3.1 milliseconds
              orbicularis oris - amplitude 1.5 millivolts
                                 duration 3.0 milliseconds

EMG - no denervation potentials
      For voluntary contraction - 2 - 3 motor unit potentials were observed
      in all of the muscles tested above.

CONCLUSION: Left facial nerve lesion. It seems that the number of motor
neurons available to supply the left facial muscles is markedly decreased
(probably 2 - 3) which is not enough for a useful contraction. It is
interesting to note that the interference pattern observed in the right
orbicularis oris is slightly decreased, suggesting a decreased number of
motor units.

Left extensor digitorum brevis was also tested. Denervation potentials with
no voluntary motor unit potentials were observed. Left temporalis was
normal at rest and during maximal contraction.

_____ M.D.
Jairo A. Puentes, M. D.
DEPARTMENT OF PHYSICAL MEDICINE
EMG REPORT

Batchelor, Gayle
Inpatient 239A Annex
21-31-49

FIGURE 36–11. Electromyographic report ten years after multiple surgical procedures and prior to a muscle transposition.

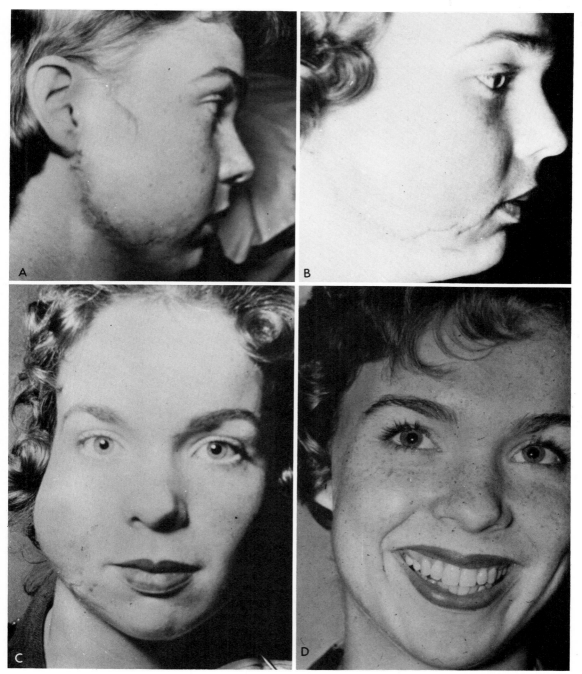

FIGURE 36–12. Immediate repair of the facial nerve and parotid duct transected at its origin by a shelving windshield laceration which avulsed almost half of the face. The main buccal and marginal mandibular branches were transected. Note the presence of the classic pseudocyst of the parotid despite a catheter in the gland and duct. *D* shows the final result.

Illustration continued on the following page.

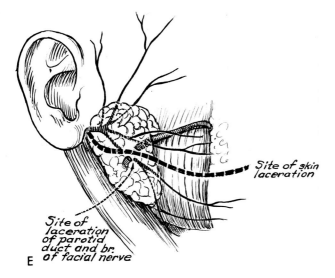

Site of skin
laceration

Site of
laceration
of parotid
duct and br.
of facial nerve

E

FIGURE 36–12 *Continued. E,* Sketch of the operative exposure of a transected facial nerve branch and Stensen's duct.

Surgery of the Facial Nerve

For the past half century the restoration of facial expression and emotional movements has been possible in a high proportion of cases by direct nerve suture. However, after 80-odd years of research, the experimental use of blood vessel segments to bridge a nerve gap is the only reported successful bridging of a nerve gap by non-nerve tissue (Woodruff, 1960). The astounding reports of Belyakova (1968), who used tantalum wire to replace nerves for the conduction of impulses, have not been corroborated by other investigators as yet.

INTRATEMPORAL SURGERY

The difficulty in reaching the facial nerve within the temporal bone was overcome with the development of mastoid surgery in the last decade of the nineteenth century. In 1894, after lifting the nerve out of the facial canal, because of destruction of bone, Alt suggested decompression. Sydenham (1909) laid a piece of silkworm gut into a defect between the nerve ends, with an alleged satisfactory result. Ney (1922) reported a safe surgical approach to the facial canal, and Bunnell (1927) reported the successful result of an intratemporal suture of the facial nerve. The right-angled course of the nerve was altered by removal of the vaginal process of the temporal bone, giving approximately 8 mm ad-

ditional nerve length, sufficient to permit a direct end-to-end suture, with an excellent recovery 17 months later.

Excision of the parotid gland relaxes the length of the facial nerve distal to the stylomastoid foramen by 1.5 cm, but nerve grafts are preferable to rerouting of the facial nerve for end-to-end suture, because of the interference of the blood supply to the nerve which such a procedure entails. Bridging a defect in a nerve by a nerve graft was first attempted by Philipeaux and Vulpian (1870); Letievant (1873), Albert (1885), and Mayo Robson (1889) followed suit. Ballance and Duel described nerve grafting in the fallopian canal in 1932, but the first reported graft had been done by Bunnell in 1930 using a 6-cm tribranched autogenous graft from the sural nerve. Ballance and Duel did not use sutures but relied on coagulation of plasma at the nerve ends to hold them in position. Although an autogenous sensory nerve was found to be as satisfactory as a predominantly motor nerve, subsequently Duel found it advantageous to utilize predegenerated nerve grafts from patients with the same blood group and believed that the results with such allografts were as satisfactory as with autografts and that the operation could be performed despite presence of gross infection. Many reports followed the original papers of Duel and Ballance, including those of Tickle (1945), Collier (1949), and Sullivan (1952). The practice of using degenerated grafts or allografts was discarded in favor of fresh autografts. Extensive experimental and clinical experience in the treatment of facial paralysis caused Ballance to regard the nerve graft procedure as the treatment of choice for intratemporal facial nerve injuries, which it remains to the present.

Technical developments in sutures and instruments, as well as the operating microscope, have contributed to the superb results of present-day intratemporal facial nerve surgery, as exemplified by the work of Kettel (1953) and Cawthorne (1956), the result of fruitful collaboration betweeen neurologist and otologist.

Technical details of nerve junctures and grafts are further discussed in Chapter 76.

EXTRATEMPORAL NERVE REPAIR

A system of routine examination in all cases of facial trauma will permit more frequent primary repair of facial nerve lacerations with minimal permanent deformities and will necessitate fewer delayed repairs with the attendant tedious dissection. That diffuse fibrosis of the paralyzed facial muscles can occur through delay is usually recognized. Less readily appreciated by those surgeons counseling delay is that fibrosis of the distal end of the nerve can obliterate the pathways for the growing neurofibrils. Recent experimental evidence has been provided by Hastings and Peacock (1973).

Despite statements to the contrary, nerve repair is best done at the time of primary repair of the facial laceration if the patient's general condition permits (Fig. 36–12). At the time of primary repair, the elasticity of the nerve permits closure of minor gaps without nerve grafts; in late repair, dissection of the scar may well cause severance of minor branches and vascular damage. If paralysis is not noticed until after the laceration has been closed, reexploration should be done as soon as the wound is sufficiently soft and the patient's general condition is adequate. However, because of the posterior innervation of the facial muscles and the ready spontaneous regeneration in terminal nerve branch sections, there is a certain percentage of satisfactory recovery of facial muscle function despite the frequent repair of lacerations of the face associated with seventh nerve section by simple reapproximation of the wound edges without regard to the nerve damage. Although often evident in clean windshield and razor injuries (Converse and Goodgold, 1959), in regard to the buccal branches, spontaneous regeneration is not to be counted upon.

Immediate Repair. There is a rapid diminution of response to faradic stimulation of the peripheral end of the cut nerve. This response becomes nil after 48 hours (Tickle, 1936); hence, after the third day only careful and outlined dissection will permit identification of small branches—a fact which emphasizes the urgency of early exploration, immediate identification of the nerve ends, and direct suture or grafting.

However, the long-held belief that repair of a seventh nerve injury must be accomplished within one year, after which atrophy of muscles and degeneration of nerve would make it impossible, has been contradicted by Conley (1973). He has demonstrated that long after one year the distal trunk of the nerve is readily identifiable and the muscles supplied by the facial nerve are not totally atrophic.

With adequate light, hemostasis, and fine, flexible instruments, the nerves can be delicately handled and the sheaths not stripped. The field is kept moist; Teflon- or plastic-coated retractors, forceps, and needle holders are used for microsurgery; and Teflon tapes are used to avoid bruising or stripping the blood supply. Braided silk sutures, commonly used to retract nerves, will tear the delicate peripheral vascular trunk.

NONSUTURE TECHNIQUE IN FACIAL NERVE ANASTOMOSIS

Rapid suture of fine, hairlike, peripheral branches of the facial nerve is limited by the tedious microsurgical techniques. The ideal approximation of the moist, viable sheaths of fine nerves would be best accomplished by a nonreactive, adaptable, flexible, and permeable cement. A combination of nonreactive materials to coapt the ends and form an adhesive, nonconstrictive, yet close-fitting tube to channel subsequent neurofibrillar growth and to provide stability during the regenerative process was tested experimentally and clinically (Freeman, 1969). Micropore adhesive tape (a nonwoven fabric of viscous rayon coated on one side with an adhesive copolymer of iso-octylacrylate and acrylic acid) can be adapted for neural coaptation, will not significantly impair the flexibility of the neural structures, and does not kink or compress. The fabric is porous and permeable to tissue or fluids. The simplest procedure and one of the least reactive—the Micropore tape tube—has been clinically used for nerve end approximation, for nerve crossing, and for nerve grafting. However, the adhesive nonsuture technique has been discontinued by most surgeons at the present time because of foreign body reaction and increased fibrosis (Anderl, 1976).*

Clinical Application. A 1.0- by 0.5-cm strip of Micropore tape, or "Steri-strip," is placed with the adhesive side up in a completely dry bed in the position selected for the reunion of the nerve ends. The carefully dried proximal nerve end is set in the center of the tape; the distal end is placed on the tape so as to abut exactly the proximal end as viewed through a magnifying (5 ×) operating microscope or binocular lens. A second strip of tape, the adhesive side down, is placed over the first and compressed. This forms a tube around the tiny nerve branches which extends 0.25 cm on each side of the nerve junction. In several nerves, the slightly longer strip is placed under the juncture, rolled over the aligned nerve ends, and compressed to adhere to itself and thus form a tube. The edges of the tape are clamped not closer than 2 mm on each side of the severed nerve end, and the excess is resected (Fig. 36–13). If there is little tension and the closing wound movements are minimal, the bond will prove to be sufficiently adhesive to maintain the position of the nerve ends for adequate cellular structural continuity and to allow regrowth of the neurofibrils. It will also prevent the ingrowth of connective tissue into the suture site, an event which might lead to a neuromatous tangle.

Technique of Nerve Grafting by the Adhesive Tube Technique.   Single and cable nerve grafts

---

*The technique has been generally given up in favor of suture using the operating microscope (see Chapter 76) (J.M.C.).

are similarly coapted by the adhesive tube method. The dried distal and proximal ends of the interrupted nerve are placed in the center of the individual strips of tape, the gap between the nerve ends is measured, and the graft is selected. The ends are dried, the proximal end of the graft is coapted to that of the nerve by the first adhesive tape strip, and the distal end of the graft is aligned with the distal end of the nerve by the second strip. The covering strips are applied and the excess tape trimmed. If the circulation of the graft bed and its cover are adequate, there should be no concern for the revascularization of the short end of the graft covered by the tape, which is porous and permeable to fluid penetration.

SUTURE TECHNIQUE IN FACIAL NERVE REPAIR

The use of 8–0 or 10–0 monofilament nylon microsurgical suture with a delicate needle (as previously mentioned) adds little trauma, provided the nerve or nerve graft is thicker than the needle. The technique facilitates the position and alignment of the multiple segments of a graft, permits stabilization for accurate tailoring, and aids in orientation of the nerve stumps. This is helpful in a moist, irregular field frequently filled with multiple moving hands. The alignment sutures offer a feeling of security when larger nerves or cable grafts are coapted and the author prefers to use tape alone for the finer filaments. The tape tube prevents the interposition of scar tissue and helps channel the regenerating fibrils into the distal Schwann tubes, especially when knuckling of the divided

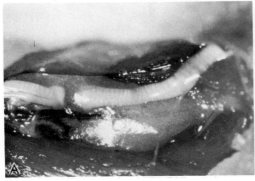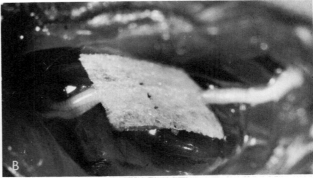

FIGURE 36–13.   Technique of micropore adhesive tube. *A,* Section of nerve. *B,* The proximal and distal stumps are applied to the adhesive surface of the tapes with the two nerve ends in perfect apposition. Another layer of tape is applied so that the nerve stumps are enclosed between the two leaves, which are then molded about the nerve and are encased in a tube. The excess tape is trimmed to within 3 mm of the nerve. (From Freeman, B. S.: Non-suture techniques in facial nerve anastomosis. *In* Conley, J. (Ed.): Plastic and Reconstructive Surgery of the Face and Neck. Vol. 2. Stuttgart, George Thieme Verlag, 1972.)

fibers occurs after the not infrequent retraction of the nerve sheath. During the past three years, the author has been utilizing a modification of the intraneural neurorrhaphy of Snyder and associates (1968) in larger nerves to stabilize the graft and the nerve ends.

A specially prepared (Ethicon) 6–0 polypropylene suture on a fine caliber needle inserted 5 mm proximal to the transection is directed centrally down the nerve to the cut end. The needle is reinserted and guided through the central fibers of the distal stump or nerve graft and either is directed through the graft to the distal stump, where it exits about 5 mm distally, or exits directly through the distal stump. Small microvascular clamps (nicknamed "bulldogs") stabilize the ends of the suture along the nerve while the tape is being applied. The ends of the suture are secured to the ends of the tape cylinder by a stitch and a half hitch or are tied together over the tube of tape. There is little additional reaction following this type of suture (Fig. 36–14).

Microsurgical Fascicular Nerve Grafting. Millesi (1967) has advocated a technique of microsurgical fascicular nerve grafting (see also Chapter 76) to avoid connective tissue proliferation at the juncture site as occurs when the

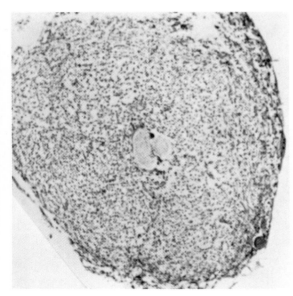

FIGURE 36–14. The minimal microscopic reaction in a nerve junction three weeks after a fine monofilament suture has been placed through the center for purposes of positioning. (From Freeman, B. S.: Non-suture techniques in facial nerve anastomosis. *In* Conley, J. (Ed.): Plastic and Reconstructive Surgery of the Face and Neck. Vol. 2. Stuttgart, George Thieme Verlag, 1972.)

nerve is repaired under tension. The sural nerve serves as a source of autogenous nerve grafts. The sural nerve is cut into pieces slightly longer than the length of the defect and placed individually between corresponding facial nerve fasciculi or groups of fasciculi. Under microscopic vision, a single 10–0 nylon suture is usually sufficient to maintain approximation between the transected ends of the nerve and the sural nerve graft. The technique is discussed further in the section on Cross-Face Nerve Transplantation in Facial Paralysis (p. 1860).

Fascicular Nerve Grafting. Fascicular nerve grafting of the facial nerve has been practiced and is suggested as a procedure to be utilized prior to resecting the main facial nerve trunk at the time of removal of a malignant parotid tumor (Apfelberg and Gingrass, 1973). The procedure is commenced by exposing the main trunk, separating the nerve into fasciculi, and stimulating the fasciculi to identify the distal branches. After completion of the resection, individual nerve grafts are placed between the fasciculi and the appropriate peripheral branches.

The operating microscope may offer an advantage over the simple technique used in Figure 36–13, in which after isolation by electric stimulation, the slender peripheral or distal branches were tagged for later juncture with a branched greater auricular nerve graft without contamination of the cancer field (Fig. 36–15).

Apfelberg and Gingrass (1973) performed fascicular dissections of the facial nerve in cadavers and animals. They were able to trace the major fasciculi proximally, and obtained mimetic function when fascicular grafting was done in animals. They suggested that if the facial nerve is to be sacrificed (as for malignant parotid tumors), a preliminary fascicular dissection should be done and followed by a fascicular graft. Conley (1975) reviewed the fascicular anatomy of the facial nerve trunk (extratemporal) and suggested that the anterior fasciculi be oriented in nerve grafting so as to serve the lower face, and the posterior fasciculi to serve the upper face.

Since World War II, neurosurgeons, in particular, have maintained that secondary or delayed repair of nerve disruption would be physiologically preferable to immediate repair, even in the best circumstances. This has been disproved by a study of the collagen accumulation on peripheral nerve sections by Hastings and Peacock (1973), who showed that the same amount of collagen accumulated at the nerve end whether the nerve was repaired or

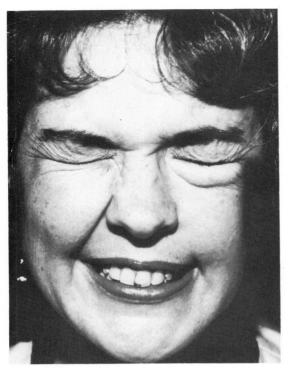

FIGURE 36–15. Result six months after resection and nerve grafting secondary to the primary closure of the wounds. The patient is showing voluntary motion. The left nasolabial fold is less well defined. There has been no recurrence twelve years after resection of the tumor.

not. The same study showed that ascorbic acid reduced the accumulation of collagen in sectioned nerves—hence, the reduced amount of scarring and obstruction of neurofibrillar regrowth.

Armamentarium for nerve anastomosis. In nerve suture or grafting, the operating microscope is of great value; however, the 5.25 binocular loupes seem adequate when dealing with the larger trunks. Nylon 8–0 or 10–0 sutures, suitably lubricated by drawing them through

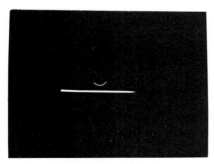

FIGURE 36–16. Ethicon atraumatic nerve sutures: BV-5 microsurgical needle (upper) and S.T. 4 taper straight "skewer" needle. Radiograph of exact size.

subcutaneous fat, are swaged to a fine caliber needle of like dimension and length (Fig. 36–16); a Castroviejo needle holder, razor knife, fine scissors, and jeweler's forceps, both straight and angled, as well as extremely delicate hooks, have aided the somewhat tedious technique.

The results of anastomosis, by suture or graft, may provide only for mass muscular motions and may not offer the fine emotional delicacy of individual muscle motions. However, the results are infinitely preferable to those obtained by the reconstructive procedures described later in the text.

FACIAL NERVE GRAFTS

Preoperative Considerations. When resection of the facial nerve may be necessary in the course of surgery, whether intracranial, intratemporal, or extratemporal, a careful evaluation of the probability of nerve resection should be made, and a detailed plan for either immediate or staged replacement of the nerve should be outlined. Repair of the facial nerve can be accomplished by short-circuiting grafts (Fig. 36–17). Restitution of the continuity of the facial nerve between its origin from the pons to the facial musculature is feasible (Dott, 1958).

Approach. The surgical approaches to the trunk of the facial nerve are many and varied. Elective exposure is by a preauricular incision around the ear lobe and across the mastoid, curving downward across the sternocleidomastoid muscle in a transverse crease. After the flaps are raised, a cleavage plane is found between the cartilage of the auditory canal and the mastoid posteriorly, and the parotid capsule, which will allow the posterior parotid margin to be elevated anteriorly. The facial trunk and its enveloping fascia are found under the sternocleidomastoid muscle. The stylomastoid foramen is located above the origin of the posterior belly of the diagastric muscle on the mastoid. The removal of a segment of a long overhanging mastoid process is not difficult and can simplify the exposure. The exposed tympanomastoid fissure can also point to the stylomastoid foramen, which is 6 to 8 mm beneath its "drop-off" point. Another method is the exposure of a peripheral branch by a routine preauricular parotidectomy incision, elevating the flaps and identifying any of the branches, which can be followed proximally to the trunk.

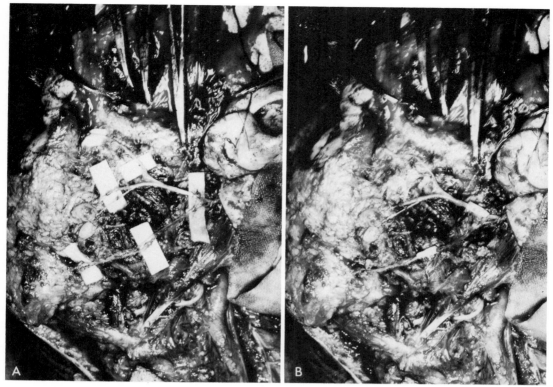

FIGURE 36–17. Autogenous nerve graft following radical resection of the parotid gland and facial nerve. Note the tape and suture anastomosis. *B,* The tape has been tubed. (From Freeman, B. S.: Adhesive anastomosis technics for fine nerves. Am. J. Surg., *108*:529, 1964.)

Choice of Grafting Procedure. Obviously the result of each attempt at grafting depends upon the particular problem, the individual surgical technique, the postoperative care, the age of the patient, and the length of the follow-up. Facial nerve repair by using a segment of the sensory cervical plexus, incorporating the greater auricular nerve with the main trunk or branches of the segments of C3 or C4, is generally used, although the sural nerve has also served as a donor site. Filaments of the nerve graft have been placed directly into muscle, without direct nerve approximation, with return of muscle function as a result of this procedure (Cardwell, 1938).

In the selection of the donor nerve and type of graft, the cross section of the graft, or grafts, should be at least equal to that of the nerve to be replaced. The donor nerve should be constant in position and readily accessible, either through the same incision or through one that does not involve a pressure area; the resultant sensory defect should be minimal in quantity and extent. The sural nerve and the external saphenous nerve are advocated by many; the greater auricular or one of the cutaneous branches of the cervical plexus, which are available without requiring an additional operative site, is preferred by the author.

The grafts should lie in a healthy, well-vascularized bed from which all scar tissue should be excised. The alternative of bypassing a scar by using a longer graft rather than passing the nerve through relatively avascular tissue should be considered.

There is some shrinkage in a long graft, and a graft at least 15 per cent longer than the defect would ordinarily require should be used. When the nerve stumps are resected, as for end-to-end anastomosis, it is advisable to avoid mobilizing the proximal segment extensively, to prevent disturbing the longitudinal branches of the vasculature. It is important to resect the distal neuroma; fibrosis in the distal stump can be responsible for failure of the procedure. Moreover, resecting the distal stump does not strip the vasculature and merely entails the use of a longer graft. The avoidance of forcible retraction and suture tension as a stimulus to fibrosis is quite important (see Chapter 76).

Ballance and Duel (1932) have shown that sensory and motor nerves function equally well for the purpose of transporting the axons as long as they are of a suitable size.

Even in the presence of infection, nerve grafts have healed well with good functional results. Inadequate resection of scar tissue in the proximal and distal ends of the nerve, post-operative hemorrhage, poor vascularization, lack of stabilization of the graft, and crude technique are the factors responsible for the largest number of poor results. It has been suggested that pre-degenerated grafts are firmer, easier to suture, and heal more rapidly. This question has been discussed by Dott (1958) and by Bentley and Hill (1936); most authors favor fresh autografts.

Nerve Rerouting. Restitution of the continuity of the facial nerve between its origin from the brain stem and the facial musculature by means of a graft was first attempted by Dott (1958) (see also Drake, 1960). Its applicability is in the surgery of acoustic neuromas; in cases of intrapetrous damage of the facial nerve in which the lesion extends proximally to the geniculate ganglion; when the petrous bone is disorganized by disease or injury so that the facial canal and nerve cannot be clearly identified, i.e., in comminuted fractures, osteomyelitis, and tuberculous mastoiditis; or if exploration for decompression or grafting has failed.

The facial nerve is exposed by a unilateral cerebellar approach, and a sural cutaneous nerve graft, 15 cm long, is sutured to the severed proximal end, brought out through the craniotomy opening, and tunneled to the posterior surface of the parotid gland, where the excess is curled up.

Ninety days later (allowing time for the nerve fibers to traverse the length of the graft and arrive at its distal end), the distal few centimeters of the graft are unraveled, the facial nerve is exposed at the stylomastoid foramen and a second nerve suture completed between the distal end of the graft and the distal stump of the facial nerve. Recovery of tone has been noted three to six months after the final nerve suture and movement observed two months later.

Preservation of the facial nerve during operations for acoustic neuroma has not been a uniformly successful venture, not only because of the difficulty of preserving the nerve during the tumor resection, but also because of the need for destroying the remaining tumor cells in the internal acoustic meatus. The nerve is commonly preserved carefully and then damaged by resection of the remaining tumor in the internal acoustic meatus. Microscopic control during surgery tends to prevent this in modest sized and smaller tumors.

Nerve Crossing. The description of this technique is largely of historical interest. The inaccessibility of the facial nerve along its intracranial and intratemporal course necessitated detours in the earlier techniques for treatment of facial palsy. Drobnik, in 1879, sutured the peripheral end of the divided facial nerve to the central end of a branch of the spinal accessory nerve and wrapped gold foil around the suture. In 1895, Ballance sutured the trunk of the divided facial nerve to a niche cut from the spinal accessory nerve; after seven years the only movement in the face occurred in association with elevation of the shoulder. Manasse (1900) showed histologic evidence of regeneration after suturing the spinal accessory or hypoglossal to the facial nerve in dogs. Kennedy, in 1901, successfully performed a human spinofacial anastomosis, with coordinated movements of the face two years afterwards. Cushing (1903) used a spinofacial anastomosis and Ballance (1924) performed a glossopharyngeal-facial nerve anastomosis, as well as an anastomosis of the glossopharyngeal and descendens hypoglossi to the facial nerve.

Nerve crossing and anastomosis are applicable in lesions of the facial nerve proximal to the geniculate ganglion, such as those following resection of acoustic neuromas in which the Dott operation had not been carried out. When the proximal end of the nerve is obscured by crushing, scar, infection, or ablation, hypoglossal-facial nerve anatomosis has been of value. This can be attempted only when the distal nerve and the muscles are in good physiologic condition. A review of patients subjected to hypoglossal-facial anastomosis showed good muscle tone, with symmetry at rest or with quiet smiling. Although Greenwood (1958) and others would not perform a nerve crossing later than a year and a half after the onset of paralysis, McKenzie and Alexander (1950) obtained good results in a patient operated upon after a lapse of 2½ years. Similarly, Conley, Hamaker and Donnenfeld (1974) have demonstrated return of facial muscle function following nerve grafts performed many years after the onset of facial paralysis.

In spite of atrophy and paralysis of half the tongue, speech may be relatively normal. However, Evans (1974) reported that 7 of 20 patients (35 per cent) had residual dysarthria. Excessive facial movement while talking and eating has occurred but can be controlled by reeducation; trick movements can overcome some of the mass or associated movements. The deformity is less and the results seem somewhat better when the twelfth nerve has been used than when the accessory or eleventh nerve has been utilized as the motor nerve. The hypoglossal nerve has more resting tone and improves the appearance of the face at rest. Some patients

learn to develop a habit pattern that allows normal smiling and voluntary closing of the eyes.

The practical details are shown in the sketches (Fig. 36–18), and the operative photograph (Fig. 36–19) shows the surgical procedure performed through the vertical incision of Greenwood. It would be well to substitute a gently curving incision starting 2.5 cm above the tip of the mastoid process and extending down along the cervical crease below the angle of the mandible to the level of the upper border of the thyroid cartilage. The facial nerve is exposed at the stylomastoid foramen; two fine sutures are placed on either side of the nerve; the nerve is sectioned and the distal cut end covered with moist cottonoid. The hypoglossal

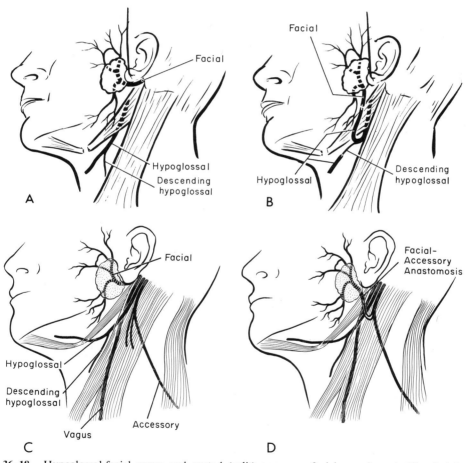

FIGURE 36–18. Hypoglossal-facial nerve and parted (split) accessory-facial crossing. *A,* The facial nerve as it emerges from the stylomastoid foramen, and *B,* its relationship to a hypoglossal-facial nerve anastomosis. Note that the major trunk of the hypoglossal nerve is attached directly to the distal end of the facial, while the considerably smaller decendens hypoglossi is sutured to the distal trunk of the twelfth nerve. *C,* Branches of the accessory nerve to the sternomastoid muscle split from the major trunk to the trapezius, and *D,* anastomosis of the individual sternomastoid smaller branches to the distal trunk of the facial.

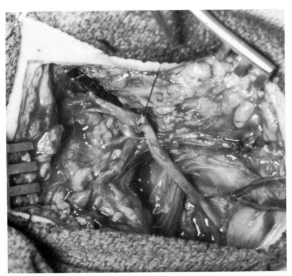

FIGURE 36–19. Hypoglossal-facial nerve anastomosis. With both nerves outlined and with accurate measurements, the nerve juncture can be accomplished without tension, as is seen in the operation by Greenwood (1958).

nerve is exposed on opening the carotid sheath; the sutures are placed as far distally as possible and the nerve sectioned distal to the suture placement. The two sutures are then retracted gently and the proximal end of the hypoglossal nerve and the peripheral end of the facial nerve are coapted and the apposing sutures tied.

After nerve crossing there is a certain amount of "hetero-innervation," when the reinnervated units are connected with different fibers from the ones which originally supplied them. Despite readjustment, movements can be quite uncoordinated. In addition, associated movement and contracture of the muscles newly innervated by fibers from the donor nerve are accompanied by contraction of the synergists of the muscles supplied by these fibers prior to operation. Mass movements, or contractures of several sets of fibers, are caused by axons branching in the reinnervated nerve, with muscle fibers in different muscle bundles innervated by branches of the same axon. However, by developing trick movements some of the disability is overcome, and adjustment of voluntary reactions to compensate for these simple derangements can be accomplished (Fig. 36–20). Only 25 per cent of the patients of Petti and Conley (1972) had return of some mimetic and volitional motion after nerve crossing, and the authors admitted that the result was "basically a mass movement." In Evans' (1974) review of hypoglossal-facial anastomosis, only 4 of 20 patients were pleased

with the results, with no patient being symmetrical during expressive movements.

Partial nerve crossing, as opposed to total nerve crossing, has been used in the hypoglossal-facial juncture, apparently with some good results. This is accomplished by partially dividing the hypoglossal nerve and suturing the neural flap to the distal stump of the facial nerve. Love (1962) suggested anastomosis of a partially divided accessory nerve to the facial nerve and reported an excellent result. Love continued this technique until his retirement, during which time he wrote the author that his results were *all good*. Bragden and Gray (1962) used a similar technique with the spinal accessory nerve.

Junction of the phrenic nerve to the facial nerve had been tried decades ago, resulting in peculiar resting facial twitches. Hardy, Perret, and Myers (1957) have reported a group of phrenicofacial nerve junctures done for facial palsy with apparently minimal physiologic disability in 8 out of 11 patients despite permanent hemidiaphragmatic paralysis in all but two. After a six-month delay, there was return of facial motion with good resting tone and symmetry. The procedure was considered contraindicated in patients with pulmonary disease unless phrenic nerve avulsion was indicated for pulmonary disease. In a review of the patients, Perret (1967) reported recovery of tone in all patients treated by phrenicofacial crossing, but noted that conspicuous asymmetry appeared with deep inspiration or expiration, coughing, whistling, or loud talking. He reported that patients had difficulty in learning to take a deep breath while smiling.

Following resection of a major branch of the facial nerve for tumor involvement, the ramus colli (to the platysma) has been sectioned and the proximal end sutured to the distal end of the divided buccal and marginal mandibular branches. Despite the disparity in size, for the cervical branches are very delicate, the end results, after a delay of six to twelve months in two cases, have been good. This procedure should be considered when a submaxillary tumor or involvement of a prevascular submaxillary lymph node in a radical neck dissection requires sectioning the marginal mandibular branch.

Most authors do not at present favor nerve crossing operations. The presence of intact facial muscles is now regarded as an indication for cross-facial nerve transplantation (see subsequent section). Patients who have undergone a previous nerve crossing procedure which had preserved muscle tone are also candidates for

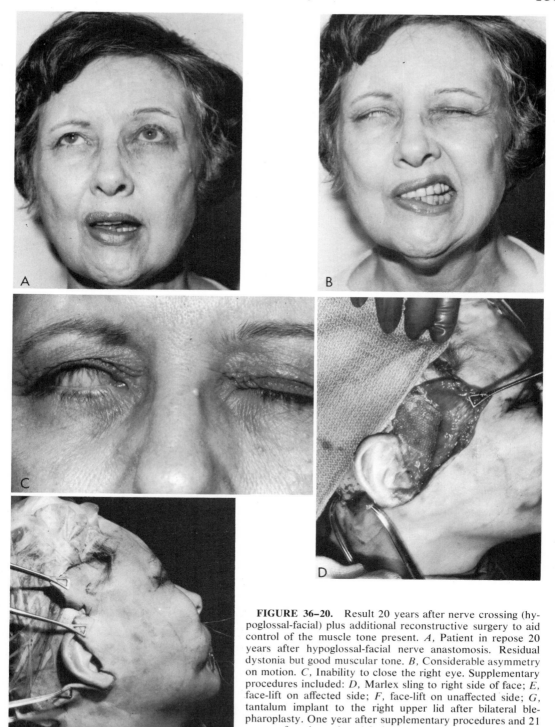

FIGURE 36–20. Result 20 years after nerve crossing (hypoglossal-facial) plus additional reconstructive surgery to aid control of the muscle tone present. *A,* Patient in repose 20 years after hypoglossal-facial nerve anastomosis. Residual dystonia but good muscular tone. *B,* Considerable asymmetry on motion. *C,* Inability to close the right eye. Supplementary procedures included: *D,* Marlex sling to right side of face; *E,* face-lift on affected side; *F,* face-lift on unaffected side; *G,* tantalum implant to the right upper lid after bilateral blepharoplasty. One year after supplementary procedures and 21 years after hypoglossal-facial anastomosis, the patient is shown at rest (*H*), blinking (*I*), and during forced lid closure (*J*) and spontaneous emotion (*K*).

Illustration continued on the following page.

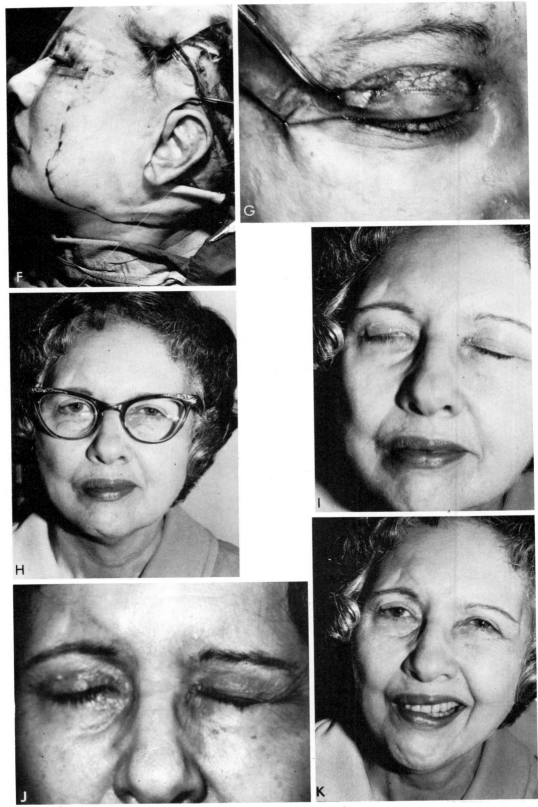

FIGURE 36–20. *Continued.*

cross-facial nerve transplantation for the restoration of some expressive and emotional movements.

Cross-Face Nerve Transplantation. Smith (1971) attempted "micronerve" transfers from the normal to the palsied side to restore facial control and symmetry.

In three patients with unilateral facial paralysis of various lengths of time, a nerve autograft, averaging 9 cm in length, was used to connect the paralyzed muscles to their corresponding "normal" muscles on the opposite side of the face. The buccal and zygomatic nerve branches were rerouted and reconnected by this technique. A bilateral 5-cm incision paralleling but 2 cm lateral to the nasolabial fold allowed the identification of a neural plexus (branches of zygomatic and buccal portions) at a point 1.5 cm below the malar prominence. Stimulation of this plexus on the normal side resulted in contraction of the infraorbital portion of the orbicularis oculi muscle, the small muscles of the nose (procerus and nasalis), and the muscles controlling the corner of the mouth and upper lip (quadratus labii superioris, zygomaticus, and levator anguli oris).

On the normal side, nerve branches going to the orbicularis were divided distal to the plexus. On the paralyzed side of the face, one or two nerve branches were divided proximal to the plexus and connected by the sural nerve graft across the upper lip between the two incisions. Anastomoses between the sural graft and nerve branches on each side were made under microsurgical control of 10 to 16 power, with the use of "skewer" sutures through the nerves, which were removed a week following surgery.

Postoperatively, improvement in facial symmetry became evident at three to six months. In all three cases some controllable muscle contraction was gained in the initially paralyzed orbicularis oculi and the zygomaticus, quadratus, and levator muscles.

Cross-face nerve transplantation has also been used by Anderl (1973). (A section on cross-face nerve transplantation follows later in the chapter.)

RECONSTRUCTION IN FACIAL PALSY

The aim in facial reconstruction is to restore, first, an adequate appearance when the face is at rest, symmetry during voluntary motion, and, if at all possible, retention of a satisfactory appearance during the balanced and controlled expression of emotions. Emotions are expressed by movements and positions of various furrows and facial landmarks—the eyebrows, the mouth, the nose, the lids, and the nasolabial folds.

Patients with facial paralysis, in whom nerve damage is irreparable or in whom the innervation of the paralyzed musculature cannot be restored by nerve suture, grafting, or cross-face nerve transplantation, should be offered some form of reconstructive static and dynamic aid. The reconstructive techniques used are:

Static
Suspension by:	a) Fascia
	b) Dermis
	c) Silastic rubber
Stabilization by:	a) Dermal flaps
	b) Marlex
	c) Bone fixation

Dynamic
Muscle transfer	a) Temporalis
	b) Masseter
	c) Digastric
	d) Sternocleidomastoid
	e) Muscle grafts (free)
Inorganic motors	a) Metal spring (upper lid)
	b) Silastic bands—lip and lid
	c) Lid weights
	d) Lid magnets

Sphincteric Reconstruction
Orbital	a) Canthoplasties
Oral	b) Buccal-oral reconstruction
Nares	c) Septal corrective surgery

Control of Antagonist Muscles
	a) Neurectomy
	1. Temporary, chemical
	2. Permanent, surgical
	b) Myomectomy

Face-lift Operations
	a) Modified cheek plasty
	b) Blepharoplasty
	c) Nasolabial excision
	d) Supraorbital excision and brow lift
	e) Temporal lift
	f) Labial and mucosal excisions

Surgical Formation of Folds and Wrinkles
	a) Construction of nasolabial fold
	b) Forehead furrows

Mechanical Aids
	a) Toothpick in the mouth
	b) Tape
	c) Pipe

The theoretical results of each procedure and what can be accomplished by judiciously combining techniques are as follows:

Suspension   → Static Control (Uplift)

    +   ⎧ Voluntary

Muscle Transfers   → ⎨ Dynamic Action

    +   ⎩ Neurotization

Control of Antagonists → Balance and Symmetry
    +
Skin Excisions   → Symmetry and Balance
    ↓
Partial Emotional Balance

Fascial slings give excellent static support; muscle transfers offer some voluntary motion and a possibility of neural reanimation, as well as static support.

Muscle Transfers

Muscle transfer entails the transposition of the whole, or a portion, of the belly of the muscle with an *adequate blood* and *nerve supply*. The insertion or the origin of the transplant is transferred.

The transposition of muscles innervated by the trigeminal nerve is by far the most popular of the muscle transposition techniques. In transferring muscle, the static deformity must be corrected, the muscle must not be overstretched, and its line of pull must be sufficiently long in a relatively straight direction to function.

Muscle transfer was first used in facial paralysis by Lexer (1908), when the anterior half of the masseter muscle was split and transferred to the muscles of the upper and lower lips. Temporalis strips similarly attached to the upper and lower eyelids were also used.

Numerous variants of muscle transfer have been reported, and even the paralyzed buccinator muscle has been transferred to the normal masseter (Morestin, 1915). The static support of fascia, added to the masticatory muscle transfer, was a later development.

A transferred muscle, after proper reeducation, can provide gross movement and at the same time support the paralyzed structures and thus combine both *static and dynamic* pull. In addition, there is evidence that neurotization of paralyzed, but healthy, superficial muscles of

expression has taken place through the arborization of motor nerves from the fifth cranial nerve to the end plates of these superficial muscles.

The masseter muscle is best used to give motion to the lower half of the face. Transplantation of the temporalis muscle, aided by a tendon or fascial slip, gives a more energetic arc of motion, but the angle of pull is more nearly upward than posteriorly. The temporalis muscle is best suited to lend support and dynamic action to the eyelids, pulling more nearly backward with a slight upward tilt when used to move the lower face, the lips, and the nasal sphincters.

Edgerton (1967) has reported using the anterior belly of the digastric muscle to replace the inferior lip depressors. A few cases have been reported (Horton and associates, 1971) of the use of the transplanted sternocleidomastoid muscle in facial paralysis.

Certain technical points about muscle transfers should be emphasized. The blood and the nerve supply must remain intact. The muscle flaps should be adequately broad, not only for support but also for motion and to pull against thickened, often fibrosed, subcutaneous tissues and musculature. The tension must be carefully adjusted so that the muscle action is mechanically efficient; yet, tautness should not be excessive so as to cause ischemia and death of the muscle fibers. Lastly, angulation of the muscle flap, whether over the zygoma or a fascial hammock, must avoid circulatory embarrassment of the muscle. The wide band of severed muscle contains many nerve fibrils for ingrowth into the exposed denervated facial muscles.

The hypothesis of neurotization, or the physiologic phenomenon of the invasion of nerves from the masseter or temporal muscle transplants into the facial muscles, was first advanced by Lexer and Eden (1911). Reinnervation of muscles by neurotization requires that the muscles have not yet undergone degeneration and atrophy. The phenomenon can occur, therefore, only in patients with facial paralysis of recent origin.

Erlacher (1914), in an experimental study, demonstrated regeneration of a paralyzed muscle by neurotization. He paralyzed the biceps muscle by severing the musculocutaneous nerve, and then implanted flaps from the pectoralis and deltoid muscles into the paralyzed muscle. According to his observation, reactivation of the degenerating muscle occurred as the result of the ingrowth of nerves from the functioning muscles. Other observers have noted movements in adjacent groups of muscles which formerly showed no movement, and movements in muscles located at a distance from the attachment of the transplanted muscle bundles. Owens (1951) revived the hypothesis expressed by Lexer and Eden (1911) and Halle (1933) of the possibility of reinnervating the paralyzed muscles by the transposition of muscular strips containing filaments of the fifth cranial nerve.

Neurotization in Muscle Transplantation. Reinnervation of transplanted muscle has been studied by electromyography and by histochemical techniques, and denervated muscle flaps have been shown to be reinnervated by the ingress of new nerve fibers and to have regained normal function after a period as long as three to eight years after total denervation (Thompson and Pollard, 1961). Thompson (1971a, b) has also demonstrated muscular neurotization of free muscle transplants from normal host muscle (see section on Autogenous Muscle Grafts).

Muscle contraction in previously denervated facial muscles following masseter and temporalis muscle transplantation can be detected by careful postoperative observation. Correlated electromyographic studies of the facial muscles showing an increasing number of motor units discharging with increasing muscular effort have caused many surgeons to agree with Owens (1951) that reinnervation occurs from the nerves in the transplanted muscle. Muscles denervated for several years have been biopsied and the motor end plates have been identified by noting localized areas of cholinesterase activity showing the essential configuration of motor end plates; these areas are probably indicators of the presence of innervated functional skeletal muscle elements. Moreover, the author has found normal striated muscle fibers without gross atrophy (but with some microscopic fibrosis) in denervated facial muscles when they are exposed many years later for the plication of the elongated and stretched muscles, a procedure which has not proved to be of value.

Masseter Muscle Transfer Combined with Fascial Suspension. Transposition of the masseter muscle is performed through either the intraoral or extraoral approach, and under local or general anesthesia. Extraoral incisions heal well and give better access to the musculature, and general anesthesia relaxes the muscle so that the technique can be more accurate. Intraoral incisions give poor exposure and make the dis-

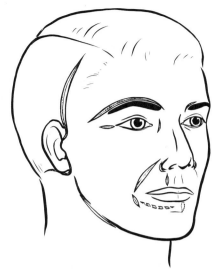

FIGURE 36–21. The usual incisions employed for placement of fascial strips or tendons preliminary to muscle transfer or in lieu of them. The incisions invariably leave little scarring. For masseter transfer the indicated cervical incision under the mandibular margin is used. Intraoral incisions for placement of circumoral fascial strips are made in the labial sulci; the mucosal incision for section of the antagonistic muscles of the lower lip is shown as a dotted line.

section laborious. The potential contamination of fascial grafts, often used in association with muscle transfers, can be another complicating factor.

TECHNIQUE. Exposure of the lower border of the mandible is made through a submandibular incision. The assistant's hand on the cheek retracts the lax submaxillary skin superiorly so that the scar will lie under the mandible. The skin incision (Fig. 36–21) continues directly to the lower border of the mandible to expose the insertion of the masseter muscle. The superficial surface of the masseter is cleared, the fascial covering is elevated from the anterior half, and the branches of the anterior facial vein and external maxillary artery are ligated. The periosteum of the mandible is incised and freed along the inferior border for approximately two-thirds the length of the insertion. Subperiosteal elevation of both the superficial and deep portions of the masseter from the mandibular ramus with an elevator permits elevation and detachment of the anterior two-thirds by splitting the muscle fibers and incising the subjacent periosteum for about two-thirds of its vertical length. A dry surgical field will often permit identification of the motor nerve entering posteriorly and branching in the upper third. A study of the anatomy of the masseter muscle and its clinical use in facial paralysis was reported by de Castro Correia and Zani (1973), who suggested separate levels of muscle dissection for the superficial and deep muscle fibers. However, a careful posterior separation, parallel to the muscle fibers, should be all that is required. The split should be no more than 4 cm from the inferior border. If more length is required, the entire masseter should be freed and advanced forward.

A nasolabial fold incision provides access for careful elevation of the skin over the superficial muscles around the angle of the mouth and lips, and permits the removal of redundant skin. Broad exposure of the superficial muscles allows attachment of the wide divided end of the masseter muscle flap to the underlying orbicularis oris muscle by white Dacron sutures. The position of the angle of the mouth is overcorrected both laterally and superiorly. In closing, multiple 5–0 white Dacron sutures attach the masseter muscle to the dermis at the nasolabial fold to mimic the musculodermal insertion and thus accentuate the fold.

A strip of fascia lata, usually combined with a muscle transplant, allows adjustment of the direction of the muscle pull. A broad strip of fascia is secured to the anterior edge of the masseter muscle and its covering fascia at the angle of the mouth and is then brought posteriorly and superiorly to the temporal fascia or around the zygomatic arch (Figs. 36–22, 36–23, and 36–24). Caution must be exercised in tightening either the muscle or the fascia. Tissue that is sutured too tensely will either dehisce or necrose. The terminal 2.5 cm of the fascia is split so that the upper tongues extend into the upper lip and the lower strips into the lower lip, both sufficiently broad and adequately tacked down to forestall eversion of the lips (so common when thin strips of fascia or tendon are used) (see Fig. 36–34, *C*).

In children, because of the delicacy of the musculature and because the majority are usually not seen until atrophy and fibrosis of the muscles are advanced, a circumoral fascial strip or a Marlex patterned strip, or, most recently, a felted implant (Proplast) is usually placed at least five weeks prior to the muscle transfer (Figs. 36–23 and 36–25). The technique involves removing a 20-cm strip of fascia lata, 0.5 cm wide, from the thigh and using the intraoral incisions shown in Figure 36–34, *A*, circling the orbicularis oris muscle. A Brand tendon puller, somewhat modified to fit the size of the child, or a Blair or Frackleton fascia needle, dissects the passage through the submucosa and muscle for the ribbon of fascia. The free end exits from the incision on the unaffected side, and the oral fissure is adjusted to a normal or overcorrected level. The fascia is sutured to the muscle at the angle of the mouth on the palsied side and a knot tied and secured by white silk to itself and to the overlying muscles. Upon muscle transfer some six weeks later, the purse-string is opened on the unaffected side by excising the fascial knot through an intraoral incision (see Fig. 36–34, *A*).

The high rate of complications following the use of inorganic implants is emphasized on page 1819.

If a face-lifting operation is required, the preauricular incision can be extended downward past the angle of the mandible and forward to a point immediately in front of the anterior border of the masseter. A typical face-lift incision with its posterior extension into the scalp may provide adequate exposure (Converse, 1974). When grafts of fascia,

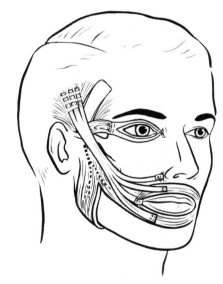

FIGURE 36–22. Masseter muscle transfer. The transfer of part of the masseter muscle directly to the orbicularis oris muscle with or without a previously inserted circumoral fascial strip. Note the position of the motor nerve to the muscle. A segment of temporalis muscle based from below is transferred directly to the orbicularis oculi muscle, together with the attached strip of covering temporalis fascia inserted as a circumorbital loop. The fascial strip for static and directional support is tacked to the underlying muscle and is woven into the temporal fascia. The drawing shows only one-half of the muscle transferred. The anterior two-thirds of the muscle are usually transferred. On occasion, the entire masseter is freed and transposed.

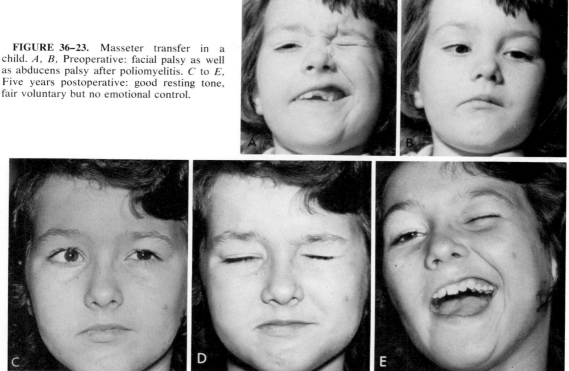

FIGURE 36–23. Masseter transfer in a child. *A*, *B*, Preoperative: facial palsy as well as abducens palsy after poliomyelitis. *C* to *E*, Five years postoperative: good resting tone, fair voluntary but no emotional control.

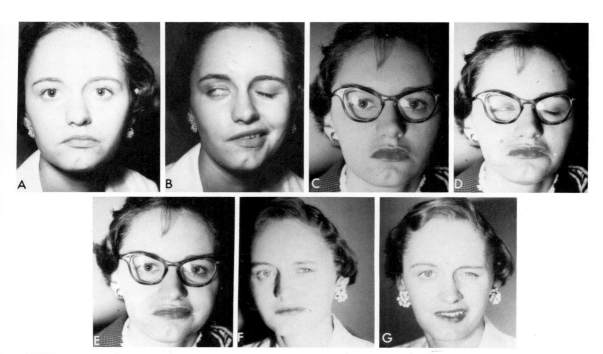

FIGURE 36–24. Complete unilateral facial paralysis after resection of an acoustic neuroma. *A*, *B*, Preoperative. *C* to *E*, Fair voluntary control, and mild emotional control, after masseter muscle transfer. *F*, *G*, Several years later. Note the wide palpebral fissure, which indicates the need for a lateral tarsorrhaphy or a temporalis fascial sling.

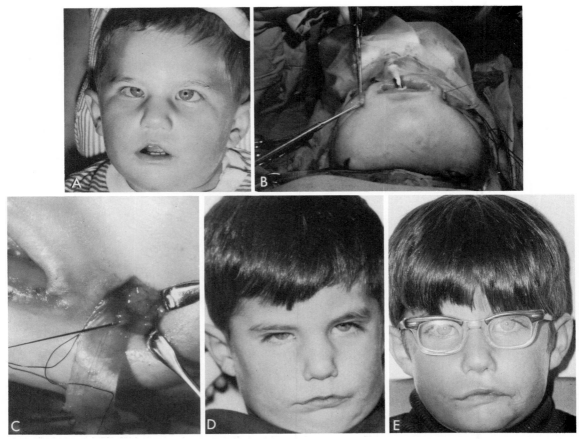

FIGURE 36–25. Möbius syndrome: correction of oral sphincter by masseter muscle transfer. *A,* Lack of orbicularis oris sphincter, causing constant drooling. *B,* Circumoral fascia lata band for attachment to free half of the masseter muscle bilaterally. *C,* Close-up view showing suture fixation of the masseter muscle and autogenous fascial band. *D,* Postoperative appearance three years later. *E,* Demonstration of sphincteric control.

dermis or cartilage, or inorganic materials are implanted, irrigation with Ringer's solution together with an antibiotic (0.5 g of neomycin and 10,000 units of bacitracin in 250 ml of Ringer's solution) is routine. Drainage is avoided to prevent ascending infection.

A split collodion gauze hammock, formed by attaching two Y's from opposite infra-auricular areas, splints the lips and cheek and yet permits access to the mouth. This is maintained for ten days. Additional pressure is placed on the cheek, and the patient is given a liquid diet for ten days.

Temporalis Muscle Transfer

FACIAL TRANSFER. Temporalis muscle transfer to the eyelids, the ala of the nose, the upper and lower lips, and the commissure of the mouth is a dynamic, controlled reconstruction with bony fixation and muscular and dermal attachments which can be secondarily readjusted. Although the technique has varied little over the past years, the technique has been employed increasingly in older patients. With the exception of children with Möbius syndrome (see Fig. 36–25) and specific lower lip paralyses, the massive temporalis muscle transfer is used by the author to the exclusion of all other muscle transfers, and the results have been uniformly gratifying.

Technique (Fig. 36–26). Through an extended face-lift incision (see Fig. 36–21), the temporalis fascia is exposed and raised superiorly along with the pericranium and inferiorly as far as the zygomatic arch. A quadrilateral fan-shaped flap approximately 8 to 10

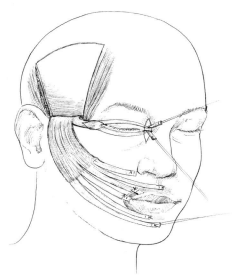

FIGURE 36–26. Temporalis transfer with muscular aponeurotic extensions to the eyelids, the ala of the nose, the lips, the oral commissure, and the lower lip. Note the loop around the muscle bundles and medial canthal tendons, and the "pull-through sutures" to the contralateral side.

lines of the muscle fibers also narrow, and is deepened bluntly through the fibers to the temporalis fossa to avoid cutting the deep temporal nerves which are branches of the anterior division of the mandibular nerve (fifth cranial nerve).

The pericranial-muscle-aponeurosis mass is dissected until it rolls down freely. Dissection with a special periosteal elevator (Fig. 36–27) allows the branches of the nerve to be felt rather than seen; denervation must be avoided. The dissected muscle complex falls over the zygomatic arch. The aponeurosis is incised over the arch and is elevated from the muscle mass. Should the pericranial-aponeurotic attachments seem tenuous, reinforcing mattress sutures are inserted into each of the major segments of the muscle belly: the anterior third, to restore the orbital sphincter; an inferior slip of aponeurosis to the ala of the nose (the nasal sphincter); and the posterior two thirds, to restore the oral sphincter (Fig. 36–28).

The preauricular extension of the temporalis incision is necessary in older individuals with facial sag and permits open dissection of the entire face to the nasolabial incision. This incision provides excellent exposure for hemostasis and complete separation of the skin from the underlying tissues, allowing a direct pull of the muscle without angling, torsion, or twisting. From incisions in the circumorbital

Text continued on page 1816

cm in width is outlined, and the upper incision is made 1 cm above the junction of the temporalis fascia and the pericranium. The lateral incision through the fascia is extended inferiorly *almost* to the zygomatic arch, becoming narrow as the

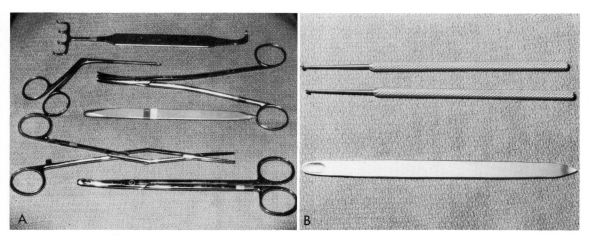

FIGURE 36–27. Instruments used in muscle transfers, muscle grafts, and fascial suspension. *A,* (Top to bottom), "cat's paw" retractors, fine tendon or fascia passers, face-lift scissors, periosteal elevator with sharp curved edge on one end and pointed "pick" on the other end, "alligator" double-action tendon, fascia, and muscle passers, and slotted dissecting scissors. *B,* Muscle dissector and periosteal elevator used in temporalis and masseter muscle transfers and free muscle grafts. Above are the balled hooks for nerve elevation.

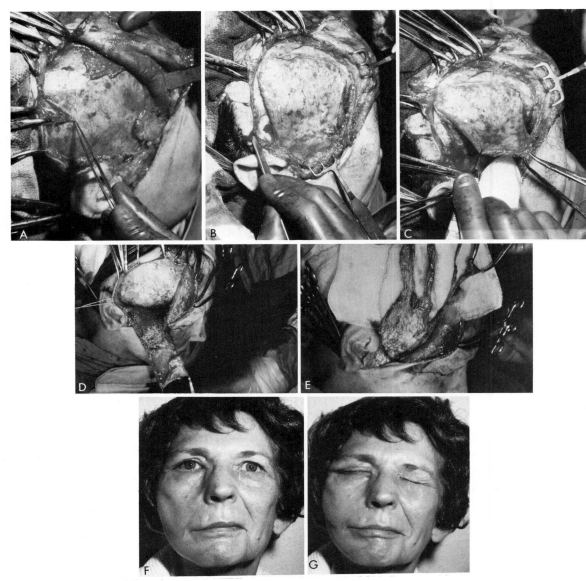

FIGURE 36–28.   Multiple steps in the early (14 days postoperative) rehabilitation of a 60 year old female with loss of function of the seventh, eighth, ninth, tenth, and twelfth cranial nerves. *A* to *G*, Dynamic reconstruction by massive temporalis muscle transfer. *A*, Beginning separation and elevation of the temporal fascia; the pericranium is connected to the temporal fascia and the muscle flap. *B*, Outlining the dissection of the muscle flaps with inferiorly based pedicles. *C*, Elevating the muscle and stripping the pericranium. *D*, Transferring the muscle inferiorly and checking the distance. *E*, Outlining the three major sections for the circumorbital area, the upper lip and nasal areas, and the angle of the mouth and circumorbital extension. Postoperative appearance: relaxed *(F)* and in contraction *(G)* showing control of periorbital and perioral sphincters.

Illustration and legend continued on the opposite page.

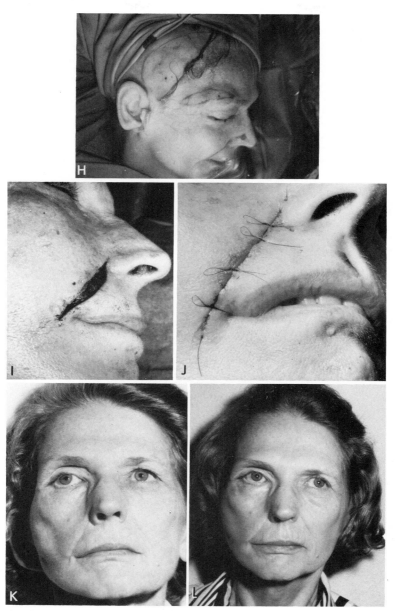

FIGURE 36–28 *Continued. H* to *L*, Auxiliary "cosmetic" techniques. *H*, Outline of brow-lift and formation of naso-labial fold on the paralyzed side. *I*, Formation of a dermal subcutaneous flap following excision of the epidermis. *J*, Closure with subcuticular and cuticular sutures to form a nasolabial fold. *K*, Postoperative view. Note the minimal scarring and improved facial balance. *L*, Appearance two years later following a face-lift operation on the contralateral side.

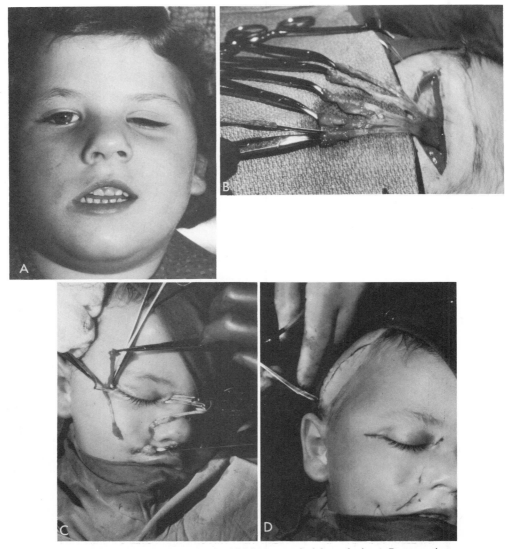

FIGURE 36–29.   Temporalis muscle transfer in a child for upper facial paralysis. *A*, Preoperative appearance. *B* to *D*, Technique. *B*, Temporalis muscle and temporal fascia delivered and five segments isolated. *C*, Slips of temporal fascia eased through tunnels by tapes. *D*, Closure.

Illustration continued on the opposite page

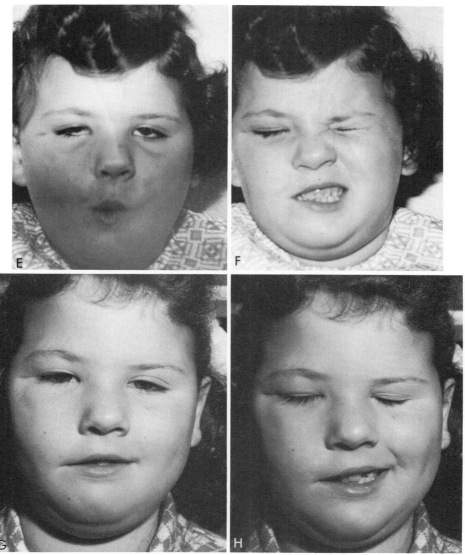

FIGURE 36–29 *Continued.* *E* to *H*, Postoperative appearance. *E, F*, Three months postoperative. *G, H*, Three years postoperative; note complete closure of lid.

region, the nasolabial fold, and along the ala of the nose, the skin is elevated to the points of insertion of the muscle. The lid insertions are described later in the text. In addition, a thin band of aponeurosis is wound around the insertion of the angular head of the quadratus labii superioris and fixed to the fibrous tissue of the nasal ala.

The aponeurosis of the lower two-thirds of the muscle-aponeurotic complex is divided into three parts, of which the upper and lower bands are again divided, thus allowing insertion of a superior slip across the midline to the contralateral orbicularis oris muscle and a branch to the apex of Cupid's bow (where the lip normally elevates for a sneer). The central segment is looped through the tissues near the commissure of the oral fissure. The aponeurosis of the inferior mass is again divided; the upper slip is inserted into the junction of the lateral and middle thirds of the paralyzed lower lip (the insertion of the quadratus labii inferioris to the orbicularis), and the inferior slip crosses the midline to the unaffected side. Except in the very young, it has rarely been necessary to add segments of fascia to elongate the strips. However, should there be undue tension, bands of fascia lata or aponeurosis are employed.

The technique of attachment is similar in both the dynamic and the static types of operation. The strip is wrapped around a band of residual muscle, secured to it by a Dacron mattress suture, and the distal end stretched medially by a pull-out mattress suture except at the oral commissure where it is looped around the muscle. On the lips and nasal area the distal free end of the fascia is secured to the undersurface of the dermis so that the final attachment simulates the insertion of a facial muscle of expression to the skin, with the hope of providing some degree of expression and curving of the lips on motion.

The author has used this technique in patients up to 60 years old. Follow-up results evaluated by means of preoperative and postoperative motion pictures as well as those of Rubin (1974) have encouraged the application of this technique on any patient for the initial treatment when the patient's condition permits the operation to be done under general anesthesia. Figures 36–28 and 36–29 show the preoperative, operative, and postoperative photographs of two patients representing the range in age of the patients.

EYELID TRANSFER. The temporal fascia is exposed and cleared to a point well above the temporal line. A strip 1.5 cm wide is outlined from the zygomatic arch to the parietal bone, and parallel vertical incisions outline the strip for 1 cm, extending through the pericranium above. This is transected by a deep horizontal cut, allowing the pericranium to be stripped down to the muscle attachment to the bone. By continuing the dissection along the pericranium, after splitting the muscles and incising the pericranium along the same vertical incisions, somewhat wider at the base to about 1 cm above the arch, a combined segment of muscle, fascia, and pericranium is freed from the bone. If the cut end of the fascia is carefully lifted from the muscle and elevated gently, it will usually remain attached at the temporal line. Nonetheless, it is safer to secure this attachment by two mattress sutures of Dacron. Figure 36–30 is a photograph of the temporalis muscle-fascia attachment with a sketch of the technique.

From the lateral canthal incision a tunnel is dissected through each lid, close to the eyelid margin, to a slightly curved vertical nasal incision. The medial palpebral tendon is exposed. The fascia is divided into two thin strips which are individually threaded through the tunnels, one to the upper, the other to the lower lid, brought under the canthal tendon, crossed, and tightened so that the upper lid overlaps the lower by about 2 or 3 mm; they are then sutured to each other and to the tendon. If the medial canthal tendon is tenuous, the nasal periosteum should be used as a point of anchorage, using two silk mattress sutures. Through the lateral incision, the exposed portion of the orbicularis oculi muscle is freed from the skin both superiorly and inferiorly and coapted over the exposed temporalis muscle transfer. Multiple fine 6–0 white silk sutures are used to attach the temporalis muscle to the palsied orbicularis oculi muscle.

A pressure dressing is maintained for a week or ten days and released for routine eye cleansing. After that time, the eye will open, and control of movement will be slowly obtained by practice.

SEGMENTAL LOWER FACE ELEVATION IN PARTIAL PARALYSIS. Occasionally it is necessary to replace or strengthen a levator of the upper lip, such as following a zygomatic muscle palsy. A similar strip of muscle and fascia with nerve and blood supply intact can be brought down. Figure 36–31 is an example of a segmental temporalis muscle transfer.

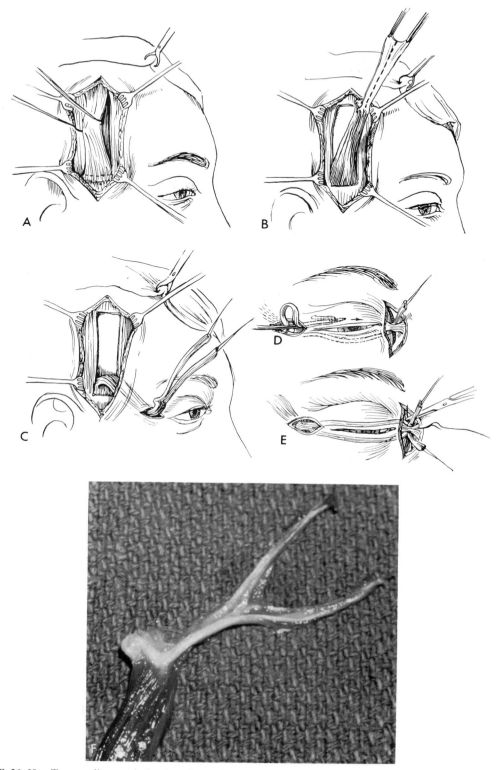

FIGURE 36–30. Temporalis muscle-fascia unit used as a circumorbital sling and motor unit. Gillies technique as modified by Andersen (1961). Inset shows segment of temporal muscle and its attachment to the temporal fascia. (This attachment may be tenuous and should be reinforced with Dacron sutures.)

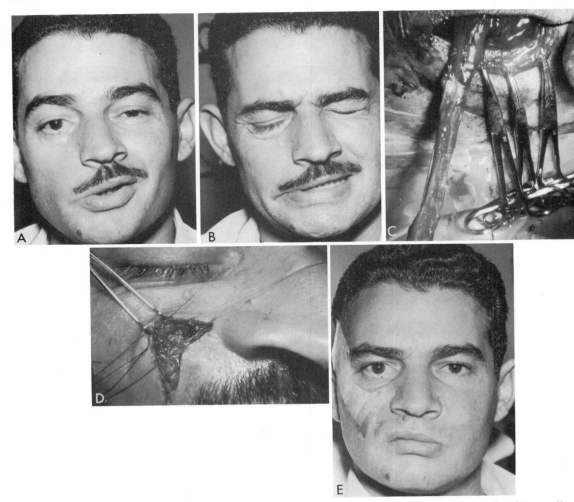

FIGURE 36–31. Segmental temporalis muscle transfer for correction of permanent partial right facial (upper lip and nose) palsy. *A,* Preoperative appearance on speaking. *B,* Voluntary action of facial muscles. *C,* Isolation and release of temporalis muscle segment and fascia. *D,* Attachment to underlying muscles and to the dermis through a nasolabial incision. *E,* Postoperative splinting maintained for three weeks. Note essential overcorrection.

The transfer of temporalis muscle and temporal fascial strips from the parietal region to the orbicularis oculi sphincter, and of masseter muscle to the orbicularis oris sphincter, involves transposing a complete motor unit, with nerve and blood supply intact, to a mechanically efficient position. Awkward or clumsy transfer may impair the original innervation and blood supply, with consequent trophic changes in the muscle, resulting in a static rather than a dynamic support. Careful isolation of a neurovascular pedicle will result in active functional units. This is extremely important when transposing major portions of the muscle.

Reanimation of the Frontalis Muscle. Adams (1946) advocated using a frontalis muscle flap from the unaffected side for reanimation, but the results have not been satisfactory. The technique of occipitalis muscle and galea transfer (Viñas, Jager and Viñas, 1973) is an interesting innovation.

Temporalis Muscle Tendon and Coronoid Process Transfer. Through an intraoral incision, McLaughlin (1952) detached the coronoid process and, by means of fascial strips, attached the temporalis muscle insertion to the angle of the mouth (Fig. 36–32). A modification of this method was used for the patient shown

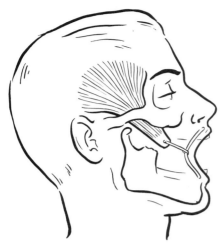

FIGURE 36–32. Temporalis tendon transfer to the circumoral region. The detached coronoid process is connected by a tendon graft to the orbicularis oris muscle.

in Figure 36–33. A variant of this technique has been advocated in children by Champion (1958).

Free Muscle Grafts. The technique of free autogenous muscle grafts is discussed in detail in a later section of the chapter.

Inorganic Implants

Static methods to relieve distortion employ the suspension of paralyzed facial muscles by various materials, varying from aluminum, bronze, wire, and silk to stainless steel and tantalum. There are advocates for the use of nonreactive plastic tapes of polyethylene, Teflon, or Silastic with or without either Marlex or Dacron mesh reinforcement and/or bonded polyurethane foam for organizational tissue attachments. Early results with these materials may prove to be excellent. Experience over a

FIGURE 36–33. Patient with unilateral facial paralysis. *A, B,* Preoperative photographs. *C, D,* Following a procedure similar to that shown in Figure 36–32. (Courtesy of Dr. M. Spira, U. S. Veterans Administration Hospital, Houston, Texas.)

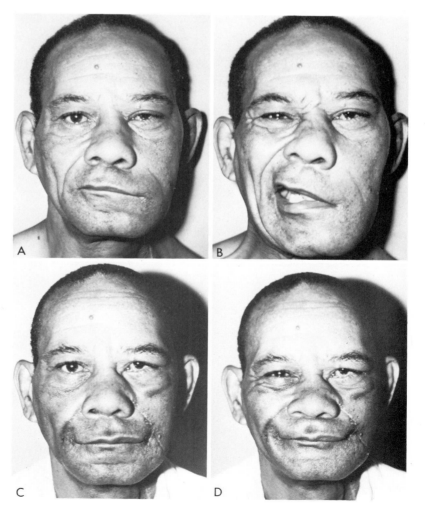

period of 30 years has led to a distrust of inorganic material placed in a position of suspension or tension in superficial locations. The reviews of Bäckdahl and D'Alessio (1958) and Conway (1958) should be consulted before one embarks on the use of inorganic materials for facial suspension.

Transplants of Dermis

Strips of dermis of width and length comparable to that of strips of fascia inserted in the same manner have a tendency to stretch more and make it more difficult to predict the amount of postoperative stretching. Dermis and lyophilized fascia are more liable to stimulate fibrous proliferation than autogenous fascia, for they fragment and disintegrate early. Postoperative subcutaneous infections are higher with dermal implants than with fascia, because saprophytic infection carried into the repaired field is manifested many days or weeks after the operation rather than in the usual 12 to 36 hours after operation (Pick, 1949). Nonetheless, dermis can be and is still used in an occasional patient.

Fascial Transplants

The use of autogenous fascia for blepharoptosis was initiated by Payr and applied to the treatment of facial paralysis by Stein (1913). However, it was Blair's advocacy (1926) of the suspension of paralyzed facial muscles by fascia lata bands that popularized the method. The technique varies considerably with the individual problem, but a modified fascial sling has proved of value as a method of primary treatment in older adults and as an adjunct method while waiting for the functional results of nerve crossings, grafts, or nerve end approximations. It is also used in association with muscle transplants and the resection of contralateral muscles, and it is helpful in prolonging the effects of skin excisions, face-lifts, and blepharoplasties.

Removal of Fascia Lata. A 5- × 20-cm sheet of fascia is obtained from the lateral aspect of the thigh using two parallel, 2.5-cm, transverse incisions (see Chapter 9). Sufficient mobilization of the skin allows dissection of the fascial band from the underlying muscle and overlying subcutaneous tissue by means of long, curved, slender scissors. Direct exposure of the longitudinal parallel incisions is obtained distally, and an unfrayed rectangle of nontrau-

matized fascia of the desired size is removed. No attempt is made to close the herniation of muscle belly through the defect. The fascial sheet is kept moist in a saline-soaked sponge. The skin is closed and an elastic pressure dressing prevents fluid collection. The Masson type of fascial stripper removes a large segment of fascia via a single small incision if the cutting edge is kept sharp. The Castroviejo stripper has a guillotine at its distal end which facilitates removal of the fascial strip.

Vasconez (1972) claimed that wide strips of fascia lata with broad attachments to the cheek and lips are superior to the thin fascial bands as originally advocated by Blair (1926).

When a tendon transplant is needed, as for the McLaughlin procedure, Brand's technique for removing the plantaris muscle and tendon is preferred; previously an extensor tendon of the lesser toes was used.

STAGE I—CIRCUMORAL FASCIA LATA BAND. If the paralysis is of excessively long standing, a strip of fascia 0.5 to 0.75 cm wide is introduced into the orbicularis oris muscle or its remnants to circumscribe the mouth through four small external incisions, one at each of the angles and slightly to the side of the midline, and one each for the upper and lower lips. The strip is threaded through a blunt fascia needle carrier or scissors which are perforated near the tip of the blades. The fascial strip is introduced through the perforation after the scissors have established a tunnel through the tissues of the lip, from the unaffected side around the mouth, as shown in Figure 36–34, *A*, coming out again on the unaffected contralateral side. The free ends are crossed and the lips manipulated to "a position of optimal symmetry," to be fixed there with interrupted silk sutures joining the orbicularis muscle to the fascial loop. The loop is closed by a knot which is secured by a suture.

Postoperatively, double-tailed collodion gauze splints are placed, one on each side of the mouth, each overlapping the other, to maintain a buttonhole splint dressing for ten days to two weeks. Fascia-muscle healing is not complete until after five weeks, and a second stage should be deferred until that time.

SECOND STAGE FASCIA LATA TRANSPLANT. The approach is through a routine preauricular temporal face-lift incision, aided by a nasolabial incision, or, when resection of excess skin is not necessary, by way of an incision within the temporal hairline and a nasolabial incision. The skin is completely undermined over the paralyzed muscles of the face and upper and lower lips to the angle of the mouth. If the

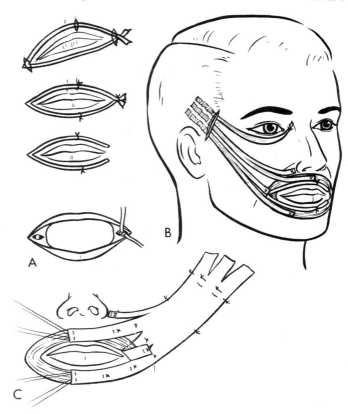

FIGURE 36–34. Fascia lata suspension. *A*, Placement of a circumoral fascial strip. Inserted via extraoral or buccal incisions, the loops are tightened on the unaffected side to elevate the paralyzed angle of the mouth. The knotted attachment at the unaffected commissure is excised after five weeks. The lowermost sketch shows the oral incisions for insertion of the circumoral band of fascia after it has been threaded through and knotted, prior to the suturing. *B*, The fascial sling to the lower lid is secured at the nasal periosteum. The lateral end is attached to the temporal fascia. The fascial band is attached through a temporal incision to the orbicularis oris. The three tails for attachment at both insertions are shortened for clarity. *C*, The typical fashioning of a fascial ribbon for adequate support using three tails for insertion: one for each lip well past the midline and one folded around the dissected orbicularis oris muscle. The similarly tailed lateral end is woven into the temporal fascia or tacked securely to the adjacent periosteum.

paralysis is of long standing, a strip of fascia should be inserted at least a month or more previously, so as to become firmly attached. The terminal 3 cm of the 5- × 20-cm fascial sheet is cut into thirds, with the central segment of the trident somewhat blunted or trimmed. Multiple mattress sutures of 4–0 Mersilene or silk anchor the insertion to the superficial muscles and to the fascial circumoral strip (see Fig. 36–34).

A more accurate result usually can be obtained by splitting the upper segment into three sections and tacking an individual strip to the undersurface of the dermis at the ala of the nose, one at the curve of Cupid's bow, and the third strip under the philtrum on the contralateral side. The lower segment is similarly split, attaching one strip to the commissure, a second to the undersurface of the dermis of the lateral third of the lower lip, and a third to the contralateral side. Alternatively, a segment of skin can be de-epithelized and used as a dermal flap, secured to the periosteum of the zygoma, for additional support.

A subcutaneous channel at least 2.5 cm in width is made in the cheek between the temporalis fascia and the nasolabial fold incision. The fascial strip is brought through, and the angle of the mouth is drawn laterally and up slightly above the level of the opposite angle. The tightened fascial band is woven through the temporalis fascia, tacked to it, reversed, and sutured to itself by nonabsorbable mattress sutures. Prior to closure of the nasolabial incision, redundant skin may be excised. A row of fine white nonabsorbable sutures attaches the dermis of the rolled lateral or proximal margin of the incision directly to the fascia. Nylon sutures close the undercut cutaneous layer after irrigation of the operative field through the temporal incision.

In most adults the orbicularis oris muscle is still of sufficient bulk and strength that the central fascial strip of the trident can be looped around the muscle belly and secured to itself by mattress sutures of nylon. The upper and lower strips are attached to the muscle of the upper and lower lips, respectively, to a point just past the midline, as well as to the previously inserted circumoral fascial loop. As shown in Figure 36–34, the closed loop on the unparalyzed side is now opened by incising it at the unaffected commissure, thus opening the oral commissure, check-reined during the previous few weeks.

If secondary adjustment of tension is needed, an incision under local anesthesia and a careful dissection of the temporal end of the fascial band permit tightening it.

THE USE OF NARROW STRIPS OF FASCIA LATA. Slings fashioned of narrow fascia lata strips are of value in a debilitated patient when the undermining necessary for extensive procedures is contraindicated. They are especially suitable in facial paralysis secondary to a stroke in an elderly individual. The method offers considerable support and aid, and can be done under local anesthesia with minimal incisions.

NARROW RIBBON TECHNIQUE USING FASCIAL LOOPS. Through a small temporal incision, using a Blair fascia needle, a fascia lata strip is brought down to a nasolabial incision at the angle of the mouth. The atrophied orbicularis oris muscle is dissected; the strip of fascial band is looped about it and is returned to the temporal region by the same instrument. The two ends of the fascial ribbon are threaded through muscle bundles or through the temporalis fascia. The fascia lata is made quite tight, and the elevation of the angle of the mouth is sufficiently *overcorrected* to compensate for later sagging.

Additional strips may be placed in the upper and lower lips or used to support the cheek by introducing the threaded instrument deep into the cheek tissues. The lax subcutaneous tissue and atrophic musculature can be elevated by multiple strips placed above and below the angle of the mouth, incorporating the atrophic subcutaneous and muscular tissue of the cheek, and again the loops can be sutured or woven into the temporalis fascia.

Under local anesthesia, modified excisions of the redundant skin prior to skin closure can be combined with the loops of fascia brought around the corner of the mouth and to the upper and lower lips. As mentioned previously, although the circumoral fascial strip procedure, described in Figure 36–34, tends to limit the opening of the mouth, later excision of the knot opens the unaffected angle of the mouth. Intraoral incisions present the theoretical disadvantage of contamination by oral secretions and subsequent infection, but such problems have been avoided by irrigation of the wound with an antibiotic solution prior to closure.

Relaxation of the suspended facial tissues occurs after a number of years and requires exposure and tightening of the slings and excision of the excess facial skin.

FASCIAL STRIPS IN THE PARALYZED EYELID.

The attachment of a fascial strip for support of the lower lid is achieved in the following manner. A tunnel is made between the skin and the underlying orbicularis oculi muscle from a small transverse incision lateral to the lateral canthus to a gently curved vertical incision at the nasal angle, close to the lid margin. The medial canthal tendon is dissected and provides a point of attachment for a strip of fascia lata approximately 3 mm wide which is looped under the tendon to be sutured to itself by two silk mattress sutures. If this point of fixation seems too fragile, the end of the fascia is tacked to the nasal periosteum above the canthus. A continuation of the tunnel is extended posteriorly to a temporal incison which exposes the temporal fascia. The anterior auricular muscle and its envelope must not be mistaken for the heavy fascia covering the temporalis muscle. The ribbon of fascia is looped through a fascial lattice and reversed after snugging up the lid to a somewhat overcorrected position (but still insufficient to cause eversion of the lid). The posterior end is woven into the temporal fascia to which it is secured with multiple silk mattress sutures.

Fascia or tendon grafts require the avoidance of excessive tension and scarring to prevent necrosis and infection (Fig. 36–35). Staging of the procedures to allow the tendon or fascia to become sufficiently adherent at the insertions lessens the chances of an avulsion or a pull-out by the motor unit, or even by the continuous increase of tension caused by scar contraction in the transplant. A typical case is illustrated in Figure 36–36, which also shows the results of a five-year follow-up.

HEALING OF FASCIAL AND TENDON TRANSFERS: A COMPARISON. Fascial strips and tendons heal in a similar fashion and require postoperative care and after-treatment not unlike that for tendon repair and replacement in the hand. Rest and compression are indicated in the immediate postoperative phase, and attempts to move the fascial strip or tendon during the third week increase the fibroplastic reaction. Continuous tension by opposing muscles or gravity should not be permitted before the fourth week and preferably not until the fifth week. Therefore, tension should be relieved by appropriate splinting for a full five-week period. As this is difficult in the mobile face in which spastic antagonists cause stress and pull, a temporary or even a permanent partial paralysis must be induced on the contralateral side either by neural section, by neural block, or, preferably, by selective myectomy. To summarize: as tendon motions prior to the third week increase the

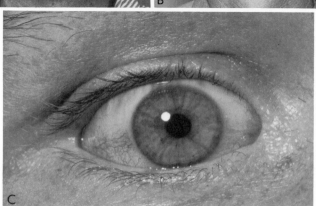

FIGURE 36–35. Fascial sling and medial canthoplasty in complete right facial palsy. *A,* Before operation. *B,* After the fascial sling and the medial canthoplasty. *C,* Close-up of the eye to show the result obtained by the medial canthoplasty.

fibroplastic reaction, the face should be covered by a compressive dressing and immobilized. Reeducation, although necessary, should not commence until after the fifth week.

Reconstruction of the Lax Oral Sphincter in Facial Paralysis

Buccal and labial mucosal protrusion, cheek biting, inability to propulse food, and drooling in patients with long established facial paralysis are due to *buccinator* muscle palsy, pressure ballooning of the cheek, stretching and thinning of the mural elements (including the fibrous muscle), persistent mucosal edema, and subsequent diastasis. Early surgical correction will prevent these complications. Excision

of the redundant mucosa, repair of the diastasis with properly secured fascia or a polypropylene mesh patch, and a layered mucosal closure have been of value. The oral sphincter is strengthened and its continuity is reestablished if one obtains a firm posterior attachment for the elastic mesh (or nonelastic fascia) at the pterygomandibular raphé or at the anterior border of the ramus of the mandible and a secure anterior attachment at the oral commissure, with extensions to the unaffected side of the upper and lower lips. At this time, the excess vermilion and labial mucosa can be excised to reduce the prolapsed and hypertrophied inner and exposed surfaces of the lips.

TECHNIQUE. Under local anesthesia, the parotid duct is located and a spindle- or leaf-shaped area of mucosa is excised (Fig. 36–37).

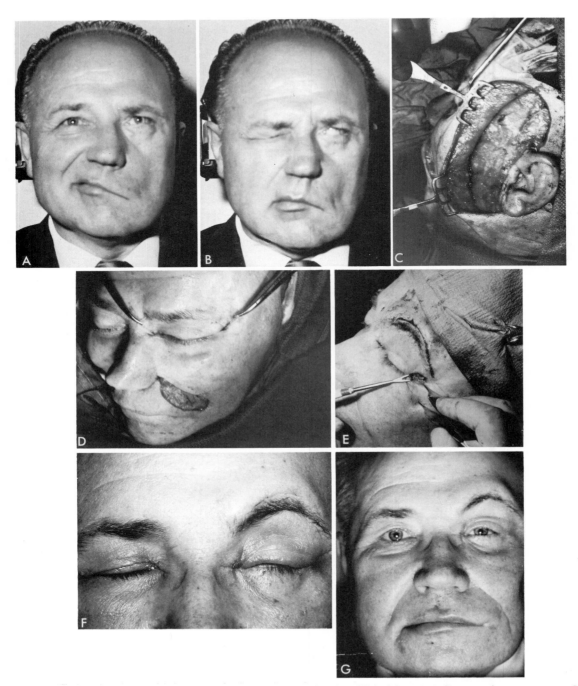

FIGURE 36–36. Repair of facial paralysis by a fascial sling via a face-lift incision. *A, B,* Preoperative appearance. *C,* Securing the fascia by weaving it into the temporalis muscle. *D,* Secondary procedures. Preparation of the dermal flap from redundant skin and placment of a Silastic band through the lower lid for elevation and support. *E,* Fixation of the dermis flap to the malar bone and brow-lift. *F, G,* Postoperative appearance five years later. The overcorrection of the brow is still present, and the eyelid does not completely close; the cornea is protected.

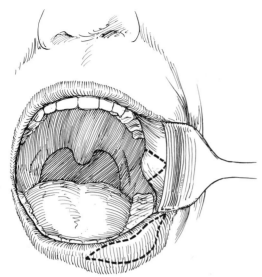

FIGURE 36–37. Excision of the redundant and hypertrophied buccal and labial mucosa afford access to the underlying musculature for repair of the diastasis. (From Freeman, B. S.: Late reconstruction of the lax oral sphincter in facial paralysis. Plast. Reconstr. Surg., *51*:144, 1973. Copyright ©1973, The Williams & Wilkins Company, Baltimore.)

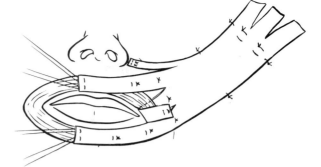

FIGURE 36–38. Method of attachment of the fascia lata or Marlex mesh by nonabsorbable mattress sutures at the pterygomandibular raphé (rather than at the mandible). The central slip of the anterior end is wrapped securely around the orbicularis oris muscle at the oral commissure. The inferior and superior slips are secured temporarily by pull-out mattress sutures to the undersurface of the dermis. (The optional small strip to the ala is secured firmly.) Insertion can also be made to the mandible.

Stainless steel wire is threaded through two drill holes in the anterior ridge of the body of the mandible and is used as a mattress suture to secure a 2.5-cm band of either fascia or Marlex mesh to the ramus. The anterior portion of the band of mesh or fascia is then drawn forward through a dissected submucosal tunnel, tightened, and sutured at the corners to the adjacent soft tissues to allow the tunnel to remain open.

The anterior end of the band is slit into three slips (Fig. 36–38). The central slip encircles the freed commissure, and it is tightened and securely fastened around the orbicularis muscle.

The superior and inferior slips of the fascia (or mesh) are advanced through dissected subdermal tunnels in the respective lips, where they are temporarily secured by pull-out mattress sutures to prevent their withdrawal or slippage. Later fibrous ingrowth causes firm adhesions and scar contracture completes the sphincter.

The redundant, everted vermilion and labial mucosa are tailored as necessary with transverse or vertical excisions. For five weeks the

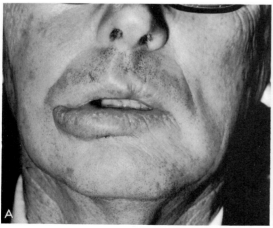
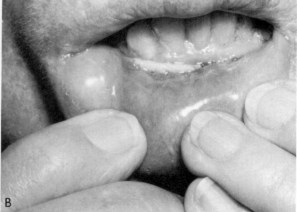

FIGURE 36–39. Complications after tight fascial sling. *A*, Mucosal protrusion but adequate control of the lip. *B*, Exposed fascia attached to the contralateral side. Complication was secondary to rubbing against a projecting canine tooth and partial anesthesia resulting from fifth cranial nerve damage.

cheek is splinted with a broad band of fine mesh gauze secured by collodion.

The only complication of the technique has been pressure erosion of the mucosa against projecting cuspid teeth exposing the tight Marlex band or the fascia (Fig. 36–39). A snug insertion of only the central band at the palsied commissure, allowing the upper and lower strips to lie more loosely and form their own fibrous attachments, has prevented subsequent mucosal erosion (Fig. 36–40).

Removal of Antagonistic Muscle Pull

Supplementary methods of aiding unilateral facial paralysis are many and varied. Niklison (1956) and Curtin, Greeley, Gleason and Braver (1960) contended that in facial paralysis the unaffected side is not normal. Increased tonus with its resultant overaction of the "normal" half, unopposed by the functionless atonic paralyzed muscles, results in gross imbalance. The surgical strengthening of the weakened side

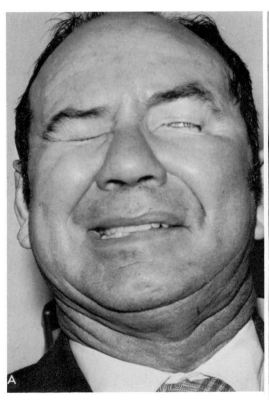
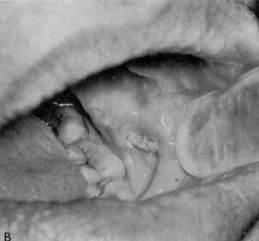
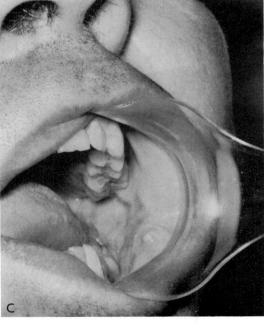

FIGURE 36–40. Complications after sphincteric reconstruction: buccal exposure of the fascial sling because of fifth cranial nerve anesthesia and grinding of molar teeth. *A,* Five years postoperative fascial sling. *B,* Exposed fascia through a buccal opening. *C,* View of smooth buccal surface two years after closure. (From Freeman, B. S.: Late reconstruction of the lax oral sphincter in facial paralysis. Plast. Reconstr. Surg., *51*:144, 1973. Copyright ©1973, The Williams & Wilkins Company, Balitmore.)

must be aided by release of the overactive muscular contractions of the nonparalyzed side, to permit healing without tension on the paralyzed side and to assist in restoring a better balance with the side of the face that has undergone the operative procedures.

Neurectomy. Attempts to section the intact facial nerve were made as early as the first quarter of the nineteenth century, when John Bell, the elder brother of Sir Charles Bell, offered to section the branches of the facial nerve of the intact side in a case of Bell's palsy. In Charles Bell's casebook, there is a note of an operative procedure suggested by the elder John Bell, a practicing surgeon in Rome—segmental resection of the branches of "the nerve" on the sound side. Interpreted by the younger man as a proposed section of the contralateral trigeminal nerve, the operation was deprecated and the patient dismissed (Gordon-Taylor and Walls, 1958).

Others advocated a *temporary* paralysis induced by drugs to release the pull and aid the healing tissues on the paralyzed side following surgery. This resulted in bilateral epiphora, increased difficulty in mastication, and muffled speech. Nonetheless, facial expressions were no longer distorted, and the patients approved of the results.

NEURECTOMY OF THE MARGINAL MANDIBULAR BRANCH. Temporary neural block by chemical means (alcohol, ammonium salts, or long-acting oily base local anesthetic agents) or neural crush should be performed by *direct* exposure of the nerve rather than by the relatively blind injection guided by faradic stimulation, as advocated by Gillies and Millard (1957). A precise approach is the method of Marino (1953), who places the patient under general anesthesia and, using a small 1-cm vertical incision between the angle of the jaw and the anterior border of the sternocleidomastoid muscle, exposes the branches of the mandibular marginal branch on the unaffected side. The nerve is isolated and held by blunt nerve hooks. Using a small nerve stimulator with a bipolar electrode, the branch innervating the contralateral muscle involved is checked.

A neurectomy of about 0.5 cm in length is done for unilateral paralysis of the nerve to the depressor muscles of the lower lip. This is preceded by an injection of 2 ml of local anesthetic solution (2 per cent Xylocaine) at the angle of the mandible to block the nerve and check the result of the interruption of nerve conduction. If the trial is satisfactory and the muscle balance is improved, the procedure is performed under general anesthesia, with anticipated good results.

NEURECTOMY OF THE TEMPORAL BRANCH. Neurectomy of the temporal branch to the opposing frontalis muscle will prevent horizontal frown lines but not the vertical fold or pull. As in the neurectomy of the marginal mandibular branch, preliminary testing with an injection of a local anesthetic solution (2 per cent Xylocaine) in the temporal area just behind the hairline will aid in the outline of the branches involved. Through an incision 2.5 cm above the lateral canthus and just within the hairline (at right angles to the transverse incision usually used for the temporal approach to a zygomatic fracture), the nerve branch or branches are found over the temporalis fascia, elevated, and stripped by a nerve hook, and a 1 cm segment is resected. The nerve to the procerus-corrugator segment also supplies a portion of the orbicularis oculi muscle via the zygomatic branches, or arcades, and segmental myectomy, as outlined below, should be done as well. A more precise approach would be the method of *partial neurectomy,* suggested for facial spasms by Greenwood (1946).

Myectomy. Selective myectomy or weakening of the muscles of the nonparalyzed side, rather than the interruption of the continuity of the facial nerve, provides improved and more permanent facial balance after a muscle transplant on the paralyzed side has contributed some facial muscular action.

The muscles most frequently causing distortion during speech, emotion, and associated actions are the quadratus labii superioris, the depressor labii inferioris, and the zygomaticus. Infrequently the risorius, caninus, and triangularis muscles are specifically spastic and warrant surgical intervention. A study of which muscle or muscle groups are responsible for the distortion permits these to be isolated and sectioned and varying amounts of muscle tissue to be resected. This procedure can be of special interest in the partial palsies often seen in patients who have had poliomyelitis or in segmental paralysis not amenable to surgical neurorrhaphy or grafting. *An accurate and complete muscle power inventory and diagnosis is important to restore functional balance in repose, voluntary activity, and spontaneous emotional action.*

Weakening of the action of antagonistic contralateral muscles is combined with facial suspension by fascia, tendon, or muscle; skin excision by a partial face-lifting operation; elliptical excision of supraorbital, infralabial, and nasolabial facial sag; and the neutralization of antagonistic muscles by neurectomy of the marginal mandibular branch and the temporal branches of the facial nerve.

Alleviation of the spastic, antagonistic muscles on the nonpalsied side has aided symmetry in action, both voluntary and emotional. For example, to correct excessive upward deviation of the opposite side of the face during a smile, the zygomaticus muscle is outlined at the angle of the mouth. The fibers, which spread up and out and become deeper superiorly, are isolated under the subcutaneous tissue and retracted for about 2 cm from the relatively diffuse origin of the muscle to its insertion into the orbicularis oris. Careful dissection exposes the tiny nerves which enter the muscle from the undersurface. It is a simple procedure to remove a segment from 1 to 2 cm in length, depending on the age of the patient.

Deviation of the philtrum to the opposite side and the upward pull of the cheek can be lessened by resecting a segment of the quadratus labii superioris muscle, as well as a short segment of the orbicularis oris at this area. The fine silk ligatures around the muscle bundles allow a careful dissection and facilitate accurate and complete exposure of the muscles.

Abnormal depression of the lip during labial speech, simulating a sneer, can be corrected either by neurectomy of the marginal mandibular branch or by isolating the quadratus labii inferioris through the mucosa and removing a segment of the muscle. The muscle outline is marked during forceful speech. The lip is everted, the mucosa incised, the muscle isolated and sectioned, and the mucosa closed.

An intraoral approach is adequate for the depressor muscles. After everting the lip, a mucosal flap is elevated, and the quadratus muscle together with the triangularis and the associated segments of the orbicularis oris are outlined. The muscles, isolated from the skin and mucosa are clipped and tied, and resected. The mucosa is closed with 5–0 catgut sutures.

The incision to expose the zygomaticus or the quadratus labii superioris (the levators) is placed in the nasolabial fold. The stouter and thickened muscles are outlined, and, after careful dissection, a 2-cm segment of muscle tissue is removed. Hemostasis by electrocoagulation is followed by approximation of the incised tissues.

Elevation and spasm of the contralateral forehead and eyebrow can be adjusted by myectomy. Through an incision of 2 cm or less at the upper median border of the eyebrow, the corrugator and procerus muscles are exposed, isolated, and resected. Since the procerus, frontalis, orbicularis oculi, and corrugator muscles act synergistically, a small median segment of the conjoint muscle of the first three muscles, which covers the corrugator muscle, is removed. The skin of the forehead is undermined and elevated from the frontalis muscle. This may result in redundant supraorbital and forehead skin, and the excess tissue is excised in a crescent, as advocated by Bames (1957) for forehead wrinkles. The supraorbital vessels and nerves pass deep to the corrugator muscle and can be avoided, but a note of caution should be offered. Hemostasis is essential. A pressure dressing is applied to the forehead lightly enough to avoid excessive compression of the skin against the frontal bossae but sufficient to obliterate the dead space and avoid postoperative edema.

The supraorbital scars may be diminished by later dermabrasion, but this is rarely necessary.

Plication or shortening of the paralyzed elevators, suggested by Niklison (1956), should be mentioned for completeness. The attenuated muscles are not suitable for dissection and plication. Although stapling the muscles rather than suturing them has prevented tearing, they lack the strength of transplants. Instead of being plicated, the muscles are spread out over the surface of the masseter or temporalis transfers with the hope that tone will return by neurotization.

Excision of Redundant Skin

Removal of redundant skin and edematous or fibrosed, thickened, subcutaneous tissue is of special interest in young adults with longstanding paralysis or older persons in whom the palsied muscles rapidly accelerate signs of aging. Excess skin is removed by the techniques routinely used for the alleviation of the excess skin of the aged. Since the object of the operation is not to regain a younger appearance but to approximate the nonparalyzed half of the face, a face lift of limited scope is indicated.

As outlined in Chapter 37, the incision is preauricular, extending superiorly to the temporal area (up to the parietal area when a temporal muscle transfer is indicated) and inferiorly and posteriorly around the ear lobe, along the retroauricular fold to and across the mastoid to the nuchal hairline. Although most surgeons prefer a pretragal incision, an incision a few millimeters behind the tragus heals as well, if closed without tension, and leaves a less

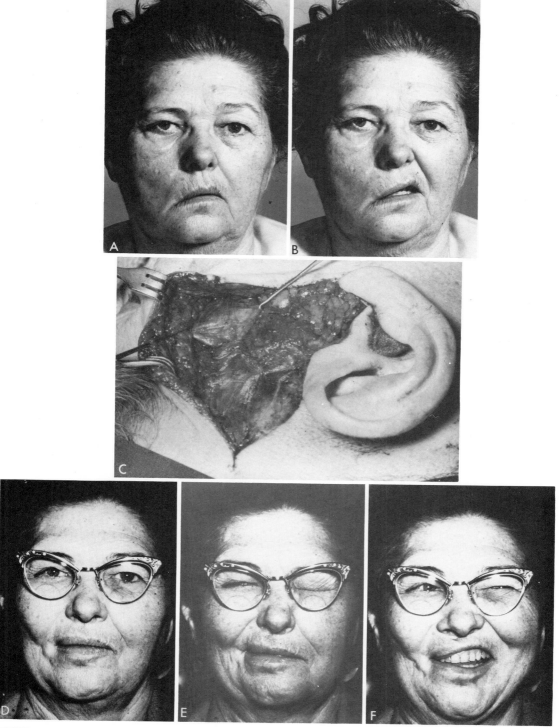

FIGURE 36–41. Combined approach in facial palsy. Preoperative, operative, and postoperative photographs of a patient with facial paralysis after an operation for removal of an extensive acoustic neuroma, resulting in total facial palsy. *A, B,* The despondent preoperative patient. *C,* At the time of surgery, via a face-lift incision, a broad fascial band is transplanted. *D* to *F,* Six months after the operation and after resection of the contralateral antagonist muscles.

conspicuous scar. The superficial undermining is extended to the nasolabial fold where a second incision is made. In palsy of long standing, excess tissue at the nasolabial fold is present and should be removed as an ellipse. Alternatively, the dermis could be retained and used as a static levator attached to the malar bone or used to form a new nasolabial fold. The necessary undermining is done. Hemostasis by 6–0 silk ties and pinpoint electrocoagulation must be complete, for drainage should not be used when fascial grafts are buried.

Upon completion of the procedure the undermined flaps are rotated superiorly and posteriorly, the necessary triangles to permit precise closure are excised, the subcutaneous tissues are deeply secured to the fascia over the mastoid and in the temporal region, and the wound is closed (Fig. 36–41). The nasolabial closure must be first done or excessive tissue excision may cause increased tension, poor healing, and the possible loss of the fascial transplant or the transferred muscle. An attempt is made to establish a new nasolabial fold by forming an adhesion along the proposed fold between the dermis of the lateral or posterior edge and the underlying fascia and muscle. This is done by inverting the posterior dermal margin with a row of mattress sutures of buried 6–0 silk; after undercutting, the skin edges are approximated with 5–0 nylon sutures. The fold is maintained by accentuating the fold when applying the collodion strips.

Joseph's (1931) procedure for excision of redundant forehead skin, together with the excision of a supraorbital crescent elevates the displaced eyebrow (Bames, 1957). This has been improved (Castañares, 1964) by suturing the inferior edge of the dermis to the pericranium with nonabsorbable sutures. Simple excision of redundant skin, subcutaneous tissue, and muscle has been extended by Berger, Slaughter, and Lansa (1961). After outlining all the redundant skin at the nasolabial fold, excision of skin, subcutaneous tissue, and muscle down to the mucosa results in an immediate improvement (Fig. 36–42). No other measures are used in conjunction with this procedure, which results in improvement, if only temporary, in a limited group of patients.

As with any static procedure, further skin excision will be necessary; as the patient ages, relaxation of the suspended tissues progresses, and secondary operative procedures are indicated.

CHOICE OF CORRECTIVE PROCEDURE

The choice of the corrective procedure is dependent on a detailed analysis of the etiology of the condition, the rate of clinical progress, the status of the deformity, the patient's age, and the overall prognosis. No one routine method can offer the efficacy of a *multiple technique approach* modified to suit the end desired and progressively achieved over a period of time.

There are but few procedures proposed for the alleviation of the signs of facial paralysis that have not been of some value in certain cases. None, however, with the possible exception of an early nerve repair or graft, is suitable for all patients. The selection of the procedure or procedures to be applied to the individual patient is not merely a matter of trial and error but a selection based on analysis of the deformity and on knowledge of the usual results in the surgeon's hands and the requirements, capabilities, and physical condition of the patient. A thorough analysis of the deformity is necessary for the selection of one or several of the multiple procedures

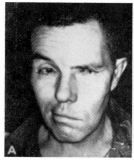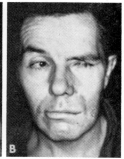

FIGURE 36–42. Nasolabial excision. Long-standing facial paralysis aided by a wide resection of the redundant facial tissues via a nasolabial fold incision. (Courtesy of Dr. Jack Berger.)

which can aid the patient. Factors under consideration include the degree, extent, and longevity of the paralysis, as well as the age, life expectancy, and overall general health of the patient. His occupation, emotional balance, and social activities must also be considered. The procedures to be considered must be gauged as to their efficacy in the individual with regard to all of the above conditions. A 72 year old debilitated stroke victim should not be subjected to reconstructive surgery by a massive muscle transfer, multiple antagonistic muscle resections, or lift and brow procedures, but more properly the surgeon should employ simple, nontraumatic techniques, the results of which, although possibly transient, can effect early improvement. Conversely, muscle transfers and surgical relaxation of contralateral muscle spasticity are more suited for a child with a partial facial paralysis with innate learning abilities. In the healthy, middle-aged adult with irreparable loss of the facial nerve, neural and muscle transfers and the panoply of techniques are available to return him to active status and to restore his mental equilibrium. In *young adults,* a total temporalis muscle transfer to the eyelids and face is aided by a selective myectomy of the antagonist muscles.

In *children,* if neural repair is no longer possible and in those cases of partial paralysis secondary to poliomyelitis or partial nuclear agenesis, surgical intervention should be started before school age (Champion, 1958). The procedures should be done in stages to prevent overcorrection and to avoid the destructive effect of tension on the delicate and attenuated structures. The external approach for a masseter transplant to the orbicularis oris muscle is preferred, reinforced by a preliminarily placed circumoral fascial band. The temporalis muscle is reserved for the paralyzed eyelids should a tarsorrhaphy be inadequate.

In *elderly patients,* a modified face-lift, a fascial transplant, and an overlapping tarsorrhaphy are followed at a later stage by excision of the contralateral spastic muscle antagonists for an effective emotional and physical rehabilitation.

COMPLICATIONS OF RECONSTRUCTIVE PROCEDURES

Complications are those encountered in the use of grafts of fascia or flaps of muscle through-out the body. The grafts may stimulate excessive reaction, contract, pull loose, or become infected. Similarly, the muscle flaps may be overstretched, or their vascular supply may be interrupted by edema, excessive tension, and kinking around a turn or over a bony prominence, or they may be strangulated by a fascial strip.

Subcutaneous hematoma should be immediately evacuated, even if it is necessary to open the entire incision in the operating room under anesthesia. Fixation of the tissues by late fibrosis or secondary infection may follow and obliterate facial movements and prevent secondary procedures.

In the presence of active infection, in addition to the usual methods of treatment, the grafts are removed.

Adequate postoperative splinting should prevent the pulling out of fascial bands or muscular attachments if they have been placed under an adequate amount of tension. If despite these safeguards the transferred muscle pulls loose, an extra autogenous fascial extension should bridge the gap before the tissue is sufficiently organized to hamper the dissection.

The most obvious and usual deficiency is inadequate excursion, and probably the commonest cause is adhesion. Because the extension of the muscle is insufficient, the muscle is restricted in range, and full motion cannot be restored; tenolysis should not be considered until after the tendon is well healed and the excursion and reeducation instituted. A second cause of failure of motion is loss of continuity due to dehiscence at either the proximal or distal junction. Similarly, after exploration and resuture, a five-week rest should elapse prior to instituting graduated active motion.

In patients with partial facial paralysis in whom elastic mesh is used, the splinting mesh may prevent stretching during the period of healing. Yet these may pull out, as have taut wire fixations at the distal end of the reconstructed sphincter.

The possibility of severance of a facial nerve branch when treating a partially paralyzed side is real, and one must watch out for the tiny branches, especially when attempting a masseter muscle transfer in a child. Section of the motor branch to the masseter muscle can occur if the section of the flap is carried too high; spontaneous nerve regrowth may remedy this complication.

Nonetheless, the good results observed in some patients may be explained by the return of function or regrowth of the nerve as long as

18 months after total loss of function after tumor ablation. This is especially true after the removal of large temporal lobe tumors, and the nerve, not well exposed at the time of surgery, is splayed but not totally severed.

Excessive resection of the contralateral muscles has not been seen, but inadequate hemostasis is the commonest cause of undue swelling.

Conley (1976) has expressed the opinion that muscle ablation on the contralateral side has not proved to be of great value from a practical point of view.

An occasional complication of myectomy on the contralateral side is the development of a facial tic (Edgerton, 1967) similar to that seen following the healing of wounds in which peripheral branches of the facial nerve have been severed (Converse and Coburn, 1971).

SPECIAL PROCEDURES IN FACIAL PARALYSIS

Surgical Simulation of Wrinkles. Surgical formation of facial wrinkles is achieved by the deliberate placing of an incision so that the healed, and possibly stretched, scar will simulate a natural crease, fold, or furrow, and by fixation of the dermis to the underlying muscle transplants. The purposeful fostering of "scar healing" in incisions placed to represent wrinkles corresponding to those on the nonparalyzed side of the face is another method (Frackelton, 1952). The incision is allowed to heal spontaneously. Although this is considered of value on the bland, smooth, palsied forehead, it would seem preferable to reduce the wrinkling on the unaffected side to match the youthful appearance of the paralyzed half by the technique of sectioning the corrugator conjoint muscle complex and freeing the skin from the frontalis muscle.

Correction of Palpebral Deformities and the Relief of Epiphora. Paralysis of the orbicularis oculi muscle or lagophthalmos involves all three of the portions of the muscle, i.e., the pretarsal, the preseptal, and the orbicular, and its early correction is important. The tight closure of the eye is lost, the lower lid droops away from the globe and becomes everted, and impaired drainage, pooling, and epiphora add to the classic houndlike eye.

Kazanjian and Converse (1974) have outlined the variety of reasons for epiphora in facial paralysis. "The paralyzed orbicularis muscle cannot dilate the lacrimal sac; due to the relaxation of the eyelid, the punctum is not in contact with the eyeball and is often stenosed; the caruncle which is exposed by the lagophthalmos becomes hypertrophied; the tear lake lies in the middle of the sagging lid and away from the canthi; increased lacrimal secretion due to exposure. . . . Interference with normal drainage leads to increased loss of tears by evaporation, thus the need for increased activity of the lacrimal gland."

Methods are available for both temporary and permanent palsies. A grouping of techniques may be established to include: (1) various medial and lateral canthoplasties (Figs. 36–43 and 36–44; (2) passive elevation of the lid by fascial Silastic bands or slings or a dermal flap; (3) temporalis muscle transfer; (4) tensing the flaccid cheek by a face-lifting operation and corrective blepharoplasties; (5) improving drainage by dilatation of the punctum and increasing the size of the punctum of the canaliculus. Effective techniques are illustrated and are simple and rapid. The McLaughlin overlapping lateral tarsorrhaphy outlined in Figure 36–45 is preferred. It does not preclude a later temporalis muscle transfer after the method of Gillies and Millard (1957), as modified by Andersen (1961), and illustrated in Figure 36–30. Temporalis muscle transfer is effective but can produce a backward distortion of the lateral portions of the lids, a distinct limitation of the technique.

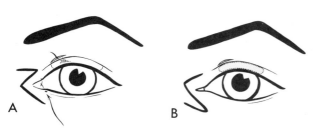

A   B

FIGURE 36–43. Medial canthoplasty for correction of epiphora. Z transposition flaps *(A)* roll back the exposed, everted punctum *(arrow)* into contact with the globe and narrow the area of exposed caruncle and the canthus, producing an effective functional and cosmetic improvement *(B)*. The incision in the upper lid along the creaseline, through skin and muscle, permits a channel to be developed into which is slipped a suitable weight. The weight, which overcomes the relaxed levator and allows the eye to close, can also stretch the thin, atrophic skin, making a corrective blepharoplasty advisable.

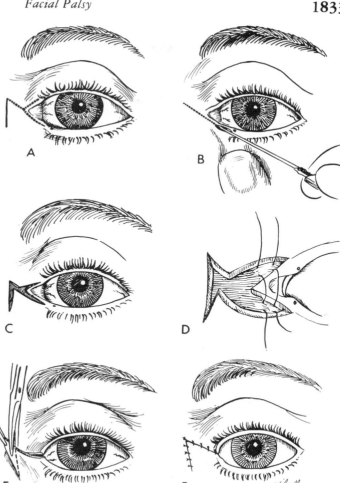

FIGURE 36–44. Medial canthoplasty which places the everted punctum against the globe and tightens a moderately sagging lower lid. *A*, The outline of the incisions. *B*, A probe is placed in the canaliculus in order to avoid severing this structure. *C*, After completion of incisions. *D*, The edges of the medial canthus are sutured by means of inverting sutures. *E*, Traction is placed on the skin flap, and excess skin is removed. *F*, The skin incision is sutured. (From Kazanjian and Converse.)

A useful and relatively simple method is the dermal flap technique (Edgerton and Wolfort, 1969). The lateral portion of the skin of the lower lid is deepithelized, and a dermal flap is prepared and introduced into a subcutaneous tunnel lateral to the palpebral fissure, placed under traction, and sutured to the periosteum.

In neglected cases, dilatation of the punctum is valueless. Formation of a triangular new ostium is more successful and permanent. This is

FIGURE 36–45. Lateral tarsorrhaphy. By removal of a triangle of the conjunctiva of the upper lid and of the skin and cilia of the lower lid, two tarsal surfaces are approximated with a mattress suture. This effectively narrows the palpebral fissure, elevates the lower lid sufficiently for protection, yet maintains an acceptable cosmetic result with a minimum of surgery.

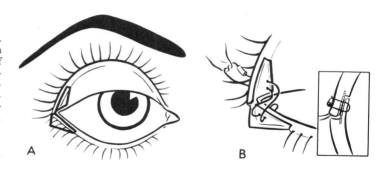

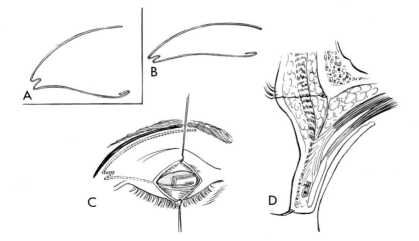

FIGURE 36–46. The palpebral spring in the treatment of paralysis of the eyelid (technique of Morel-Fatio). *A, B,* Stainless steel wire formed in the shape of a "W." *C,* Dacron felt covering over the doubled lower end. Note incisions. *D,* Cross-sectional view. (Figs. 36–46 to 36–48 after Morel-Fatio.)

merely an enlargement of the punctum by a sharp pair of scissors, cutting a 2-mm triangle out of the sides of the duct.

Eversion must be corrected by one of the adjunct procedures shown, so that the new opening drains the lake adequately. The fascial sling is described earlier in the chapter in the section describing fascial transplants; the temporalis muscle transfer is discussed in the section on muscle transfer.

In facial paralysis involving the orbicularis oculi muscle, gravity acts to close the eye when the levator muscle relaxes in sleep. Two original methods for the correction of the upper palpebral paralysis use metallic implants to compensate for the muscular deficiency. Morel-Fatio and Lalardrie (1962) used a stainless steel wire spring inserted into the upper lid. Increasing the weight of the upper lids by metallic implants is an alternative.

Palpebral Spring for Lid Palsy: The Technique of Morel-Fatio (1974). A round, 0.3-mm stainless steel wire formed into a figure "W" (Fig. 36–46, *A*) is measured directly on the lid at the time of surgery. The upper arm of the spring and the upper portion of the central bend of the "W" are fixed to the orbital aponeurosis with eight small caliber Teflon sutures. The lower branch of the spring is set in place under the muscles through a vertical incision of the muscles. A most important innovation, as compared with the original description, is the method of attaching the lower branch of the spring to the lid. It was the experience of many surgeons that sutures through the lower spring eventually tore through the

muscles. Therefore, the distal end of the lower branch is *not* sutured. Alternatively, it is bent on itself so that the "U"-shaped end of the wire lies in front of and directly on top of the tarsus at the junction of the inner and outer two-thirds. A small space (5 × 4 mm) corresponding to the size of the doubled end is pre-

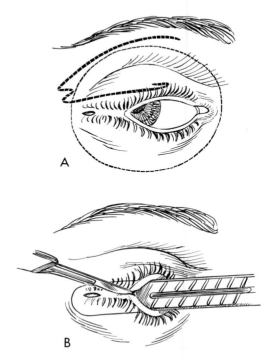

FIGURE 36–47. The use of the palpebral spring when a tarsorrhaphy is present. *A,* Initial position of the spring. *B,* Tarsorrhaphy is divided at a later date.

pared. A flattened sheet of Dacron felt is folded over the doubled lower end and is cut to fit exactly the 5- × 4-mm space. A suture can be placed through the Dacron to maintain the wrap, which is then buried beneath the muscles and closed by fine sutures. The lower border of the Dacron envelope is placed no closer than 3 mm from the ciliary border. The skin incision is closed separately. As will also be seen in the drawings (Fig. 36–47), should a tarsorrhaphy be in position at the time of surgery, the spring is set in place, and a month later adjustment of the spring may be completed and the tarsorrhaphy taken down. As Morel-Fatio (1974) stated, "the spring must exactly fit the dimensions of the orbit and lid, as well as its curvature (both vertical and horizontal) which must accurately correspond to the eyeball shape. It is difficult to adjust perfectly and this can only be done by a surgeon in the operating room" (Fig. 36–48). The clinical application of the Morel-Fatio spring is illustrated in Figure 36–49.

Morel-Fatio (1975) reported his results in 72 cases: 27 secondary operations were required; 11 complications occurred (5 springs broke; 2 springs were extruded; infection occurred in 4 cases); in 5 cases the spring was deliberately removed. Guy's (1974) experience, using a slightly different technique, is the following: in a series of 24 patients, 6 were removed; 8 required minor adjustments, and 18 were still functioning after three years.

Upper Lid Loading in Lagophthalmos. Increasing the weight of the upper lid permits the lid to fall when the levator is relaxed. A submuscular tantalum implant has been utilized by the author for the past 30 years, in patients with temporary and permanent lagophthalmos caused by facial paralysis, both as a single procedure or in conjunction with complementary procedures such as tarsorrhaphy. The operation is simple; the implant can be changed or removed as an office procedure.

Accentuation of gravity by a weight in the lid was described by Sheehan (1927) in his book, *Plastic Surgery of the Orbit*, in which he recommended the use of stainless steel mesh in the upper lid. During World War II tantalum, which is malleable, became available. It is nonreactive, can be readily fashioned during the operation, and has proved to be useful. The upper lid weight is increased by implanting a tantalum strip of 0.75 g. Cronin achieved similar results with a lead strip. Nonetheless, the

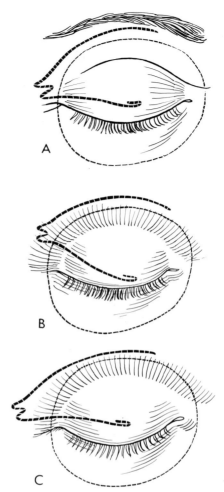

FIGURE 36–48. Some abnormalities of the spring requiring adjustments. *A*, Projection of the spring on the lid and limits of the orbital rim. *B*, The external "W" is high and the inferior branch is vertical, limiting the opening of the lid and possibly causing extrusion. *C*, The "W" is placed too far laterally; the range of motion is limited in opening and in closing; a fold appears above the lateral canthus.

various implants of gold seem to provide a better color match for white patients and have been commercially prepared* (Jobe, 1974). The author's preference is given to a somewhat larger prosthesis easily fashioned by a dental laboratory (Fig. 36–50). Nonetheless, the atrophic skin and muscle may sag, and the excess skin often requires later adjustment by blepharoplasty.

---

*Heyer Schulte Corporation.

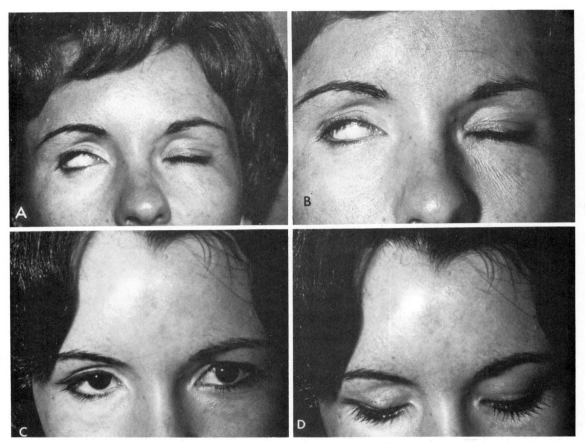

FIGURE 36–49. Morel-Fatio spring. *A*, Preoperative appearance. *B*, Close-up preoperative appearance. *C*, Postoperative—eyes opened. *D*, Postoperative—eyes closed. (Courtesy of Dr. D. Morel-Fatio.)

Through a transverse incision in the supratarsal fold extended to the tarsus, a pocket is dissected to the lid margin. A piece of tantalum plate (0.4 mm thick and measuring 8 mm × 15 mm) is folded on itself, bent to conform to the curvature of the globe, and, with its sharp edges filed smooth, is inserted into the pocket, and the wound is closed (Fig. 36–51). Atrophy of the muscle, stretching of the skin, and aging all combine to cause skin redundancy. Because

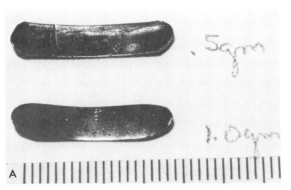
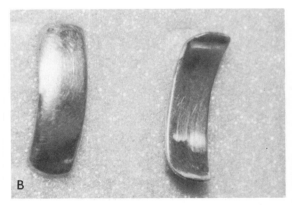

FIGURE 36–50. Upper lid implants. *A*, Implants hand-fashioned in the operating room out of tantalum. *B*, Gold implants weighing approximately 1.0 gram. The former can be altered; the latter cannot be changed.

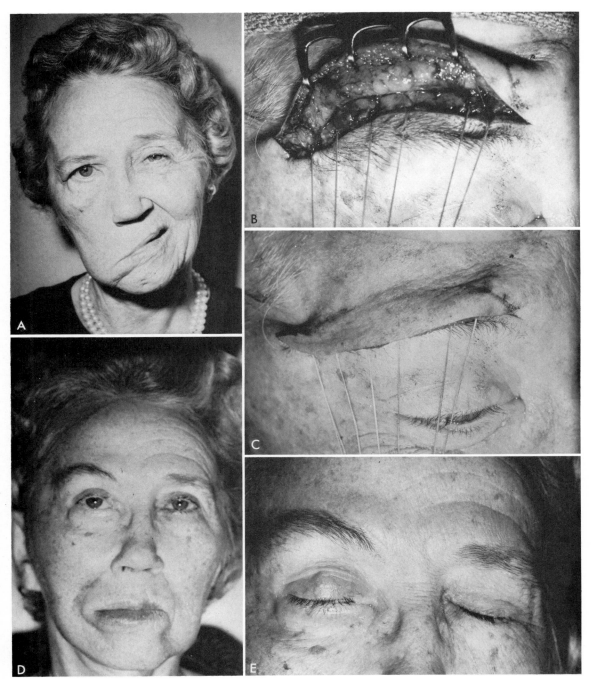

FIGURE 36–51. Upper lid weight, lower lid Silastic suspension, brow-lift, and fascial sling to the face and lips. *A,* Twenty years untreated, unilateral facial paralysis. *B,* Brow-lift—the dermis is secured to the pericranium. *C,* Brow-lift—the redundant tissue of the forehead is excised. *D,* After a lower lid Silastic band suspension, an upper lid weight, a brow-lift, and a massive fascial implant (in repose). *E,* Eyelids closed.

of these factors a submuscular, supratarsal, and supralimbal implant insertion is indicated for a continued satisfactory result. A simple skin excision blepharoplasty may be necessary several years later.

The technique is associated with some problems: unreliability in the recumbent position and differences in lid weights required by individual patients. Long-term evaluation of the method is also lacking.

Lid Magnets. Mühlbauer, Segeth and Viessmann (1973) have implanted two miniaturized, siliconized curved magnets beneath the orbicularis muscle near the upper and lower eyelid margins. The tarsal plates prevent erosion of the rods into the conjunctival sacs. The magnetic force employed in the open eye position for the double magnet system was 200 to 300 m p, and this corresponds to the lost muscle tone of the orbicularis muscle, thus preventing upper lid retraction, corneal irritation and epiphora. Normal lid opening is maintained by the intact levator mechanism.

Initially the lid magnets are taped to the lid margins to determine the ideal magnet force. When this is established, the lid magnets are implanted under local anesthesia.

Silastic Rod Reconstruction of the Paralyzed Eyelid. Preliminary to, or in place of, static or dynamic support, elastic support of the paralyzed lower lid can be obtained by using a narrow Silastic band or rod secured to the nasal periosteum, threaded through the lower lid, and fastened to the lateral orbital periosteum and temporal fascia.

In patients with partial and complete paralysis of the lower lid, the simple band elevates the lateral aspect of the lid, holds the lid conjunctiva against the globe, and improves the appearance. All of the prostheses eventually break, and this is not to be regarded as a permanent reconstructive procedure (Freeman, 1969).

This rapid procedure can be accomplished at the completion of a prolonged operation for unilateral facial paralysis to maintain the normal upward slant of the lower lid (from the inner canthus outward), to bring the lid margin and punctum in contact with the bulbar conjunctiva, and to redirect the flow of tears medially. The procedure, initially used to produce tunnels for later dynamic support of the face, to lessen adhesions, and to increase the excursion after muscle transplant, resulted in temporary

improvement in lid elevation. Despite the author's distrust for superficially placed inorganic material under tension, the technique is selected for older patients who require associated extensive reconstructive operations and for younger patients as an elastic assist with partial paralysis of the lower lid.

Technique. With the patient's head erect, the normal positions of the lateral canthus and of the nasal attachment of the lid are marked. While the local anesthetic is taking effect, the punctum is dilated, and a small lacrimal probe is inserted into the canaliculus; this is left in place during surgery.

A 1-cm incision in the crease lines of the lateral nasal wall allows dissection through the orbicularis muscle to the periosteum. A similar incision over the upper portion of the lateral orbital rim, above the lateral canthus, is also extended to the periosteum. A submuscular pocket, or tunnel, from incision to incision is dissected, through which a narrow (1.5 mm O.D.) Silastic rod is threaded. Two 5–0 Prolene sutures firmly secured to the nasal periosteum are tied over the rod, and similar sutures are inserted into the periosteum at the lateral orbital rim (and occasionally in the temporal fascia as well). The band is carefully tensed so that the lid hangs correctly; the sutures are serially tied over the Silastic rubber rod. The wounds are irrigated and closed.

One must avoid cutting the Silastic tube or rod with the suture, causing extensive tension (which would press the lid too tightly against the globe), and damaging the canaliculus while burrowing. The patient is told of the probability of later surgery and of the necessity of later substitution of the Silastic rod by autogenous tissue.

A word of caution as to the potential physical changes in the Silastic rod is necessary. Spontaneous fracture has occurred, and section of the medial canthal tendon has been observed. This latter complication necessitates attachment to the nasal bone through drill holes.

CIRCUMORBITAL SILASTIC STRING RECONSTRUCTION OF THE ORBICULARIS SPHINCTER. Arion (1972) has been able to maintain the orbicularis sphincter with a circumorbital Silastic string, and his technique has been modified by Wood-Smith (1973), as shown in Figure 36–52.

TECHNIQUE. After infiltration with local anesthesia, a horizontal incision is made in the lateral canthal area over the lateral orbital rim;

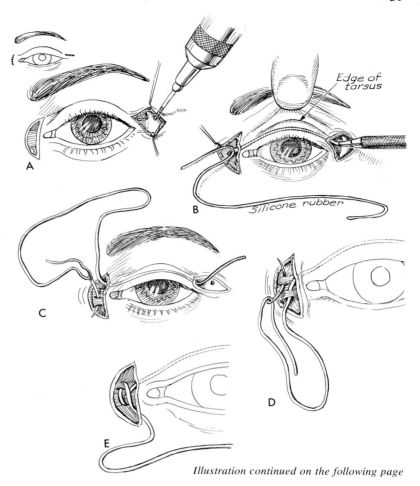

FIGURE 36–52. Construction of an orbicularis sphincter by a circumorbital Silastic string—technique of Arion (courtesy of Dr. D. Wood-Smith). Illustrations show a technique of threading a fine Silastic band around the lids. The band is sutured to the medial canthal tendon and secured to the lateral orbital rim by a dacron suture passed through a drill hole. The technique is performed under local anesthesia, as the cooperation of the patient in adjusting tension is essential. The small vertical incision over the medial canthal tendon and the small horizontal incision over the lateral orbital rim are closed with fine nylon sutures. Note the special instrument used to pass the Silastic string through the upper and lower eyelids. (From Kazanjian and Converse, 1974.)

Illustration continued on the following page

a vertical incision is made over the medial canthal tendon, and the latter is skeletonized (Fig. 36–52, *A*). The Silastic string is passed through the upper lid after a special instrument is passed in a subcutaneous position at the edge of the tarsus (Fig. 36–52, *B*). With a Mayo needle the Silastic string is interwoven in the medial canthal tendon (Fig. 36–52, *C, D, E*) and later passed in a subciliary position through the lower eyelid (Fig. 36–52, *F*). Both ends are secured to a Dacron suture passed through a drill hole in the lateral orbital rim (Fig. 36–52, *G, H*) after adjustment of tension is made with the cooperation of the patient. The wounds are approximated with 6–0 nylon sutures.

Rousso (1975) reported a 15 per cent incidence of extrusion at the medial canthus as well as loosening and breakage of the prosthesis. Wood-Smith (1976) stated that 9 per cent of the prostheses require removal and replacement.

EXTERNAL MECHANICAL SUPPORT FOR FACIAL PARALYSIS

External mechanical aids, while employed by the ancients, find little application in the present day. A restraining hook set in the depressed angle of the mouth can be supported from a loop around the ear, by a leather, plastic, or plaster headdress, or a dental attachment. Similar elevators for lids can be attached to eyeglasses. Bands of adhesive strapping, or collodion strips, presently used postoperatively to splint the facial muscles, have been advocated for lifting the everted ptotic lower lid, or for restraining the edematous, sagging lip. These temporary measures are inferior to the simple surgical maneuvers suggested earlier in the text.

Appliances are of value at times, and mention should be made of the Chicago lawyer

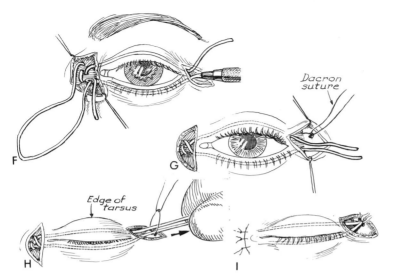

Dacron suture

Edge of tarsus

FIGURE 36–52 *Continued.*

who effectively disguised his lower facial paralysis with a tightly clenched pipe jutting out of the angle of his mouth; the female dentist who never relinquished her long cigarette holder; and the East Texas farmer with the matchstick toothpick in his molars for 25 years, obscuring a pronounced facial paralysis.

In general, mechanical support is useless and harmful for the skin, does not prevent the overstretching of the paralyzed muscles, and is of little practical importance. Occasionally in excessive tearing in older people, the severe epiphora can be alleviated by supporting the lower lid with strapping, or oral drooling can be helped by elastic strapping of the mouth.

UNUSUAL RESIDUALS OF FACIAL PARALYSIS

Injury to the facial nerve proximal to the geniculate ganglion may misdirect fibers, which normally would be directed to the submaxillary gland through the chorda tympani nerve, to the lacrimal gland through the greater superficial petrosal nerve. As a result of this change, the patient lacrimates when eating. This phenomenon, known as the "crocodile tear" syndrome, or *paradoxical lacrimation,* can be treated by dividing the greater superficial petrosal nerve (Boyer and Gardiner, 1949).

Spasmodic contraction of the muscles of the face is observed infrequently after lacerations of the facial nerve, but may be rather severe and most marked around the angle of the mouth, or the eyelids. This is often observed when recovery after nerve injury is delayed and imperfect. The spastic twitching may be rhythmical, but is usually irregular and increased by excitement and fear. Ehni and Woltman (1945) described the condition, and Greenwood (1946) outlined the surgical treatment by partial selective neurectomy.

It has been shown that not all of the axons at the proximal end of the damaged nerve regenerate and that each regenerating axon subdivides into several fibers. The orientation of these fibers differs frequently from the original pattern (Young and Sanders, 1942). This phenomenon accounts for the mass action and irregular action of the involved facial muscles, as well as the synergistic action of unrelated muscles which can occur after severance and repair.

Autogenous Muscle Grafts in the Reconstruction of the Paralyzed Face

NOEL THOMPSON, F.R.C.S.

The principles of free autogenous skeletal muscle grafting are discussed in Chapter 11. There are three prerequisites: prior denervation of the muscle, intimate contact with the host muscle for neurotization of the muscle graft, and preservation of full fiber length of the muscle graft.

TREATMENT OF EYELID PARALYSIS

Ipsilateral Temporalis Muscle Reinnervation of the Graft. The procedure is simple and effective in relieving disabling epiphora and corneal exposure. Because the resulting eyelid closure is unrelated to closure of the contralateral unaffected eyelids, it is reserved for elderly or infirm patients. Using a preauricular-temporal incision on the paralyzed side of the face, the temporalis muscle is exposed after reflecting the anterior skin forward and widely raising the temporal fascia (Fig. 36–53). By blunt, subcutaneous, scissors dissection from within the wound, the eyelid margins are undermined to allow the tendons of two of the bellies of a previously denervated extensor digitorum brevis muscle graft to be passed subcutaneously to reach the medial canthal tendon. At this point, through a small medial canthal incision, the two tendons of the transplant are firmly anchored to the canthal tendon by nonabsorbable sutures. The two muscle bellies of the transplant are aligned so that the higher belly pulls on the lower lid and vice versa. The muscle grafts are sutured in direct contact with the exposed fibers of the tem-

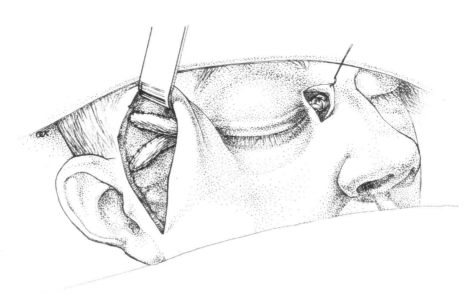

FIGURE 36–53. The use of grafts of the extensor digitorum brevis muscle, applied to the temporalis muscle on the paralyzed side. Reinnervation of the grafts after three to six months results in the restoration of eyelid closure in response to temporalis muscle contraction. (From Thompson, N.: Treatment of facial paralysis by free skeletal muscle grafts. Transactions of the Fifth International Congress of Plastic and Reconstructive Surgery. Australia, Butterworth, 1971.)

1841

poralis muscle. Positioning of the graft is planned to produce slight positive tension on the tendons inserted into the adjacent eyelids. The temporal wound is sutured with drainage.

Contralateral Orbicularis Oculi Muscle for Reinnervation of Graft.

If voluntary, synchronous, and bilateral closure of the eyelids is desired, the tendons of the transplant acting on the paralyzed eyelids must be activated by a muscle graft innervated by the normal (contralateral) orbicularis oculi muscle. In such a case, because of the delicacy of the neuromuscular mechanism being reconstructed and the maximal mechanical efficiency desired, it is essential that both the muscle and the tendon of

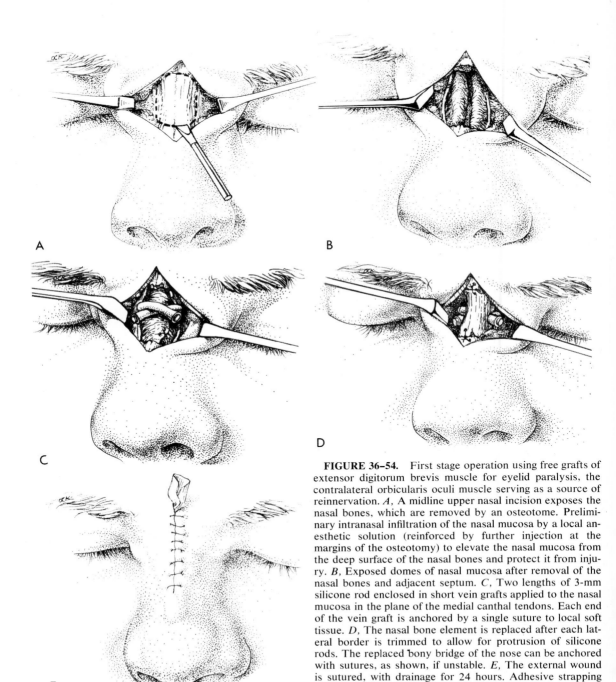

FIGURE 36–54. First stage operation using free grafts of extensor digitorum brevis muscle for eyelid paralysis, the contralateral orbicularis oculi muscle serving as a source of reinnervation. *A*, A midline upper nasal incision exposes the nasal bones, which are removed by an osteotome. Preliminary intranasal infiltration of the nasal mucosa by a local anesthetic solution (reinforced by further injection at the margins of the osteotomy) to elevate the nasal mucosa from the deep surface of the nasal bones and protect it from injury. *B*, Exposed domes of nasal mucosa after removal of the nasal bones and adjacent septum. *C*, Two lengths of 3-mm silicone rod enclosed in short vein grafts applied to the nasal mucosa in the plane of the medial canthal tendons. Each end of the vein graft is anchored by a single suture to local soft tissue. *D*, The nasal bone element is replaced after each lateral border is trimmed to allow for protrusion of silicone rods. The replaced bony bridge of the nose can be anchored with sutures, as shown, if unstable. *E*, The external wound is sutured, with drainage for 24 hours. Adhesive strapping retains a light dressing.

the transplant should function in the plane of the eyelids.

In the first stage, which is completed at the time of denervation of the extensor digitorum brevis muscle of the foot, removal of the nasal bony bridge and the subjacent septum and preparation of a bed for the transplanted tendons are also completed (Fig. 36–54). This was originally achieved (Thompson, 1971) by replacing nasal mucosa at this site by a small,

median forehead, subcutaneous island flap, as used by Converse and Wood-Smith (1963) for the repair of upper nasal defects. With increasing experience, this has proved unnecessary. By carefully infiltrating the mucosa intranasally with local anesthetic solution in the region of the bony nasal bridge and adjacent septum, one can almost invariably preserve the nasal mucosa intact. Even if it is damaged, it is to such a limited degree that it can readily be

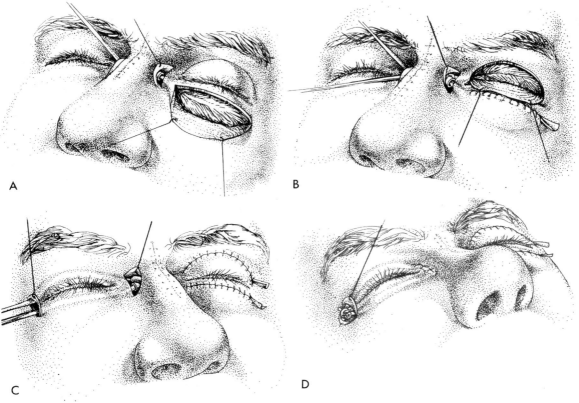

A

B

C

D

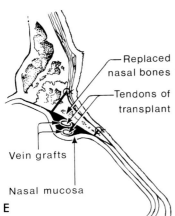

Replaced nasal bones

Tendons of transplant

Vein grafts

Nasal mucosa

E

FIGURE 36–55. Second stage operation: transplanting the extensor digitorum brevis muscle grafts to the contralateral orbicularis oculi muscle for reactivation of the paralyzed eyelids. *A,* The lower eyelid skin and underlying orbicularis oculi muscle (on the unparalyzed side) are reflected as a composite musculocutaneous flap. Any underlying fat deposits are removed, and the muscle graft of extensor digitorum brevis is sutured directly to the orbicularis oculi muscle. Its associated tendon is railroaded through one of the transnasal grafts after the silicone rod spacer is removed. *B,* The upper eyelid is similarly managed by raising the orbicularis oculi muscle with the skin flap and by suturing the belly of the muscle graft to it. The two tendons of the graft are crossed where they lie inside the vein grafts behind the nasal bone. Both muscle grafts are drained. *C,* The two tendons of the graft are passed subcutaneously along the eyelid margins on the paralyzed side; the upper tendon lies at the upper border of the tarsal plate, and the lower tendon lies at the margin of the lower eyelid. *D,* Anchoring the tendon of the grafts to the lateral canthal tendon of the paralyzed eyelids. *E,* Diagrammatic sagittal section showing the tendons of the transplants lying inside the ensheathing vein grafts (after removal of the silicone rod spacers), behind the replaced nasal bones, and lying on the nasal mucosa.

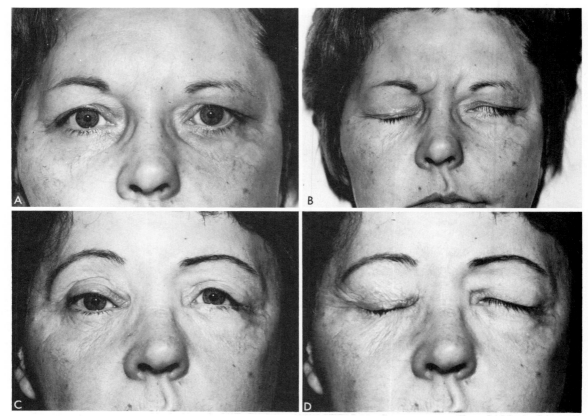

FIGURE 36–56. Woman, aged 42. Complete left facial paralysis of 15 years' duration. Lateral tarsorrhaphy had been done earlier. *A*, Preoperative (repose). *B*, Preoperative (on closing the eyes). *C*, Postoperative, five years after transplantation of the extensor digitorum brevis muscles to the eyelids and release of the tarsorrhaphy. At rest. *D*, Five years postoperative. Voluntary eyelid closure.

repaired by one or two absorbable sutures. Two short lengths of silicone rod (3 mm in diameter) are used as "spacers" for future replacement by the tendons of the grafts; in the past these have been ensheathed in a tube of silicone sheet. However, experience has shown that, if this sheet is left permanently as a sheath for the future tendons, the graft is susceptible to late infection. At the suggestion of Hakelius (1973), the silicone tubes have been replaced by two small vein grafts, one over each silicone rod. The vein grafts are obtained by stripping 10-cm segments of the long saphenous vein from the ankle region at the same time as the extensor digitorum brevis muscles are denervated.

At a second stage two weeks later, when the extensor digitorum brevis muscle is removed from the foot for transplantation to the face, the skin and underlying orbicularis oculi muscle are reflected downward as a musculocutaneous flap from each eyelid on the normal side (Fig. 36–55). Any herniation of orbital fat through the orbital septum is removed. In each eyelid, a suitable muscle graft is sutured to the orbicularis oculi, and the associated tendons in continuity are passed through the transnasal vein grafts after removal of the silicone rods. By blunt subcutaneous dissection along the paralyzed eyelid margins, they are anchored under slight but definite positive tension to the lateral canthal tendon on the paralyzed side. The larger muscle graft is applied to the lower eyelid on the normal side to act on the upper eyelid of the paralyzed side. A patient who underwent this procedure is illustrated in Figure 36–56.

TREATMENT OF ORAL PARALYSIS

Reconstruction of the Oral Sphincter. Using the palmaris longus muscle and its associated tendon (or a combination of multiple bellies of the extensor digitorum brevis muscle together

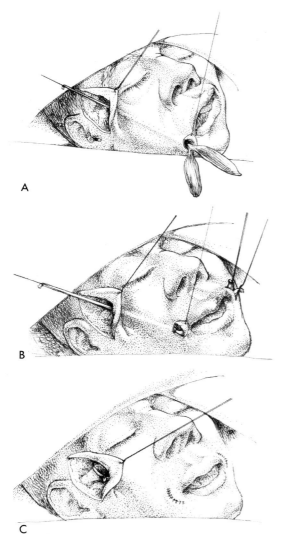

tendon is preserved. A preauricular-temporal incision on the paralyzed side is employed to obtain access to the zygomatic arch. By blunt scissors dissection, a subcutaneous tunnel is made to reach a small skin incision at the angle of the mouth; through this tunnel the tendon of the palmaris longus muscle transplant is advanced into the temporal wound. A similar technique is used to undermine widely the skin of the upper and lower lips in a plane superficial to the orbicularis oris muscle, from the angle of the mouth on the paralyzed side to the contralateral angle, where a third small skin incision is made. Each half of the muscle transplant is drawn subcutaneously along the full extent of each lip in order to surround the oral aperture completely. The muscles are firmly sutured with nonabsorbable sutures to the deep tissues at each angle of the mouth; this maneuver preserves normal tension in the muscle graft, even when traction is exerted upon the associated tendon. The two perioral incisions are closed, and the distal end of the palmaris longus tendon is slung around the zygomatic arch, firmly tightened to overcorrect the sagging facial musculature on the paralyzed side, and solidly anchored in position. Drainage of the muscle grafts is by a suction drain inserted down the track of the tendon and into the lips (or, alternatively, small local drains inserted through the oral angular incisions) for 48 hours. Pressure upon the grafts by external adhesive strapping is maintained for five days. Reinnervation of the transplanted muscle occurs from the orbicularis oris muscle of the normal side and progressively advances along the length of the transplant on the paralyzed side.

The reanimation of the face reconstructed following excision of maxillofacial cancer evidently represents a useful application of the autogenous free muscle graft. This technique applies particularly to reconstruction of the eyelids and mouth (Fig. 36–58).

Reconstruction of Totally Paralyzed Elevators of the Angle of the Mouth. Reconstruction of the elevators of the angle of the mouth may be most readily achieved by applying the muscle graft to the ipsilateral temporalis muscle, passing its attached tendon subcutaneously so that it can be attached to the oral region at the paralyzed angle of the mouth (usually by splitting the terminal tendon and passing it subcutaneously along the upper and lower lips before suturing it to the musculature of the unparalyzed lips just beyond the midline).

FIGURE 36–57. The use of a graft of palmaris longus muscle with its tendon to reconstruct the oral sphincter in a case of unilateral right facial paralysis. *A,* The palmaris muscle belly is split and its tendon in continuity brought up to the zygomatic region on the paralyzed side. *B,* Each half of the palmaris muscle belly is passed subcutaneously along the full width of the upper and lower lips to encircle the mouth in contact with the orbicularis oris muscle. The muscle graft is anchored deeply at each angle of the mouth. *C,* The suspensory palmaris tendon is secured to the zygomatic arch. (From Thompson, N.: Treatment of facial paralysis by free skeletal muscle grafts. Transactions of the Fifth International Congress of Plastic and Reconstructive Surgery. Australia, Butterworth, 1971.).

with a plantaris or long toe extensor tendon), the muscle belly of the transplant is split longitudinally in the line of its fibers into two equal halves (Fig. 36–57). The attachment to the

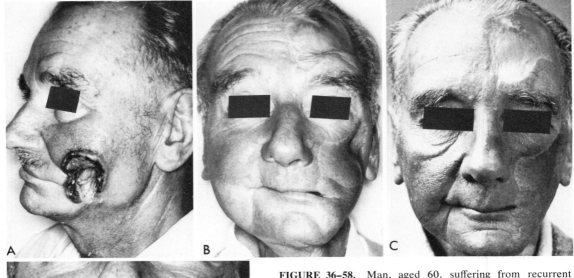

FIGURE 36–58. Man, aged 60, suffering from recurrent buccal carcinoma with a bucco-oral fistula and radionecrosis of the left mandible. *A*, Preoperative appearance. *B*, Appearance following radical excision of the left cheek, including lateral one-third of the mouth, left hemimandibulectomy, partial left maxillectomy, and block dissection of neck with simultaneous repair of the soft tissue using a temporal-forehead flap as buccal lining and upper chest flap as covering. A rib graft was later used to reconstruct the left mandible. Incompetence of the oral sphincter with severe dribbling persisted. *C*, Appearance following dermis-fat graft to correct the cheek contour two years after a muscle graft (with tendon sling to the left zygomatic bone) to reconstruct the oral sphincter. *D*, Appearance on pursing lips. Complete control of dribbling.

Although positive animation of the paralyzed angle of the mouth usually results, its elevation is produced by contracting the temporalis muscle (as during mastication), producing a bizarre and uncoordinated movement of the mouth region as a whole. It is therefore preferable to restore activity of a less vigorous but more bilaterally symmetrical character by the somewhat more complicated method that uses the cross-zygomaticus muscle graft (Fig. 36–59). Synchronous elevation of the angles of the mouth, as in smiling or grimacing, can be achieved to an appreciable degree by harnessing contraction of the zygomaticus major muscle on the normal side to produce elevation of the paralyzed angle of the mouth, using a palmaris longus muscle-tendon free graft for the purpose.

A nasolabial incision is used to gain access to the zygomaticus major and levator anguli oris muscles of the normal side, and a small incision is made at the angle of the mouth on the paralyzed side. The palmaris longus muscle is sutured in direct contact with the zygomaticus muscles of the normal side, the musculotendinous junction being firmly anchored to the angle of the mouth region by buried sutures. From this point blunt scissors dissection is used to prepare a subcutaneous tunnel traversing the width of the upper lip to reach the angle of the mouth region on the paralyzed side, where the tendon extremity is firmly anchored.

When reinnervation of the muscle graft has occurred approximately three months later, at a second operation a nasolabial incision is used on the paralyzed side to gain access to the already inserted tendon near the paralyzed angle of the mouth. The tendon is advanced to a drill hole in the zygomatic process of the maxilla by a small tendon sling (of plantaris or toe extensor tendon), which is tightened to overcorrect slightly the sag of the paralyzed musculature. The tendon sling is best inserted during a separate procedure after muscle graft reinnervation

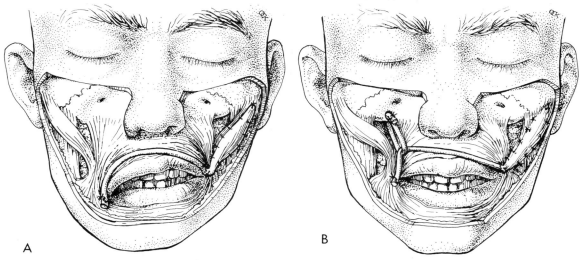

FIGURE 36–59. The "cross-zygomaticus" muscle graft to restore movement to the paralyzed angle of the mouth. Two operations are required after the initial denervation of the muscle graft. *A*, Stage 1. Palmaris longus muscle graft sutured to the zygomaticus muscles of the (left) normal side and its tendon railroaded subcutaneously to be anchored to the deep tissues at the paralyzed (right) angle of mouth. *B*, Stage 2. The palmaris longus tendon is advanced up to a drill hole in the maxilla by another tendon graft to elevate the paralyzed right angle of the mouth and allow transmission of the pull from the reinnervated muscle graft.

has occurred in order to limit adhesion formation between the palmaris tendon and the tendon sling.

It should be noted that the degree of movement restored to the paralyzed oral angle is inevitably limited due to the complexity of the mechanical arrangements necessarily made for the transmission of traction from the normal to the paralyzed side (Fig. 36–60).

Reconstruction of Partially Paralyzed Elevators of the Angle of the Mouth. In cases of in-

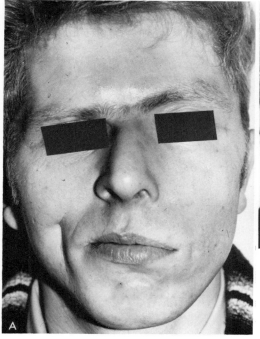

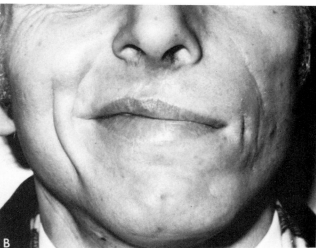

FIGURE 36–60. Man, aged 28, with congenital left-sided facial paralysis (complete). *A,* Preoperative, at rest. *B,* Postoperative, three years after "cross-zygomaticus" transplantation of the palmaris longus muscle to restore elevation to the angle of the mouth. On smiling, there is a degree of symmetrical, bilateral animation.

completely recovered Bell's palsy, it is not unusual to have persistent weakness of the elevators of the angle of the mouth on the affected side. If clinical examination (accompanied by electromyographic investigation in cases of doubt) shows survival of contractile activity in the levator anguli oris and zygomaticus muscles, these muscles may be reinforced by applying to them a muscle graft of extensor hallucis brevis. The graft gives static support to the drooping angle of the mouth as the tendon is passed subcutaneously to be anchored to the temporal fascia. In such a case, reinnervation of the muscle graft occurs from a host muscle which is itself partially denervated. However, improved muscle activity at the graft site becomes demonstrable by electromyography after three to six months.

Hakelius (1974) reported that in 23 of 28 free autogenous muscle grafts performed according to the technique of Thompson, facial muscle function was restored to a satisfactory degree.

Harii, Ohmori and Torii (1976) have presented preliminary results with a free gracilis muscle transplant with microneurovascular anastomosis for the treatment of facial palsy.

Reconstruction of the Face Through Cross-Face Nerve Transplantation in Facial Paralysis

HANS ANDERL, M.D.

A true reanimation of the face following facial paralysis can be accomplished, in the event of a definite break in continuity, only through reconstruction of the facial nerve by means of a nerve suture, or in the case of a nerve defect, through a nerve graft. This has been repeatedly confirmed by numerous authors since the report of Bunnell in 1927 (Martin, 1931; Ballance and Duel, 1932; Bunnell, 1937; Lathrop, 1953, 1956; Conley, 1957; Wullstein, 1958; Miehlke, 1960a, b, 1961; Miehlke and Buske, 1967; Pulec, 1966, 1969; House and Crabtree, 1966; Fisch, 1969).

Even with this type of surgical treatment, a natural reanimation of the face is not always totally possible and certainly cannot be accomplished by substitute operations.

For this type of nerve reconstruction, the facial nerve roots must be intact and the muscle must be capable of regeneration.

The method developed by Dott (1958) for extreme cases of facial palsy involves a major procedure, with extratemporal nerve transplant bridging following trepanation and intracranial anastomosis. Moreover, the validity of the preoperative judgment as to the usability of the facial nerve roots is uncertain, especially after removal of large neuromas of the eighth nerve (Olivecrona, 1967). The spinocervical anastomoses, with hypoglossal, spinal accessory, and glossopharyngeal cranial nerves, which are still recommended because of the relative simplicity with which they can be performed, can activate the paralyzed muscles and occasionally achieve facial symmetry.

Arbitrary innervation, however, almost always results in unnatural facial muscle action and loss of normal facial expression.

The satisfactory results obtained in the reconstruction of peripheral nerves with microsurgical techniques (Smith, 1966; Millesi, Ganglberger and Berger, 1967; Hakstian, 1968), as well as a few positive experiences with bridging of nerve defects over a wide distance (Sanders, 1954; Martin and Helsper, 1957; Seddon, 1972), have encouraged an attempt to reinnervate the paralyzed muscles by means of intermediate nerve grafts from the various fascicles of the nerve on the unparalyzed side.

The delicate peripheral branching of the fascicles is easily identified and demonstrated and fascicular suturing is possible when the operating room microscope is used. It has been shown that, in the treatment of facial twitches and spasms (Clodius, 1970), entire rows of nerve end branches can be severed without visible functional loss of facial muscles. Indeed, recurrences are not uncommon and thus emphasize the unique regenerative ability of the facial nerves (Conley, 1957).

Experience has shown that, for the performance of such transfacial "cross-face" nerve transplants in facial paralysis, a certain amount of weakening of the muscles of the healthy side is sometimes preferred. This weakening by means of myotomy or myectomy of various muscle groups has been recommended (Niklison, 1956). The basic principle underlying the procedure consists of redirecting a sufficient part of the reservoir of intact nerves from the healthy side toward the paralyzed side by way of nerve transplants.

The most important facial muscle functional zones are supplied in the following manner: (a) a nerve transplant for the orbicularis oculi across the frontal muscles and across the upper portion of the orbicularis oculi; (b) two nerve transplants for the corner of the mouth across the orbicularis oris; and (c) a nerve transplant for the quadratus labii inferioris across the chin muscles.

Smith (1971) first utilized the "cross-face" nerve graft principle. For reconstruction of the facial nerve, he routed a sural nerve transplant through the upper lip from the healthy to the paralyzed side. Two fascicles from the oral plexus on the healthy side were anastomosed with the transplant via a central percutaneous pull-out wire which was threaded through the nerve. The anastomoses on the paralyzed side were accomplished with the buccal plexus in a similar manner. Three to six months after surgery, a certain amount of improvement in the paralysis, especially in terms of facial symmetry, was noted.

Scaramella (1971) used the buccal branch of the facial nerve for anastomosis of a nerve transplant, which he directed via a submandibular route to the other side and connected with the stem of the facial nerve.

ANATOMICAL CONSIDERATIONS

The procedure involves only the peripheral parts of the buccal and zygomatic branches

and, if indicated, a branch of the marginal mandibularis (Kullmann and Cody, 1969). The final area of distribution on the healthy side and location of the main branch of the nerves corresponding to these areas on the paralyzed side are important factors for a successful nerve transplant.

Furthermore, in cross-face nerve transplantation certain sensory branches of the trigeminal nerve, especially the infraorbital, buccal, zygomaticofacial, mentalis, and the above-described juncture with the intact facial nerve, must be taken into consideration (Lathrop, 1953). The positions of the single main branches of the facial nerve, the form of the final distribution, and the plexus formation with the trigeminal nerve vary considerably and cannot be standardized. This problem presents difficulties with localization and dissection (McCormack, Cauldwell and Anson, 1945). After their emergence from the parotid gland, two to three branches usually reach the masseteric fascia directly below the subcutis and accompany the parotid duct to the periphery (the duct can be found on an imaginary line drawn between the antitragus and the corner of the mouth). One to 2 cm anterior to the nasolabial fold, the buccal branches ramify upward and downward into the mouth muscles and en-

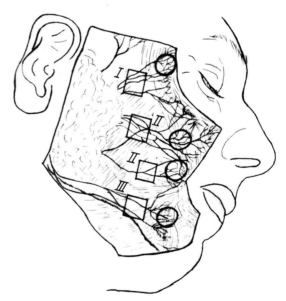

FIGURE 36–61. Main branches of the facial nerve with peripheral area of distribution: I. zygomatic, II. buccal, III. marginal mandibular. The circles indicate the area of juncture of the facial nerve fascicles with the fascicles of the transplant on the unaffected side. The squares indicate the connections of the main branches of the facial nerve with the transplant on the paralyzed side of the face.

ter into an anastomosis with the zygomatic branch in 80 per cent of patients (McCormack and coworkers, 1945; Dingman and Grabb, 1961); in 5 to 12 per cent of patients they combine with the marginal mandibular branch.

The fascicles to be selected for the mouth-cheek connection on the healthy as well as on the affected side are shown in Figure 36–61.

The zygomatic branches, in a formation of two to three parallel and adjacent fine caliber nerves, proceed after emerging from the parotid over the anterior aspect of the zygomatic bone directly under the subcutis in the direction of the upper lateral orbital rim. Single branches supply the orbicularis portion of the lower lids. The interfascicular plexus formation begins approximately above the zygomaticofrontal suture, and at this site the fascicles selected for connection to the healthy side will be principally found (Fig. 36–62).

The marginal mandibular branch in its anterior segment lying on the mental side of the facial artery is always double-layered, so that both nerves lie one above the other and above the lower margin of the mandible. The upper segment of the nerve mainly supplies the orbicularis muscle of the lower lip, while the deeper-lying branch supplies the quadratus labii inferioris and the mentalis muscle.

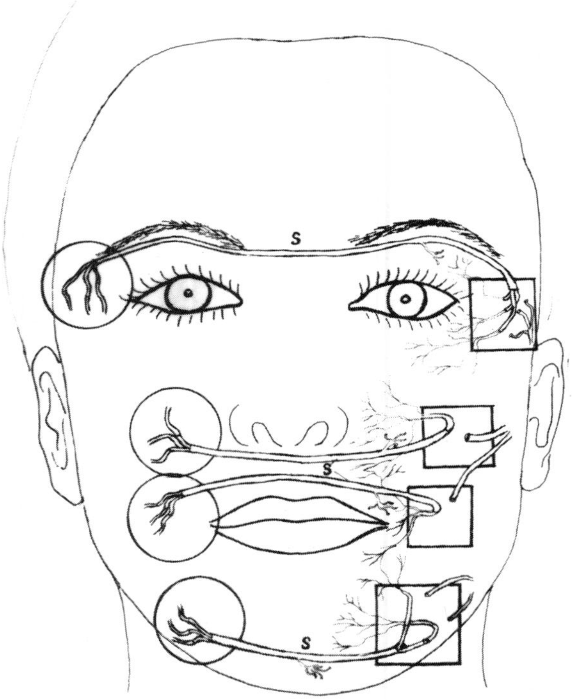

FIGURE 36–62. Position of the single nerve grafts with anastomoses on the unaffected side (circles) and on the paralyzed side (squares) of the face.

OPERATIVE PROCEDURE

A knowledge of and experience with microsurgical techniques are requisite for cross-face nerve grafting (see Chapter 76). This technique permits the location of the facial nerve fascicles and precise anastomoses which fulfill the following criteria: (1) to produce intact and smooth cut edges of the fascicles; (2) to produce tight contact of the nerve endings; (3) to use a limited number of sutures; (4) to

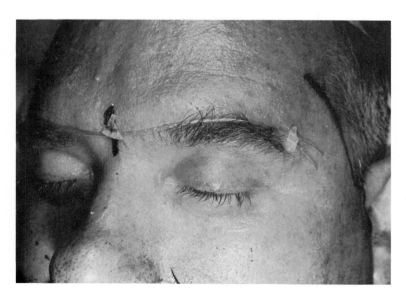

FIGURE 36–63. Incisions and the position of the sural nerve graft (tagged with a suture). In order to take advantage of additional direct neurotization of the orbicularis oculi muscle, the transplant is displaced directly below the eyebrow on the upper portion of the muscle.

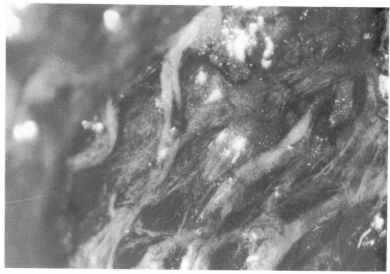

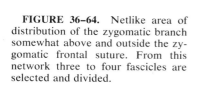

FIGURE 36–64. Netlike area of distribution of the zygomatic branch somewhat above and outside the zygomatic frontal suture. From this network three to four fascicles are selected and divided.

achieve stabilization of the anastomoses; (5) to attain complete freedom from tension at the juncture site (Millesi, Ganglberger, and Berger, 1967).

For a fascicular anastomosis, it is sufficient in most cases to use a single perineural suture (10 to 11–0 monofilament nylon), so that the junction is strong enough, yet the draining plasma can cause the relaxed adjacent nerve endings to adhere to each other (see Chapter 76).

The sural nerve is suitable for use as a transplant, since with its two to four small fascicles it is thin and long, and it leaves behind almost no functional deficit in the region of its sensory supply.

ANATOMICAL REQUIREMENTS

Reanimation of the Orbicularis Oculi Muscle. For the reanimation of the orbicularis oculi muscle, the distribution area of the zygomatic branch on the healthy side is identified (Figs. 36–62, 36–63, and 36–64).

The selection of three to four fascicles of the orbicularis nerve is accomplished by applying a drop of 1 per cent local anesthesia with a No. 24 needle to the perineurium of the selected fascicles and noting localized absence of response to faradic stimulation. If, after stimulation of the complete nerve branch, one can still note other proximal muscle contractions in the

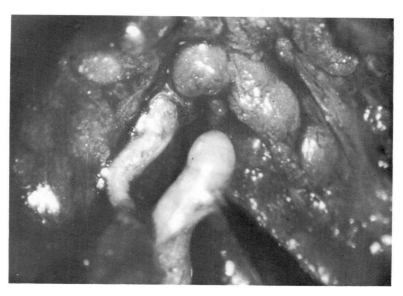

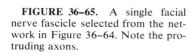

FIGURE 36–65. A single facial nerve fascicle selected from the network in Figure 36–64. Note the protruding axons.

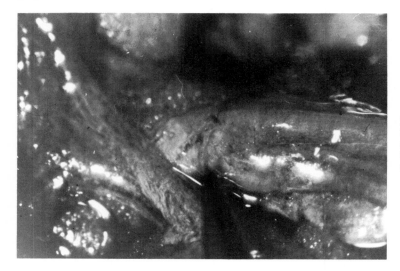

FIGURE 36–66. Anastomosis of a facial nerve fascicle with a fascicle of the sural transplant on the nonparalyzed side of the face. The solitary suture (10–0 nylon) lies on the back of the plane of the picture.

area of supply, the tested fascicle can be severed. In this manner three to four fascicles are located and obtained for the anastomosis (Fig. 36–65). The lower portion of the frontalis and/or the upper muscle fibers of the orbicularis oculi are tunneled bilaterally, and a sural nerve transplant (15 to 17 cm) is inserted in the same directional course as in the leg (see Fig. 36–62). The distal ends are marked with a colored suture in the subcutis of the paralyzed side directly above the zygomatic arch for future identification. The prepared fascicles on the healthy side are connected with the transplant in the described manner (Fig. 36–66). Four to six months after the initial procedure, the transplant is connected with the zygomatic branch on the paralyzed side of the face

after amputation of the transplant neuroma, a sign of successful regeneration (Figs. 36–67 and 36–68).

Reanimation of the Mouth and Cheek Muscles. The reanimation of the paralyzed mouth and cheek muscles is effected by two grafts from the peripheral area of the buccal branch of the healthy side (Fig. 36–69). Three or four fascicles are demonstrated approximately 1 cm behind the nasolabial fold above the bottom edge of the crista zygomatico alveolaris. About 1 cm caudal from these fascicles, three to four additional fascicles are exposed. Two tunnels are fashioned through the muscles of the upper lip, and a sural nerve transplant (13 to 15 cm) is inserted in each. The distal ends should be

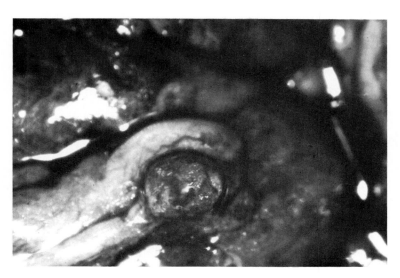

FIGURE 36–67. Tumorlike neuroma on the ends of the sural transplant on the paralyzed side of the face.

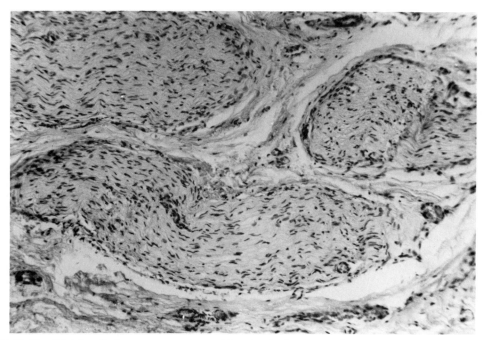

FIGURE 36–68. Distal end of a nerve transplant with a developing amputation neuroma with entwined nerve fiber bundles and connective tissue. Hematoxylin-eosin, × 100.

positioned as closely as possible to the anterior border of the parotid gland. They are also marked with a colored suture through the skin. The upper end of the transplant should lie approximately 1 cm above an imagined line running from the corner of the mouth to the tragus; the lower end should lie 2 cm beyond.

The anastomoses with the main branches of the buccal segment of the paralyzed side are

also performed four to six months later. The preparation of the paralyzed buccal branches of the facial nerve is facilitated by the introduction of a probe into the parotid duct via the mouth.

Reanimation of the Muscles Supplied by the Marginal Mandibularis. The graft from the marginal branch of the healthy side can origi-

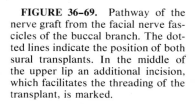

FIGURE 36–69. Pathway of the nerve graft from the facial nerve fascicles of the buccal branch. The dotted lines indicate the position of both sural transplants. In the middle of the upper lip an additional incision, which facilitates the threading of the transplant, is marked.

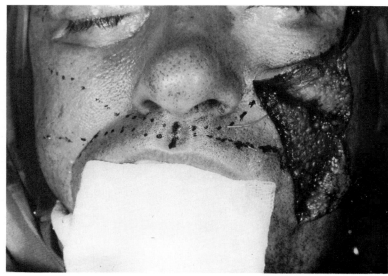

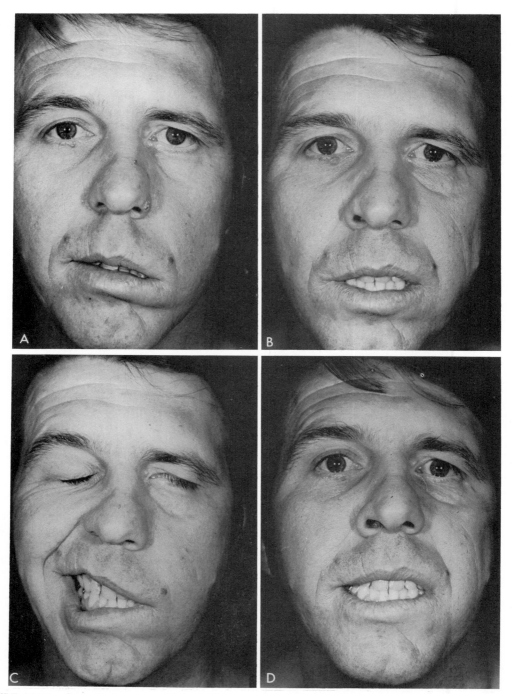

FIGURE 36–70. Cross-face nerve grafting. *A*, Thirty-one year old man with left-sided facial paralysis (repose). *B*, Appearance (repose) eight months after surgery. *C*, Preoperative appearance on voluntary contraction (Morel-Fatio spring in place in upper lid). *D*, Postoperative appearance on voluntary contraction.

Illustration continued on the following page.

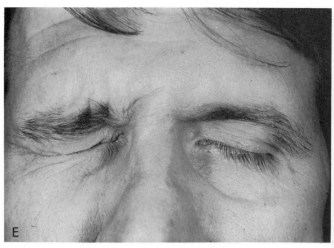
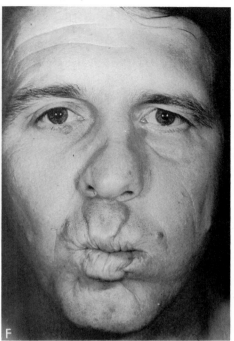
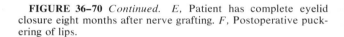

FIGURE 36–70 *Continued.* *E,* Patient has complete eyelid closure eight months after nerve grafting. *F,* Postoperative puckering of lips.

nate from the fascicles of the final area of distribution of both marginal branches.

Both branches of the marginal segment distal to the crossover point of the facial artery should be located on the paralyzed half of the face and, after an appropriate time period, should be connected with the transplant.

The transplantations in the eye and mouth region can be undertaken at the same time. Clinical results are illustrated in Figure 36–70.

Cross-Face Nerve Grafting in Combination with Free Nerve-Muscle Transplantation. If a cross-face nerve graft was performed without success because of muscle atrophy, the sural nerve transplants which have regenerated from the healthy side should be connected with a free nerve-muscle transplant (Freilinger, 1975). The reinnervation of this muscle would result from neuromuscular neurotization and not from muscular-muscular neurotization, which is the method advocated by Thompson (1971). All of the different preparations and requisites for a free muscle transplantation are done in the manner recommended by Thompson earlier in the chapter.

One important difference lies in the fact that the nerve leading to the muscle must be accurately prepared to obtain an intact unit. The other is characterized by different positioning in the area where the new function is expected, because only the factors of tension and power of the muscle are essential.

There have been successful reports of a combined method of cross-face nerve grafting and free nerve-muscle transplants (Millesi, 1974; Freilinger, 1975). Because the sural nerve transplants are anastomosed on the healthy side with selected facial nerve fascicles to reinnervate a corresponding muscle function on the paralyzed side, the free nerve-muscle transplantation connected with such a sural nerve permits the return of differential function, e.g., lid closure, elevation of the mouth, and so forth. The techniques are illustrated in Figures 36–71 and 36–72. The optimal position of the muscle in regard to the distribution of power and tension can be established only after additional clinical experience.

Cross-Face-Nerve Transplantation in Combination with Muscle Transposition. As free nerve-muscle grafts have the disadvantage of losing a considerable amount of fibers and must be followed by another operation, it might be preferable to use muscle that is already available, such as the temporal and masseter muscle. The method of muscle transposition has already been described earlier in the chapter, and provides adequate dynamic support to the lips and sufficient eyelid closure. The impulse for the muscle movement is not a

MUSCULAR NEUROTIZATION

Intimate contact between host muscle + muscle contact

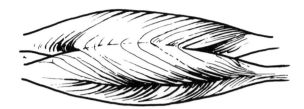

NEURAL NEUROTIZATION

Nerve to nerve suture

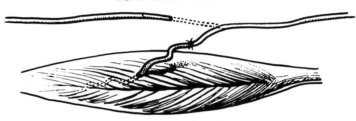

Nerve implantation into the muscle

with Cross face nerve implantation

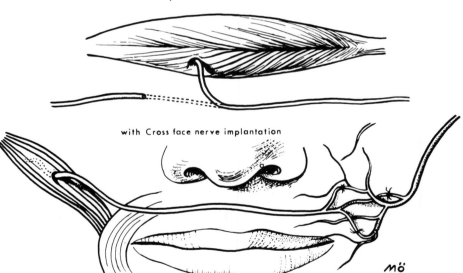

FIGURE 36–71. Schema of muscular and neural neurotization. Muscular neurotization requires intimate contact between the host muscle and muscle graft. Neural neurotization of the muscle can be accomplished either by nerve-to-nerve suture or by direct implantation of the nerve into the muscle. The lowest drawing shows cross-face nerve grafting in combination with muscle transplantation. (Courtesy of Dr. G. Freilinger.)

physiologic one, because the innervation originates from the trigeminal nerve. In order to receive specific innervation from the facial nerve, that part of the masseteric or temporal nerve leading to the transposed muscle can be severed, and connected with a corresponding cross-face nerve graft from the unaffected side. The transposed masseter will thus be innervated by buccal branches, and the temporal muscle will receive innervation from the zygomatic branches of the facial nerve of the contralateral side (see Figs. 36–73 and 36–74).

Before muscle transposition and anastomoses of the trigeminal nerve to the sural nerve, it is necessary to perform cross-face nerve transplantation about four to six months earlier. By so doing, the axons from the healthy side have already grown through the transplant, and can proceed at once into the nerve of the masseter and temporal muscles. The procedure on the healthy side is similar to that already described.

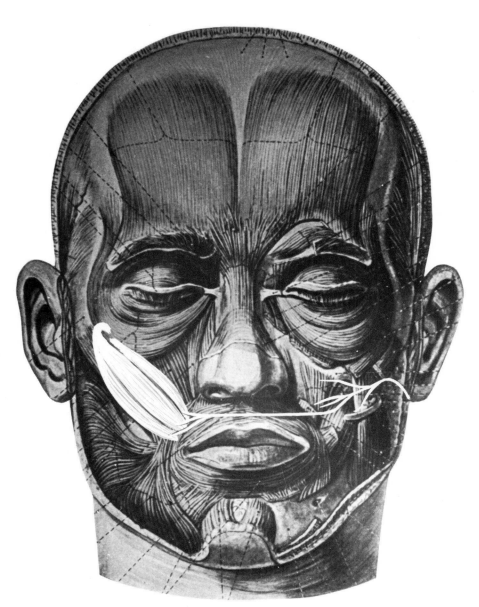

FIGURE 36–72. Cross-face nerve grafting in combination with free muscle transplantation to correct right-sided facial palsy. (Courtesy of Dr. G. Freilinger.)

On the paralyzed side, after separation of the masseter and temporal muscles, the trigeminal nerve can be identified without difficulty, especially when the microscope is used. The frontal portion of the nerve leading to the muscle that is to be transposed is severed and anastomosed with the fascicles of the sural graft. If there is a sural fascicle in excess, it can be implanted directly into the muscle.

The indication for this procedure is a facial palsy of long duration.

INDICATIONS FOR SURGERY

If, after clinical and electrical examination, a severance of the facial nerve is present and all

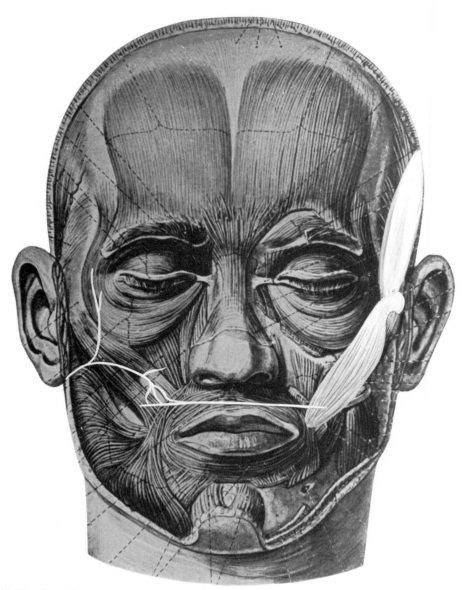

FIGURE 36–73. Cross-face nerve grafting in combination with temporalis muscle transposition to correct left-side facial palsy. (Courtesy of Dr. D. Freilinger.)

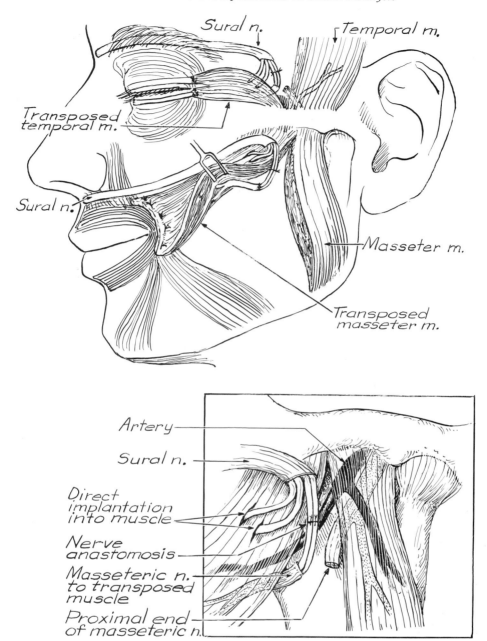

FIGURE 36–74. Cross-face nerve transplantation in combination with temporal and masseter muscle transposition for restoration of the eyelid and oral sphincters, respectively. Sural nerve grafts have previously been inserted across the brow region and upper lip. The inset shows anastomoses of some of the sural nerve fascicles to the nerve of the masseter muscle; the residual fascicles are implanted directly into the transposed muscle.

possibilities of primary nerve repair or transplantation are not feasible, cross-facial nerve grafting can be considered. A requisite for this procedure is that no serious degeneration of the muscle as yet exists, i.e., definite signs of fibrillation must be present on electromyographic study (Buchthal, 1962, 1965; Rosenfalck and Buchthal, 1962; Taverner, 1965a).

In the nerve as in the muscle, conditions for regeneration remain optimal for several months after nerve division. After approximately four to six months, the nerve sheath begins to shrink; the neurons and muscle cells atrophy and are overgrown by connective tissue. Because of the associated degenerative process, reconstruction can be considered only in rare cases after 18 months (McCabe, 1970; Seddon, 1972).

Since the axon budding occurs at the rate of 0.5 to 3 mm per day (Seddon, 1972), with a nerve transplant length of 13 to 15 cm, it is necessary to provide a three- to four-month interval between the first and second surgical phases. This delay must consequently be considered in terms of calculated muscle degeneration when determining expediency and scheduling of the cross-facial nerve graft.

The question is often raised as to whether it would be better to perform the procedure in addition to or at the same time as other palliative reconstructive measures in facial nerve paralysis with little probability of regeneration, in order to prevent progressive degeneration of the facial muscles. The same question pertains to unfavorable facial nerve repair, since any time lost following the repair may exceed the critical interval with regard to the regenerative ability of the paralyzed muscles. One should, therefore, consider the possibility offered by available nerve anastomosis on the paralyzed side in such patients and also consider carefully the unquestionable advantage offered by cross-face nerve grafting.

An unfavorable condition for cross-face nerve grafting is scarring resulting from reconstructive surgery. This can greatly complicate the dissection and can lead to poor positioning of the sural nerve transplant.

Nylon suspension of the cheek should be avoided in all cases being considered for nerve grafting. On the other hand, Silastic membrane and lid spring implants cause no residual scarring, are nondisruptive, and can be recommended as intermediate measures in association with nerve grafting (Wilflingseder and Anderl, 1971; Anderl, 1972). The indication for nerve grafting is also reduced because of the length of the surgical procedures, a point

which demands careful selection of patients in terms of their general physical condition.

NERVE ANASTOMOSIS

The greatest danger for a nerve anastomosis is the proliferation of connective tissue, which either impairs the budding of axons in the distal nerve stump or renders it completely impassable. This complication is more likely to occur if the requirements already quoted for an optimal nerve suture are not followed during the operating procedure. After nerve interruption, the epineurium is considered the most potent site of connective tissue formation and should be resected 0.5 to 1 cm back from the section point (Millesi, Ganglberger and Berger, 1967). This technique, which is used in the repair of peripheral nerves in the extremities, is generally superfluous in the area of peripheral sections of the facial nerve, since these end branches show a large number of fascicular structures. In order to protect the anastomoses from invasion by surrounding connective tissue, sheaths were constructed using millipore membrane (Campbell, 1961), grids of collagen or collagen tubes (Braun, 1966), and polyethylene cylinders (Miehlke, 1960). These techniques did not prove satisfactory, since the foreign bodies caused increased scarring, with strangulation and interruption of axon budding.

Suture material also stimulates increased scar formation. For this reason, fixation of the anastomoses was attempted with acrylic adhesive (Freeman, 1965; Perl and Wagner, 1965). However, localized areas of necrosis frequently occurred under the surfaces of adhesion, and these adhesives were found to be unsuitable for nerve repairs.

Since a strong contact in the area of the nerve stumps is produced by the adhesive power of the plasma exuding from the wound surfaces, it was shown that, if there is complete freedom from tension, a single fascicular suture of 10 to 11–0 monofilament nylon suffices. An additional adhesion with autologous or homologous plasma and/or fibrin suspension is therefore not required (Medawar and Young, 1940; Tarlow and Boernstein, 1948). After covering by skin closure, the anastomosed nerves are securely positioned in the adipose tissues of the invading connective tissue. The cutaneous incisions should be made in the main skin lines and should always be placed 1 to 2 cm to the side of the planned site of anastomosis.

THE CHOICE OF NERVE TRANSPLANTS

As has been shown in clinical experience and experimental examination of animals, thin autografts are superior to allografts and preserved nerves. This finding is especially valid in the bridging of larger defects (Sanders, 1954; Nigst, 1969; Millesi, Berger and Meisal, 1972; Seddon, 1972). The delicacy of the tissue structure in the area of the facial nerve limits the possibilities of revision, with exclusion of reinnervation to a greater extent than in extremity nerve surgery. Because of these reasons, the cross-face nerve graft can hardly be repeated; consequently, the use of allografts with a questionable likelihood of success is a definite risk.

CHOICE OF FASCICLES AND NERVE BRANCHES

A considerable problem exists in the selection of peripheral nerve branches on the paralyzed as well as on the healthy side, since shunts from sensory nerves, such as the trigeminal branches, would be worthless for muscular reinnervation. Therefore, sensory fascicles must not be anastomosed.

Even on the healthy side, the differentiation of nerves into sensory and motor fascicles is not assured with testing by electrical stimulation. Utilization of indirect stimulation is not possible on the paralyzed side because of nerve degeneration. In addition, anastomoses of sensory nerve branches of the infraorbital, the buccal, the zygomatic-facial, and the mental nerve with facial nerve branches can lead to error in the selection of nerve connections on the healthy side. By electrical stimulation of the sensory nerves, the stimulus can be further conducted to motor fibers, and a muscle response is obtained. Furthermore, after the connection of such presumed "motorized nerve fascicles" to the transplant, the number of remaining available nerve fibers capable of regeneration of the paralyzed muscle is reduced.

After exploration of the facial nerve branches on the healthy side of the face, nerve fibers only in sufficient numbers for reinnervation of the paralyzed side may be severed, so that a noticeable impairment of the healthy side does not result. A minimum of three to four fascicles in the eye region, six to eight fascicles in the mouth region, and two to three fascicles in the marginal mandibular branch region seems adequate without resulting apparent loss of motor function. In the area of peripheral supply of the buccal branch, a larger branch can be severed for the connection without fear of a functional deficit. Such a thick fascicle can usually be found under and lateral to the insertion of the alar base of the nose. The efficacy of the anastomoses, reported by Smith (1971), of only two fascicles from the buccal complex of the healthy side and only one nerve transplant in trying to reinnervate the muscle of the cheek and eye region is questionable. The differential functions of eyelid closure and/or the blinking reflex demands increased and specific nerve connections. Additionally, interruption of the majority of the buccal branches on the healthy side could definitely lead to functional impairment of the mouth and cheek muscles.

In the author's opinion, a critical factor in the cross-face nerve graft procedure is the presence of a double anastomosis (Holmes and Young, 1942); experience has shown that an interval of four to six months is required for axon budding through the cross-face nerve graft.

The axonal growth can be continually monitored by electromyography and clinically and visually diagnosed by the formation of a neuroma. A one stage anastomosis carries with it the danger of scarring in the anastomoses on

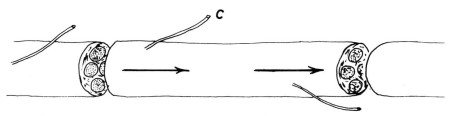

FIGURE 36–75. Detached sural nerve segment transplanted to the calf area. *C* represents a severed cutaneous branch. The arrows designate the directional course.

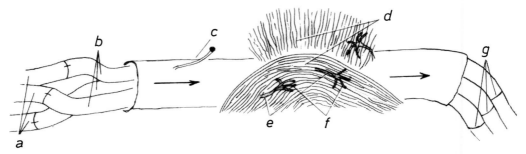

FIGURE 36–76. Anatomical directional course of the sural nerve and the frontalis and orbicularis muscles following a cross-face nerve graft. *A*, Intact fascicles of the facial nerve. *B*, Fascicles of the sural nerve graft. *C*, Cutaneous branch of the sural nerve graft. Note terminal neuroma. *D*, Frontalis and orbicularis oculi muscles. *E*, Cutaneous branch of the sural transplant ingrowth into the muscles. *F*, Budding axons with newly formed motor end-plates. *G*, Fascicles of the zygomatic branch of the facial nerve.

the paralyzed side. Complications in nerve transplantation within the extremities can be corrected through revision and a new anastomosis, but such a technique would hardly be possible in the facial area.

If a free nerve-muscle transplantation is planned, it is of great value to have already functioning nerve fibers from the healthy side in the sural transplant. The reinnervation of the free muscle transplant will be quicker because the intervening gap can be bridged in a shorter time, therefore reducing atrophy of the muscle graft.

NEUROTIZATION

If the facial branches are difficult to demonstrate, as on the paralyzed side in the area of the eye or in small children, the fanlike branched ends of the fascicles of the transplant can be directly implanted into the muscle. With this type of implantation, a muscle reinnervation can be expected, based on experimentation, clinical experience (Steindler, 1915, 1916; Erlacher, 1915; Hoffmann, 1951; Aitken, 1965; Thompson, 1971), and personal obser-

vation. These nerve implantations should also, as in the case of the anastomoses, be performed in two stages. The delay enables the proliferating axon, after resection of the neuroma, to bud into the muscle fibers on the free end of the transplant where they either reactivate already existing motor end-plates or generate new ones.

A partial neurotization in the paralyzed muscle corresponding to the position of the nerve transplant has already been observed by the author. The nerve transplant was implanted into the muscle in the original proximal-to-distal direction (Figs. 36–75 and 36–76), so that the "cutaneous branches" which originate within the nerve transplant could grow into the muscle fibers and reinnervate them. Based on these considerations, strict attention must be paid to the anatomical directional course of the nerve transplant. In contrast, in nerve transplantation in the extremities, the nerve is anastomosed in the reverse direction (Fig. 36–77); that is, the original distal transplant end is joined to the fascicle of the proximal nerve stump, in order that the above-mentioned erroneous budding from the cutaneous branches will be avoided so as not to incur a decrease in the number of axons at the distal anastomosis.

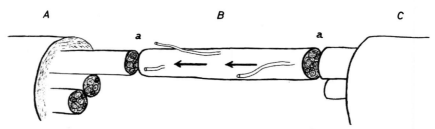

FIGURE 36–77. Interfascicular nerve graft in the extremities. *A*, Proximal nerve stump. *B*, Nerve graft. *C*, Distal nerve stump. *a*, Fascicular juncture. Arrows show the directional course of the sural nerve graft.

RESULTS

In the cross-face nerve grafts, especially after bridging of large distances, a final result can only be expected after two years. For objective evaluation of the method, a pre- and postoperative electromyogram is of primary importance; this study will establish the irreversible paralysis of the facial nerve and will document the ability of the transplant to conduct a stimulus after surgery is performed.

Therefore, electrical potential must be detectable from the reinnervated muscles of the originally paralyzed side after spontaneous innervation, as well as after direct stimulation of the facial nerve branch on the unaffected side. Through monitoring with electromyography, a spontaneous regeneration of the facial muscle, which can occur through fibers of the trigeminal nerve, can be eliminated. The restitution of muscle function through the trigeminal nerve after division of the facial nerve in the region of the parotid has been observed as a rare phenomenon by some authors (Conley, 1955; Martin and Helsper, 1957).

These phenomena were also observed in experimental studies on dogs (James, Karlar, Kensey and Meagher, 1960). Reinnervation from the contralateral side (Buchthal, 1965), probably over neighboring muscles, was described and verified through electromyography. The presence of a neuroma on the transplant end and excitability response on the healthy side after antidromic nerve stimulation are criteria which allow an estimation of prognosis. With surgical techniques that achieve optimal nerve budding, the clinical result is dependent to a great extent on the muscle volume capable of reinnervation.

After nerve suturing or, more often, after nerve transplantations to the facial nerve, uncontrolled movements of different facial portions occasionally accompany gradual rehabilitation. This phenomenon occurs especially with more centrally located lesions, as numerous pathways are available for the budding nerve fibers to follow, causing the nerve fibers to arrive in a region peripheral to the original innervational area.

As Förster (1937) has already described, the periphery dictates the intensity of movement in the cortex of the brain. This is shown in the course of muscle regeneration by an increasing subordination of previously defective muscle function to a directed formation of volition.

By the reanimation of the face through cross-face nerve grafting, the same muscle groups on the other side of the face will be predominantly innervated. However, because of the short observation period and the inadequate number of cases, it still cannot be determined if a separated innervation of both facial halves is possible in every case.

In one of our patients it was noticed that, at the beginning of reinnervation after four months, an attempt to elevate the healthy corner of the mouth was accompanied by a movement in the lower eyelid of the paralyzed side. This phenomenon subsequently disappeared.

From the beginning of the paralysis until complete recovery, intensive electrical therapy and physiokinetic therapy before a mirror are essential for the acquisition of directed movement (Förster, 1916; Zülch, 1956). The value of electrophysiotherapy in retarding advancing muscle atrophy is still disputed (Förster, 1937; Gutmann and Young, 1944; Taverner, 1965b; Kettel, 1965).

These therapeutic measures appeared completely rational and were therefore employed. The patients were treated, on an average, three times weekly with exponential current at a strength of 20 to 60 milliamperes, whereby each muscle group received a two- to three-minute dosage.

It is difficult to classify results in facial paralysis because, in addition to the functional criteria, there are also esthetic aspects. Techniques that have been used over a short period of time are difficult to evaluate, as nerve regeneration may take two or three years to be completed. The results obtained are the following: in five patients the result was very good; they showed symmetric active movements of the eyelids and of the perioral muscles, and regeneration appears to be progressing further; three patients showed satisfactory regeneration, but the follow-up period is too short to be conclusive; one patient showed poor regeneration; in two patients, no regeneration has occurred.

The reasons leading to failure were:

1. Advanced muscle atrophy before and during the course of treatment.

2. Preparation of an insufficient number of fascicles of the facial nerve on the healthy side of the face.

3. Insufficient or defective anastomosis of the transplants to the main facial branch on the paralyzed side.

4. Inadvertent anastomosis of the transplants to sensory (trigeminal) branches on the healthy side as well as on the paralyzed side.

5. Foreign bodies and scars from previous reconstructive operations in the region of the nerve anastomoses.

6. Surgical and microsurgical technical errors.

7. Neglect of pre- and postoperative electrical and active physiotherapy.

REFERENCES

Adams, W.: The use of the masseter, temporalis and frontalis muscles in the correction of facial paralysis. Plast. Reconstr. Surg., *1*:216, 1946.

Aitken, J. T.: Problems of reinnervation of muscles. Progr. Brain Res., *14*:232, 1965.

Albert, E.: Einige Operationen an Nerven. Wien. Med. Presse, *26*:1285, 1885.

Anderl, H.: A simple method for correcting ectropium. Plast. Reconstr. Surg., *49*:156, 1972.

Anderl, H.: Nerventransplantation bei Facialisparese (eine neue Methode). Presented at the Annual Meeting of the Swiss Society for Plastic and Reconstructive Surgery, Zurich, 1972.

Anderl, H.: Reconstruction of the face through cross-face nerve transplantation in facial paralysis. Chir. Plast. (Berl.), *2*:17, 1973.

Anderl, H.: Personal communication, 1967.

Andersen, J. G.: Surgical treatment of lagophthalmos in leprosy by the Gillies temporalis transfer. Br. J. Plast. Surg., *14*:339, 1961.

Apfleberg, D. B., and Gingrass, R. P.: Funicular nerve grafting of the facial nerve. Surg. Forum, *24*:513, 1973.

Arion, H. G.: Dynamic closure of the lids in paralysis of the orbicularis muscle. Internatl. Surg., *57*:48, 1972.

Bäckdahl, M., and D'Alessio, E.: Experience with static reconstruction in cases of facial paralysis. Plast. Reconstr. Surg., *21*:211, 1958.

Ballance, C.: Results obtained in some experiments in which the facial and recurrent laryngeal nerves were anastomosed with other nerves. Br. Med. J., *2*:349, 1924.

Ballance, C., and Duel, A. B.: The operative treatment of facial palsy by the introduction of nerve grafts into the fallopian canal and by other intratemporal methods. Arch. Otolaryngol., *15*:1, 1932.

Bames, H. O.: Frown disfigurement and ptosis of eyebrows. Plast. Reconstr. Surg., *19*:337, 1957.

Beahrs, O. H., Judd, E. S., and Woodington, G. F.: Use of nerve grafts for repair of defects in the facial nerve. Ann. Surg., *153*:433, 1961.

Bell, C.: On the nerves, giving an account of some experiments on their structure and functions, which leads to a new arrangement of the system. Trans. R. Soc. Lond. (Phil.), *3*:398, 1821.

Belyakova, L. V.: Employment of tantalum in reconstructive intracanal surgery of the facial nerve. Arch. Otolaryngol., *88*:104, 1968.

Bentley, F. H., and Hill, M.: Experimental surgery and nerve grafting. Br. J. Surg., *24*:368, 1936.

Berger, J., Slaughter, W., and Lansa, F.: Personal communication, 1961.

Blair, V. P.: Notes on the operative correction of facial palsy. South. Med. J., *19*:116, 1926.

Blunt, M. J.: The blood supply of the facial nerve. J. Anat., *88*:520, 1954.

Boyer, F. C., and Gardiner, W. J.: Paroxysmal lacrimation and its surgical treatment. Arch. Neurol. Psychiatr., *61*:56, 1949.

Bragden, F. H., and Gray, G. H.: Differential spinal accessory—Facial anastomosis with preservation of function of trapezius. J. Neurol., *19*:981, 1962.

Braun, R. M.: Comparative studies of neurorrhaphy and sutureless peripheral nerve repair. Surg. Gynecol. Obstet., *122*:15, 1966.

Buchthal, F.: Electromyogram: Its value in diagnosis of neuromuscular disorders. Wld. Neurol., *3*:16, 1962.

Buchthal, F.: Electromyographie in paralysis of the facial nerve. Arch. Otolaryngol., *81*:463, 1965.

Bunnell, S.: Suture of the facial nerve within the temporal bone with a report of the first successful case. Surg. Gynecol. Obstet., *45*:7, 1927.

Bunnell, S.: Surgical repair of the facial nerve. Arch. Otolaryngol., *25*:235, 1937.

Bunnell, S.: Summation of papers on management of facial paralysis. Arch. Otolaryngol., *55*:417, 1952.

Byars, L. T.: Preservation of the facial nerve in operations for benign conditions of the parotid area. Ann. Surg., *136*:412, 1952.

Campbell, J. B.: Microfilter sheaths in peripheral nerve surgery: A laboratory report and preliminary clinical study. J. Trauma, *1*:139, 1961.

Cardwell, E. P.: Direct implantation of free nerve grafts between facial musculature and facial trunk. Arch. Otolaryngol., *27*:469, 1938.

Castanares, S.: Forehead wrinkles, glabellar frown and ptosis of the eyebrows. Plast. Reconstr. Surg., *34*:406, 1964.

Cawthorne, T.: The contribution of surgery to the problems of neurology. Br. Med. Bull., *12*:143, 1956.

Champion, R.: Re-animation of facial paresis in children. Plast. Reconstr. Surg., *22*:188, 1958.

Clodius, L.: Discussion of: Myographie in der Facialis und Handchirurgie, by A. Struppler. Chir. Plast. Reconstr., *8*:10, 1970.

Clodius, L.: Die Lymphographie und Isotopendiagnostik in der plastichen chirurgie. Chir. Plast. Reconstr., *8*:37, 1970.

Collier, J. J.: The present position of facial nerve surgery. Ann. Otol. Rhinol. Laryngol., *58*:686, 1949.

Collier, J.: Re-animation in facial paralysis. Br. J. Plast. Surg., *5*:243, 1953.

Conley, J. J.: Facial nerve grafting in treatment of parotid gland tumors. Arch. Surg., *70*:359, 1955.

Conley, J. J.: Facial rehabilitation following radical parotid gland surgery. Arch. Otolaryngol., *66*:58, 1957.

Conley, J. J.: Facial nerve grafting. Arch. Otolaryngol., *73*:322, 1961.

Conley, J. J.: Techniques of extratemporal facial nerve surgery. *In* Miehlke, A. (Ed.): Surgery of the Facial Nerve. W. B. Saunders Company, Philadelphia, 1973.

Conley, J. J.: Salivary Glands and the Facial Nerve. Georg Thieme Verlag, Stuttgart, 1975.

Conley, J. J.: Personal communication, 1976.

Conley, J. J., Hamaker, R. C., and Donnenfeld, H.: Long-standing facial paralysis rehabilitation. Laryngoscope, *84*:2155, 1974.

Converse, J. M.: Facial paralysis. *In* Kazanjian, V. H., and Converse, J. M. (Eds.): Surgical Treatment of Facial Injuries. 3rd Ed. Baltimore, Williams & Wilkins Company, 1974.

Converse, J. M., and Coburn, R. J.: The twitching scar. Br. J. Plast. Surg., *24*:272, 1971.

Converse, J. M., and Goodgold, J.: Referred to by Kazanjian and Converse (1974).

Converse, J. M., and Wood-Smith, D.: Experiences with

the forehead island flap with a subcutaneous pedicle. Plast. Reconstr. Surg., *31*:521, 1963.

Conway, H.: Muscle plastic operations for facial paralysis. Ann. Surg., *147*:541, 1958.

Craig, M.: Face Saving Exercises. New York, Random House, 1970.

Curtin, J. W., Greeley, P. W., Gleason, M., and Braver, D.: A supplementary procedure for the improvement of facial nerve repair. Plast. Reconstr. Surg., *26*:73, 1960.

Cushing, H. W.: The surgical treatment of facial paralysis by nerve anastomosis. Ann. Surg., *37*:641, 1903.

Davis, R. A., Anson, B. J., Budinger, J. M., and Kurth, L. E.: Surgical anatomy of the facial nerve and parotid gland based upon a study of 350 cervico-facial halves. Surg. Gynecol. Obstet., *102*:385, 1956.

de Castro Correia, P., and Zani, R.: Observacoes Anastomicas Sobre o Nervo Masseterico. Sua aplicacao a Tecnica da Mioplastia Comm. Masseter no Tratamento da Paralisia Facial, Univ. de Sao Paulo, 1954. Plast. Reconstr. Surg., *52*:370, 1973.

Dingman, R. O., and Grabb, W. C.: Surgical anatomy of the mandibular ramus of the facial nerve based on the dissection of 100 facial halves. Plast. Reconstr. Surg., *29*:266, 1962.

Dott, N. M.: Facial paralysis—restitution by extrapetrous nerve graft. Proc. R. Soc. Med. Lond., *51*:900, 1958.

Drake, C. G.: Acoustic neuroma—Repair of facial nerve with autogenous grafts. J. Neurosurg., *17*:836, 1960.

Drobnik: Ueber die Behandlung der Kinderlaehmung mit Funktionstheilung und Funktionsübertragung der Muskeln. Dtsch. Z. Chir., *43*:473, 1896.

Edgerton, M. T.: Surgical correction of facial paralysis: A plea for better reconstruction. Ann. Surg., *165*:985, 1967.

Edgerton, M. T., and Wolfort, F. G.: The dermal-flap canthal lift for lower eyelid support. Plast. Reconstr. Surg., *43*:42, 1969.

Ehni, G., and Woltman, H. W.: Hemifacial spasm and review of 106 cases. Arch. Neurol. Psychiatr., *53*:205, 1945.

Erlacher, P.: Über die motorischen Nervenendigungen. Z. Orthop. Chir., *34*:561, 1914.

Erlacher, P.: Direct and muscular neurotization of paralyzed muscles. Experimental research. Am. J. Orthop. Surg., *13*:22, 1915.

Evans, D.: Hypoglossal-facial anastomosis in the treatment of facial palsy. Br. J. Plast. Surg., *27*:251, 1974.

Field, W. S.: Personal communication, 1971.

Fisch, U. P.: Operations on the facial nerve in oto-neurosurgical operation. *In* Yasargil, M. G. (Ed.): Microsurgery. Stuttgart, Thieme, 1969, p. 208.

Förster, O.: Die Schussverletzungen der peripherene Nerven und Behandlung. Z. Orthop. Chir., *36*:310, 1916.

Förster, O.: Facialisclahmung. Band 3, S. 594, Berlin, 1937.

Frackelton, W. H.: Surgical creation of wrinkles. Plast. Reconstr. Surg., *9*:565, 1952.

Freeman, B. S.: Adhesive anastomosis technics for fine nerves: Experimental and clinical technics. Am. J. Surg., *108*:529, 1964.

Freeman, B. S.: Adhesive neural anastomosis. Plast. Reconstr. Surg., *35*:167, 1965.

Freeman, B. S.: An immediate combined approach for rehabilitation of the patient with facial paralysis. Plast. Reconstr. Surg., *37*:341, 1966.

Freeman, B. S.: Silastic rod sling to elevate the paralyzed lower lid. Plast. Reconstr. Surg., *44*:401, 1969.

Freeman, B. S.: Non-suture techniques in facial nerve anastomosis. *In* Conley, J. (Ed.): Plastic and Reconstructive Surgery of the Face and Neck. Vol. 2. Stuttgart, George Thieme Verlag, 1972a, p. 92.

Freeman, B. S.: Techniques for sphincteric control in facial paralysis. *In* Conley, J. (ed.): Plastic and Reconstructive Surgery of the Face and Neck. Vol. 2. Stuttgart, George Thieme Verlag, 1972b, p. 103.

Freeman, B. S.: Late reconstruction of the lax oral sphincter in facial paralysis. Plast. Reconstr. Surg., *51*:144, 1973.

Freeman, B. S.: Comparative long-term results following reconstruction of the palsied face, neural, muscular, and suspensory: conclusions and indications. Presented at the Sixth International Congress of Plastic and Reconstructive Surgery, Paris, August 25, 1975.

Freeman, B. S., Perry, J., and Brown, D.: Experimental study of adhesive surgical tape for nerve anastomosis. Plast. Reconstr. Surg., *43*:174, 1969.

Fyfe, A.: A System of the Anatomy of the Human Body. 3rd Ed. Edinburgh, J. Pillans & Sons, 1814.

Freilinger, G.: A new technique to correct facial paralysis. Plast. Reconstr. Surg., *56*:44, 1975.

Gilliatt, R. W., and Taylor, J. C.: Electrical changes following section of the facial nerve. Proc. R. Soc. Med., *52*:1080, 1959.

Gillies, H. D., and Millard, D. R., Jr.: The Principles and the Art of Plastic Surgery. Boston, Little, Brown & Company, 1957.

Gordon-Taylor, G., and Walls, E. W.: Sir Charles Bell. Baltimore, Willians & Wilkins Company, 1958.

Greenwood, J., Jr.: The surgical treatment of hemifacial spasm. J. Neurosurgery, *3*:506, 1946.

Greenwood, J., Jr.: Address to Houston Society of Plastic Surgeons, 1958.

Gutmann, E., and Young, J. Z.: Reinnervation of muscle after various periods of atrophy. J. Anat., *78*:15, 1944.

Guy, C. L.: Palpebral spring. *In* Kazanjian, V. H., and Converse, J. M.: Surgical Treatment of Facial Injuries. 3rd Ed. Baltimore, The William and Wilkins Company, 1974, p. 1281.

Hakelius, L.: Personal communication, 1973.

Hakelius, L.: Transplantation of free autogenous muscle in the treatment of facial paralysis. A Clinical study. Scand. J. Plast. Reconstr. Surg., *8*:220, 1974.

Hakelius, L., and Stalberg, E.: Electromyographical studies of free autogenous muscle transplants in man. Scand. J. Plast. Surg., *8*:211, 1974.

Hakstian, N. R.: Funicular orientation by direct stimulation. J. Bone Joint Surg., A-*50*:1178, 1968.

Halle, D.: Die Beseitigung der Entsellung bei Facialislähmung. Rev. Chir. Plast., May 3, 1933.

Hardy, R. C., Perret, G., and Myers, R.: Phrenicofacial nerve anastomosis for facial paralysis. Neurosurgery, *14*:400, 1957.

Harii, K., Ohmori, K., and Torii, S.: Free gracilis muscle transplantation with microneurovascular anastomosis for the treatment of facial paralysis. Plast. Reconstr. Surg., *57*:133, 1976.

Hastings, J. C., and Peacock, E. E.: Effect of injury, repair, and ascorbic acid deficiency on collagen accumulation in peripheral nerves. Surg. Forum, *24*:516, 1973.

Hoffmann, H.: A study of the factors influencing innervation of muscles by implanted nerves. Aust. J. Exp. Biol. Med. Sci., *29*:289, 1951.

Holmes, W., and Young, J. Z.: Nerve regeneration after immediate and delayed suture. J. Anat. (Lond.), *77*:63, 1942.

Horton, C. E.: Special Problems of Facial Paralysis in Childhood: The Use of the Sterno-Cleidomastoid Muscle. Plastic Surgery in Infancy and Childhood. Philadelphia, W. B. Saunders Company, 1971, p. 322.

House, W. F., and Crabtree, J. Z.: Surgical exposure of petrous portion of seventh nerve. Arch. Otolaryngol., *81*:506, 1966.

Huber, E.: Evaluation of Facial Musculature and Facial Expression. Baltimore, Johns Hopkins University Press, 1931.

James, A. G., Karlan, M., Kensey, D. L., and Meagher, J. M.: Spontaneous regeneration of the seventh nerve. Arch. Surg., *81*:223, 1960.

Jobe, R. P.: A technique for lid loading in the management of the lagophthalmos of facial palsy. Plast. Reconstr. Surg., *53*:29, 1974.

Joseph, J.: Nasenplastik und sonstige Gesicht Plastik. Leipzig, C. Kacitzsch, 1931, pp. 498–842.

Kazanjian, V. H., and Converse, J. M.: The Surgical Treatment of Facial Injuries. 3rd Ed. Baltimore, Williams & Wilkins Company, 1974.

Kennedy, R.: "Nerve Crossing." Trans. R. Soc. Lond. (Phil.), *194*:127, 1901.

Kent, G. C., Jr.: Comparative Anatomy of the Vertebrates. 2nd Ed. St. Louis, Mo., C. V. Mosby Company, 1969.

Kettel, K.: Om den säkaldte rheumatiske facialisparese set fro it kirurgisk synspunkt. Ugesk. Laeger, *115*:353, 1953.

Kettel, K.: Surgical treatment in atraumatic facial palsies. J. Laryngol. Otol., *73*:491, 1959.

Kettel, K.: Surgery of the facial nerve. Arch. Otolaryngol., *81*:523, 1965.

Kline, D. G., and DeJonge, B. R.: Evoked potentials to evaluate peripheral nerve injuries. Surg. Gynecol. Obstet., *127*:1239, 1968.

Krarup, B.: Electro-gustometry: A method for clinical taste examinations. Acta Otolaryngol., *49*:294, 1958.

Kullman, G., and Cody, D.: The anatomy of the facial nerve. Minn. Med., *52*:213, 1969.

Langworth, E. P., and Taverner, D.: The prognosis in facial palsy. Brain, *86*:465, 1963.

Lathrop, F. D.: Affections of the facial nerve. J.A.M.A., *152*:19, 1953.

Lathrop, F. D.: Surgical repair of facial nerve: Technique. Surg. Clin. North Am., *36*:583, 1956.

Letievant, E.: Traité des Sections Nerveuses. Paris, Baillère et Fils, 1873.

Lexer, E.: General Surgery: A Presentation of the Scientific Principles upon which the Practice of Modern Surgery Is Based. New York, D. Appleton & Company, 1908.

Lexer, E., and Eden, R.: Über die chirurgische Behandlung der peripheren Facialislähmung. Beitr. Klin. Chir., *73*:116, 1911.

Love, J. G.: Surgical treatment of facial paralysis—A modification of spinofacial anastomosis. Proc. Staff Meet. Mayo Clin., *37*:404, 1962.

Love, J. G.: Personal communication, 1970.

McCabe, B. F.: Facial nerve grafting. Plast. Reconstr. Surg., *45*:71, 1970.

McCormack, L. J., Cauldwell, E. W., and Anson, B. J.: Surgical anatomy of the facial nerve with special reference to the parotid gland. Surg. Gynecol. Obstet., *80*:620, 1945.

McHugh, H. E., Sowden, K. A., and Levitt, M.D.: Facial paralysis and muscle agenesis in the newborn. Arch. Otolaryngol., *89*:131, 1969.

McKenzie, K. G., and Alexander, E.: Restoration of facial functions by nerve anastomosis. Ann. Surg., *132*:411, 1950.

McLaughlin, C. R.: Permanent facial paralysis. Lancet, *2*:647, 1952.

Manasse, P.: Ueber Vereinignung des N. Facialis mit dem N. Accessorius durch die Nervenpropfung (Greffe Nerveuse). Arch. Klin. Chir., *62*:805, 1900.

Marino, H.: Paralysis of the muscles of the chin. Surgical treatment. Surg. Gynecol. Obstet., *96*:433, 1953.

Martin, H., and Helsper, J. T.: Spontaneous return of function following surgical section or excision of the seventh cranial nerve in the surgery of parotid tumors. Ann. Surg., *146*:715, 1957.

Martin, R. C.: Intratemporal suture of the facial nerve. Arch. Otolaryngol., *13*:259, 1931.

Maxwell, J. H.: Repair of the facial nerve after facial laceration. Trans. Am. Acad. Ophthalmol., *58*:733, 1954.

Mayo, H.: Anatomical and Physiological Commentaries. London, T. & G. Underwood, 1822–3.

Medawar, P. B., and Young, J. Z.: Fibrin suture of peripheral nerves: Measurement of rate of regeneration. Lancet, *11*:126, 1940.

Miehlke, A.: Die Chirurgie des Nervus Facialis. Berlin, Urban und Schwarzenberg, 1960a.

Miehlke, A.: Über den chirurgischen Wiederaufbau des Gesichtsnerven nach extratemporaler Laesion. Dtsch. Med. Wochenschr., *85*:506, 1960b.

Miehlke, A.: Extratemporale Facialischirurgie. Z. Laryngol. Rhinol., *40*:338, 1961.

Miehlke, A.: Surgery of the Facial Nerve. Philadelphia, W. B. Saunders Company, 1973.

Miehlke, A., and Buske, A.: Die operative Freilegung der mittleren Schadelgrube und das Porus acusticus internus zur Behandlung interlabyrintharer Laesionen des N. facialis. Chir. Plast. Reconstr., *3*:37, 1967.

Millesi, H.: Zum Problem der Überbrückung von Defekten peripherer Nerven. Wien. Med. Wochenschr., *9/10*:182, 1968.

Millesi, H., Berger, A., and Meisal, G.: Experimentelle Unterschungen zur Heilung durchtrennter Nerven. Chir. Plast. (Berl.), *1*:174, 1972.

Millesi, H., Ganglberger, J., and Berger, A.: Erfahrungen mit der Mikrochirurgie peripherer Nerven. Chir. Plast. Reconstr., *3*:47, 1967.

Morel-Fatio, D.: Personal communication, 1974.

Morel-Fatio, D.: Round-table discussion at Sixth International Congress of Plastic and Reconstructive Surgery, Paris, 1975.

Morel-Fatio, D., and Lalardrie, J.-P.: Contribution à l'étude de la paralysie faciale: le ressort palpébral. Ann. Chir. Plast., *7*:275, 1962.

Morel-Fatio, D., and Lalardrie, J.-P.: Utilization d'un "anti-ressort" dans le traitément de ces Fams Ptosis palpebreaux. Ann. Chir. Plast., *13*:170, 1968.

Morestin, H.: Section du facial, du lingual et du maxillaire supérieur par le même projectile; tentative d'amélioration de la paralysie faciale par anastomoses musculaires. Bull. Soc. Chir. Paris, *41*:1370, 1915.

Mühlbauer, W. D., Segeth, H., and Viessmann, A.: Restoration of lid function in facial palsy with permanent magnets. Chir. Plastica (Berl.), *1*:295, 1973.

Ney, K. W.: Facial paralysis and the surgical repair of the facial nerve. Laryngoscope, *32*:327, 1922.

Nigst, H.: Chirurgie des peripheren Nerven. Z. Unfallmed. Berufskr., *62*:199, 1969.

Niklison, J.: Contribution to the subject of facial paralysis. Plast. Reconstr. Surg., *17*:276, 1956.

Niklison, J.: Facial paralysis: Moderation of nonparalysed muscles. Br. J. Plast. Surg., *18*:397, 1965.

Olivecrona, H.: The surgical treatment of intracranial tumors. *In* Handbuch der Neurochirurgie. Bd. 4, vieter Teil, S. 192. Berlin, Springer-Verlag, 1967.

Owens, N.: Preliminary report on the development of neuromuscular junctions in cases of facial paralysis followed by masseter muscle transplantations. Plast. Reconstr. Surg., *6*:345, 1950.

Owens, N.: Surgical treatment of facial paralysis. Plast. Reconstr. Surg., *7*:61, 1951.

Perl, J., and Wagner, R.: Intrathoracic phrenic nerve repair. J. Internatl. Coll. Surg., *44*:171, 1965.

Perret, G.: Results of phrenicofacial nerve anastomosis for facial paralysis. Arch. Surg., 94:505, 1967.

Petti, G., and Conley, J. J.: Hypoglossal-facial nerve crossover in the treatment of facial paralysis. *In* Conley, J. J., and Dickenson, J. T. (Eds.): Plastic and Reconstructive Surgery of the Face and Neck. New York, Grune & Stratton, 1972.

Philipeaux, J. M., and Vulpian, A.: Les essais de greffe d'un tronçon de nerf lingual entre les deux bouts de l'hypoglosse. Arch. Physiol. Norm. Path., 3:618, 1870.

Pick, J. F.: The Surgery of Repair. Vol. 2. Philadelphia, J. B. Lippincott Company, 1949, p. 617.

Pulec, J. C.: Total decompression of the facial nerve. Laryngoscope, 76:1015, 1966.

Pulec, J. C.: Facial nerve grafting. Laryngoscope, 79:1562, 1969.

Rhoton, A. L., and Lineweaver, W.: Personal communication, 1976.

Robson, A. W. M.: A case of successful nerve grafting. Trans. Clin. Soc. Lond., 22:120, 1889.

Rogers, B. O.: Bilateral congenital facial paralysis (palsy): The Möbius syndrome. *In* Converse, J. M. (Ed.): Reconstructive Plastic Surgery. Philadelphia, W. B. Saunders Company, 1964, p. 1286.

Rosenfalck, P., and Buchthal, F.: Studies on fibrillation potentials of denervated human muscle. Electroencephalogr. Clin. Neurophysiol. (Suppl), 22:130, 1962.

Rosenthal, A. M.: Electrodiagnostic testing in neuromuscular disease. J.A.M.A., 177:829, 1961.

Rousso, M.: Round-table discussion at Sixth International Congress of Plastic and Reconstructive Surgery, Paris, 1975.

Rubin, L. R.: The anatomy of a smile: Its importance in the treatment of facial paralysis. Plast. Reconstr. Surg., 53:384, 1974.

Sammarco, G. J., Ryan, R. F., and Longenecker, C. G.: Anatomy of the facial nerve in fetuses and stillborn infants. Plast. Reconstr. Surg., 37:566, 1966.

Sanders, F.: The preservation of nerve grafts. *In* Ciba Foundation Symposium, London, 1954, p. 175.

Scaramella, L.: L'anastomosi tra i due nervi facciali. Arch. Ital. Otol. 82:209, 1971.

Seddon, H. J.: Report on Peripheral Nerve Injuries in World War II. Medical Research Council Special Report Series #282. Her Majesty's Stationery Office. London, 1954.

Seddon, H.: Surgical Disorders of the Peripheral Nerves. London, Livingstone, 1972.

Shapiro, H. H.: Maxillofacial Anatomy. Philadelphia, J. B. Lippincott Company, 1954.

Sheehan, J. E.: Plastic Surgery of the Orbit. New York, MacMillan, 1927.

Sheehan, J. E.: Progress in correction of facial paralysis with tantalum wire and mesh. Surgery, 27:122, 1950.

Slaughter, W. B.: Observation of the Later Stages of Nerve Regeneration. Dept. of Anatomy, University of Nebraska, Omaha, 1935.

Smith, J. W.: Microsurgery of peripheral nerves. Plast. Reconstr. Surg., 33:317, 1964.

Smith, J. W.: Microsurgery: Review of the literature and discussion of microtechniques. Plast. Reconstr. Surg., 37:227, 1966.

Smith, J. W.: A new technique of facial animation. Trans. Vth Internatl. Congr. Plast. Surg. Australia, Butterworths, 1971, p. 83.

Snyder, C. D., Webster, H. D., Pickens, J. E., Hines, W. A., and Warden, G.: Intraneural neurorrhaphy: A preliminary clinical and histological evaluation. Ann. Surg., 67:691, 1968.

Stein, A. E.: Die kosmetische Korrektur der Fazialislaehmung durch freie Faszienplastic. Muenchen. Med. Wochenschr., 60:1370, 1913.

Steindler, A.: The method of direct neurotization of paralyzed muscles. Am. J. Orthop. Surg., 13:33, 1915.

Steindler, A.: Direct neurotization of paralysed muscles: further study of the question of direct nerve implantation. J. Orthop. Surg., 14:707, 1916.

Sullivan, J. A.: Recent advances in the surgical treatment of facial paralysis and Bell's palsy. Laryngoscope, 62:449, 1952.

Sunderland, S.: Funicular suture and funicular exclusion in the repair of severed nerves. Br. J. Surg., 40:580, 1952.

Sydenham, F.: Treatment of facial paralysis due to mastoid disease or to the mastoid operation. Br. Med. J., 1:1114, 1356, 1909.

Tarlow, I. M., and Boernstein, W.: Nerve regeneration: A comparative experimental study following suture by clot and thread. J. Neurosurg., 5:62, 1948.

Taverner, D.: Electrodiagnosis in facial palsy. Arch Otolaryngol., 81:470, 1965a.

Taverner, D.: Treatment of facial palsy. Arch. Otolaryngol., 81:489, 1965b.

Taverner, D., Kemble, F., and Cohen, S. B.: Prognosis and treatment of idiopathic facial (Bell's) palsy. Br. Med. J., 4:581, 1967.

Thompson, N.: Autogenous free grafts of skeletal muscle. A preliminary experimental and clinical study. Plast. Reconstr. Surg., 48:11, 1971a.

Thompson, N.: Treatment of facial paralysis by free skeletal muscle grafts. Trans. Vth Intnatl. Congr. Plast. Reconstr. Surg. Melbourne, Butterworths, 1971b, pp. 66–82.

Thompson, N., and Pollard, A. C.: Motor function in Abbe flaps. Br. J. Plast. Surg., 14:66, 1961.

Tickle, T. G.: The after care of surgery of the facial nerve. Ann. Otol. Rhinol. Laryngol., 45:7, 1936.

Tickle, T. G.: Surgery of the facial nerve in 300 operated cases. Laryngoscope, 55:191, 1945.

Vasconez, L. O.: Personal communication, 1972.

Viñas, J. C., Jager, E., and Viñas, J. M.: Treatment of facial paralysis with a transfer of the occipitalis muscle and galea aponeurotica. Presented at the Society of Ophthalmic Plastic Surgeons, Dallas, 1973.

Wilflingseder, P., and Anderl, H.: Indications for intermittent, palliative surgical measures and long-term results with alloplasties in facial paralysis. Arch. Ital. Otol., 82:268, 1971.

Woodruff, M. F. A.: The Transplantation of Tissues and Organs. Springfield, Ill., Charles C Thomas, Publisher, 1960.

Wood-Smith, D.: Encircling Silastic band for paralysis of the orbicularis oculi muscle. Presented at the Society of Ophthalmic Plastic Surgeons, Dallas, Texas, September 16, 1973.

Wood-Smith, D.: Personal communication, 1976.

Wullstein, H.: Die Methode der Kekompression des N. facialis vom Austritt aus dem labryinth bis zu dem aus dem Foramen stylomastoideum ohne Beeintrachtigung des Mittelohres. Arch. Ohr. Nas. Kehlk.-Heilk., 172:582, 1958.

Young, J. Z., and Sanders, F. K.: The degeneration and reinnervation of grafted nerves. J. Anat., 76:143, 1942.

Zülch, K. J.: Wert der konservativen Behandlung für die Restitution der gestörten Facialisfunktion. Fortschr. Kiefer. Gesichtschir., 2:132, 1956.

CHAPTER 37

ESTHETIC SURGERY FOR THE AGING FACE

CARY L. GUY, M.D.,
JOHN MARQUIS CONVERSE, M.D.,
AND DANIEL C. MORELLO, M.D.

Aging suggested wisdom in antiquity, and this attitude persists in many nonindustrialized countries today. With the development of modern industrial society and the competition for employment, as well as the contemporary emphasis on youth, beauty, and success, patients have sought means of removing or lessening the signs of growing older, an unwelcome contrast to the smooth physiognomy of youth. In response, various types of cosmetic or esthetic operations were devised beginning early in the twentieth century. Rogers (1971a, b) has reviewed the history of cosmetic surgery.

The American Medical Association has provided a definition of cosmetic surgery as "that branch of surgery which is done to revise or change the texture, configuration, or relationship with contiguous structures of any feature of the human body which would be considered by the average, prudent observer to be within the broad range of 'normal' and acceptable variation for age and ethnic origin, and in addition, is performed for a condition which is judged by competent medical opinion to be without potential for jeopardy to physical or mental health."

Patients may be moved to seek corrective surgery for signs of aging by a desire for self-improvement or by a desire to preserve a relatively youthful appearance. These quests may also reflect a desire to be a useful member of society after the arbitrary age of retirement.

HISTORICAL BACKGROUND

The first American surgeon to publish a paper on esthetic surgery was Miller, whose article was entitled "The excision of bag-like folds of skin from the region about the eyes" (1906). Miller, an unethical practitioner about whom Rogers (1971a) has written in detail, published one year later (1907), in collaboration with his wife, another paper with the first photograph showing the lines of incision in the lower eyelids for removal of a crescent of excess skin. Another American, Kolle, included in his book on *Plastic and Cosmetic Surgery* (1911) the first easily understandable illustrations of lower eyelid incisions for the removal of loose skin.

Many early practitioners were poorly trained in surgery, but Bourguet, an ophthalmologist practicing in Paris, was well trained in his field and described the design of small crescentic or angular incisions for corrective blepharoplasty in 1919. In 1924 he described his technique for the excision and correction of protruding palpebral fat pockets and in 1925 published "before and after" photographs of patients who had undergone this type of operation. Dupuis and Rees (1971) have provided some historical notes on blepharoplasty.

The vast number of men who were facially disfigured during World War I and the remarkable achievements of surgeons in rehabilitating many of them attracted surgeons who had been trained in the techniques of reconstructive surgery to the field of cosmetic surgery.

Passot, who had received part of his training under Morestin (who inspired Gillies; see Chapter 1), published a paper in 1919 in which he described various types of small skin incisions and excisions considered useful for the removal of excess facial skin. Passot later wrote a number of books, mostly intended for the lay public and undoubtedly used for patient recruitment. Another surgeon who described operations for face lifting at about that time was LaGarde (1925).

Holländer of Berlin wrote in 1932 that he had performed a face lift operation in 1901, and that this type of operation had been completely unknown prior to that time. Dissatisfied with the results of excision of isolated pieces of skin, he gradually developed a more extensive procedure. He made an incision extending from the temporal area downward in the preauricular fold, around the lobe of the ear and along the hairline. A similar incision extending from the temporal region into the preauricular region and under and behind the earlobe was demonstrated in the United States by Bettman in 1919. He showed "before and after" photographs of a patient who had submitted to a face lift operation and published them in 1920.

In the textbook *Die gesamte Wiederherstellungschirurgie* ("The Complete Reconstructive Surgery"), a remarkable compendium of reconstructive surgical procedures published in 1931, Lexer also stated that he had performed a face lift operation in 1906. He described the technique that he subsequently employed: S-shaped excisions of skin in the temporal area, in the preauricular region, at the insertion of the earlobe, and in the postauricular and scalp areas. After excising the redundant skin, Lexer anchored the subcutaneous tissue to the periosteum of the mastoid. He stated that the simple closure of small skin incisions without undermining the skin, as performed in his day by many so-called "cosmetic surgeons," would not result in long-lasting improvement.

Other operations for face lifting were published by Joseph in 1921 and 1928. Frühwald (1922) described operations similar to those of Joseph with minor modifications. During this period other surgeons who published books on cosmetic surgery were Hunt (1926) and Nöel (1926); the latter was one of the first to emphasize the psychologic aspects of cosmetic surgery.

The importance of esthetic surgery of the face to psychologic well-being and vocational success was only slowly recognized by the medical profession at large. Operations to correct nasal deformities were more quickly accepted because many of these deformities were associated with functional problems that required correction in conjunction with the rhinoplasty procedure. On the other hand, it is true that esthetic surgery in its early stages was performed most often by unqualified, and often unscrupulous, surgeons who used unethical means such as newspaper advertisements to recruit their patients. Paraffin injected subcutaneously (Gersuny, 1900) was used until the late 1920's to smooth out the wrinkled face despite innumerable complications, such as migration of the inorganic material and the development of paraffinomas.

Even into the 1930's recognition of the significance of esthetic surgery was hampered by lack of understanding on the part of the medical profession. The world-renowned surgeon von Bergmann, Lexer's teacher, publicly ridiculed Joseph's rhinoplastic operations as pandering to the vanity of patients. Some of the surgeons did not enjoy a high standing in the medical profession. Moreover, many books were published for the benefit of the lay public and were not regarded as ethical.

The history of cosmetic surgery has been reviewed in considerable detail by Rees and Wood-Smith (1973).

AGING OF THE FACE

Aging of the skin usually parallels aging of the body, an ineluctable biological phenomenon. The facial skin, however, being exposed to sunlight and other extraneous factors, is apt to show signs of aging more rapidly than unexposed areas (see Fig. 37–6).

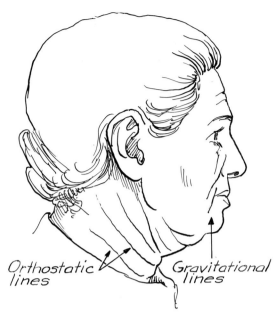

FIGURE 37–1. Orthostatic and gravitational lines of the face and neck.

Aging of the face varies from person to person because of life style, illnesses, environmental influences including exposure to sunlight, and many other factors, among which heredity plays an important role. Although changes wrought by aging and the relative stages of deterioration are extremely variable, there are certain elemental alterations which are generally accepted by most investigators. The morphologic changes culminate in a classic picture of old age. The pink, soft, warm, translucent, resilient skin of youth is transformed to a dull, yellowish tan, scaly, atonic, and opaque covering with a predisposition to lentiginous and other benign, precancerous, or cancerous lesions: seborrheic keratoses, senile seborrheic hyperplasia of Jadassohn, senile hemangioma, lentigo maligna of Hutchinson, and basal cell, basosquamous cell, or squamous cell carcinoma (Mihan, 1962).

Skin Folds and Wrinkles. The folds and wrinkles of the aging face may be divided for purposes of orientation into orthostatic, dynamic, gravitational, and combination types.

Orthostatic lines are natural furrows which may be present at birth or become apparent later as the infantile panniculus adiposus disappears. These lines do not represent a true manifestation of the aging process but are mentioned only because of their plastic surgical significance. They are due to skin excess, which is required over certain areas for the purpose of flexion and extension. They are found over the posterior and anterolateral aspects of the neck and are generally arranged in a transverse curvilinear or intersecting fashion; they usually number from one to three (Fig. 37–1).

Dynamic lines develop as a result of the repetitious right angle pull on the skin by the muscles of expression. The time of development and the number of dynamic lines vary considerably. The first dynamic lines to develop are those of the forehead, usually beginning in adolescent years as a result of the action of the frontalis muscle (Fig. 37–2). These lines vary in position, number, depth, and continuity. They generally occupy a transverse, superiorly convex, curvilinear position extending from the anterior margin of the temporal fossae across the forehead, arching over the supercilia, and arching upward over the mid-forehead region. Once developed, they usually become progressively more evident in repose.

The next dynamic lines to develop usually appear in the twenties as a result of contraction of the orbicularis oculi muscles (Fig. 37–3, *A*). These are the primary lines of expression of the lateral canthal areas, commonly referred to as "crow's feet" or "laugh lines." They vary in position, number, and depth, extending in a

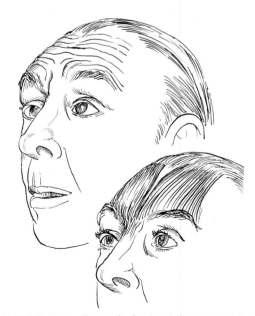

FIGURE 37–2. Dynamic forehead lines caused by the contraction of the frontalis muscle.

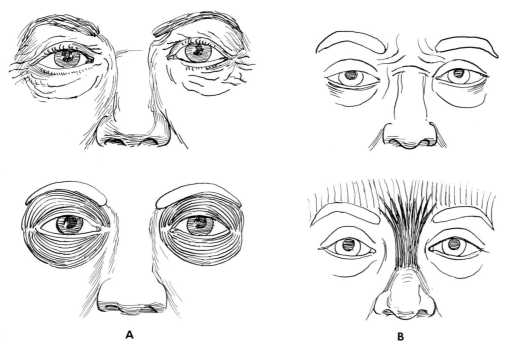

FIGURE 37–3. *A*, Dynamic lateral canthal and eyelid lines caused by the contraction of the orbicularis oculi muscle fibers. *B*, Dynamic vertical glabellar lines caused by the contraction of the paired corrugator supercilii muscle fibers. The dynamic horizontal lines at the root of the nose are caused by the contraction of the procerus muscle fibers.

radial, fanlike fashion from the lateral canthal regions in irregular lengths. Secondary lines directed obliquely downward develop later; these curvilinear lines extend laterally from the lower eyelid toward the zygoma. The lines are caused by the interplay of the contracting fibers of the orbicularis oculi muscles.

In Occidentals and approximately 50 per cent of Orientals, the supratarsal folds of the upper eyelids represent dynamic manifestations of the attachment of the skin to the aponeurosis of the levator palpebrae superioris muscle (see Chapter 28).

As a result of gravitional as well as dynamic influences, the nasolabial folds become accentuated. They represent the area of junction of the skin of the lip, which is tightly bound to the underlying orbicularis oris, and the more loosely bound skin of the cheek over the buccal fat pad. The folds result mainly from the pull of the infraorbital and zygomatic fibers of the quadratus labii superioris and of the zygomaticus and risorius muscles. The nasolabial folds appear to arise from the superolateral aspect of the alar cartilages and extend downward and obliquely in varying lengths and

depths, terminating usually about 1 cm lateral to the oral commissures; they may also continue downward to the lower border of the mandible, helping to form the anterior margin of the later developing "jowl." The nasolabial folds may become quite deep in repose.

The glabellar frown lines develop at variable ages, depending largely on the expressive habits of the individual (Fig. 37–3, *B*). These vertical lines are caused by the action of the paired corrugator supercilii muscles. The lines vary in number, depth, length, and regularity. They are usually curvilinear, originating from the lower border of the medial aspect of the corrugators, coursing nasally to the lateral margins of the root of the nose to curve upward as straight lines across the glabella, and terminating in the lower portion of the mid-forehead region. Often one or more central straight vertical lines develop, which are apt to be more evident in repose and can extend as high as the forehead hairline.

The horizontal frown lines in the area of the root of the nose are usually relatively inconspicuous (Fig. 37–3, *B*). They consist of short transverse furrows, irregular in depth and

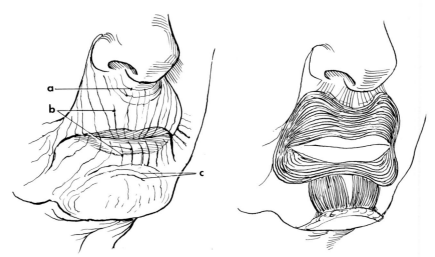

FIGURE 37–4. *Left,* Horizontal lines below the columella are caused by the contraction of the depressor septi nasi muscles (*a*). The dynamic circumoral lip lines are caused by the contraction of the orbicularis oris muscle fibers (*b*). Lines and dimplelike depressions develop in the chin as a result of the contraction of the mentalis muscles (*c*). *Right,* Anatomy of the involved muscles.

length, ranging in number from one to three, and they owe their presence to the action of the procerus muscle.

Horizontal lines below the columella result from the contraction of the depressor septi muscle (Fig. 37–4, *a*). Beginning usually in the fifth decade of life, circumoral lines in the upper lip and later in the lower lip are common in females (Fig. 37–4, *b*). These lines result from the contractural pull of the orbicularis oris muscle. They are situated in a vertical plane and are irregular in number, length, and depth.

Irregularly dispersed "dimplelike" depressions over the surface of the chin line develop as a result of the dynamic effect of the mentalis muscle (Fig. 37–4, *c*). These depressions are not found in all individuals, but they may be extremely prominent in some.

Gravitational lines develop insidiously and are variable in their time of onset. Usually they become apparent after age 40 and progress in accordance with the effect of gravity on the atonic skin. Histologic changes occurring within the skin and subcutaneous tissue, together with dynamic furrows and the atrophy of the facial bony architecture associated with the loss of teeth and alveolar process, result in a loose, unpadded skin covering which falls in dependent folds at the mercy of gravity (Fig. 37–5). The gravitational lines are manifest throughout the face and neck and appear to

originate from the underlying bony prominences (orbital rims, zygoma, and mandible). The upper eyelid skin becomes horizontally redundant and tends to fall in loose folds over the cilia, especially in the lateral third of the eyelids. Later, the superciliary skin drops below the superior orbital rim and increases the redundancy of the upper eyelid skin. Similar changes occur in the skin of the lower eyelids. Both upper and lower eyelids may be affected by protrusion of orbital fat beneath the septum orbitale, resulting in additional puffiness and bagginess of the lids. As age advances, the orbital fat may atrophy, causing the ocular globes to appear more deeply set within the orbits.

Owing to the gradual loss of subcutaneous fat, especially in the buccal fat pad, the cheeks become sunken and the skin hangs in redundant vertical folds from the zygoma and lower border of the mandible to form the characteristic "jowl" (Fig. 37–5, *A*). As a result of generalized atrophy, interlacing secondary lines develop over the entire facial and cervical skin, notably the cheeks, lips, chin, pretragal region, posterior cervical region, and anterior base of the neck. Later even the nasal skin and earlobes are involved. Secondary furrows may develop parallel to the nasolabial folds, originating at the oral commissures and coursing inferiorly toward the lateral aspect of the chin. These lines are caused in part by the pull of

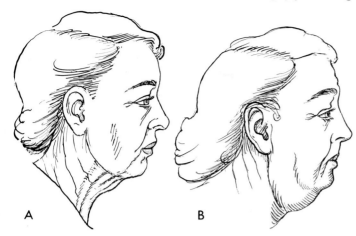

FIGURE 37–5. Gravitational lines. *A,* Submental vertical skin folds ("turkey gobbler" neck). *B,* Double chin caused by the accumulation of submental fat.

the depressor muscles around the mouth, but are more attributable to the gravitational effect.

The neck responds in a different manner. The effect of gravity is to accentuate the horizontal orthostatic lines and to form vertical submental folds. The horizontal orthostatic lines become exaggerated and permanent in repose. Secondary interlacing lines gradually develop over the posterior cervical region, particularly in men, resulting in the "leatherneck" appearance.

The pull of the decussating fibers of the medial portion of the platysma muscles within the substance of the skin itself may form two long, vertical, "turkey gobbler" folds when the submental fat pad is not present to fill the intervening space (Fig. 37–5, *A*). The folds hang from the lower margin of the mandible bilaterally, often overlapped by the "jowls," and extend vertically inferiorly and medially to end over the tendinous sternal heads of the sternomastoid muscles. The submental region may undergo a paradoxical change in individuals in whom a familial tendency results in the development of an excessive amount of submental fat, which is not necessarily related to obesity (Fig. 37–5, *B*).

Gonzalez-Ulloa and Flores (1965) described changes in physiognomy occurring with aging and emphasized the atrophy of adipose tissue. They stated that the general atrophy of the tissues weakens the supporting structures of the eyelids (the orbicularis oculi muscle and the septum orbitale) and produces protrusion of orbital fat in the eyelids.

Gonzalez-Ulloa, Simonin, and Flores (1971) used cephalometric-like radiographs to assess the changes associated with aging in the face and neck. They charted the gravitational changes of the eyebrows, the oral commissure, and the cervical tissue. The acute change in the eyebrows usually occurred between 25 and 40 years of age; the maximal rate of descent of the labial commissure occurred after the age of 50 years; and the rate of descent of the cervical tissues (the angle of incidence of the neck in reference to the facial plane) was greatest between 35 and 55 years of age.

TEXTURE. The fine scaliness, dryness, and inelasticity of the aging skin associated with loss of the rebound phenomenon and lack of tonus are the result of the degenerative process. The textural changes are not uniform; wrinkling is more conspicuous on the exposed areas of the face and dorsum of the hands than on the unexposed portions of the body.

Histologic and Histochemical Characteristics of Aging Skin. Freeman (1971) summarized the changes associated with aging in unexposed skin:

Epidermis
    Thinning is questionable
    Greater cellular variation
    Fewer, more variable, melanocytes
Dermis
    More hydroxyproline
    More insoluble collagen
    Less soluble collagen
    Collagen is more resistant
    Elastin is less extensible
    Less hexosamine, acid mucopolysaccharides
Appendages
    Eccrine sweat glands—fewer and less responsive
    Apocrine sweat glands—greater variation
    Hair follicles—fewer and more irregular
    Sebaceous glands—less sebum

THE EPIDERMIS. Freeman (1971) failed to demonstrate a statistically significant difference with age in the thickness of buttock skin (unexposed to solar radiation) of individuals 25 to 76 years old. Gonzalez-Ulloa and Flores (1965) reported a decrease in thickness of the exposed epidermis, primarily the basal layer. Prunieras (1973) studied epithelial regeneration as a function of age and demonstrated a slackening of the growth of keratinocytes with aging.

Katzberg (1952) and Andrew (1962) described increasing mitoses in senile skin in the human and in the experimental animal. After age 50 the number of mitoses remains constant (Katzberg, 1952) and may even decrease (Baker and Blair, 1968). Nevertheless, there is progressive rounding and vacuolization of the cells of the stratum germinativum with flattening of the cells of the stratum granulosum and the stratum spinosum (Johnson and Hadley, 1964). With aging there may be an actual growth decline in the epidermal cells, and according to Maciera-Coelho (1973), this may be due to an increased sensitivity to cell crowding caused by an impairment in the control of ribosomal ribonucleic acid synthesis. Andrew (1962) also described greater variations in the size and appearance of the nuclear and cytoplasmic elements of aged skin.

Fitzpatrick, Szabo, and Mitchell (1965) found that the number of dopa-positive cells in human epidermis decreases with aging. Although the dopa-positive cells may represent both the functional and nonfunctional melanocytes, there is nonetheless an overall diminution in the number of epidermal melanocytes with aging. Epidermal melanocytes are larger in senile skin than in young skin, probably owing to functional hypertrophy.

THE DERMIS. Collagen fibers appear to swell, then later to fragment and atrophy, with basophilic cytoplasmic degeneration. The rate of synthesis of collagen parallels that of skin growth, and the changing rate causes a diminution in the amount of new (soluble) collagen and a concomitant increase in mature (insoluble) collagen (Rasmussen, Wakim, and Winkelman, 1965). Collagen is continually being synthesized throughout life, but its metabolic activity, both synthesis and degradation, decreases with aging (Pinto, 1974). Collagen fibers become progressively thicker until the age of 20 years, with minimal increase thereafter. The maturation of collagen is associated with an increase in intermolecular cross linking, which makes the collagen more resistant to degradation (see Chapter 3). The end result of increased cross linking among collagen molecules could be impaired diffusion of oxygen and waste products between cells and resultant impairment of homeostasis (Fleischmajer, Perlish, and Bashey, 1973).

Knowledge of changes in elastin is less certain. Pinto (1974) stated that elastin fibers increase in number and thickness throughout life, and Sams and Smith (1965) demonstrated a fivefold increase in the elastin content of human skin from fetal to adult life. The lipid content of the dermis is unchanged with aging (Pearce and Grimmer, 1973). In a simultaneous study of cutaneous and vascular specimens from the same individuals, Bouissou, Pieraggi, Julian, and Blazy (1973) suggested that there may be a parallel between cutaneous and vascular aging, especially of the aorta.

The loss of elasticity of aged skin has been shown to be associated with homogenization of the ground substance and an increase in fibrous connective tissue rather than with elastin degeneration. Although elasticity decreases, tensile strength actually increases. The tone of the skin, on the other hand (expressed by the rebound phenomenon), is decreased because of changes in the collagen fibers and ground substance, and because of atrophy of the arrectores pilorum muscles. Progressive fragility and sclerosis of papillary and reticular vascular plexuses and glomeruli occur. Paradoxically, Ellis, Montagna, and Fanger (1958) showed that with advancing age the complexity of the blood supply around the sebaceous glands increases in proportion to the number of lobulations as well as the size of the glands. The interconnections of the blood capillaries among all of the cutaneous glands and hair follicles are particularly abundant in the aged.

Cauna (1965) showed that the receptor organs of the dermis undergo variable changes; pacinian corpuscles increase in size with aging, and Meissner's corpuscles decrease in number but increase in length with resultant lobulation and coiling. Free nerve endings undergo the least change with age. The changes in receptor organs may signify a morphologic adaptation to change environmental stimuli or physiologic requirements. The dermal ground substance undergoes minimal change with aging, with a small decrease in hexosamine and acid mucopolysaccharides.

THE APPENDAGES. Eccrine sweat glands become dilated with flattened epithelium and evidence of a decreased rate of sweating and a decreased response to epinephrine and Mecholyl

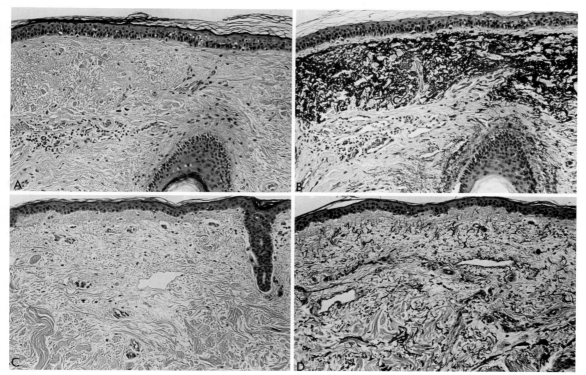

FIGURE 37-6. Changes in aging skin in a 60 year old white male. *A*, Skin with long-term sun exposure. Note the accumulation of elastotic material in the dermis, as shown by special elastin stain in *B*. Contrast *A* with *C*, taken from the buttocks which had received no sun exposure. Note the diminution of elastotic material, as shown in *D* (elastin stain of same section). (Courtesy of Dr. A. B. Ackerman, Skin and Cancer Unit, New York University Medical Center.)

(Silver, Montagna, and Karacan, 1965). Some of the eccrine glands undergo complete involution, reducing the absolute number. Montagna (1965) has described considerable morphologic variation in the the apocrine glands with aging in young adults. Oberste-Lehn (1965) cited a decrease in the number and an increase in the irregularity of hair follicles with aging. Pochi and Strauss (1965) concluded that the aging of the sebaceous gland in man is primarily influenced by endogenous androgens in males. Montagna and Parakkal (1974) ascribed the control of sebaceous secretions in the female to a combination of ovarian and adrenal androgens and noted the antagonistic role of progesterone.

THE SUBCUTANEOUS TISSUE. With advancing age the subcutaneous adipose tissue decreases in thickness, particularly in the face, with atrophy of the buccal fat pad and its temporal extension. The bony architecture of the skull, face, and spine also shows signs of atrophy which accentuate the physiognomic changes.

Freeman (1971) concluded that "it is increasingly apparent that the cutaneous changes giving rise to the connotation of old age are due more to environmental influences than to senescence alone." He cited chronic sun exposure as the most significant factor in the process (Fig. 37-6). There is flattening of the epidermis with disappearance of the rete ridges in exposed skin (Montagna, 1965), whereas in unexposed skin there is preservation of the rete ridges, even in the elderly. The dermal papillae are flattened, and the basement membranes are shortened in sun-damaged skin; this is seen as a decrease in the size of the dermis. These changes are partially reversible; Gerstein and Freeman (1963) transplanted sun-damaged skin to unexposed areas and demonstrated partial improvement of the cutaneous architecture. Damage by exposure to the sun has been demonstrated in the skin of 25 year olds with heavy sun exposure (Smith, 1963). Maciera-Coelho (1973) agreed that ionizing radiation appears to accelerate the aging process.

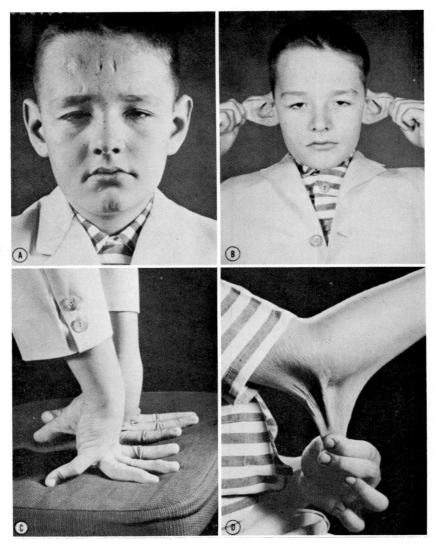

FIGURE 37–7.   A patient with Ehlers-Danlos-syndrome. *A*, Widened scars on the forehead. *B*, Ease with which the ears can be stretched from the head. *C*, Hyperextension of the joints. *D*, Typical hypoelastic skin. (From Rees, T. D., Wood-Smith, D., and Converse, J. M.: The Ehlers-Danlos syndrome. Plast. Reconstr. Surg., *32*:39, 1963. Copyright 1963, The Williams & Wilkins Company, Baltimore.)

The Ehlers-Danlos Syndrome. This syndrome is characterized by hypoelastic skin (Fig. 37–7). There may be hyperextension of joints, and the patients often demonstrate the acrobatic positions they are able to assume. Rees, Wood-Smith, and Converse (1963) have shown that, because of what appears to be faulty collagen maturation found in this syndrome, surgical treatment has resulted in prolonged wound healing and disappointing cosmetic results. Rybka and O'Hara (1967) noted that hemorrhage from large vessels was the most frequent serious complication of this syndrome. Beighton and Bull (1970) reported that the scars are often darkly pigmented or telangiectatic, and that fleshy, heaped-up pseudotumors sometimes develop in relation to the scars. The problems encountered with surgery relate to increased tissue fragility, and for this reason corrective surgery in patients with this syndrome is often not recommended.

The characteristics of the Ehlers-Danlos syndrome vary in their severity. In some patients with hypoelastic skin, a face lift operation may be performed with the understanding that it may be necessary to perform more than one operation in order to obtain a satisfactory result.

Diseases of Premature Aging. Three diseases that may represent examples of premature aging are of importance to the plastic surgeon: cutis laxa, progeria, and Werner's syndrome.

Cutis laxa is a rare hereditary disorder involving skin and connective tissue. It is inherited as an autosomal recessive trait. The onset of the disease is usually in childhood, and there is a decrease in the number and size of elastin fibers with fragmentation and disruption of their normal arrangement (Dingman, Grabb, and Oneal, 1969). This results in a severe degree of gravitational skin folding with associated abnormalities such as inguinal and ventral hernias, bowel and bladder diverticula, pulmonary emphysema, congenital heart disease, and aneurysms of the great vessels. The skin is loose, not hyperelastic, and the joints are normal. Goltz and associates (1965) have proposed that there is a deficiency of elastase inhibiting substance which is related to decreased serum copper levels, but measurements of serum and urine copper in several cases to date have been inconclusive. Dingman, Grabb, and Oneal (1969) stated that repeated rhytidectomy and blepharoplasty are indicated in these patients, since the skin changes appear to become less severe as age increases, and the patient derives considerable benefit from these procedures.

Progeria, also inherited as an autosomal recessive trait, is a generalized disease without evidence of endocrine deficiency. There is growth retardation with premature closure of the epiphyses, balding, loss of subcutaneous fat, arteriosclerosis or arterial calcification, cardiac disease, and a shortened life span. The onset is in childhood, and the changes occur rapidly. There does not seem to be any indication for plastic surgical treatment of the facial deformities of progeria.

Werner's syndrome is another rare disorder thought to be related to the aging process (Fleischmajer and Nedwich, 1973). It is also inherited as an autosomal recessive trait. The onset is during early adult life, with the appearance of shortened stature, high-pitched voice, cataracts, a tendency to mild diabetes mellitus, muscle atrophy, osteoporosis, premature arteriosclerosis, and a high incidence of associated neoplasms. There are also baldness, aged facies, and both hypo- and hyperpigmentation. The most characteristic feature is the appearance of scleroderma-like indurated patches of skin. The patients also have a microangiopathy similar to that of diabetes, which makes elective surgical procedures contraindicated.

ESTHETIC SURGERY OF THE FACE: PREOPERATIVE CONSIDERATIONS

The patient consults the surgeon for a variety of motives. The motive may be a simple one: the desire to improve his appearance. The motivation may be quite different, however (see Chapters 21 and 22), and it is important to make the patient understand that corrective surgery will not necessarily solve such problems as the threat of losing a job because of the signs of aging or recapturing the affections of an unfaithful spouse.

Overweight patients should be advised to lose weight. The patient should be carefully questioned concerning any type of physical disability. Medical problems should be completely evaluated. Allergies to drugs and medications should be checked. It is also important to find out what medication the patient may be taking on a regular basis. Aspirin is one of the most frequently used medications, and a patient taking the drug should be advised to discontinue the medication two weeks prior to the operation (see p. 1923). This latter precaution minimizes the danger of excessive bleeding during or after the operative procedure. In patients who are unusually apprehensive, tranquilizing medication will be needed.

The quality of the result the patient can expect to obtain is related to many factors, but one of the most important is the quality of the patient's skin. While the resiliency of the skin of the face is not directly related to the patient's age, a patient in the fifth decade has a more favorable prognosis and a better and more durable result than a patient of advanced age with loose, atonic, and sun-damaged skin.

THE ESTHETIC BLEPHAROPLASTY

"Blepharochalasis" was coined by Fuchs (1896) from two Greek words to designate relaxation of the eyelids. The term is inappropriate because excess eyelid skin may be present without "relaxation" of the eyelids. In older people relaxation of the eyelids, the lower eyelid in particular, is a frequent deficiency leading to senile ectropion. It is caused primarily by a loss of tonicity of the orbicularis oculi muscle. "Dermachalasis," the term used by Fox (1952) to indicate the condition characterized by protruding orbital fat, is also inappropriate, as its etymology suggests relaxation of the skin. The term "baggy eyelids" expresses in the vernacular the condition of the eyelid characterized by relaxation of the septum orbitale, protrusion of orbital fat, and excess aging skin; it is far from an elegant term, but at least it is not pretentious. The patients often refer to "pockets," "bags," "pouches," or "fat pads" under the eyes and to "hanging" skin of the upper eyelids.

Esthetic or corrective surgery of the eyelids is performed for two specific indications: (1) excess skin of the eyelids, which may reach such proportions in older patients that it obstructs vision when the skin of the upper lid folds downward over the eyelashes; and (2) protrusion of orbital fat caused by relaxation of the septum orbitale. The fat is most visible in the medial canthal area of the upper eyelid (but the protruding fat may extend along the whole length of the upper eyelid) and in three areas in the lower lid, medial, central, and less frequently lateral. These areas of protruding fat are frequently referred to as herniated fat, ordinarily an inappropriate term. However, in exceptional cases in older patients, erosion of the septum orbitale has been observed, and orbital fat is actually herniated through the septum.

Two types of patients request corrective blepharoplasties. In the first group are patients who show protruding fat at an early age but may not consult a surgeon until their late twenties or early thirties when the fatty protrusions have become more conspicuous. The condition described by Dupuytren (1839) and Sichel (1844) is usually hereditary and is caused by a congenital weakness of the septum orbitale. The deformity has been described as being present in members of the family for several generations (Panneton, 1936). In the second group loss of elasticity causes the eyelid skin to fall in folds over the lines of expression of the eyes, and in patients of advanced age a noticeable change of skin texture, in the form of a crepey characteristic, complicates the deformity.

Many patients do not "see their own eyes." They may request only a face lift operation because of relaxation of the skin of the face and neck. Upon examination it is observed that the major deformity is in the eyelids. It is sometimes more diplomatic to point out the eyelid problem to the patient while examining the patient's photographs at the time of the second visit. It is obvious that if the patient undergoes a successful face lift operation, the contrast between the rejuvenated face and the aged appearance of the eyelids will cause the patient to return for a second operation.

The eyes are the most expressive features of the human face. For this reason errors in the technique of eyelid surgery are immediately manifest. Improper placement of the incisions and excessive removal of skin or orbital fat are common causes of round and expressionless eyes.

There are many other causes of baggy eyelids. These include edema from cardiovascular disease or allergies, thyrotoxic exophthalmos (see Chapter 28), and hypothyroidism. Appropriate medical consultations are indicated, and the underlying medical conditions should be evaluated and treated.

Anatomy. The anatomy of the eyelids is described in Chapter 28. The important anatomical structures to be considered in performing a cosmetic blepharoplasty are the levator palpebrae superioris muscle and aponeurosis in the upper eyelid, the septum orbitale, and the orbicularis oculi muscle. In the area of the lateral canthal raphé, the orbicularis oculi fibers are intimately connected with the skin, and sharp dissection is required to separate skin from muscle. As the dissection proceeds over the pretarsal and preseptal portions of the orbicularis oculi muscle, the dissection is effected with greater ease, because the skin is less adherent to the muscle. A second point to recall is that the characteristics and thickness of the skin change at the orbital rim, as shown in Chapter 28 (Fig. 28–13). Whereas the skin of the eyelids is the thinnest in the body, a transition occurs at the orbital rim to the thicker skin of the face.

Classification of Eyelid Deformities Requiring Esthetic Blepharoplasty. Castañares (1976) has provided this classification:

Blepharochalasis (Fig. 37–8, *A*) is characterized by loss of elasticity and relaxation of the lid skin. The skin becomes thin, wrinkled, and redundant as a result of aging. Visual obstruction may result.

Dermachalasis (Fig. 37–8, *B*), first described by Sichel in 1875, also affects middle-aged and older individuals who develop hypertrophy of the upper eyelid skin. The skin is no longer intimately connected to the orbicularis oculi muscle and hangs over the ciliary margin when the patient raises the upper eyelid. This condition is to be distinguished from the deformity pro-

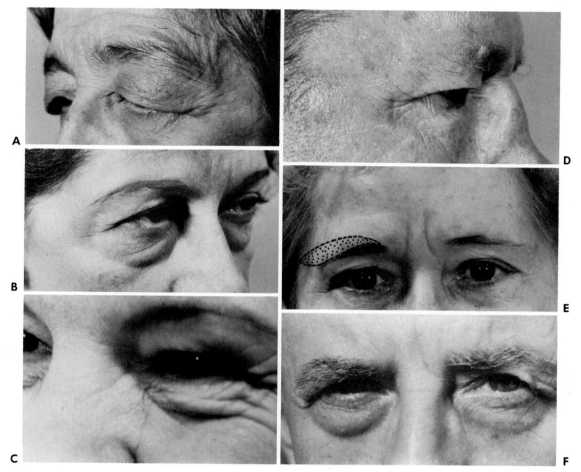

FIGURE 37-8. *A*, Blepharochalasis. *B*, Dermachalasis. *C*, Protrusion of orbital fat. *D*, Hooding of the upper eyelids caused by ptosis of the eyebrows. *E*, Hypertrophy of the orbicularis oculi muscle. *F*, Combination of the deformities shown in the preceding photographs. (Courtesy of Dr. Salvador Castañares.)

duced from protrusion of orbital fat. The term "ptosis adiposa" employed by Sichel is a misnomer, as the condition is a "pseudoptosis" caused by the thickened skin.

Protrusion of orbital fat (Fig. 37–8, *C*). This is the major cause of deformity of the eyelids requiring blepharoplasty. "Herniation" is an inaccurate term, since the proptosis of the orbital fat is the consequence of the relaxation of the septum orbitale which normally retains the fat in the orbital cavity. The orbital fat protrudes beneath the septum orbitale; the eyelids lose their smooth contour owing to the "bags" or "fat pads" under the preseptal portion of the orbicularis oculi muscle and the skin. A herniation of orbital fat through the distended, atrophic, and thin septum orbitale is an exceptionally rare observation in aged patients.

It is generally accepted that the orbital fat is distributed in two areas in the upper lid (medial and central) and in three areas in the lower lid (medial, central, and lateral). These collections of orbital fat (or compartments) are separated by tenuous septa.

Hooding of the upper eyelids caused by ptosis of the eyebrows (Fig. 37–8, *D*). Ptosis of the eyebrows is a component of the generalized ptosis of the aging facial tissue: relaxation of the skin and stretching of the musculature. This condition cannot be corrected by eyelid surgery alone. A brow-lifting operation consisting of an elliptical supraorbital resection of skin is often required.

Hypertrophy of the orbicularis oculi muscle (Fig. 37–8, *E*). A horizontal bulge of the orbicularis muscle occurs in individuals who habitually squint while in the sun or for functional reasons (myopic patients). The muscle flap technique (see Fig. 37–13) is particularly suited to correct this deformity.

Combination of any of the above-described conditions (Fig. 37–8, *F*). Two or three of the deformities described may be present.

Preoperative Examination. The type of operation varies from the all inclusive corrective blepharoplasty involving resection of skin and protruding fat from the upper and lower eyelids to lesser operations, such as removal of unilateral protruding orbital fat in a young patient or a minor trim of the upper and lower lid skin.

The condition of the patient's vision should be checked by having the patient read a chart. The patient may be unaware of a non-seeing eye and the surgeon may be accused of causing the blindness after the operation has been performed.

In assessing the problem the following factors should be considered and described to the patient:

1. The amount of excess skin of the upper and lower eyelids.

2. The amount and distribution of the orbital fat.

3. The character of the skin and degree of elastic degeneration as shown by fine (crepey) or obvious wrinkling or the presence of edema.

4. Pigmentation of the lids and the usual gradual increase of pigment toward the lid margins.

5. The presence of a skin lesion, such as a papilloma or xanthelasma, and its amenability to inclusion in the routine excision.

6. Asymmetry of the eyes, especially in their shape and the degree of retraction upon opening of the upper lid.

7. Protrusion of the globe or exophthalmos, in which case excessive resection of the skin may result in corneal exposure.

8. The degree of "scleral show" between the iris and the lower lid margin. An unusual amount of sclera may show below the cornea in a relatively young patient as a congenital condition. In the older patient this is a sign of weakness of the orbicularis oculi muscle and incipient senile ectropion. Plicating the lower lid transversely between the thumb and the index finger in its lateral (temporal) third will indicate the extent of the looseness of the lid. The patient should be warned that a wedge excision may be required to tighten the lid and thus prevent ectropion and eversion of the inferior lacrimal punctum (see Chapter 28, p. 871).

9. Ptosis of the brow and prominence of the supraorbital rim.

10. Scars from previous surgery or accidents.

11. Prolapse of the lacrimal gland.

12. The presence of blindness or other ophthalmologic problems.

13. Anatomical variations associated with race, age, or individual characteristics, such as the absence of a supratarsal fold, prominence of the medial canthal tendon, and epicanthal folds.

14. Ptosis or levator muscle weakness. It is important to verify that the patient does not have a slight degree of ptosis of one upper lid.

The patient may not be aware of the discrepancy between the two upper lids but will become very much aware of such a discrepancy after the operation.

Photographs. The two halves of the face are asymmetrical. Photographs will demonstrate disparities in size and shape of the eyes prior to the surgical procedure.

The importance of preoperative photographs has been stressed in Chapter 1. Black and white photographs taken by a professional medical photographer provide the surgeon with detailed information. They are useful in assessing the patient's defects and in defining them to the patient. A full understanding should be reached with the patient concerning the degree of improvement to be achieved by corrective surgery. Several consultations are helpful in determining if a patient is realistic in his request or if the expectations are beyond attainment.

As well as documenting the problems for which the patient has consulted the surgeon, photographs record incidental lesions such as nevi, keratoses, and blemishes that have been overlooked, ignored, or denied by the patient. In addition, they are useful to the surgeon in preoperative planning of surgical procedures. In cases of doubt concerning the efficacy of the result, the photograph is an infallible psychologic (and medicolegal) document; postoperative photographs should also be obtained.

To be able to refresh one's memory with the photographs on the night before surgery is an asset. In the operating room, the patient is in a recumbent position. Either he is under general anesthesia with an endotracheal tube and its inevitable distortions or there is local distortion caused by infiltration of an anesthetic solution. Preoperative photographs are therefore invaluable.

Anesthesia. The operation is performed under either local or general anesthesia, depending on the preferences of the surgeon and the patient and on the available expertise. If local anesthesia is selected, the patient is sedated preoperatively. The type of preoperative medication varies according to the individual surgeon's preference. A formula similar to that administered to the patient undergoing a corrective rhinoplasty is the following. The patient is ensured of a restful night's sleep by the prescription of Seconal or Dalmane. On the day of surgery the formula is the following:

two hours preoperatively, 15 mg Valium by mouth; one hour preoperatively, 20 mg Pantopon and 20 mg chlorpromazine (Thorazine), 0.2 mg scopolamine, all administered by intramuscular injection. The dosage of the medications must be varied according to the patient's age, size, and general health. If additional sedation is required, diazepam (Valium) is administered intravenously in the operating room. This degree of sedation would not be advisable if the surgery were done in an outpatient facility.

Demerol given in small doses intravenously will often sedate the restless patient. However, excessive dosages of intravenous medication cause anoxia and restlessness. Oxygen administered through a catheter and insufflated into the nasopharynx ensures adequate oxygenation. Narcan is an effective antagonist to the respiratory depressant effect of narcotics.

The local anesthetic of choice is 1 per cent lidocaine solution with 1:50,000 epinephrine solution. The injection of the anesthetic solution is done only after careful outlining and marking of the operative plan.

Planning the Operation. The placement of suture lines in the eyelids is of such importance that the planning and marking of the lines of incision must be done with the utmost care. It is often advisable to outline the incisions on the patient the night before the operation, with the patient opening and closing his eyes while in a sitting position. If the outlining of the incisions is to be done in the operating room, the head end of the operating table can be elevated, placing the patient in a semi-sitting position. Thus, the true excess of skin can be more accurately determined.

Technique of the Esthetic Blepharoplasty

Skin Marking. It is important to outline the intended lower lid incision before that of the upper lid (Fig. 37–9). The outline is made just below the ciliary margin and extends from the punctum medially to the lateral canthus, where it is extended into a horizontal "crow's foot." The lateral extension of the incision will depend on the amount of skin to be removed.

When the segment of skin to be removed from the upper lids is being outlined, the lowermost ink line is placed below the upper border of the tarsus and the supratarsal fold, so

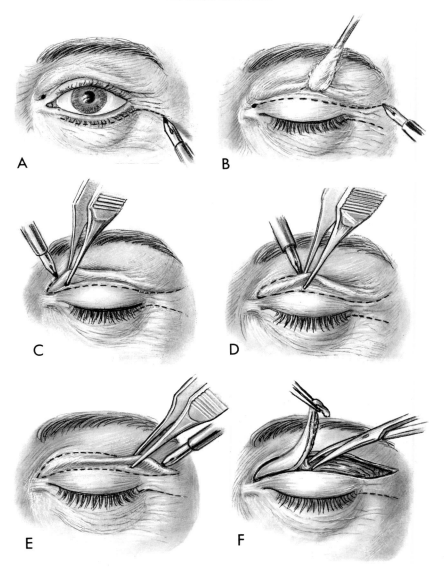

FIGURE 37–9. Technique of the esthetic blepharoplasty: the upper lid. *A,* The subciliary line of incision is drawn with a lateral extension into a line of the crow's feet. *B,* Slight upward retraction of the eyelid skin tenses the skin over the tarsus. The upper border of the tarsus can then be identified. The line of the incision is outlined along, or slightly below, the upper border of the tarsus, and its lateral extension is into one of the lines of the crow's feet. Note that the lines of incision for the upper and lower lid have an interval of skin between them. This is important to preserve lymphatic drainage and to avoid complications, such as the formation of a lateral epicanthal fold and a dimunition in the horizontal dimension of the palpebral fissure. *C,* The upper line of the incision is outlined by the "pinch" technique. The skin is pinched until the excess skin has been determined. *D,* Outlining the segment of skin to be removed from the upper lid is continued. *E,* Outlining of the upper lid segment is completed. *F,* The outlined segment of skin is removed after infiltration with a local anesthetic solution.

that when the incision is sutured, the resulting line will be in the supratarsal fold. Slight upward traction on the skin compensates for the loose skin in the aged patient (Fig. 37–9, *B*). The medial end of the line should be placed along the upper border of the medial canthal tendon (Fig. 37–9, *B*). If it impinges on the tendon, a linear contracture similar to an epicanthal fold may develop.

An equally important precaution is to avoid transgressing the frontier between the thin eyelid skin and the thicker nasal skin for fear

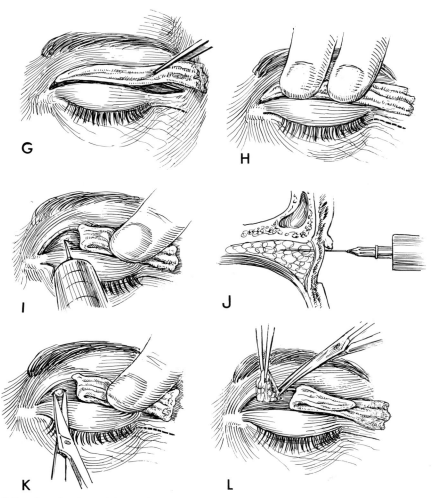

FIGURE 37–9 *Continued.* *G, H,* After excision of the skin of the upper lid, an epinephrine-soaked sponge is placed over the raw area, and two saline-soaked sponges are placed over the orbital area. At this point the operator continues with the surgical procedures on the contralateral upper eyelid. After completion of the excision of the skin on the contralateral eyelid, the epinephrine sponge is removed, and any bleeding vessels are electrocoagulated with jeweler's forceps. *I,* When the patient is operated upon under local anesthesia, it is necessary to inject a small amount of anesthetic solution through the orbicularis oculi muscle and the septum orbitale in order to remove the protruding orbital fat without causing undue pain. *J,* Sagittal section showing the penetration of the needle through the orbicularis oculi muscle and the septum orbitale into the orbital fat. *K,* A buttonhole opening is made at the medial canthus separating the fibers of the orbicularis oculi muscle and the septum orbitale. Note that the assistant exerts slight pressure over the orbital contents in order to facilitate extrusion of the orbital fat. *L,* Yellow and white fat are *gently* teased out through the opening. Scissors divide the septa between the lobes of fat to facilitate extrusion of the fat.

of producing another linear contracted scar. Placing the line too far above the medial canthal tendon results in a scar that is visible when the eye is open. The lateral aspect of the outlined area is equally important and is placed so that the suture line upon closure will lie within a natural skin fold of the "crow's feet." *It should never extend below the level of the canthus* (Fig. 37–9, *B*).

After this line is traced, the amount of skin to be removed is determined by picking up the excess skin with forceps in several places and completing the ink outline (Figs. 37–9, *C, D, E*). The extension of the incision laterally will depend on the amount of skin to be removed. More skin removal will require a longer incision.

The lateral rim of the orbit is located by

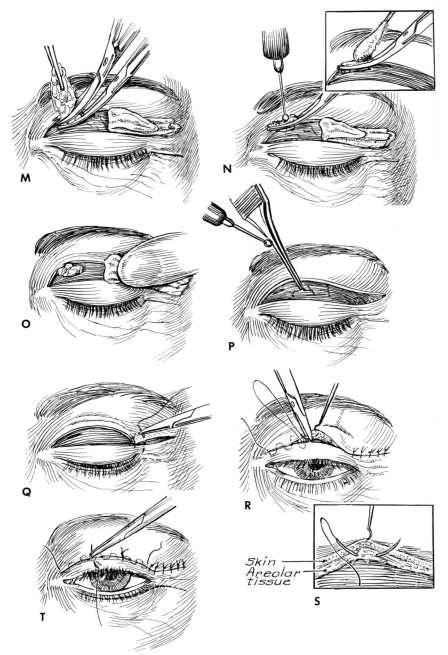

FIGURE 37–9 *Continued.*   *M,* After an adequate amount of orbital fat has been extruded, the fat is clamped close to the orbicularis oculi muscle, and the excess fat is divided with scissors. *N,* The remaining cuff of orbital fat over the curved hemostat is electrocoagulated. The orbital fat is wiped with a cotton applicator to remove the excess coagulated tissue (inset). *O,* Additional pressure is applied over the orbital contents to verify that more fat does not need to be removed. *P,* Final hemostasis is performed prior to closure of the wound. *Q,* The lateral portion of the defect is closed by 6–0 interrupted sutures. The first suture is placed at the lateral canthus after a slight amount of lateral traction has been exerted in order to avoid a pucker at the lateral end of the defect. *R,* The wound edges of the eyelid defect are closed by a continuous subcuticular suture. *S,* The position of the needle in the areolar tissue beneath the dermis. *T,* One or two interrupted sutures are placed to reinforce the subcuticular suture. A continuous running suture is an equally effective means of closing the wound.

pressing a finger along its periphery. This structure delimits the frontier between the eyelid skin proper and the thicker skin of the temporal area. In younger patients, when possible, it is advisable to avoid extending the line of incision lateral to the rim, because a scar in this area can remain noticeable for an extended period of time (see Fig. 37–12, p. 1890). In the older patient with loose tissues and indented crow's feet, the lateral extension rapidly becomes relatively inconspicuous. The design of the outline of excess skin to be resected varies according to the individual's requirements.

The upper and lower incisions should be equal in length in order to avoid puckering at one end of the suture line.

The Upper Eyelids. The lids are infiltrated immediately beneath the skin with a conservative amount of local anesthetic solution, and the skin is removed (Fig. 37–9, *F*). The dissection of the skin from the underlying muscular plane is usually started laterally where the skin is more firmly bound to the peripheral portion of the orbicularis oculi muscle. The dissection is done with a scalpel or scissors. As the dissection proceeds more medially, the skin separates more easily. Hemostasis by punctate electrocoagulation can be minimized by applying an epinephrine-soaked gauze or sponge to the denuded area (Fig. 37–9, *G, H*), which is left in place while the skin is removed from the contralateral lid. A large moistened gauze compress is applied over the orbital area.

Similar procedures are performed on the contralateral upper lid. After the excision of the skin, the attention of the surgeon is returned to the original eyelid. The gauze compress and epinephrine-soaked sponge are removed. Often their will be little or no bleeding. Punctate coagulation with jeweler's forceps will eliminate small bleeding points.

Protruding orbital fat is most often conspicuous in the medial canthal region. Slight pressure over the lid onto the ocular globe causes the fat to protrude and become manifest. The epinephrine-soaked gauze is reapplied, leaving the medial canthal area exposed (Fig. 37–9, *I*). The medial fat of the upper lid is removed after infiltration of a small amount of anesthetic solution, the needle piercing the septum orbitale (Fig. 37–9, *I, J*). With gentle compression of the globe the muscle and septum orbitale are pierced with small fine-pointed scissors (Fig. 37–9, *K*). The fat is teased out gently with forceps by sniping the fine connective tissue bands between the lobes of fat (Fig. 37–9, *L*).

The extruded fat is clamped and resected with scissors, a small cuff of fat being left (Fig. 37–9, *M*) which can be cauterized without touching the clamp (Fig. 37–9, *N*). The remaining coagulated fat is wiped from the clamp with an applicator (Fig. 37–9, *N* [inset]). The presence of additional fat can be determined by pressure on the globe (Fig. 37–9, *O*). Generally the more medial portion of the fat is lighter in color and appears to be separate from the yellow fat. Hemostasis is completed with jeweler's forceps and electrocoagulation (Fig. 37–9, *P*). The amount of orbital fat removed from each lid is then compared.

Most patients show protruding fat medially; less frequently, fat has protruded in the more lateral portion of the lid, obliterating the orbitopalpebral fold. The procedure for the removal of fat in this area is similar to that employed for the removal of fat in the medial canthal area. Care must be taken to perforate the septum orbitale below the supraorbital rim so as to avoid injury to the levator which sweeps downward toward the tarsus.

Prior to suturing the skin, Converse and Rogers (1976) have used a technique which is effective to obtain symmetry of the supratarsal folds. The upper border of the tarsus is identified. Jeweler's forceps are used to pinpoint electrocoagulate the tissues immediately above the tarsus. The eyelid skin adheres to the electrocoagulated supratarsal line. The technique has often obviated the need for more complicated operations such as supratarsal fixation (see p. 1895).

The lateral portion of the incision is closed with interrupted 6–0 nylon sutures which extend to a point just medial to the lateral canthus (Fig. 37–9, *Q*). In older patients the closure of the lateral portion of the excised area is begun, the skin being placed under slight lateral traction. In the younger patient, if the excised area has not transgressed the orbital rim, slight medial traction when the first sutures are being placed will avoid a pucker at the lateral porton of the suture line. The remaining incision is closed with a running subcuticular 5–0 nylon suture (Fig. 37–9, *R, S*) or a continuous running 6–0 nylon suture. In the older patient with thin atrophic eyelid skin, a more efficient closure can be achieved with interrupted sutures or a continuous running suture. If the sutures are removed two or three days after the operation, epithelial tunnels do not form. A few interrupted sutures are usually required even though adequate skin approximation is obtained (Fig. 37–9, *T*).

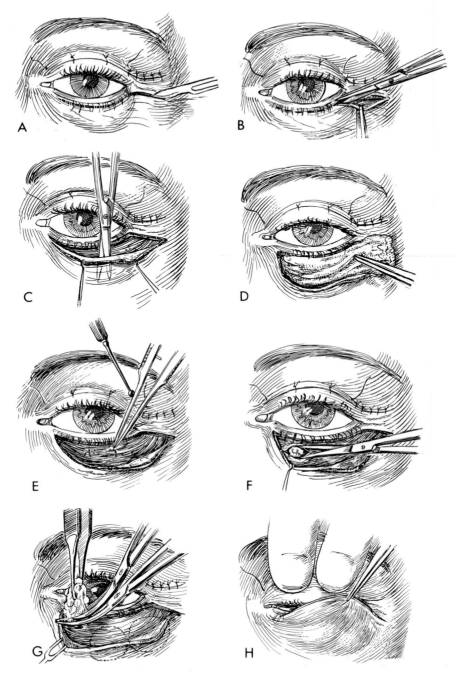

FIGURE 37–10.   Technique of the esthetic blepharoplasty: the lower lid. *A*, An incision is made through the skin at the lateral extension of the outlined incision. *B*, The subciliary incision is made with sharp pointed scissors. *C*, Careful dissection of the skin from the orbicularis muscle is done under direct vision with sharp pointed scissors. *D*, An epinephrine-soaked sponge is placed under the undermined skin. At this point a similar operation is performed on the contralateral lower eyelid. *E*, After completion of the operation on the contralateral eyelid, the skin is retracted, and bleeding vessels are electrocoagulated. *F*, Pressure is exerted upon the orbital contents after the opening has been made through the orbicularis oculi muscle and the septum orbitale. The scissors perforate the septum orbitale immediately above the infraorbital rim. The drawing demonstrates an opening of the medial fat pocket. *G*, The extruded fat is clamped with a curved hemostat and will be resected as shown in Figure 37–9, *M*. Electrocoagulation of the remaining cuff of fat is done as shown in Figure 37–9, *N*. *H*, The central and lateral fat pockets are indicated. Fat will be removed from the central pocket and sparsely from the lateral pocket.

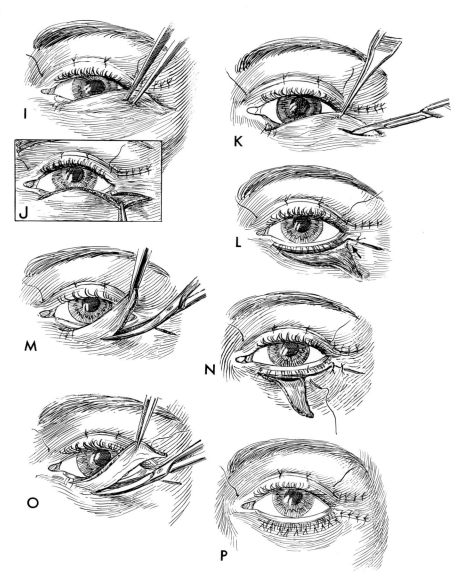

FIGURE 37–10 *Continued.* *I*, The skin is raised in an upward and lateral direction, and verification is made that sufficient fat has been removed and that there is no remaining adherence of the orbicularis muscle to the skin. *J*, Traction is exerted on the skin flap to show the position of the border of the eyelid. *K*, An incision is made at the level of the subciliary incision. *L*, After the flap is outlined by the incision in *K*, it is raised and retracted downward. A suture closes the lateral portion of the wound. *M*, Eyelid skin is resected over the more medial aspect of the eyelid. *N*, A suture is placed to approximate the eyelid to the subciliary incision. *O*, The eyelid skin is excised along the remaining portion of the lid. Note that the excised skin does not extend medially to the lower lacrimal punctum. *P*, The operation is completed after the placing of 6–0 interrupted nylon sutures.

The Lower Eyelids. An incision is made with a knife lateral to the lateral canthus (Fig. 37–10, *A*), and the subciliary incision is completed through the skin with sharp scissors (Fig. 37–10, *B*). The incision should not be extended beyond the lower lacrimal punctum for fear of producing a slight degree of eversion of the punctum, sufficient to result in annoying epiphora, even though it may last for only a short time after the operation.

Separation of the skin from the orbicularis oculi muscle is done laterally by careful sharp scissors dissection to separate the attachments of the peripheral portion of the muscle, which is intimately attached to the skin in this area as part of the lateral canthal raphé. Adequate lateral undermining is essential to prevent upward displacement of the lateral subcutaneous tissue upon advancement of the skin flap. Separation of the skin from the muscle in the remainder of the lower lid is more easily performed under direct vision, as the skin is less adherent to the muscle (Fig. 37–10, *C*). Hemostasis is obtained with epinephrine-soaked sponges placed under the skin (Fig. 37–10, *D*). The contralateral lower lid is operated upon in a similar fashion. Pinpoint electrocoagulation, if required, completes the hemostasis (Fig. 37–10, *E*).

The fat is removed from the three compartments or "pockets." Barker (1976) has injected the three compartments with a solution of methylene blue and demonstrated that they are separated by tenuous septa, thus confirming the original findings of Castañares (1951). For practical purposes the three areas are referred to as "fat pads": medial, central, and lateral. The amount of fat to be removed varies from none to large quantities. Just as fat can be left behind, ruining an otherwise good result, *too much* fat can be removed, giving a hollowed out, cadaverous look with excessive sclera visible below the cornea, "*scleral show,*" which is usually attributed to excessive skin removal, another cause of this complication (the "white eye" syndrome). Taking an excessive amount of orbital fat, particularly in thin individuals, causes the infraorbital rim to protrude, giving the orbital area a "sunken eye" enophthalmic appearance.

The fat pads are opened with small pointed scissors which spread the fibers of the preseptal portion of the orbicularis muscle and perforate the septum orbitale (Fig. 37–10, *F*). The fat protrudes spontaneously, or a moderate amount of pressure is applied on the upper lid and ocular globe. The ends of the scissors are spread, thus opening the compartment; the extruded fat is grasped with a hemostat (Fig. 37–10, *G*). The cuff of fat is clamped, the excess resected with scissors, coagulated, and wiped as in the removal of the upper lid fat (see Fig. 37–9, *N*). By advancing the undermined skin and by using gentle pressure on the globe, additional fat can be detected and removed (Fig. 37–10, *H*).

Once the fat is removed, the most important step remains: resection of the excessive skin. Expertise, caution, and meticulous care are essential. The skin is advanced upward and laterally, with careful attention to the position of the lower lid (Fig. 37–10, *I*), which can easily be altered by lashes under the flap or by inadvertent tension which distorts the lid position.

A number of maneuvers have been described to avoid the removal of too much skin. Rees (1968) advocated gentle pressure on the globe, which elevates the lid slightly, if the patient is under general anesthesia. If local anesthesia is being used and the patient can cooperate, the patient can look up or open his mouth. Removing too much skin, with resultant ectropion, *must* be avoided. The key to success is the removal of the precise amount of skin to avoid ectropion or "scleral show."

The flap is everted (Fig. 37–10, *J*), and the lateral excess is removed by outlining a flap with either scissors or a knife (Fig. 37–10, *K*). To maintain the direction of the advanced skin flap, a 6–0 nylon suture is placed to anchor the flap to the lid (Fig. 37–10, *L*). The remaining excision follows by gently spreading the skin upward and laterally. *No tension* is exerted at this stage; the flap is elevated, the subciliary skin incision being kept in view. The skin is trimmed to fit and is then carefully approximated with interrupted 6–0 nylon sutures (Fig. 37–10, *M* to *P*). A continuous suture with nylon has a tendency to cause a purse-string type of ruffling unless precautions are taken to avoid this complication.

The eyes are open at the completion of the surgery because of paralysis of the orbicularis oculi muscles caused by the local anesthetic agent. To protect the eye from drying, an ophthalmic ointment is applied after irrigation of the conjunctival sac.

Gentle pressure bandaging of the eyes and use of an occlusive suture have been recommended in the past to reduce oozing and edema and prevent hematoma. However, the application of ice compresses to the eyes in a sedated patient who is resting quietly in bed with the head elevated allows the surgeon to examine the eyes, is a safer procedure, and avoids the discomfort and anxiety associated with an occlusive dressing. The most important advantage to avoiding a compressive dressing is that a complication such as a retrobulbar hemorrhage with proptosis of the eye cannot be hidden. In addition, a compressive dressing in the presence of a retrobulbar hemorrhage is the principal cause of blindness as a result of increased intraocular and intraorbital tension; the orbital tissues cannot expand, as they are restricted by the compressive dressing.

The sutures in the lids including the subcuticular suture are removed on the second or third day, leaving only some sutures in the thicker skin lateral to the canthus. If these are removed along with the lid suture, it is advisable to support the lateral incision with strips of paper tape.

During the first postoperative days, the patients are advised to apply ice compresses over the eyelids. The compresses have a soothing effect. Patients are advised to limit their activities until the edema and ecchymosis have disappeared. Cosmetics can be used after ten days but must be removed carefully.

Figure 37–11 shows a patient who underwent the procedure illustrated in Figure 37–9 and 37–10.

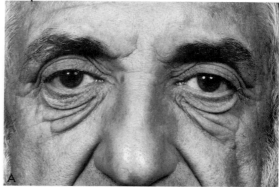
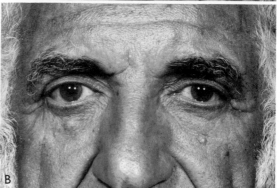

FIGURE 37–11. *A*, Male patient, 55 years old. Preoperative appearance. *B*, Postoperative views four years after the operation performed according to the technique illustrated in Figures 37–9 and 37–10.

Upper Eyelid Blepharoplasty: Technical Details. In the older patient it is often necessary to transgress the anatomical frontier between the thin eyelid skin and the thicker periorbital skin at the lateral orbital rim in order to remove a large area of excess skin and achieve a satisfactory correction (see Fig. 37–9). The sutured lateral extension placed in a fold of the "crow's feet", usually present in older patients, gradually becomes inconspicuous. In the above description of the technique of blepharoplasty, emphasis was placed on limiting the area of the skin excision to the eyelid proper, whenever possible. By avoiding a scar in the thicker skin lateral to the orbit, only an inconspicuous, often invisible linear postoperative scar remains if the area of skin to be excised is correctly outlined.

The design of the upper eyelid outline should be done with the patient in a sitting up position. If the patient is heavily sedated, cooperation is inadequate. The outline is marked with Bonney's blue or a marking pen the evening before the operation. With the patient's full coopera-

tion, the eyelids are opened and closed and carefully studied. The upper border of the tarsus is readily identified by gently retracting the skin of the lid upward or by exerting slight downward traction on the lid. The outline is made along the upper border of the tarsus. A fold is usually seen sweeping up from the lateral end of the outline toward the lateral orbit rim (Fig. 37–12, *A*). The ink outline is made (Fig. 37–12, *B*). The pinch technique illustrated in Figure 37–9, *C* to *E*, provides the outline of the upper incision. The skin is then excised. If the upper and lower outlines are of equal length, the wound edges are approximated without puckering of the skin at either end of the suture line.

The Muscle Flap Technique. In the esthetic blepharoplasty described in Figures 37–9 and 37–10, the skin of the lower eyelid is separated from the orbicularis oculi muscle. In the muscle flap technique, the line of cleav-

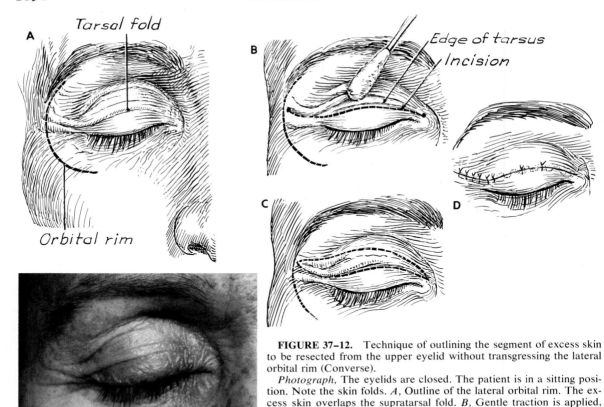

FIGURE 37–12. Technique of outlining the segment of excess skin to be resected from the upper eyelid without transgressing the lateral orbital rim (Converse).

Photograph, The eyelids are closed. The patient is in a sitting position. Note the skin folds. *A,* Outline of the lateral orbital rim. The excess skin overlaps the supratarsal fold. *B,* Gentle traction is applied, raising the skin and identifying the superior border of the tarsus. An ink outline is drawn immediately below the upper border of the tarsus. *C,* Outline completed by the pinch technique. *D,* Suturing completed.

age is situated between the orbicularis oculi muscle and the septum orbitale. The operation appears to have been originally devised by Sheehan; he taught the technique to McIndoe (1960), who used the muscle flap routinely in performing a blepharoplasty. Beare (1975) also uses the technique routinely. In 1967 Beare listed the advantages of the muscle flap technique as follows: (1) the technique causes less ecchymosis; (2) ectropion is less likely to occur; (3) the plane of dissection is covered by a layer of normal tissue; and (4) one can perform a secondary operation through the classic approach, separating the skin from the orbicularis muscle through tissues that have not been scarred by a previous operation.

The muscle flap technique is particularly indicated in younger patients with protruding orbital fat, and when hypertrophy of the orbicularis oculi muscle causes an unsightly protrusion.

An incision which extends through the skin and orbicularis muscle is made in one of the folds lateral to the lateral canthus (Fig. 37–13, *A*). It is continued with scissors through the skin and the orbicularis muscle at the subciliary level. It is essential in this operation to avoid extending the incision as far as the lower punctum. Cutting through the orbicularis muscle at this level interferes with the lacrimal pump function of the muscle and may lead to a troublesome postoperative period of epiphora (Fig. 37–13, *B*). The subciliary incision having been completed through the skin and the muscle, the lower lid is raised by means of two sutures (Fig. 37–13, *C*). The pretarsal portion of the orbicularis oculi muscle is carefully dissected from the tarsus, and the preseptal portion of the orbicularis oculi muscle is raised from the septum orbitale, which is now exposed (Fig. 37–13, *C*). The three areas where orbital fat protrudes under the septum orbitale can be seen under direct vision (Fig. 37–13, *D*). Stab incisions are made to remove the protruding fat. After careful hemostasis the excess skin is

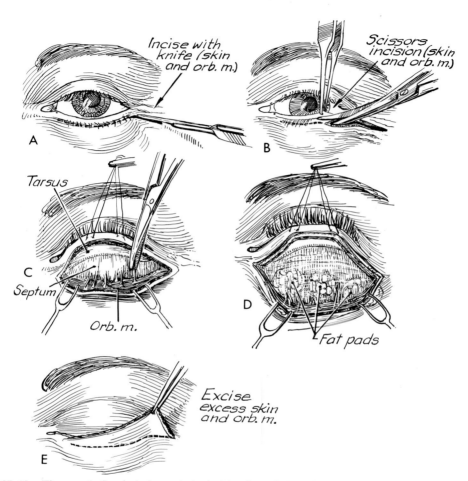

FIGURE 37–13. The muscle flap technique. *A,* An incision is made lateral to the lateral canthus in one of the folds of the crow's feet. *B,* The incision is extended medially through skin and muscle. The subciliary incision through the skin and muscle is continued with scissors to a point lateral to the lacrimal punctum. *C,* Sutures (or eyelid hooks) are placed to raise the lower lid and facilitate dissection. The tarsus is exposed. The preseptal portion of the orbicularis oculi muscle is dissected from over the septum orbitale. *D,* The septum orbitale is exposed, and the orbital fat is seen to protrude beneath it. *E,* The excess skin and orbicularis muscle are excised. When the subciliary incision is being sutured, it is often necessary to resect some of the underlying orbicularis muscle in order to thin the border of the flap so that the skin flap is better adapted to the subciliary skin.

The muscle flap technique is also indicated to correct orbicularis oculi muscle hypertrophy (see p. 1880). Occasionally the hypertrophy results in a transverse bulge near the orbital rim, which may be misinterpreted as fat pads. In such cases the skin should be dissected from the muscle before the muscle is dissected from the septum orbitale.

removed along with the attached orbicularis oculi muscle (Fig. 37–13, *E*), and the subciliary incision is carefully sutured.

Although the technique is employed as a routine procedure by some surgeons, others are of the opinion that it should be reserved for patients of the younger age group with congenital protruding fat and for patients of the older group who require moderate skin removal. It is also indicated to remove excess orbicularis oculi muscle which causes an unsightly ridge which is accentuated when the patient smiles. This condition may require, in addition, dissection of the skin from the orbicularis muscle and adjustment of the muscle to the eyelid border.

In the older patient with degenerated, relaxed, and ptotic skin, the muscle flap technique would require the removal of an excessive amount of orbicularis oculi muscle. In such patients, the technique shown in Figures 37–9 and 37–10 is preferable.

Variations in Technique. The standard technique employed at the Institute of Reconstructive Plastic Surgery as illustrated in Figures 37–9 and 37–10 varies according to the design of the surface area of skin that must be excised from the upper lids in order to obtain a satisfactory result and also according to individual preferences in technique.

One variation consists of undermining the skin of the lower eyelid by subcutaneous blunt dissection instead of by dissection under direct vision. Another variation in technique is to incise the orbicularis muscle for the exposure of the septum orbitale and the fat pads. This technique requires suturing the edges of the incised orbicularis muscle.

The amount of undermining of the skin of the lower lid varies according to the extent of the deformity. Sufficient undermining should be done to avoid inadvertent plication of the orbicularis oculi muscle, which would result in the formation of an unsightly ridge.

Removal of the protruding orbital fat through the conjunctival approach is an alternative technique in the young patient with the hereditary type of deformity. The technique is relatively simple: the lower eyelid is retracted downward until the infraorbital rim of the orbit protrudes in the depth of the lower fornix. Stab incisions through the conjunctiva and septum orbitale and slight pressure over the upper eyelid and ocular globe cause the orbital fat to protrude through the openings in the conjunctival sac. The orbital fat is clamped; excess fat is resected, and the cuff of orbital fat is coagulated. The remainder of the fat is reintegrated behind

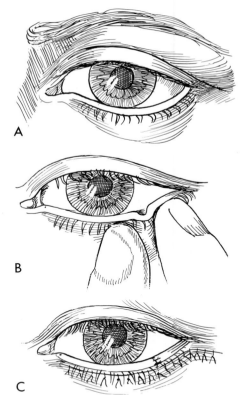

FIGURE 37–14. Diagnosis of incipient senile ectropion. *A,* Slight downward droop of the lower lid. *B,* When the lateral third of the lower lid is pinched and folded upon itself, the laxity of the lid becomes apparent. *C,* Reestablishment of an adequate horizontal dimension of the lower lid following V-excision combined with an esthetic blepharoplastic operation.

the septum orbitale. In most cases, however, the removal of a sizable amount of fat leaves a moderate excess of eyelid skin. Because of this the muscle flap technique described in Figure 37–13 is generally preferable.

As mentioned earlier in the text, older patients with incipient senile ectropion and relaxation of the orbicularis oculi muscle are extremely susceptible to postoperative ectropion after the excision of even a moderate amount of eyelid skin. Laxity is obvious when the lid is pinched between the index finger and thumb (Fig. 37–14). Two procedures are available to avoid this complication.

The first technique can be employed in patients with extreme excess of skin falling in folds combined with large fat pockets. This variation involves making the skin incision in the lower lid at a lower level. The skin over the tarsus remains undisturbed, and thus the leverage effect upon the tarsus, which produces the ectropion as a result of the excision of the skin through a subciliary incision, is avoided. In the older patient, the lower incision leaves an inconspicuous scar.

The second technique involves tightening the lower eyelid by excising a wedge of orbicularis oculi muscle, tarsus, and conjunctiva after the skin of the lower eyelid has been raised and the protruding fat removed. Rees (1971) has emphasized the importance of shortening the horizontal dimension of the eyelid in order to prevent postoperative ectropion. The excision is performed in the lateral third of the eyelid. The technique of wedge excision of the eyelid has been described in Chapter 28 (see Fig. 28–23). The removal of excess eyelid skin is then accomplished as illustrated in Figure 37–10.

Complications of the Esthetic Blepharoplasty

Transient Complications. Epiphora is caused by edema or by the temporary paralysis of the orbicularis oculi muscle following injection with the local anesthetic solution. These subside in a short while; persistence of epiphora is suggestive of overzealous removal of skin or injury to the canaliculus at the time of surgery. Troublesome epiphora from a slight eversion of the punctum may occur if excess skin is removed below the lower lacrimal punctum.

The eversion may correct itself and the punctum return to its position of contact with the lacrimal lake. In other cases the epiphora persists, and release of the eversion by incising the subciliary scar and adding a small skin graft taken from the upper eyelid will remedy this complication.

Transient diplopia can be caused by temporary paralysis of an extraocular muscle due to the injection of a local anesthetic solution or by edema of the conjunctiva. The most commonly injured extraocular muscle is the inferior oblique, because of its proximity to the medial fat pad.

Corneal abrasion or conjunctival irritation occurs occasionally and may be due to operative trauma or to corneal or conjunctival desiccation. Periodic instillation of saline solution will protect the cornea during the operation. When a blepharoplasty is performed in conjunction with a face lift operation, desiccation of the corneas may occur if the eyelid procedure is performed first and is followed by the cervicofacial procedure. The eyelids, temporarily paralyzed by the local anesthetic agent, remain open, exposing the corneas to desiccation by the operating room lights. Careful surgical technique and periodic instillation of saline solution into the conjunctival sacs, followed by the application of

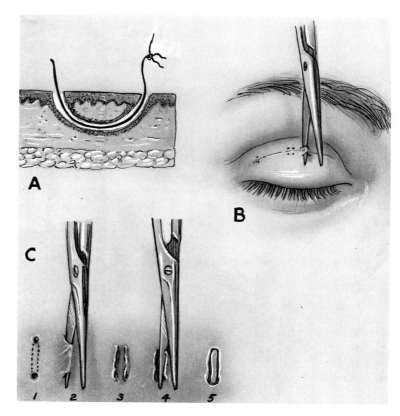

FIGURE 37–15. The marsupialization of epithelized tracts following esthetic blepharoplasty. *A*, The epithelized tract along the suture. *B*, Fine pointed scissors are placed through the tunnel. *C*, The stages in the marsupialization, opening the tunnel and resecting the edges of the tunnel. (From Converse, J. M.: Clinical note: Treatment of epithelized suture tracts of the eyelid by marsupialization. Plast. Reconstr. Surg., *38*:576, 1966. Copyright 1966, The Williams & Wilkins Company, Baltimore.)

ophthalmic ointment to the eyes after the completion of the operation, decrease the incidence of this complication. If the patient complains of corneal irritation following the operation ("scratchy feeling," "sand in the eye," pain), the cornea should be stained and the abrasion identified and treated under the supervision of an ophthalmologist. Search for a foreign body (an eyelash or small piece of suture material) should always be routine in such cases.

Postoperative Complications

MINOR COMPLICATIONS. Conjunctival hemorrhage is uncommon and self-limited. Ecchymosis occurs frequently, is generally self-limited, and disappears without sequelae. In some dark-complexioned patients, ecchymosis is long-lasting. This is especially true in patients with "dark circles" under the eyes preoperatively. Occasionally there is a small hematoma which requires drainage at the lateral portion of the incision. Telangiectasis and pigmentation below the line of incision in the upper lid occur in older patients and may remain permanently. In these cases Cronin (1972) has advocated an incision placed immediately above the line of the eyelashes in the upper eyelid blepharoplasty.

Inclusion cysts occur along the suture line in the upper lid. These "whiteheads" result from entrapment of epithelial cells, and enucleation is generally adequate. Epithelial tunnels develop by epithelization along a suture tract and are prevented by early removal of sutures. Treatment involves opening the tunnel by cutting the roof, thus marsupializing the tract (Converse, 1966) (Fig. 37–15). Destruction of the roof of the tunnel by electrodesiccation is another technique.

Hypertrophic scarring is rare and occurs when the resection of the excess skin lateral to the orbital rim has not followed the lines of minimal tension. It usually responds to intralesional injections of triamcinolone acetonide. Scars which may be red or thickened for a short period usually fade. Stitch abscesses, rarely seen because the sutures are removed early, are treated by the application of warm soaks.

MAJOR COMPLICATIONS. The complications listed thus far do not generally endanger the final result, whereas those that follow may.

Ptosis. Ptosis may be either temporary or permanent. Temporary ptosis may be due to overzealous use of electrocoagulation or to the insertion of sutures in the septum orbitale and orbicularis oculi muscle (Beyer, Smith, and Buerger, 1970). Permanent ptosis is usually the result of injury to the levator muscle or section of the levator aponeurosis and will require a secondary repair (see Chapter 28, p. 920). In removing fat from the upper eyelid, the surgeon must penetrate the septum orbitale above the levator aponeurosis to avoid injuring this structure (see Fig. 37–16). Lagophthalmos is common after blepharoplasty but usually corrects itself rapidly as the postoperative edema regresses.

Ectropion. One of the most serious complications of blepharoplasty is ectropion. Ectropion of the upper lid is extremely rare, while that of the lower lid is more common. Edgerton (1972) reviewed the factors in the etiology of lower lid ectropion and listed them as follows: (1) excess removal of skin; (2) suture infolding of the septum orbitale; (3) thickening and fixation of the lower lid to the orbital floor; (4) paresis or displacement of the orbicularis oculi muscle; (5) gravitational drag of the cheek; (6) upward angulation of the orbicularis muscle during the suture of the subciliary incision; and (7) excessive removal of orbital fat or hematoma. He recommended conservative early treatment (time, artificial tears, taping of the lid) and did not consider a secondary operation for a number of months. Operative procedures for the correction of ectropion are described in Chapters 28 and 33.

The minor temporary postoperative "scleral show," which is fairly commonly seen, is caused by the removal of an excessive amount of skin and fat with changes in the anatomical relationships of the lids and the globe.

As mentioned earlier, one of the frequent causes of postoperative ectropion of the lower lids in the older patient is the presence of incipient senile ectropion. Even the removal of the smallest amount of eyelid skin may cause ectropion in these patients. In such cases the previously mentioned variations in surgical technique can be used to avoid this complication.

Asymmetry of the Supratarsal Folds. Disparity in the surface area of skin removed from one lid as compared to that removed from the contralateral lid results in an asymmetrical appearance. It is often necessary, however, to remove more skin on one side than on the other. Careful evaluation of the amount of skin resection required, as illustrated in Figure 37–9, *C to E,* will ensure that, although the amount of skin resected may vary, the design of the outlined area to be resected is similar in both upper eyelids.

Asymmetry is best prevented, but it can be treated by secondary operation if indicated, ample time being allowed to elapse before the secondary procedure is performed.

Asymmetry cannot be avoided when there is a noticeable difference in the size of the orbits and ocular globes. Such abnormalities should be pointed out to the patient prior to the surgical procedure. Minor asymmetry is always present, as the two halves of the face are asymmetrical in all human beings, and this fact should also be explained to the patient.

Disparity of the level of the supratarsal folds

is one of the most frequent causes of an asymmetrical appearance.

Supratarsal fixation. As stated earlier in the chapter, in older patients the excess of upper eyelid skin may hang as a curtain downward over the eyelashes, obliterating the supratarsal fold.

The technique described on page 1885 consisting in punctate electrocagulation along the upper border of the tarsus is often effective. A number of operations have been described to

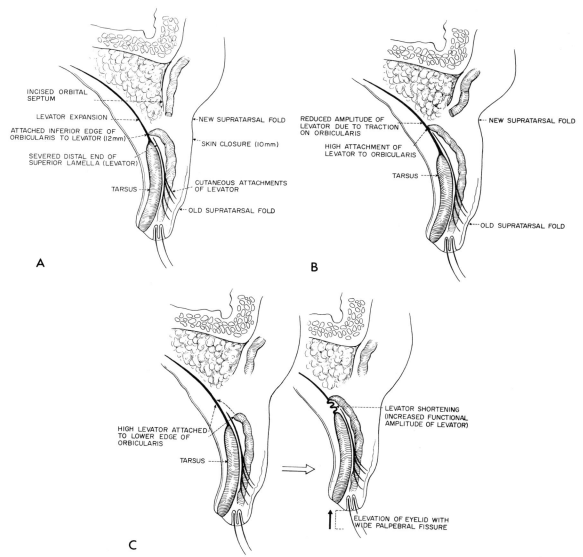

FIGURE 37–16. Supratarsal fixation. *A,* Sagittal section illustrating the correct location and relationship of the attachment of the levator aponeurosis to the inferior incised edge of the orbicularis muscle. This technique allows full and immediate function of the levator muscle and does not modify the shape of the palpebral fissure in the immediate postoperative period. *B,* When the attachment of the levator to the orbicularis muscle is made at a higher level, the amplitude of function of the levator is reduced. This results in a narrow palpebral fissure which may persist for up to three months but corrects itself at the end of that period. *C,* When a level disparity is present at the attachment of the levator aponeurosis and the orbicularis muscle, a shortening of the levator aponeurosis occurs equal to the disparity on an almost one for one basis (unlike congenital ptosis). The functional amplitude of the levator is increased and results in a shortening of the lid and a wide palpebral fissure which does not correct itself with time. (From Sheen, 1974).

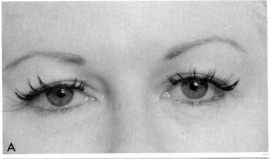

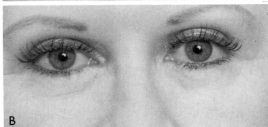

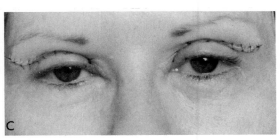

FIGURE 37–17. Supratarsal fixation. *A*, Preoperative appearance showing overhanging in the upper eyelids and loss of the lateral portion of the supratarsal folds. *B*, Postoperative result following supratarsal fixation. *C*, Early postoperative view. (Courtesy of Dr. J. Sheen.)

reestablish the supratarsal folds. These operations, which also ensure the symmetry of the two supratarsal folds, are modifications of the operations for the restoration of the absent fold in the Oriental eyelid (see Chapter 28, p. 947).

Sheen (1974) has emphasized the need for supratarsal fixation. He stresses the following points in the technique of supratarsal fixation: (1) The lower incision for the excision of redundant skin should be made exactly where the supratarsal fold should be located: 10 to 12 mm above the ciliary border (above the superior border of the tarsus; it should follow the curvature of the superior border of the tarsus). (2) The orbicularis oculi muscle should be incised 2 mm above this level. The muscle should be under normal tension and not retracted by the surgeon or his assistant. (3) Close attention should be paid to the relationship of the levator aponeurosis to the orbicularis oculi muscle. The correct relationship between these structures is illustrated in Figure 37–16, *A*, which also demonstrates the point of attachment of the inferior edge of the incised orbicularis muscle to the levator aponeurosis. Eight to ten sutures of 7–0 silk attach only small amounts of tissue between the levator and the orbicularis muscle. When the lower edge of the orbicularis muscle is attached to the levator at a higher level (Figs. 37–16, *B*, *C*), shortening of the levator aponeurosis occurs, and the patient has a palpebral fissure with increased vertical dimension. Figure 37–17 is a photograph of a patient with a satisfactory restoration of symmetrical supratarsal folds.

In the heavy upper eyelid with severely re-

dundant skin, Flowers (1975) has modified the technique of forming a supratarsal fold in the Oriental eyelid (see Chapter 28, p. 947) and Sheen's supratarsal fixation. His technique includes removing a portion of orbicularis muscle and then anchoring the skin margin to the levator aponeurosis, the tarsus, or both. This technique according to Flowers is associated with some morbidity. He has used the technique in 743 patients. Cies and Baylis (1975) placed through-and-through sutures through the eyelid in secondary operations to form a supratarsal fold.

Keratoconjunctivitis Sicca (The "Dry Eye" Syndrome). Irritative symptoms following blepharoplasty may be due to injury to the conjunctiva or cornea during surgery or to aggravation of a previous ocular problem (Swartz, Schultz, and Seaton, 1974). Other factors associated with dry eye symptoms include allergies (pollen, cosmetics), air pollution, and foreign bodies.

The dry eye syndrome occurs predominantly in women of menopausal age, in association with the use of tranquilizers, or as a part of Sjögren's syndrome. The latter consists of chronic polyarthritis, keratoconjunctivitis sicca, and atrophy of the lacrimal, salivary, and mucinous glands. The eye symptoms are the most consistent and often the initial finding. Graham, Messner, and Miller (1976) recommended the measurement of tear production prior to blepharoplasty, because keratoconjunctivitis sicca is a common, often asymptomatic, disorder of middle age, and the corrective blepharoplasty may accentuate its symptoms.

A careful preoperative history may disclose dry eye symptoms, and measurement of tear production by the Schirmer test is indicated in such patients. The test is done by placing a strip of standardized filter paper on the lower punctum and measuring the length of tear-soaked paper in five minutes. Failure to anesthetize the cornea and conjunctiva at the start of the test results in the measurement of both reflex and basal secretions, giving a false-negative rate of 15 per cent. The normal value in middle age is greater than 15 mm. Transient decreases in Schirmer test measurements have been documented in postoperative blepharoplasty patients (Graham, Messner, and Miller, 1976). Prolonged deficiency occurred in a case reported by Rees (1975a). Such decreased tear production in conjunction with normal tear evaporation can result in desiccation of the cornea with the formation of minute corneal abrasions. Irritative symptoms rapidly follow the formation of such abrasions. Other tests include the rose bengal staining test and the analysis of tear lysozyme concentration.

Topical lubricants provide satisfactory relief for most patients. When it is evident that the patient has a postoperative "dry eye," there are effective agents for the treatment of the condition. A polyvinylpyrrolidone derivative is one of the most effective wetting agents by dissolving and becoming a part of the lipid and mucoid components of the tear film. A methylcellulose derivative has the inconvenience of leaving a fine white residue on the lashes and must be instilled into the conjunctival sac more frequently than the polyvinyl-pyrrolidone drops.

Various types of ophthalmic ointments, frequently applied particularly at night, are also effective, but have the inconvenience that they impair visual function.

The physiology of tear production has been discussed in Chapter 28.

Acute Closed Angle Glaucoma. Green and Kadri (1974) have reported acute closed angle glaucoma occurring in one patient following blepharoplasty. The classic findings of pain, blurred vision, corneal edema, and a dilated pupil were present. The diagnosis was made, and treatment was successful. The authors noted that most patients undergoing blepharoplasty are women, in whom acute closed angle glaucoma is more frequent.

Retrobulbar Hemorrhage. By far the most dramatic complication of esthetic blepharoplasty is retrobulbar hemorrhage, which usually develops at the time of the injection of the local anesthetic agent in preparation for the removal of the fat pads or during their removal.

There is sudden and severe proptosis of the globe with suffusion of blood into the tissues. Usually there is no hematoma amenable to drainage, and it is difficult or impossible to identify the bleeding vessel. The process is usually self-limited, with spontaneous cessation of bleeding.

In some cases the globe becomes stony hard, and the patient experiences severe eye pain. These findings reflect a precipitous increase in intraocular pressure caused by the retrobulbar hemorrhage. The increase in pressure occurs through two basic mechanisms: (1) transmitted pressure from the increase in intraorbital contents (hemorrhage); and (2) precipitation of a condition similar to acute narrow angle glaucoma (in which outflow through the canal of Schlemm is prevented by forward pressure of the iris) (Hartley, Lester, and Schatten, 1973). These authors reported a case in which acute retrobulbar hemorrhage occurred during blepharoplasty without injection of the fat pad. Paracentesis of the anterior chamber of the eye and the use of osmotic diuretics for decompression were recommended as the treatment for acute retrobulbar hemorrhage to prevent blindness.

Loss of vision which occurs after retrobulbar hemorrhage is usually transient. Duke-Elder (1972) stated that retrobulbar hemorrhage rarely causes permanent blindness (2 of 2750 cases), and Lemoine (1973), Rees, Lee, and Coburn (1973), and DeMere, Wood, and Austin (1974) have advised against anterior chamber paracentesis with its attendant complication rates which would be higher than those of the untreated retrobulbar hemorrhage. The favored method of treatment of retrobulbar hemorrhage consists of removal of sutures to allow for decompression and conservative treatment with intravenous injections of mannitol.

The authors of this chapter reiterate that they do not employ pressure dressings following blepharoplasty. Thus direct observation is possible, and proptosis of the ocular globe and the orbital contents can occur in case of orbital hemorrhage without being camouflaged by the dressing.

Loss of Vision. Hartman, Morax, and Vergez (1962) reported optic atrophy and blindness following corrective blepharoplasty, a complication which they attributed to vascular spasm resulting from excessive traction on the orbital fat. Moser, DiPirro, and McCoy (1973) reported seven cases of unilateral blindness after surgery of the eyelid. Three cases were attributed to optic neuritis, one to optic nerve injury, two to central retinal artery and vein thrombosis, and insufficient data were available for a diagnosis in the last case. No causal relationship with preexisting diseases, drugs, anesthesia, surgical procedures, dressings, or postoperative care could be established.

DeMere, Wood, and Austin (1974) surveyed plastic and ophthalmic surgeons (98,000 operations) and found 40 cases of unilateral blindness after eyelid surgery (0.04 per cent incidence). There was no correlation with the type of anesthesia or with the use of dressings. Of interest is the finding that only 15 per cent of plastic surgeons had conducted an adequate preoperative visual examination. DeMere, Wood, and Austin recommended a preoperative ophthalmologic examination for the following reasons: (1) approximately 2 per cent of the population has amblyopia; (2) a preexisting ocular disease may be present; (3) many patients have poor vision in one eye, and some are blind in one eye. The patient may not realize these defects until after the corrective surgery and may incriminate the plastic surgeon and hold him responsible for a condition which was present prior to the surgical procedure.

Prior to the operation the patient's vision should be checked using a visual chart, first one eye being covered and then the other. The patient should also be interrogated concerning any ocular pathology. When a history of ocular pathology is obtained or any abnormality is noted after the patient has read the visual chart, the patient should be referred to an ophthalmologist for further examination.

Another possible cause of blindness after blepharoplasty is optic nerve injury from the electrocautery. Fine needlepoint cauterization and the use of newer machines which cut off when the grounding is not functioning minimize or eliminate the likelihood of this complication.

THE FACE LIFT OPERATION

Various names have been used for the face lift operation; "rhytidectomy," from its derivation, indicates the excision of wrinkles, while "rhytidoplasty" implies an operation to remove wrinkles. A number of other pretentious names have been coined and will not be mentioned. The term face lift has come into common usage; in non-English speaking countries the operation is often designated as "le lifting," "der lifting," or "el lifting"!

Preoperative Examination. The patient's attitude about his (or her) weight is an important consideration in assessing the anticipated degree of improvement and provides a clue to the patient's self-image. If the patient is overweight, the required weight loss is recommended before surgery. Considerable weight loss following surgery results in a disappointing sag of the face and neck.

Clinical observation has shown that patients who undergo cosmetic surgery for the aging face at a relatively younger age obtain a more satisfactory and durable result than patients in their late fifties or even older. The results obtained by operative procedures done by the plastic and reconstructive surgeon for the repair of deformities, including corrective rhinoplasty, are usually definitive; surgery for the aging face, however, does not provide a permanent result because the aging process continues. After a variable number of years, a secondary operation will be required. Some of the most remarkable results have been obtained in patients who, for professional reasons, have been obliged to maintain an appearance of youth.

Patients usually ask, "Doctor, how long will it last?" The answer to this question is a difficult one, as the duration of a satisfactory result is dependent upon so many factors that a precise figure cannot be given.

In older patients it is often impossible to achieve a satisfactory result in a single operation. A face lift operation may be required six months after the primary operation. Based on his evaluation of the patient, the surgeon must decide whether or not to warn the patient prior to the primary operation that a second operation will probably be necessary.

Patients with badly sun-damaged skin may require a later planing (chemical peel or dermabrasion) (see Chapter 17). A chemical peel in the perioral area and the forehead is feasible in conjunction with a face lift operation; a full-face chemical peel, however, is contraindicated in conjunction with a face lift operation.

Other considerations of importance in the preoperative assessment of the patient include: (1) the general structure of the face and neck, and the distribution of fat, whether in jowls, submental fat, or edema over the zygoma; (2) chin retrusion and the mandibular-cervical angle; (3) the skin texture, the presence of lines, crow's feet, deep nasolabial folds, circular cervical skin folds of the neck, and fine generalized lines of the skin; (4) vertical lines of the lips, more prevalent on the upper lip in females; (5) the contour of the temporal sideburn in males, and the position of the postauricular hairline in all patients; (6) the presence of scars from previous surgery or trauma; (7) pigmentation and the presence of skin lesions such as keratoses; (8) asymmetry of the face and neck.

Anatomy. The surgeon must be aware of structures encountered in the course of the operation, the facial nerve branches in particular; thus, injury to these structures is avoided.

In the thin individual lying in a recumbent position with the head turned to the opposite side, the skin protrusions formed by the anterior border of the sternomastoid muscle and the external jugular vein are often clearly visible.

The attachments of the cutaneous tissues over the temporal, cheek, cervical, and retroauricular areas vary.

The cheek area consists of two anatomically distinct portions. As in the temporal area, the preauricular and parotid-masseteric areas are covered by a deep fascia underneath which lie the superficial temporal vessels, the parotid gland, and the facial nerve. Over these areas the skin is adherent to the fascia. Anterior to the masseter muscle, the cheek wall is relatively thin. This can be observed by placing one finger inside the mouth and the other over the skin anterior to the masseter muscle. The subcutaneous tissue in this area consists of a connective tissue lamella disposed in a crisscross manner and containing a variable amount of fat. Immediately anterior to the masseter muscle is a special mass of fat that is present even in the thinnest individuals; this fatty mass, often referred to as the buccal fat pad of Bichat,* has a posterior extension between the masseter and the buccinator muscles. The buccal fat pad communicates freely with the temporal fossa and with the zygomatic fossa. The buccinator muscle is covered by a thick fascia which gradually becomes thinner, finally ending at the oral commissure as a thin lamina. Stensen's duct travels along the lateral surface of the buccinator muscle for a distance of 5 or 6 mm, perforating the muscle to penetrate through the oral mucosa. The duct is covered by the buccal fat pad. The areolar area extends to the nasolabial fold, and the skin may be raised subcutaneously by careful blunt dissection as far as the nasolabial fold. The buccal branches of the facial nerve can be avoided, as they lie at a deeper level, and the fat pad of Bichat protects the parotid duct.

In the temporal area the scalp is attached to a deep fascia to which it is adherent. The dissection of scalp tissue should always be performed below the level of the galea aponeurotica in order to prevent the destruction of the

---

*Bichat's original term was "la boule graisseuse," "the fatty ball" of the cheek.

bulbs of the hair follicles. When the dissection is being performed anterior to the scalp toward the lateral canthus, it should then become superficial and immediately subcutaneous in order to avoid sectioning of the facial nerve branch to the frontalis muscle. Furnas (1965) has described the landmarks for the temporofacial division of the facial nerve. As Conley (1976) has pointed out, the pattern of distribution varies from individual to individual (see p. 1900). Careful superficial subcutaneous dissection will also prevent injury to this superficial branch. Electrocoagulation should also be prudently used.

The superficial temporal artery, the smaller of the two terminal branches of the external carotid artery, begins in the substance of the parotid gland behind the neck of the mandibular condyle, crossing over the root of the zygoma. About 5 cm above the root of the zygoma, it divides into two branches, a frontal and a parietal. These vessels and their accompanying veins are situated immediately below the superficial layer of the temporal fascia. Careful dissection in this area, remaining superficial to the fascia, will avoid excessive bleeding from these vessels. As the dissection proceeds downward, bleeding is encountered from the transverse facial artery, which arises from the superficial temporal artery before the artery leaves the substance of the parotid gland and passes transversely across the masseter muscle. If the dissection penetrates the parotid-masseteric fascia, bleeding originates from this vessel. The middle temporal artery arises immediately above the zygomatic arch and perforates the temporal fascia. The anterior auricular branches of the superficial temporal artery are distributed to the anterior portion of the auricle. Bleeding points in the course of the dissection may originate from any of these vessels or their veins; complete hemostasis must be achieved before proceeding with the remainder of the operation.

The platysma muscle (Fig. 37–18) extends upward over the lower part of the mandible, and the superior border of its upward extension is delimited by a line extending from the tragus to the commissure of the mouth. In some cases the upper extension reaches the orbicularis oculi muscle. Beneath the platysma and its underlying fascia lie the branches of the facial nerve. The marginal mandibular branch of the facial nerve lies under the platysma at varying levels; it lies at a lower level in the living subject than in the cadaver. Subcutaneous dissection in this area should extend over the platysma in order to avoid injury to the nerve.

The incision over the mastoid process

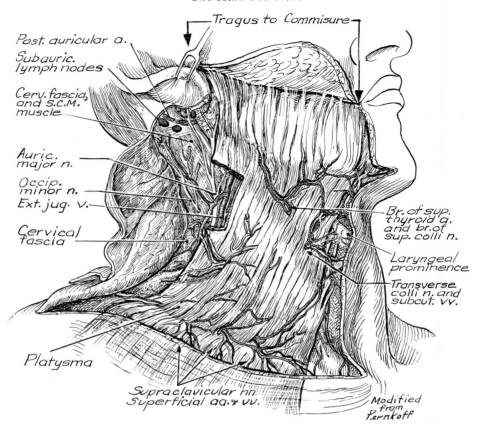

FIGURE 37–18. Anatomy of the cervical area with particular emphasis on the relationship of the platysma muscle with the subjacent structures. Note that the upward extension of the platysma reaches a horizontal line joining the tragus to the commissure of the mouth. The lower portion of the platysma arises from the fascia covering the upper portions of the pectoralis major and deltoideus muscles. Its fibers cross the clavicle and proceed upward along the side of the neck. The posterior border of the platysma has been cut out to demonstrate that the external jugular vein is located on the undersurface of the posterior portion of the platysma muscle. The anatomy of the platysma muscle as represented in the drawing differs somewhat from the description given in most anatomy books. The drawing is based upon in vivo observations by Dr. John Conley in the course of head and neck ablative operations. The reader should be reminded that in vivo anatomy varies considerably from postmortem anatomy.

should be extended down to the fascia covering the sternomastoid muscle. The dissection then proceeds downward along a cleavage plane between the fascia and the subcutaneous tissue. One of the most frequently injured structures in the course of a face lift operation is the greater auricular nerve, the largest of the superficial ascending branches of the cervical plexus. It arises from the second and third cervical nerves and winds around the posterior border of the sternomastoid muscle after perforating the deep fascia. It ascends upon the muscle beneath the platysma to the parotid gland, where it divides into anterior and posterior branches. The posterior branch provides sensory innervation over the mastoid process, the posterior aspect of the auricle and the lobe, and the lower portion of the concha. Severance of the postauricular nerve results in anesthesia of the portions of the auricle innervated by the

nerve. Another superficially situated nerve is the lesser occipital nerve, which arises from the second cervical nerve and occasionally also from the third. The lesser occipital nerve curves around and ascends along the posterior border of the sternomastoid muscle. As it approaches the cranium, it perforates the deep fascia and extends upward behind the auricle, supplying the skin and communicating with the greater occipital nerve, the greater auricular nerve, and the posterior auricular branch of the facial nerve. The lesser occipital nerve gives off an auricular branch which provides the sensory innervation of the skin of the upper and posterior portions of the auricle. Section of this nerve results in a loss of sensation in its area of distribution.

In the postauricular area and over the mastoid process, bleeding is encountered from the postauricular branch of the posterior auricular artery, a branch of the external carotid, and from the postauricular vein. This vein drains into the posterior facial vein, which receives blood from the superficial temporal vein. The posterior facial vein drains into the external jugular vein.

As the dissection proceeds downward over the fascia of the sternomastoid muscle, the subcutaneous tissue becomes looser, in contrast to the adherence of the skin over the mastoid and the upper portion of the sternomastoid muscle, where the skin is attached by a system of trabeculae to the subjacent plane. The external jugular vein, as it descends from the parotid region near the anterior border of the sternomastoid muscle, crosses obliquely to pass beneath the platysma, descending obliquely toward the supraclavicular region.

At this point in the dissection of the skin from the underlying tissues, one encounters the posterior border of the platysma. The platysma is a broad, thin muscle invested by the superficial fascia which has divided into superficial and deep layers. In most anatomy texts the platysma is represented as being too oblique. As mentioned earlier in the text, Conley has pointed out that the posterior border of the platysma is often situated in a more posterolateral position and serves as a landmark in operations upon the parotid (see Fig. 37–18). The platysma muscle has an upward extension which reaches the tragus of the auricle; the muscle extends forward, proceeding upward and medialward along the side of the neck. As it reaches the suprahyoid region, it ascends upward to the mental symphysis, where it interdigitates with the muscles about the commissure of the mouth and the lower lip. Because of the close relationship with the muscles around the oral commissure and the muscles of the lower lip, sectioning the platysma in the submandibular area can produce a weakness in the lower lip which may be erroneously interpreted as an injury to the marginal mandibular branch of the facial nerve (Conley, 1976).

At the lower border of the mental symphysis, the platysma interlaces with the platysma on the contralateral side, leaving a triangular area devoid of muscle between the medial edge of each muscle. The apex of the triangle is at the mental symphysis. The area situated between the two platysma muscles is covered by the superficial fascia lying immediately beneath the skin; beneath the superficial fascia are the two bellies of the digastric muscle, which also leave a smaller intervening triangular area. It is in this area that submental fat accumulates in predisposed individuals and skin is apt to become loose, wrinkled, and ptotic in older individuals.

It was mentioned earlier that the platysma is enclosed between two layers of the superficial fascia and is attached to the skin of the neck. The platysma is a remnant of a thin, wide band of muscle in reptiles, the primitive sphincter colli, activated by a branch of the seventh cranial nerve, which in more highly developed mammalian species has grown forward along the sides of the face to form the muscles of facial expression which also have connections with the freely movable skin (Huber, 1931; see also Kazanjian and Converse, 1974, Chapter 1). The deep surface of the platysma lies over the cervical fascia, to which it is joined by a layer of loose areolar tissue which can readily be separated by blunt dissection. The purpose of this particular anatomical arrangement is to allow the platysma to move the cervical skin without being hampered by underlying attachments.

Technique of the Face Lift Operation

Two different techniques have been developed for the face lift operation. In the first, the operation is performed entirely subcutaneously. Infiltration of a local anesthetic solution under the skin facilitates the dissection by separating the skin over the areas where it is adherent to the deep fascia: the temporal and preauricular areas and over the sternomastoid muscle. The operation is performed by separating the platysma muscle from the skin (*the supraplatysma technique*), with the patient either under general anesthesia supplemented by the subcutaneous injection of local anesthetic solution or under sedation supplemented by the infiltration of local anesthetic solution.

The second technique is the *subplatysma technique* of Skoog (1974). Regional block anesthesia is advocated. The dissection proceeds along the undersurface of the platysma muscle through the loose space between the fascia surrounding the platysma and the external cervical fascia.

The Supraplatysma Approach: The Three-point Fixation Technique. The operation may be performed under general endotracheal anesthesia without induced hypotension. Hypotensive anesthesia increases the difficulty of identifying the bleeding vessels and of obtaining complete hemostasis. If the patient is to be operated on under local anesthesia, the pre-operative medication is similar to that prescribed for the esthetic eyelid operation. The patient's hair should be shampooed on the day preceding the operation.

The patient's head is placed on a rubber doughnut-shaped pad on a neurosurgical head rest. This type of extension facilitates the surgeon's operation.

The hair is saturated with pHisoHex and combed in the temporal and postauricular area. It is then trimmed with scissors in the appropriate areas and plastered upward; if sufficiently long, it is fixed at the top of the head with a rubber band. Shaving the scalp in the temporal and postauricular areas is not necessary; trimming the hair with scissors suffices. The head is draped with a sterile towel and turned, leaving

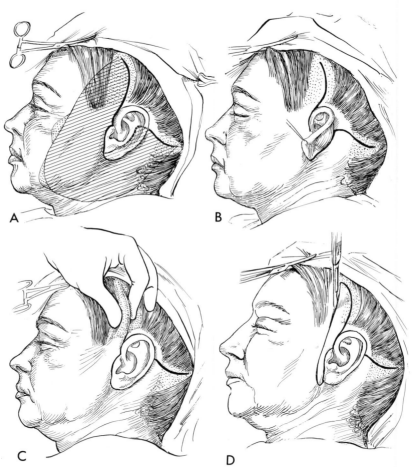

FIGURE 37–19. *The face lift operation:* the supraplatysmal approach. *A,* The shaded area illustrates the amount of skin undermining in the average face lift operation. Additional undermining varies in extent when indicated. In the older patient with loose cervical skin, complete undermining of the cervical area may be required (see Fig. 37–20). The outline of the incision is indicated. Note the curve of the incision in the temporal area. *B,* In the drawing, the temporal area and retroauricular scalp area are represented as shaved for purposes of clarifying the drawing. Shaving is not necessary. The hair can be cut sufficiently short with scissors to allow the surgeon to perform the operation. The drawing illustrates the incision made above the retroauricular fold when the ear is retracted forward. The purpose of making the incision *above* the retoauricular fold is to allow the suture line to fall into the retroauricular fold when the forward retraction of the auricle is relaxed. Note that the incision is made at the junction of the earlobe with the cheek. *C,* An estimate of the amount of temporal scalp to be resected is obtained by the "pinch" technique. The area to be excised is then outlined. *D,* A preauricular area has been outlined for excision. Note that the posterior line of excision follows the preauricular fold upward to the tragus, then curves around the tragus, thus avoiding a straight line in the preauricular area. The incision then curves around the helix and assumes a curve. The posterior curve in the temporal area, contrasting with the straight line of the anterior incision, results in an upward rotation of the skin of the cheek. The more accentuated the curve, the greater the upward rotation of the cheek tissue.

only one side of the face exposed (Fig. 37–19, *A*). It can be held in place and the hair is kept out of the field by clamping the hair and towel in the temporal area. The lines of incision are marked using the skin fold anterior to the helix as the "take-off" point (Fig. 37–19, *A, B*). The line extends into the temporal area in a curvilinear fashion, and inferiorly it curves into the groove between the helix and tragus. Thus a straight preauricular line of incision is avoided; such an incision leaves a visible scar. Inferiorly it is placed in the skin crease lying anterior to the tragus and the anterior border of the conchal cartilage. An incision behind the tragus may be employed but is not generally advisable (see variations). The marking curves under the lobe and into the postauricular crease (Fig. 37–19, *B*) to the desired height, depending on the close proximity of the postauricular hairline to the helix. It then extends posteriorly into the hair-bearing postauricular scalp in a curvilinear manner (Fig. 37–19, *B*). When the auricle is retracted, the line of incision should be placed

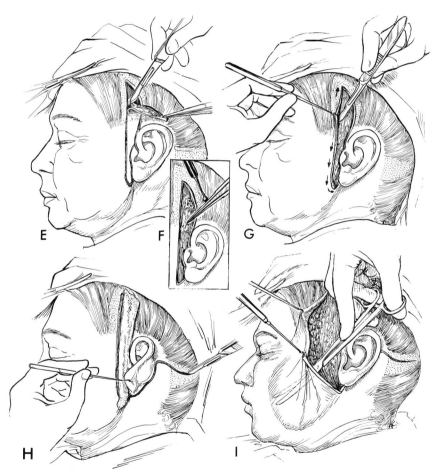

FIGURE 37–19 *Continued. E,* The excision of the scalp and preauricular segment is done by sharp dissection. The purpose of the excision of the preauricular segment is to facilitate the surgical approach to the cheek. *F,* In the temporal area, if the excision of the scalp is at a level above the temporal fascia, little bleeding occurs. Hemostasis is completed by electrocoagulation. *G,* The subcutaneous dissection is begun and will be extended along the entire length of the anterior edge of the excised preauricular segment. *H,* The preauricular raw area is covered with moist gauze. The incision is made a few millimeters above the retroauricular fold when the ear is retracted forward. The incision then curves up over the mastoid to a point immediately above the level of the upper border of the tragus and extends into the scalp. *I,* Undermining of the skin over the cheek area is done with scissors. The undermining extends over the parotid-masseteric fascia and may extend, when necessary, by blunt dissection as far as the nasolabial fold. In the temporal area the dissection proceeds foward at a level below the hair follicles in the scalp area. Anterior to the scalp, the undermining becomes immediately subcutaneous as it approaches the lateral rim of the orbit to avoid injury of the frontal branch of the facial nerve.

Illustration continued on the following page.

slightly above the postauricular crease; thus, when the auricle is released, the line falls into the crease.

In order to predetermine the amount of scalp to be removed, the preauricular facial and temporal scalp is manually advanced and plicated (the "pinch" technique) (Fig. 37–19, *C*). With experience, an estimate is obtained of the size and shape of the segment to be excised. The beginner should be conservative for fear of resecting too much scalp. The "pinch" technique also provides infor-

mation concerning the mobility of the scalp over the galea aponeurotica, important information for the determination of the amount of skin and scalp to be resected from the posterosuperior portion of the cervicofacial flap in the retroauricular area. Additional scalp can be resected, if warranted, after the undermining of the scalp and the temporal skin anteriorly. The amount of preauricular skin to be removed is also estimated and outlined with ink. Determination of the definitive amount of skin to be excised and the final contouring of the flap to

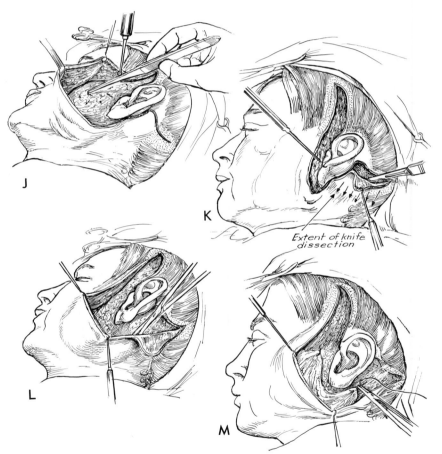

FIGURE 37–19 *Continued.* *J*, All bleeding vessels are electrocoagulated. *K*, The retroauricular portion of the operation is performed. An incision has been made down to the fascia covering the sternomastoid muscle, and the plane of dissection should be at the level of the fascia. As the skin is very adherent to the fascia in this area, sharp dissection is advisable. *L*, As the incision extends further down along the sternomastoid muscle, the attachment of the skin becomes looser, and scissor dissection is feasible. During this portion of the dissection, care must be taken to avoid injury to, or sectioning of, the greater auricular nerve, which often lies superficially over the sternomastoid muscle. The dissection is continued into the cervical area, the external jugular vein being avoided. As he proceeds with the downward dissection, the surgeon encounters the border of the platysma muscle lying over the sternomastoid muscle. As the external jugular vein lies under the platysma muscle, there is little risk of the vessel being sectioned when the supraplatysmal technique is employed. The dissection in the cervical area thus proceeds on a plane superficial to the platysma, and if the dissection is extended forward for a considerable distance, fiberoptic retractors are useful not only in providing the illumination for the dissection but also in locating bleeding vessels which are electrocoagulated. *M*, A technique of plicating the fascia.

fit the preauricular incision are completed only after the undermining and advancement-rotation of the skin in the temporal area. The pre-excision of the temporal and preauricular skin facilitates entering the plane of dissection and avoiding the superficial temporal vessels (Fig. 37–19, *D*).

Whether general or local anesthesia is used, the areas to be undermined and excised (see Fig. 37–19, *A*) are infiltrated with a solution of lidocaine (0.5 per cent) and epinephrine 1:200,000. The infiltration provides local anesthesia. It also assists in hemostasis and facilitates the dissection of the flaps. When the solution is infiltrated along the planes of dis-

section, it achieves a veritable "hydraulic dissection," facilitating the surgical dissection. The Pitkin automatic refilling syringe is particularly useful in achieving rapid infiltration of the anesthetic solution. The predetermined area of preauricular and temporal skin is resected (Fig. 37–19, *E*), and hemostasis is secured with electrocoagulation (Fig. 37–19, *F*). The scalp is dissected from the fascia in the temporal area (Fig. 37–19, *G*), and the post-auricular line is incised (Fig. 37–19, *H*). The "hydraulic dissection" is particularly helpful in facilitating a plane of dissection over the areas where the cutaneous tissues are adherent to the underlying temporal fascia, the preauricu-

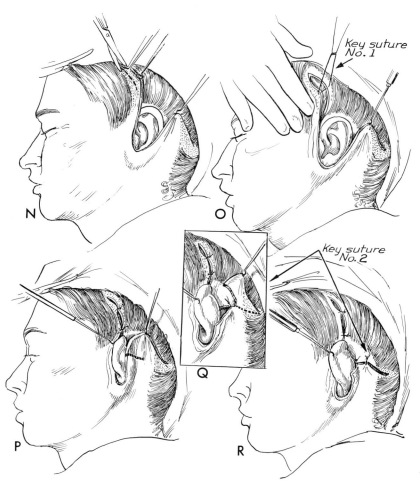

FIGURE 37–19 *Continued. N,* Traction is placed upon the anterior edge of the excised scalp area, and additional scalp is excised when required. With a sufficient amount of practice, the area to be excised can be accurately determined, and often the additional incision is not required. Note that traction is placed upon the undermined skin in an upward and posterior direction. *O,* Closure of the scalp defect is begun (key suture #1). *P,* An incision is made, the skin being maintained under traction, in order to approximate the skin to the incision over the mastoid (see *Q*). *Q,* The suture is placed in the mastoid area. The remainder of the excess skin is resected. *R,* Key suture #2 is illustrated.

Illustration continued on the following page.

lar area, and the sternomastoid muscle. After the infiltration over the sternomastoid muscle, there is little need for further infiltration, as block anesthesia of the superficial branches of the superficial cervical plexus has been achieved, and the plane of dissection in the cervical area is readily established anterior to the sternomastoid muscle.

The plane of dissection in the temporal area is established by sharp knife dissection along the plane of the temporalis fascia and below the level of the bulbs of the hair follicles. In the preauricular area the dissection extends over the parotid-masseteric fascia. Once the plane is established, dissection follows with scissors or scalpel, traction being applied with skin hooks on the skin edge as the assistant provides counteraction (Fig. 37–19, *I*). The dissection extends over varying distances, depending on the indi-

vidual case, and may reach the level of the lateral orbital rim at the lateral canthus, the nasolabial line, and the "jowl" area along the mandible (Fig. 37–19, *A*). The extent of the undermining of the cervicofacial skin is variable. In older patients extensive undermining is usually required (see Fig. 37–20). Meticulous hemostatis is secured by electrocoagulation (Fig. 37–19, *J*). The fiberoptic retractor is helpful in providing illumination of the undermined flap. Sharp dissection in the postauricular area is necessary because of the firm fixation of the postauricular flap to the fascia of the sternomastoid muscle, which is inserted by a strong tendon to the entire lateral surface of the mastoid process (Fig. 37–19, *K*). Below the level of the earlobe, dissection is resumed (Fig. 37–19, *L*) but must be done cautiously under direct vision to avoid damage to the greater auricular

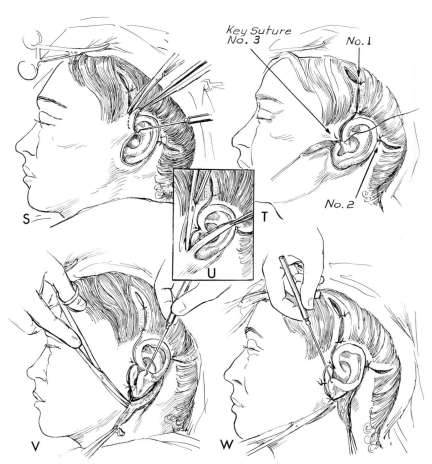

FIGURE 37–19 *Continued.* *S,* Excision of the preauricular skin is begun. *T,* The third key suture is placed immediately above the tragus. *U,* Excision of preauricular skin is continued. *V,* Careful excision around the lobe is necessary to avoid a frequent deformity seen after these operations: excessive downward traction on the earlobe. *W,* Suture of the earlobe to the skin has been completed, and the excess retroauricular skin is excised.

nerve and the external jugular vein. Bleeding is more profuse if the dissection penetrates the underlying muscle fibers. During the dissection globules or particles of fat appear and should be wiped or irrigated from the surgical field. Plication of the facial or cervical fascia or both is considered by some to have merit (Fig. 37–19, *M*). In 33 patients Tipton (1974) plicated the superficial fascia in a vertical direction in the preauricular area on one side of the face in the course of a face lift operation but did not plicate the tissues on the other side. He observed that after two years there was no observable difference between the two sides of the face. If undertaken, it should be for specific problems such as laxity of the face in the jowl or jaw line area or laxity of the neck tissues. Once hemostasis has been

ensured, plication of the fascia is accomplished with nonabsorbable sutures, avoiding "bunching up" of the subcutaneous tissues.

The undermined skin is advanced and rotated by applying traction on the temporal area upward and posteriorly (Fig. 37–19, *N*) and on the postauricular flap in a similar direction (Fig. 37–19, *N*). If the temporal flap requires more trimming, it is done at this point, and the flap is fixed in position with a suture (Fig. 37–19, *O*). This is the first point of the "three-point" fixation technique. The second point of fixation is in the postauricular area where the undermined flap is advanced in the appropriate direction, incised at the highest point of the postauricular incision, and fixed with a suture (Fig. 37–19, *O* to *R*). Once the direction of advancement is established, the amount of redun-

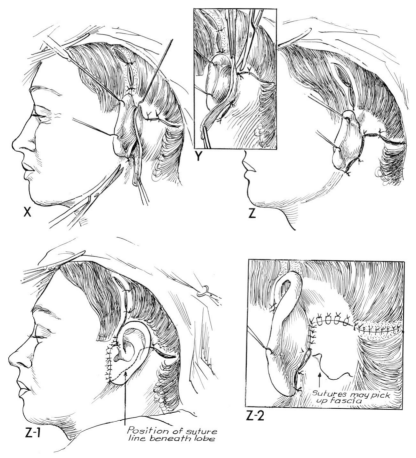

FIGURE 37–19 *Continued.* *X, Y,* The excess retroauricular skin is resected. *Z,* A few sutures are placed after the resection of the excess retroauricular skin. Note that the continuity of the hairline has been maintained. *Z–1,* The earlobe has been preserved, and the suture line lies under the earlobe, maintaining a free earlobe. *Z–2,* Suturing is being completed. Note the mattress sutures with a dermal component which eliminates suture marks. A point of technique: when the retroauricular incision is being sutured, the needle penetrates the subcutaneous fascia and occasionally the perichondrium. Interrupted sutures are illustrated; continuous running sutures are as effective in the scalp, and they save time.

dant skin is obvious; it is excised with either a knife or scissors (Fig. 37–19, Q). These two points of fixation are important since all the tension in the advancement of the cervicofacial flap is based upon cranial points of fixation. The amount of tension under which the temporal and retroauricular scalp wounds are sutured should be carefully controlled; excessive tension causes ischemia, alopecia, and hypertrophic scarring. The redundant preauricular skin is then trimmed and fitted to the preauricular incision without tension. For greater precision, it is helpful to rotate the patient's head from the laterally flexed position to a face forward position (the nose "pointing to the sky"). Definitive preauricular trimming is done to fit the flap to the prehelical incision and into the notch above the tragus; it is continued from this point for a short distance to allow the point of the flap to be fixed with a suture to the notch above the tragus (the third pont of fixation) before the remaining excision is continued to the earlobe (Fig. 37–19, S to U). Care is exercised to stay high under the lobe in order to avoid a downward drag on the earlobe, as the scar contracts (Fig. 37–19, V, W). The flap excision is completed so that the flap fits the postauricular incision without tension (Fig. 37–19, X to Z). The incisions are closed in the temporal area with interrupted (or continuous running) 3–0 or 4–0 nylon sutures, in the preauricular area with running or interrupted 6–0 nylon (Fig. 37–19, Z-1), and in the postauricular area with 4–0 nylon. Mattress sutures with an anterior dermal component are placed in the non–hair-bearing portion of the postauricular flap to avoid suture marks or cross-hatching (Fig. 37–19, Z-2). In the closure in the retroauricular groove, interrupted (or continuous running) sutures are used. In order to avoid a tendency to tent over the sulcus and allow a gutter in which blood may accumulate, the postauricular fascia is included in the suture to obliterate the dead space. It is not advisable to include the conchal cartilage in the suture because of the danger of a subperichondrial hematoma over the anterolateral aspect of the auricle and the risk of chondritis. At the completion of the operation, antibiotic ointment is spread over the suture lines. The purpose of the ointment is to keep the gauze dressing from sticking to the sutures. Gauze compresses are then rolled around the auricle to avoid compression of the auricle by the pressure dressing. Two large gauze packs filled with teased out Acrilan cotton are placed on each side of the face, and they serve to provide moderate compression

maintained by circular bandages. A suction-type drain is placed beneath the dissected cervical skin and brought out through the lower end of the scalp incision. A variable amount of blood and serum is aspirated during the first 24 hours. A moderately compressive dressing is applied, which remains in position for 48

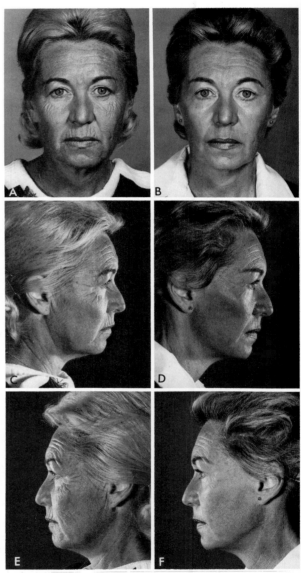

FIGURE 37–20. The face lift operation combined with a corrective blepharoplasty and a chemical peel of the upper lip. *A,* Preoperative appearance of the patient. *B,* Postoperative appearance of the patient following the blepharoplasty technique illustrated in Figures 37–9 and 37–10 and the face lift operation illustrated in Figure 37–19. During the same operative session, the patient underwent a chemical peel of the upper lip (see Chapter 17). *C, D,* Pre- and postoperative right profile views of patient. *E, F,* Pre- and postoperative left profile views of patient.

hours (for a discussion of the postoperative care without a compressive dressing, see later in the Chapter under Variations).

The technique illustrated and described in Figure 37–19 is applicable to the patient in the 40 to 50 age range with resilient skin and without submental fat or the midline "turkey gobbler neck." More extensive procedures are required in older patients with more severe ptosis of the soft tissues (see Variations).

POSTOPERATIVE CARE. Ideally the patient is hospitalized postoperatively for two days. Bedrest is encouraged for the first day, since this is the most crucial period in the development of hematoma. Visitors should be restricted. Sedatives or tranquilizers are helpful during this period. Minimal ambulation is allowed the day following surgery, and on the second postoperative day the dressing and drains are removed before the patient is discharged from the hospital. Staged removal of the sutures can be arranged on an outpatient

basis. During this period the patient will often need reassurance, and the doctor-patient relationship becomes very important.

A patient who underwent a face lift operation according to the technique illustrated in Figure 37–19 and blepharoplasty is shown in Figure 37–20. A chemical peel of the upper lip was also performed.

THE UPPER FACE LIFT OPERATION. In the younger patient the presence of an early sag of the face manifests itself in deep nasolabial folds and beginning jowls without sagging of the neck (Fig. 37–21, *A, C*). Such a condition warrants surgical correction without a complete face lift; an upper (or temporal) face lift is indicated (Fig. 37–22). The procedure is limited to dissection and undermining in the temporal and cheek areas (Fig. 37–22, *A*); an incision must be made beneath the earlobe to allow the lobe to be released from tension or displacement (Fig. 37–22, *B*).

The temporal excision is planned as in a

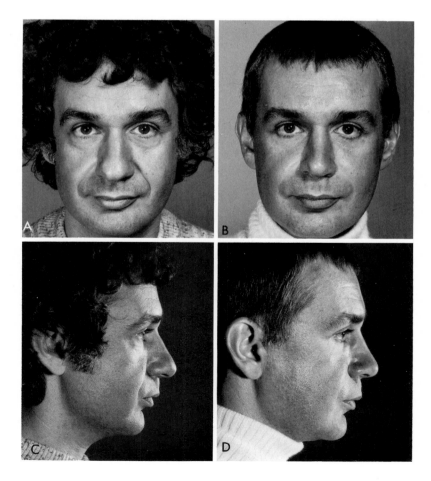

FIGURE 37–21. The upper face lift operation. *A, C,* Preoperative views of the patient. *B, D,* Postoperative views following the upper face lift operation illustrated in Figure 37–22.

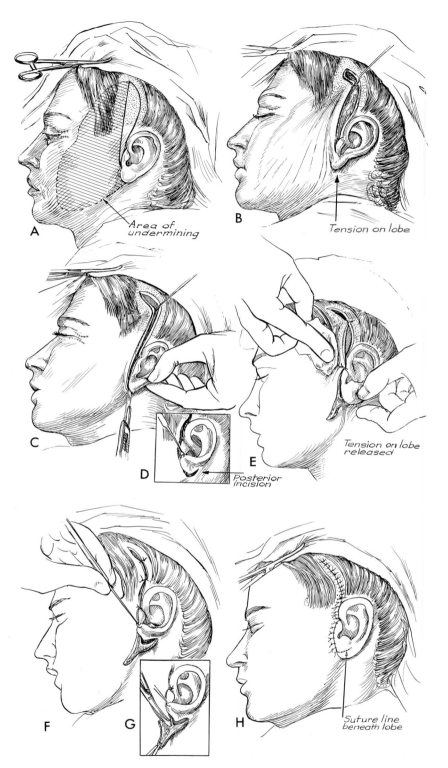

FIGURE 37–22. The upper face lift operation. *A,* Outline of the area of excision. The shaded area illustrates the extent of the dissection and undermining in the temporal and cheek areas. *B,* The tension on the lobe when the undermined facial flap is raised upward and backward. *C,* The incision around the earlobe in order to release the tension. *D,* The earlobe has been raised, showing the posterior extent of the incision. *E,* The temporal scalp suture at the point of fixation has been placed, as well as the suture above the tragal notch. The incision in front of the earlobe has been extended downward and a flap of excess skin reflected. *F, G, H,* Details of the excision of the excess skin below the earlobe and final adjustment of the lobe. The operation is completed.

face lift operation by plicating the scalp and outlining the area of the temporal tissue to be plicated (Fig. 37–22, *A*), with the proviso of being conservative and with the option for additional excision after the undermining has been completed and the superoposterior rotation of the flap is achieved. The plane of dissection is established after the temporal and preauricular tissue is excised. Once the undermining has been completed and the skin advanced (Fig. 37–22, *B*), the incision should be extended under the earlobe (Fig. 37–22, *C, D*). The skin excision is completed in the preauricular area after a key suture is placed in the temporal area (Fig. 37–22, *E*). The excision is performed down to the notch above the tragus, and another suture is placed for fixation (Fig. 37–22, *E*) before the incision is continued to and around the lobe (Fig. 37–22, *E, F, G*). The incision is closed in the same manner as in the full face lift (Fig. 37–22, *H*). A similar compressive dressing is applied as for the complete face lift operation.

The Subplatysma Approach. In the first edition of *Reconstructive Plastic Surgery* (1964), the technique of dissecting the undersurface of the platysma was advocated for the removal of redundant cervical tissue. Skoog (1974) has refined this approach (the *subplatysma technique*) and described his technique in detail.

Skoog prefers to perform the operation under sedation and regional block anesthesia. This is provided by a mandibular nerve block (transcutaneous injection) and by blocking the infraorbital nerve. The superficial cervical plexus block is obtained by injecting the anesthetic solution under the fascia along the posterior margin of the sternomastoid muscle in its midportion. The technique has the advantage of avoiding the obscuring effect of the local anesthetic solution, thus facilitating the identification of anatomical structures.

Skoog's incision extends through the temporal, preauricular, and postauricular areas and is angulated downward immediately behind the hairline. This type of incision (along the hairline) has, however, generally been abandoned because of the hypertrophic scarring which often occurs in this area. The dissection which is begun in the temporal region is extended anteriorly under the skin of the forehead and the lateral canthal region for a distance sufficient to raise the eyebrow and correct the lateral canthal region. The amount of undermining is dependent upon the subcutaneous tissue mobility. Blunt dissection is used to avoid damage to the frontal branch of the facial nerve. Undermining of the cheek is achieved by dissecting between the thin fascial layer of the subcutaneous tissue and the deep fascia of the face over the zygomatic area and over the parotid-masseteric fascia where the subcutaneous tissue is more adherent. At the level of the anterior border of the masseter muscle, the tissue layers can be easily separated by "cautiously spreading the scissors" (Skoog, 1974). The buccal fat pad is exposed, and in certain cases the parotid duct and the branches of the fifth and seventh cranial nerves are visible. Keeping the scissors immediately subcutaneous and superficial to the buccal fat pad, the surgeon may advance them as far as the nasolabial fold. After carefully undermining in a subcutaneous level toward the nasolabial fold, the surgeon can grasp the subcutaneous fascia with forceps. Backward traction is exerted on the fascia, which is sutured to the parotid-masseteric fascia. Excessive traction must be avoided, particularly in the older patient with relaxed tissues, as a kinking of the parotid duct may result in obstruction and temporary swelling of the parotid. Acute swelling of the parotid is extremely painful, and evacuation of the parotid secretions may not occur for ten days or more, during which time the patient suffers acute pain. When the dissection reaches the superoposterior border of the platysma muscle (see Fig. 37–18), the edge of the muscle is identified and freed for a distance extending approximately 3 cm. The upper portion of the freed edge of the platysma should be at least 1 cm. inferior to the lower border of the mandible to avoid the marginal mandibular branch of the facial nerve.

Anterior to the sternomastoid muscle, the dissection is extended forward on the undersurface of the platysma, in contrast to the supraplatysma technique. The external jugular vein is identified and protected. Proceeding by blunt dissection, the potential space between the fascia covering the undersurface of the platysma and the external cervical fascia is carefully undermined. The edge of the platysma with its covering skin can then be submitted to a backward traction in a posterosuperior direction until the redundant tissues of the neck have been eliminated. The edge of the platysma with its accompanying fascia is sutured to the mastoid fascia posterior to the ear lobe, care being taken to avoid including the sensory nerves in the sutures. In some cases Skoog advances the platysma muscle at the inferior aspect of the cheek where the muscle does not have a clearly defined deep fascial surface.

The cheek flap is advanced in a posterosuperior direction, and sutures are placed between the subcutaneous fascia and the parotid-masseteric fascia. Dead space is thus eliminated, and tension on the preauricular suture line is reduced. Redundant skin is then excised.

Skoog dissects as far as the lateral border of the orbicularis oculi muscle, which is exposed. The muscle is splayed out and sutured in the spread position in order to prevent excessive wrinkling at the lateral canthus. Skoog states that the orbicularis oculi may be split laterally and the cut ends separated without disturbing eyelid function.

The Supraplatysma Versus the Subplatysma Technique: Advantages and Disadvantages. The supraplatysma technique as illustrated in Figure 37–19 is the safest technique. When adequately performed, the operation is devoid of complications, particularly those involving the facial nerve. The figures on the incidence of hematoma given later in the text in Table 37–1 refer to patients operated upon by the supraplatysma technique. No information is presently available on the incidence of hematoma formation following the subplatysma technique. Surgeons who have employed this technique state that the incidence of postoperative hematoma is lower.

Caution should be exercised in approaching the platysma when performing the subplatysmal operation. The cervical branch of the facial nerve may descend lower than usual into the neck. Section of the nerve with subsequent denervation of the platysma muscle is a possible complication.

At the time of this writing it is too early to evaluate the long-term results of the subplatysma technique as described by Skoog. Because the posteriorly and superiorly exerted traction on the platysma occurs at a right angle to the fibers of the muscle, whether the muscle will eventually stretch in order to resume its former position should be seriously considered.

The distinct advantages of the subplatysmal technique (as in the muscle flap technique of corrective blepharoplasty) are the absence of ecchymosis and the diminished incidence of hematoma formation. With careful technique, injury to branches of the facial nerve is avoided. The main disadvantage of the subplatysma technique as described by Skoog is the inability to "clean up" the submental area. Some of the modifications recently introduced (see Fig. 37–27) may remedy this disadvantage.

Secondary Face Lift Operation. A repeat face lift operation is required after a certain number of years. While the initial operation relieves the patient of redundant cutaneous and adipose tissues and restores a more youthful appearance, the result is not permanent, as the aging process proceeds unrelentingly. The indications for a repeat operation vary according to the patient's personal needs or desires. The time interval between the primary and secondary operations also varies from six months to five years. In the aged patient with relaxed and inelastic tissues, a secondary operation may be indicated six months after the first. Repeat operations are indicated at variable time intervals according to each patient's individual needs.

TECHNIQUE OF THE SECONDARY FACE LIFT OPERATION. The operative procedure is similar to that described in Figure 37–19. Resection of the preauricular segment as shown in Figure 37–19 should be avoided in a secondary operation for fear of removing too much skin. In the temporal area, prudence is required, as often the excision of only a small amount of scalp is required. Resection of too much scalp results in tension, ischemia, and alopecia.

Combined Corrective Blepharoplasty and Face Lifting. Rather than submit the patient to two separate operations, it is often convenient for both the patient and the surgeon to perform the two procedures during the same operating session. Whether to perform the blepharoplasty first and the face lift operation second or vice versa is a matter for debate. When the blepharoplasty is performed first, there is an opportunity to remove remaining redundant skin by undermining from the temporal area toward the lateral canthal area. An argument in favor of doing the face lift operation first is that the patient may be checked for a possible hematoma after the completion of the blepharoplasty.

The No Dressing Face Lift. A constrictive pressure dressing is uncomfortable. When a blepharoplasty is performed during the same operative session, the tight compressive dressing tends to impede lymphatic circulation and thus increase the postoperative periorbital edema. A moderately compressive dressing is mainly protective. Neither type of dressing prevents hematoma formation.

The patient is more comfortable during the postoperative period with a dressing. The previously mentioned suction tubes (Jackson-Pratt) are placed bilaterally through the postauricular scalp wound and lie under the cervical skin. The tubes are removed after a variable amount of blood and serum is aspirated and drainage ceases.

Face Lifting in the Male Patient. There has been an increasing demand for surgery of the aging face in male patients. The results obtained in the male appear to be as satisfactory as, if not superior to, those obtained in females. The thicker skin of the male patients explains the satisfactory results. Male patients, however, seem more prone to postoperative hematoma. Hemostasis, therefore, must be meticulous.

In the face lift operation in the male, greater emphasis is given to a vertical lift. This can be obtained by accentuating the curvature of the posterior incision in the temporal region (Fig. 37–23).

The technique is similar to that described for the face lift in the female. The postauricular incision may be extended further upward and more posteriorly into the scalp in order to camouflage the scars better. One problem which arises is the recession of the sideburn, which is displaced into the preauricular area. Many patients do not object to the inconvenience of shaving this area with an electric razor. The sideburn is restored as a result of the upward lift which brings the bearded portion of the cheek into the sideburn area.

To remedy the inconvenience of the beard pattern, Baker and Gordon (1969) preserved a small strip of non–hair-bearing skin in front of the ear, placing the preauricular incision at the junction of the bearded area with the hairless skin. However, it must be emphasized that the sideburn is sacrificed in part by this technique.

A technique which involves a horizontal incision extending from one of the lateral folds of the crow's feet area to the preauricular region has been employed; the excess skin is removed in a vertical direction, and the horizontal wound is sutured (Hamilton, 1974). The retroauricular portion of the operation is performed as described above. The technique, however, can result in objectionable scars.

The Supraplatysma Technique: Variations. The technique shown in Figure 37–19 is a basic technique which can be modified according to the needs of the individual case.

The preauricular incision shown in Figure 37–19 leaves an inconspicuous scar in most patients, particularly those of the older age group. An incision extending behind the tragus

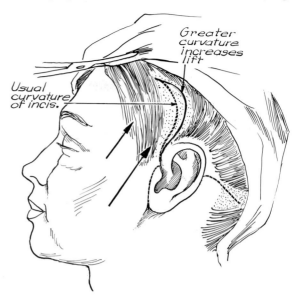

FIGURE 37–23. Accentuation of the curve of the posterior incision in the temporal area to increase the upward rotation of the cheek skin.

can be employed, but it is usually difficult to avoid a deformity of the tragus by this technique. Another technique consists of placing the incision 2 mm anterior to the border of the tragus. The skin overlying the tragus must be excised along a superficial level in order to preserve the subcutaneous tissue over the tragal cartilage. Prior to the advancement of the cheek skin over the tragus, subcutaneous tissue must be excised from the undersurface of the flap so that the skin will simulate the thin skin normally overlying the tragus. There should be no tension along the suture line, which lies very close to the border of the tragus.

Another variation is the excision of a triangle from the portion of the facial flap immediately below the hairline in the temporal area (Rees and Guy, 1971), which will produce the desired additional elevation when the skin is excessively redundant along the mandible. The technique is employed in secondary face lift operations. Another technique which places the scar behind the hairline is to accentuate the curve of the posterior incision line in the temporal area (Fig. 37–23); resection of a triangular area of scalp above the auricle is occasionally required to remove a fold of excess scalp when the extensive upward sweep of the cheek has been completed.

The amount of undermining varies according to the patient's needs. In general, a younger patient requires less undermining of the skin than an older patient. Patients in the 50 year old group and particularly those in the 60 or 70 year old group have redundant skin in the middle of the neck. Extensive undermining crossing the midline of the neck is often required (Fig. 37–24). The side to side undermining can be facilitated by making a short submental incision. When a submental lipectomy is required, the fat is removed medially in the submental area (see Fig. 37–26) and laterally superficial to the platysma muscle.

In patients with deep nasolabial folds, subcutaneous dissection extending to the fold is required. The dissection proceeds anterior to the masseter muscle, immediately subcutaneously by careful separation of the loose tissue overlying the fat pad of the cheek.

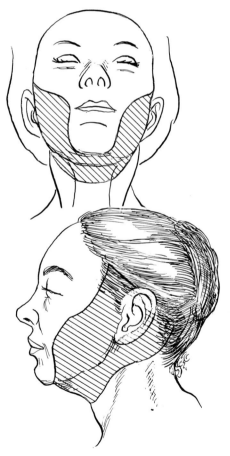

FIGURE 37–24. The extent of undermining of the skin of the cervical area in the patient with redundant skin of the midline of the neck. The undermined areas join each other in the midline.

As previously stated, the mobility of the scalp is variable; in some patients the scalp is very loose, while in others it is tight. When the amount of skin and scalp to be resected from the retroauricular portion of the cervicofacial flap is being undermined, the following maneuver is of great assistance: the flap has been undermined, hemostasis has been achieved, and the excised temporal area has been sutured; the superoposterior portion of the flap is grasped with a Kocher clamp, and tension is placed upon the flap. The tension should be parallel to the lower border of the mandible (Fig. 37–25, *A*). The assistant then advances the scalp posterior to the incision in an anterior direction. By raising the flap and examining the relative positions of the flap and the edge of the scalp incision, one can make a precise determination of the size and shape of the area of skin and scalp to be excised (Fig. 37–25, *A*). A skin hook is placed on the undersurface of the flap at the edge of the scalp incision (Fig. 35–25, *B*). The required amount of skin and scalp is then excised with a knife by extending the line of excision from the hook to the lowermost and posterior end of the scalp incision. After the excision of the excess skin and scalp, the continuity of the hairline is reestablished.

In the temporal area the superficial undermining of the skin toward the lateral canthal area varies in extent. Backward traction on the temporal flap will show whether the excess of skin in the canthal area is adequately stretched; careful superficial undermining as far as the orbital margin may be required in order to remove the excess skin in this area.

Abandonment of the vertical incision along the postauricular hairline, which was formerly employed, has eliminated the widened and hypertrophic scars frequently seen. The technique illustrated in Figure 37–19 leaves a slightly visible scar over the mastoid area. If the hairline is situated more posteriorly than usual, leaving a wider area of exposed skin in the retroauricular area, the retroauricular incision can be extended upward more vertically than in the technique shown in Figure 37–19. The scalp portion of the incision then curves downward.

Additional Operative Procedures

THE SUBMENTAL AREA. The most difficult correction in the cervical region is the reestablishment of the mandibular-cervical angle in an area which extends between the lower border of the mandible to the hyoid. It is in

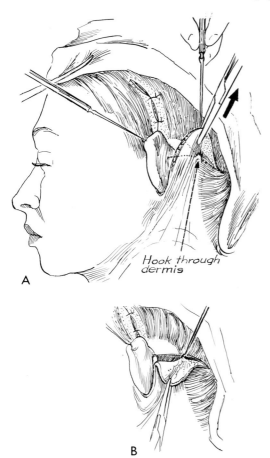

A

B

FIGURE 37–25. Technique for evaluating the amount of skin and scalp excision. *A*, The Kocher clamp exerts traction along a line parallel to the lower border of the mandible. The assistant exerts finger pressure on the scalp to advance the scalp in an anterior direction. A hook is then placed at the hairline as shown. The hook indicates where the incision should be placed for the excision. *B*, The position of the hook at the hairline.

this area that accumulation of fat and vertical wrinkling (the "turkey gobbler" deformity) occur. Frequently, in spite of the correction obtained by the face lift operation, submental fat or a "double chin" persists.

Many variations have been proposed for the surgical approach to this problem. Morel-Fatio (1964) suggested a lying down H-incision with the lower incision near the hyoid cartilage. The double advancing flaps were trimmed in the midline. Johnson and Hadley (1964) listed upright and inverted T-incisions and a variation of the Morel-Fatio H-incision, each of these involving the excision of a ver-

tical ellipse of skin with a variable amount of undermining. Adamson, Horton, and Crawford (1964) advocated excision of a wide transverse ellipse with separation and imbrication of the platysma in the midline and excision of most of the fat. They also found an average of 15 to 25 grams of submental fat in 17 adult cadavers. Millard, Pigott, and Hedo (1968) used a transverse incision with dissection of the fat as far as the thyroid cartilage. They also advocated removal of the submandibular fat through the rhytidectomy incision. Cronin and Biggs (1971) proposed a T–Z-plasty approach, emphasizing that the major excision is in the horizontal direction. They overlapped the platysma above the hyoid or performed a Z-plasty, imbricating the two edges of the platysma. Conley (1968) advocated triangular excision with T closure. Cannon and Pantagelos (1971) reported the W-plasty submental lipectomy. Weisman (1971) performed a Z-plasty on the platysma and removed fat both superficial and deep to the platysma. He noted that there is little danger of significant nerve damage in the midline. Millard and his associates (1972) reported that they had done submental or submandibular lipectomy in 63 per cent of their last 100 face lifts and that they were resecting platysma near the midline. Viñas and associates (1972) transposed the excess submental fat to the chin in the treatment of receding chin and used a tie-over bolster in the region of the lower incision.

Snyder (1974) noted that submental lipectomy is fraught with technical problems such as ridging, attributed to insufficient resection of fat, excessive removal of fat, failure to leave a layer of fat under the flap, or insufficient undermining of the area in the course of the face lift procedure. With progressive relaxation of the jowls, there is a tendency for bulges to form on each side of the area from which the submental resection has been performed. Snyder also emphasized the importance of the addition of a chin implant in patients with microgenia. Snyder (1974) believed that, in the patient with a severe "turkey gobbler" deformity, the subplatysmal dissection tends to produce a better result, obtaining greater tension across the hyoid area. Snyder has also emphasized the difficulty in obtaining a good result in the submental area with the subplatysma technique.

A technique of submental lipectomy and resection of redundant skin. Anesthesia is usually obtained by local infiltration with 1 per cent lidocaine with epinephrine. An outline is marked following the inferior border of the mandible (Fig. 37–26, *A*). It is important to follow the line of the mandible rather than the submental skin crease. The amount of tissue to be removed will determine how far the line of incision should be extended laterally. The incision is made to the muscle layer, and the area is undermined (Fig. 37–26, *A, B*). The extent of undermining is determined by the amount of fat and skin to be removed. Once the skin-fat flap has been undermined and hemostasis obtained, the flap is advanced, and the excess is excised without undue tension (Fig. 37–26, *C* to *H*). The submental fat pad is then dissected from the flap (Fig. 37–26, *I* to *K*), care being taken to leave an adequate layer of fat on the flap (Fig. 37–26, *I*) to prevent an unsightly depression and adherence of the skin in the submental area. Hemostasis must be obtained again at this point, and the wound is closed with subcutaneous absorbable sutures with attach-

ment to the mandibular periosteum to avoid a downward drift of the chin (Fig. 37–26, *L*). The skin incision is sutured (Fig. 37–26, *M*). When the submental lipectomy is done in conjunction with a face lift operation, the cervical skin should be widely undermined and the operation completed prior to the submental lipectomy (see Fig. 37–28). If the submental lipectomy is performed prior to the face-lift operation, the submental incision line is unduly elongated.

Castañares (1975) stated that he is satisfied with a technique he has used for many years. The technique consists of designing an ellipse over the submental lipectomy area, excising the ellipse of skin and fat, and suturing the wound without undermining.

Chin augmentation combined with face lifting: the cutaneous approach. A sagging neck is often associated with a weak chin, and

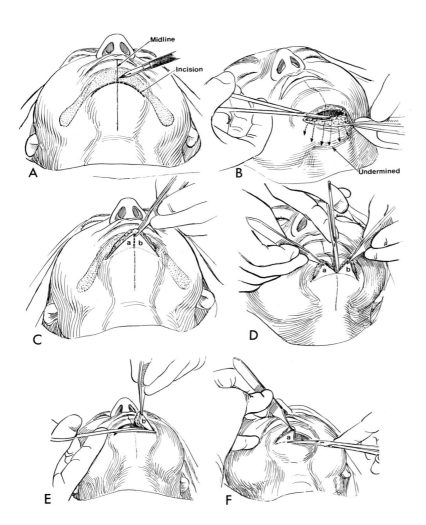

FIGURE 37–26. Technique of submental lipectomy and excision of excess skin. *A,* The mid-sagittal plane of the face has been outlined over the mental symphysis and extended into the cervical area. The outline of the incision along the posterior edge of the inferior border of the symphysis is indicated. *B,* The incision is extended down to the muscle layer. The arrows indicate the extent of the undermining along the plane of the muscle layer. The extent of the undermining depends upon the magnitude of the fat accumulation. *C,* Excess fat has been resected from under the skin-fat flap. The skin-fat flap is being advanced, overlapping the upper edge of the wound. The upper edge of the wound is indicated by the dotted line. *D,* The advanced skin-fat flap is separated into two triangular segments (*a* and *b*) by a vertical incision. *E,* The triangular flap *b* is excised at the level of the submental incision. *F,* The triangular flap *a* is resected.

augmentation of the chin with an inorganic implant performed concomitantly with a face lift operation and/or a submental skin-fat excision, or as a delayed procedure, can be helpful in achieving an optimal result. The intraoral approach has been previously described (see Chapter 30, p. 1385). The cutaneous approach provides good exposure for fixation of the implant.

Technique. The incision is outlined along the posteroinferior margin of the symphysis. Anesthesia is obtained by local infiltration of 1 per cent lidocaine and epinephrine, and the incision is extended down to the inferior margin of the mental symphysis (Fig. 37–27, *A*). The periosteum is exposed and incised for a distance just short of the length of the implant (Fig. 37–27, *B*, *C*). The periosteum is then elevated from the mental symphysis over an area wide enough only to accommodate the Silastic implant. The periosteum is left at-

tached to the most inferior aspect of the mandibular margin laterally. Care is taken to make the pocket exactly the size of the implant and to maintain the pocket directly over the mental prominence (Fig. 37–27, *D*, *E*). Since the Silastic implant is pliable, one end is inserted under the periosteum and the other can be bent to be inserted under the periosteum in the other end of the pocket (Fig. 37–27, *G*). By notching the implant in the center, one can ensure that the center is over the midline of the mental symphysis (Fig. 37–27, *F*).

If the dissection is meticulous and symmetrical, the implant almost snaps into place and cannot be moved in any direction. If there is any mobility, it is maintained by suturing the periosteum over the implant (Fig. 37–27, *H*) (even to the bone by drilling a hole along the inferior margin). The incision is closed in two layers, and only a light dressing is required. No external adhesive tape fixation is required, as

FIGURE 37–26 *Continued. G,* Sagittal section showing the position of the incision through the skin and the fat down to the muscle layer. The level of dissection is also illustrated. *H,* After the skin-fat flap is advanced. *I,* Excess submental fat is resected. *J,* Resection of the excess fat. *K,* The excess skin removed by the two triangular segments *a* and *b* and the submental fat pad are shown as specimens. *L,* Suturing of the deep layer. *M,* Closure of the skin incision has been completed.

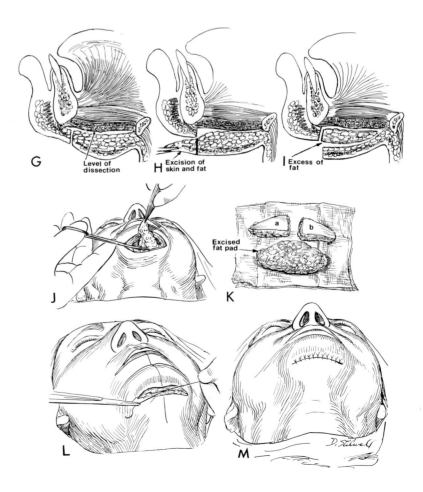

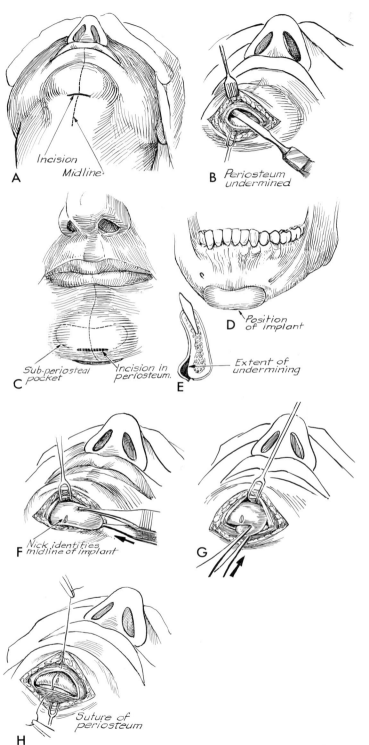

FIGURE 37–27. Technique of chin augmentation by means of an inorganic implant placed in a subperiosteal pocket through an external incision. *A*, The mid-sagittal line of the face is drawn over the chin and upper cervical area. An outline of the incision is made along the inferior border of the mental symphysis. *B*, After the incision is made through the skin and subcutaneous tissue, a shorter incision is made through the periosteum. The periosteum is raised over the symphysis, establishing a subperiosteal pocket large enough only to accommodate the inorganic implant (Silastic). *C*, The respective positions of the cutaneous incision and the incision through the periosteum. *D*, Position of the inorganic implant over the lower portion of the mental symphysis, an area of hard bone resistant to absorption. *E*, Sagittal section illustrating the extent of the undermining of the periosteum. *F*, The Silastic implant is introduced into the subperiosteal pocket. *G*, The implant is folded upon itself in order to introduce it under the periosteum on the contralateral side. *H*, The edges of the periosteum are approximated over the implant. The wound is then closed in two layers. No external pressure is necessary to prevent hematoma formation.

This technique is particularly useful in the microgenic patient who is undergoing a face lift operation. The chin augmentation assists in reestablishing a mandibular-cervical angle. The chin augmentation can also be performed in conjunction with a submental lipectomy or resection of excess skin in the midline of the neck, as shown in the technique illustrated in Figure 37–26.

the limited dissection minimizes the danger of hematoma (Fig. 37–28).

THE CERVICAL AREA. The cervical deformity of the aging individual which is a result of relaxation of skin, subcutaneous tissue, and platysma may result in a "scraggy neck" in thin patients. The subjacent musculature becomes noticeable. The medial margins of the platysma muscle which are widely separated anteriorly, forming two cords, are most conspicuous.

Various procedures have been attempted, such as the suturing of the medial borders of the platysma to each other in the submental area. This technique may result in a vertical band unless wide Z-flaps are used to imbricate the flaps from one platysma muscle into the other. Another technique involves ex-

cising the medial border of the platysma (Millard, Pigott, and Hedo, 1968). If this procedure is performed in the submandibular area, a weakness of the lower lip can be produced which is erroneously interpreted as injury to the marginal mandibular division of the facial nerve. As mentioned earlier in the chapter, the reason for the weakness in the lower lip is that the platysma muscle interdigitates with the muscles of the commissure of the mouth and also with the subcutaneous tissue and dermis (Conley, 1976).

Various techniques have been developed to improve the mandibular-cervical angle. Guerrero-Santos, Espaillat, and Morales (1974) have employed flaps of plastysma muscle which are retracted, overlapped, and sutured

FIGURE 37–28. Combined face lift operation, submental lipectomy, and chin augmentation. *A*, Preoperative appearance. Note the microgenia which is more evident in *C*. *B*, Postoperative appearance. *C*, Preoperative profile. The microgenia and the absence of the mandibulocervical angle are evident. *D*, Postoperative profile.

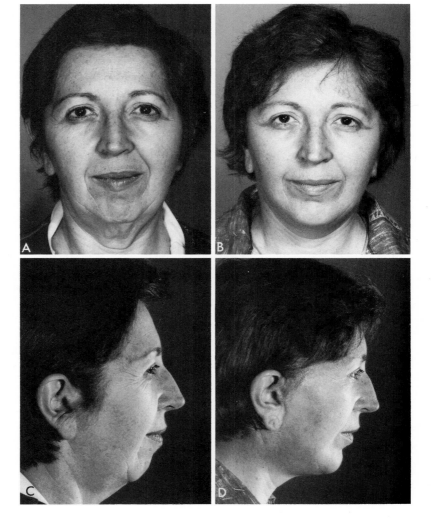

to the more posterior portion of the platysma muscle.

Another technique used to eliminate the prominent medial borders of the platysma involves excision followed by a low horizontal incision through the platysma, the incision extending from the remaining anterior border of the platysma horizontally to the posterior border. After subplatysma dissection, the muscle is retracted superiorly and posteriorly.

Peterson (1977), in order to obtain a better definition of the mandibular-cervical angle, has described the following technique: an incision is made through the parotid-masseteric fascia from the earlobe downward, and the incision is extended along the anterior border of the sternomastoid muscle. The greater auricular nerve is posterior to this line of incision and is not endangered. When the posterior border of the platysma is encountered, blunt dissection frees the undersurface of the muscle, and injury to the external jugular vein is avoided. The

platysma is then divided low in the neck through a horizontal incision approximately 5 cm below the inferior border of the mandible (Fig. 37–29, *A*). The parotid-masseteric fascia and platysma are mobilized and sutured in a posterior and superior direction. The incision extends to a point 2 to 3 cm from the anterior border of the muscle. The upper portion of the platysma is then sutured over the sternomastoid muscle resulting in a tightening of the lower portion of the cervical area. Peterson combines this technique with a submandibular resection of adipose tissue removed from the surface of the platysma (Fig. 37–29, *B*). Care must be exercised to avoid perforating the platysma under the mandibular angle to avoid injury to the marginal mandibular branch of the facial nerve.

Peterson combines the operation for mandibulocervical angle definition with imbrication of the medial borders of the platysma in association with a lipectomy (Fig. 37–29, *C*). The incision for the lipectomy is not placed immedi-

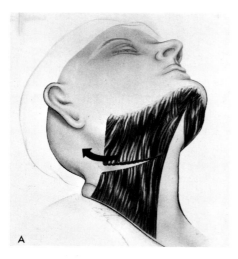

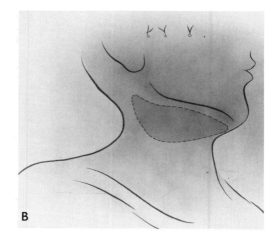

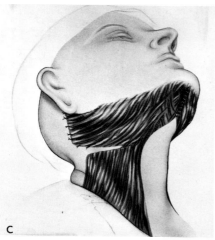

FIGURE 37–29. Peterson's technique for a definition of the mandibulocervical angle. *A,* The platysma has been divided with scissors parallel to and approximately 5 cm below the inferior border of the mandible. The anterior border of the platysma is not divided. *B,* The shaded region indicates the area of excision of fat over the superficial surface of the platysma. *C,* The platysma flap is reflected in a posterosuperior direction and sutured.

ately below the chin but rather over the area of maximum convexity of the adipose tissue, which is usually located above the level of the hyoid cartilage. A narrow elliptical skin excision is made; the widest portion of the elliptical excision is one-tenth its width (i.e., 4 mm wide, 4 cm long). The lipectomy is performed, and the platysma borders are imbricated.

The reader is reminded that a face lift operation is palliative and not definitive; it must usually be repeated after a varying period of time. At the time of this writing, it is not possible to predict whether platysma flaps will complicate the performance of a secondary operation.

JOWLS. These objectionable protrusions situated anterior to the masseter muscle along the mandible are caused by the accumulation of redundant skin and fat. Careful dissection in the immediate subcutaneous plane over the upward extension of the platysma muscle into the face and removal of fat will correct the deformity after the skin of the area has been rotated in a superoposterior direction.

DEEP FOREHEAD WRINKLES. In a patient with overactive frontalis muscles, deep furrows form as transverse folds, which are conspicuous even when the frontalis muscles are not active. When the frontalis muscles are contracted, the furrows become deeper.

The obliteration of such deep furrows by liquid silicone injections requires long-term serial injections of small volume, and the quantity of fluid required may be considerable.

A surgical approach can be employed; exposure is obtained by means of a scalp flap situated 5 cm behind the hairline in female patients. Between the pericranium and the galea aponeurotica above, and the frontalis muscles below, the scalp flap is raised to a point immediately above the supraorbital rims, thus preserving the sensory innervation of the flap. Careful symmetrical excision of strips of frontalis muscle diminishes the activity of the forehead and thus the conspicuous deep wrinkles (Skoog, 1974). The patient should be warned, however, that she may experience paresthesias and temporary loss of sensation posterior to the scalp incision.

A smooth forehead can be obtained by bilateral section of the frontalis branch of the facial nerve. Because the frontalis muscle elevates the brows, a progressive downward depression of the brows occurs. Secondary procedures are required to raise the forehead by excising scalp tissue.

GLABELLAR FROWN LINES. Frown lines are produced by the habitual contraction of the two corrugator supercilii muscles which draw the eyebrows medially, producing vertical wrinkles in the glabellar area (see Fig. 37-3). Pierce, Klabunde, and Bergeron (1947) described a technique which involved approaching the corrugator muscles through short superciliary incisions. The corrugator muscle arises from the medial end of the supraorbital arch, and its fibers pass upward and laterally between the fibers of the orbicularis oculi muscle and are inserted into the deep surface of the skin above the midportion of the orbital arch. The point of origin of the muscle near the medial end of the supraorbital arch is raised using a periosteal elevator. A portion of the root and belly of the muscle is resected. Castañares (1964) has advocated sectioning the procerus muscle transversely between two hemostats slightly above the nasofrontal angle. The procerus muscle is a small pyramidal muscular slip arising by tendinous fibers from the fascia covering the lower portion of the nasal bone and the upper part of the lateral cartilage; it is inserted into the skin over the lower portion of the forehead between the two eyebrows, its fibers decussating with those of the frontalis muscle.

Castañares (1964) has excised deep linear frown lines with satisfactory results. Borges (1973) has also excised a deep frown line and closed the wound by the W-plasty technique. Dermabrasion performed two months after healing of the resulting scar will usually render it relatively inconspicuous.

Chemical peel or deep dermabrasion is effective for the eradication of relatively superficial frown lines. Because of the thickness of the skin in the glabellar area, a deep chemical peel or dermabrasion generally heals satisfactorily after a period during which the skin is pink or even red in color.

THE DROOPING EYEBROW AND LATERAL CANTHUS. Ptosis of the eyebrows occurs in certain individuals and affects mostly the lateral portion of the eyebrow. The deformity is often accompanied by an antimongoloid slant of the lateral canthus. The cause of this type of deformity remains undetermined. It has been noted, however, that the supraorbital rim shows a downward curve in patients with this type of deformity. Various types of excisions have been proposed to raise the eyebrow. Unless they are carefully executed, objectionable scars may persist except in the older patient. Excision of skin above the eyebrow has been advocated by pinching the skin over the lateral portion of the eyebrow and estimating the amount of skin excision to be performed. Castañares (1964) has described various designs of the area to be excised. Tipton (1974) has obtained satisfactory results in older patients by excising an elliptical area of skin from the midportion of the forehead, thus raising the lateral portion of the brow. Dermabrasion at a later date results in an inconspicuous scar.

In the older patient the appearance of a drooping lateral canthus and lateral portion of the upper eyelid is caused by the pendulous fat overlying the levator aponeurosis (see Fig. 37–16). Operative procedures to restore the supratarsal fold should include excision of the fat collection lying superficial to the levator aponeurosis (see Fig. 37–16).

TRANSVERSE FOLDS AND REDUNDANT TISSUE AT THE NASOFRONTAL ANGLE. Horizontal folds develop at the nasofrontal angle at a right angle to the direction of the procerus muscle. In older patients deep folds and redundant skin are objectionable and may be successfully removed by an appropriately designed transverse excision.

Postoperative Complications of the Face Lift Operation

The face lift operation is a palliative procedure which does not ensure a permanent result; complications should be reduced to a minimum.

Minor Complications. Small hematomas are usually absorbed spontaneously. Although troublesome, they usually leave no sequelae. Areas of ecchymoses are frequent but usually resolve spontaneously. A residual brown pigmentation at the site of the ecchymosis may occasionally persist (McGregor and Greenberg, 1971). Scars may widen, especially in the temporal area hairline when the wound edges are sutured under tension. Hypertrophic scars are unusual, since the cervical hairline incision has been abandoned. In the predisposed individual, a hypertrophic scar or a typical keloid may form at the junction of the earlobe and the cheek; it is treated early with intralesional injections of triamcinolone acetonide. Infection is unusual, most infections being of the stitch abscess type. Persistent edema is also unusual and presumably is related to lymphatic stasis. Earlobe deformity occurs if the skin flap is not trimmed so that an exact fit is obtained without tension. The most common type of deformity is the excessive adherence of the lobe to the skin of the cheek (pixie ear).

Major Complications

HEMATOMA. The discussion which follows applies only to face lift operations done by the supraplatysma technique, as figures of the incidence of hematomas following the subplatysma technique are not yet available. Hematoma is by far the most frequent major complication following a face lift operation. They vary from small, discrete, undetected collections, which are discovered only after the edema has begun to subside, to massive expanding hematomas involving both sides of the face. Hematomas which demand immediate attention generally occur within the first 24 hours following the operation but can also develop later.

Usually the first sign of any significant collection of blood is pain. Since there is minimal pain following an uncomplicated face lift operation, this complaint should not be ignored. The edema associated with a hematoma is generally obvious and can be seen by simply examining the patient's face without removing the bandage. Usually there will be associated ecchymosis and often a trickle of blood seeping below the pressure dressing. A swollen ecchymotic eye or swollen lips should not be ignored any more than a complaint of pain. If there is *any* doubt, the dressing should be removed and the face examined.

A hematoma large enough to cause pain, swelling, and ecchymosis should be evacuated as an emergency procedure, as a massive collection may cause so much tension as to endanger the viability of the flap. The diminished blood supply and venous engorgement cause cyanosis of the flap and even vesiculation of the skin. Necrosis of a major portion of the distal end of the undermined cervicofacial flap may be the consequence of delay in evacuating a large expanding hematoma. The sutures should be removed and the clots evacuated immediately rather than waiting for the preparation of the operating room. The patient should be returned to the operating room, the remainder of the hematoma should be evacuated, and the bleeding should be arrested under general anesthesia.

The "silent" small hematoma can be treated later. The clots generally liquefy about the ninth to twelfth day. The liquefaction is accelerated by injections of streptokinase-streptodornase (Sk-Sd) or hyaluronidase.

According to Conway (1970), approximately half of all major face lift complications are hematomas. The incidence of large hematomas reported in the literature varies, as shown in Table 37–1.

TABLE 37-1. *Hematoma After Face Lift Operation*

AUTHOR AND YEAR	NUMBER OF PATIENTS	NUMBER OF HEMATOMAS	%
Serson Neto (1964)	170	2	1.2
Baker and Gordon (1967)	300	1	0.3
Conway (1970)	325	21	6.5
McGregor and Greenberg (1971)	524	42	8.0
McDowell (1972)	105	3	2.9
Stark (1972)	100	3	3.0
Webster (1972)	221	2	0.9
Gleason (1973)	102	1	1.0
Morgan (1973)	40	1	2.5
Pitanguy and associates (1973)	52	4	7.7
Rees, Lee and Coburn (1973)	806	23	2.9
Barker (1974)	151	2	1.3
Black (1976)	1804		2.5

Conway (1970) failed to note a significant difference in the incidence of postoperative hematomas when the operation was performed under general anesthesia compared to local anesthesia. Rees, Lee, and Coburn (1973) studied 23 expanding hematomas and noted that 20 occurred in patients who had received general anesthesia, 12 of whom had been operated upon under the hypotensive technique. They were unable to identify the hematoma-prone patient preoperatively and implicated coughing and vomiting in the etiology of hematoma. To this list may be added a compilation by Black (1976) of the incidence of hematomas in 1804 patients operated upon between 1968 and 1974 at the Manhattan Eye, Ear and Throat Hospital by the staff and the residents of the Institute of Reconstructive Plastic Surgery; the incidence of hematoma formation was 2.5 per cent.

Webster (1972) attributed a hemostatic effect to Valium (diazepam) when it was used as an adjunct to local anesthesia. He stated that Musgrave, using a similar technique, has limited the blood loss to an average of 50 ml. Roth, Saunders, Stark and DeHaan (1963) found the average blood loss using hypotensive anesthesia to be 393 ml, and that under routine general anesthesia to be 609 ml. Stark (1972), in a later followup, reported an average blood loss of 288 ml under hypotensive anesthesia.

Baker and Gordon (1967) advocated proceeding with dissection of the second side prior to closing the first side in order to verify the status of the hemostasis. Baker (1974) inspected each side 30 minutes after dissection and found more than "minimal or no bleeding" in only 11 of 60 facial halves. The question of whether drains affect the incidence of hematoma is unresolved.

Pitanguy, Pinto, Garcia and Lessa (1973) stated that the male face is more vascular than that of the female and reported four large and two small hematomas in 52 patients.

Wide undermining of the skin flaps makes hematoma formation more likely because of the greater surface area exposed and the more difficult task of finding all the bleeding vessels and ensuring hemostasis. In spite of extreme care during the operative procedure, some bleeding may unavoidably occur postoperatively. The best treatment is prevention by careful and complete hemostasis.

Dissection under direct vision with the aid of good illumination and a fiberoptic illuminated retractor provides a better opportunity of thorough hemostasis as the bleeding vessels are seen as the dissection proceeds, and hemostasis is provided immediately. The danger of delaying hemostasis is that the vessel may contract and stop bleeding momentarily only to bleed secondarily. The operator, therefore, does not have an opportunity to provide the hemostasis that he has when it is done immediately upon section of the tissues.

If the hematoma is in the preauricular area, it may be possible to roll it out with a gauze sponge into an area most favorable for its evacuation. Frequent observation and pressure dressing changes are necessary to prevent further bleeding and to ensure adequate healing.

Hematoma usually occurs unilaterally; bilateral hematoma is unusual. When it does occur, it is usually massive, and blood transfusion may be required.

Hematomas following a face lift operation have been attributed to inadequate hemostasis, inability to see the bleeding vessel because of hypotensive anesthesia or because of the vasoconstriction produced by the lidocaine-epinephrine solution, excessive absorption of aspirin, and fibrinolysis.

Aspirin and Platelet Function. From an inert particle that was once thought to be an artifact, the platelet has emerged as a dynamic and remarkable structure. Platelets are derived from megakaryocytes as detached portions of the cytoplasm, as originally hypothesized by Wright in 1906. The platelet is a complete hemostatic unit ("thrombocyte") and has several important functions in hemostasis: (a) continual maintenance of vascular integrity, (b) initial arrest of bleeding by platelet plug formation, and (c) stabilization of the plug by contributing phospholipid to the process of fibrin formation. Red blood cells will migrate through the vessel walls in large numbers and appear in the lymphatics or soft tissue as petechiae or purpura if the platelets are absent from the circulation. After vascular injury platelets adhere immediately to exposed subendothelial connective tissue structures, including collagen fibers and basement membrane. The adherence mechanism is as yet undefined, but it is inhibited by aspirin. The platelets then loosely aggregate, owing to platelet release of ADP (adenosine diphosphate), which promotes a change from the normal disc configuration to a spiny shape, thereby facilitating interaction. Concomitantly, platelets release vasoactive substances (epinephrine, serotonin, etc.), enhancing both vasoconstriction and further platelet aggregation. Platelet aggregation is a process distinct from adherence to collagen, although initiated by it.

Patients should consequently be advised to abstain from taking aspirin for a period of two weeks prior to the operation.

Fibrinolysis. An unusual cause of postoperative hematoma is increased fibrinolysis. Fibrinolysis is the body's major physiologic means of disposing of fibrin after its hemostatic function has been fulfilled (Wintrobe and associates, 1974). Fibrinolysis is the normal process of blood clot dissolution, and it results from the conversion of an inert plasma proenzyme, plasminogen, into the proteolytic enzyme, plasmin. Plasminogen is transformed into plasmin by a variety of activators which are present in many tissues (tissue activator), in the circulating blood (blood activator), in urine (urokinase), and in other body fluids. According to Astrup and Thorsen (1972), there exists in living organisms a dynamic equilibrium or hemostatic balance between fibrin formation and resolution.

Increased fibrinolysis has been associated with anxiety, exercise, and injection of epinephrine (Macfarlane and Biggs, 1946; Biggs and MacFarlane, 1947). However, such fluctuations are minor and are not known to be associated with any clinically detectable deleterious effects (Kwaan, 1972). Blood fibrinolytic activity also shows a diurinal variation, the activity being low during the night and increased during the day (Rosing and associates, 1970). Healthy individuals appear to have minor variations in the blood fibrinolytic activity without harmful consequences (Kwaan, 1972). Gross changes are encoun-

tered in a wide variety of clinical disorders, however, and these may cause excessive bleeding and even contribute to the formation of thromboembolism.

The majority of patients with acquired hypofibrinogenemia suffer from "disseminated intravascular clotting," or "consumptive coagulopathy." This is now a frequently recognized syndrome, especially in association with gynecologic disorders, e.g., retained dead fetus, amniotic fluid embolism, premature separation of the placenta. Spontaneous primary fibrinolysis is a rare disorder, but it may occur in patients without evidence of underlying disease and give rise to serious bleeding (Williams and associates, 1972). Primary fibrinolysis may also occur in patients with metastatic prostatic carcinoma, shock, sepsis, cirrhosis, and portal hypertension (Wintrobe and associates, 1974).

It is clinically important to differentiate between disseminated intravascular clotting and primary fibrinolysis, since specific treatment depends on the correct diagnosis, and improper treatment can be disastrous. At present, there is no definitive diagnostic test for distinguishing between these two entities. Disseminated intravascular clotting is relatively common, whereas primary fibrinolysis is a rare disorder (Williams and coworkers, 1972).

There is no single test or combination of tests sufficiently specific to provide a definitive diagnosis, but the tests, together with the patient's clinical picture, can indicate what the problem is and how it should be treated (Colick and Fisher, 1970).

Labile Hypertension. Berner, Morain, and Noe (1976) emphasized that anxiety and emotional stress are associated with labile hypertension, and that most postoperative hematomas occur in patients with unusually high blood pressure in the postoperative period. They were able to eliminate large, expanding hematomas by careful monitoring of blood pressure postoperatively and by controlling blood pressure elevation with chlorpromazine. Hypertensive patients under medication, in particular, should be carefully monitored in the postoperative period.

HAIR LOSS. Hair loss in the temporal area is not an infrequent complication when attention to technique is not observed. There are two technical causes of alopecia in the temporal area. The first is the superficial undermining of the scalp which injures the hair follicles and causes loss of hair. The second is closure of the wound under excessive tension with resulting ischemia in the area, loss of hair, and widening of the scar. This complication can be avoided by careful planning of the operation. The hairless areas, unless massive in size, can usually be excised a few months later. Wider areas of alopecia require hair replacement by a transposed or rotated scalp flap (see Chapter 6).

SKIN SLOUGH. Though not the most frequent complication, skin slough is probably one of the most serious. Fortunately sloughs are generally minor and occur infrequently in the postauricular area. All sloughs result from a diminished blood supply to the flap. The diminution of blood supply can be caused by (1) tension, (2) pressure, (3) underlying hematoma, (4) or too superficial dissection of the flap. All sloughs should be treated conservatively. Minor sloughs heal with amazingly minimal scarring; objectionable scars require secondary repair. Sloughing of the posterosuperior portion of the cervicofacial flap has become an unusual complication since the incision along the hairline has been abandoned. The previous technique produced an angle with a restricted blood supply which thus made the flap more susceptible to varying degrees of ischemia. When the type of incision illustrated in Figure 37–19 is employed, skin loss, either superficial or full-thickness, is exceptional. If the skin flap is raised at too superficial a level, instead of on a plane superficial to the fascia covering the sternomastoid muscle, and if tension is caused by excessive resection of skin, superficial or deep sloughing may result. The ischemia manifests itself in superficial desquamation of skin and blistering, similar to what is observed in a superficial burn. Reepithelization usually occurs but may leave in its wake superficial scarring or pigmented skin of a coarser appearance.

Full-thickness loss of skin is usually limited and heals by second intention; the healing leaves in its wake varying degrees of scarring. The main cause of extensive necrosis of skin is a large hematoma which has been left untreated for a considerable amount of time. After the cervicofacial flap has been widely undermined, revascularization of the skin also takes place rapidly through vessels growing from the underlying structures into the flap. The dermal and subdermal vessels cannot provide a sufficient vascular supply if the flap has been placed under tension by a large hematoma which separates the flap from the underlying tissues.

SUBMENTAL DEPRESSION. In the description of the technique illustrated in Figure 37–26, emphasis was placed upon avoiding the resection of an excessive amount of fat in performing submental lipectomy. The most accentuated depression occurs when so much fat has been removed that the skin adheres to the deep tissues. Attempts have been made by Wilkinson (1976) to correct this secondary deformity by plication of the digastric muscles to add bulk to the area and by improvement of the contour by means of a superiorly based dermis-fat flap.

NERVE LOSS. Facial paralysis is a serious complication following such a palliative operation as a face lift operation. Facial paralysis is fortunately extremely rare following a face lift operation, but when it occurs, it is probably the most serious complication of the operation. Total facial paralysis is extremely rare, but paralysis of a single branch of the nerve is occasionally observed. Most weakness or paralysis which occurs is transient and results from trauma to the nerve from dissection or cautery without actual severance of a branch. The local anesthetic solution can cause an alarming temporary paralysis which disappears in a few hours.

If the paralysis is transient and is due to trauma other than severance of the nerve, conduction will generally recover in a few weeks. As in most areas, prevention of nerve injury is ensured by dissecting along the proper plane.

McGregor and Greenberg (1971) reported a 2.6 per cent incidence of facial nerve injuries in their series of face lifts. This incidence appears to be high in comparison to the near absence of facial nerve injuries in the authors' series of cases. Castañares (1974) has reported the incidence of facial nerve involvement in his own series of cases. As expected, the three portions of the facial nerve which are the most exposed were the most frequently injured: the frontal branch, the buccal branches, and the mandibular branch. He stated that in all of the patients thus affected complete recovery occurred after a period varying from a few days to five months.

Castañares (1974) drew attention to the danger of performing a face lift operation in a patient who has had Bell's palsy. He cited the case of a patient who had recovered from Bell's plasy and developed a second Bell's palsy a few weeks after a successful face lift operation. The patient responded well to treatment with steroids and a stellate ganglion block.

One of the vulnerable branches of the facial nerve is the branch to the frontalis muscle; the plane of dissection should be immediately subcutaneous in order to avoid injury to this nerve when dissection is being made under the skin toward the lateral aspect of the orbit. The result of the unilateral paralysis of the frontalis muscle is an asymmetry of the forehead, the frontalis muscle on the unaffected side producing the usual transverse folds, which contrast with the smooth surface of the paralyzed side of the forehead. If recovery does not occur spontaneously, the only method of treatment presently available is section of the nerve to the frontalis muscle on the unaffected side. The entire forehead then becomes smooth. As stated earlier in the chapter, however, over a period of time a progressive drooping of the eyebrows occurs, and periodic lifting of the forehead is required through a bifrontal scalp incision.

Because of the multiple connections between the facial nerve branches which innervate the orbicularis oculi muscle, paralysis of the orbicularis oculi muscle is exceptional. The authors have observed one patient in whom the orbicularis muscle was paralyzed; nerve function recovered over a period of one year.

The buccal branches as they exit from the anterior border of the parotid gland lie over the buccinator muscle, and careful dissection in the subcutaneous plane should be observed. Because of the numerous connections between the buccal nerve branches and the branches of the fifth cranial nerve, gradual spontaneous regeneration is frequent. It is important to recall that, although nerve regeneration usually takes place without any sequelae, there is always the danger of twitching following the restoration of nerve conduction. This phenomenon is frequent following the repair of lacerations of the face ("the twitching scar") (Converse and Coburn, 1971).

The mandibular branch is another part of the facial nerve which is vulnerable. When the plane of dissection remains superficial to the platysma, however, there is little danger of injury. In contradistinction to the supraplatysmal plane of dissection, the subplatysmal dissection may proceed by blunt dissection along the anatomical cleavage plane, the surgeon staying below the mandible to protect the marginal mandibular branch.

Castañares (1974) studied various causes of paresis due to interference with the conduction of the facial nerve branches. Among these he listed excessive traction and undue stretching of the deeper tissue and pinching with forceps, particularly in the course of electrocoagulation. Electrocoagulation can be dangerous if the current is too strong and the depth of coagulation is deeper than expected. It is always wise to verify the potency of the electrocoagulation prior to using the instrument. The bleeding soft tissues should be elevated with fine jeweler's forceps, and the bleeding vessel should be coagulated to avoid possible injury to an underlying nerve. Castañares also emphasized the possible distortion of the anatomy which occurs when one or more face lifts have been previously performed and there may be extensive subcutaneous fibrosis.

INJURY TO OTHER NERVES. In the section on anatomy, the various sensory nerves exposed to injury were described. The most vulnerable is the greater auricular nerve. Injury to the greater auricular nerve, which lies under the fascia of the sternocleidomastoid muscle, may result in temporary loss of sensation of a portion of the ears, scalp, and face. During this period the patient should be advised against the wearing of compressive earrings, since trophic ulcers can develop as a result of unnoticed excessive pressure.

CHRONIC PAIN. Significant postoperative pain is unusual, and Conway (1969) estimated the incidence of prolonged pain as 2.5 per cent. The pain is usually associated with numbness and tingling and may be due to surgical injury to one or more of the cervical cutaneous nerves. Rees (1975b) has observed pain in only two patients for a period longer than three months after the operation. Converse (1975) described the case of one patient who had undergone an uneventful face lift operation and who complained of paresthesias ("crawling sensations") and pain in the cervical area for a period of six months. Guerrero-Santos, Espaillat and Morales (1974) stated that severe neck pain can occur if the platysma is plicated in association with a rhytidectomy; prompt relief follows the use of muscle relaxants.

SALIVARY CYSTS. Salivary cysts occur rarely (Serson Neto, 1964) and usually respond to aspiration and light pressure dressings.

REFERENCES

Adamson, J. E., Horton, C. E., and Crawford, H. H.: The surgical correction of the "turkey gobbler" deformity. Plast. Reconstr. Surg., *34*:598, 1964.

Alexander, J. E.: Complications of cosmetic blepharoplasty. *In* Masters, F. W., and Lewis, J. R., Jr. (Eds.): Symposium on Esthetic Surgery of the Face, Eyelids and Breast. St. Louis, Mo., C. V. Mosby Company, 1972.

Andrew, W.: Aging of the skin and related structures. *In*

Bourne, G. H. (Ed.): Structural Aspects of Aging. London, Pitman Medical Publishing Company, 1962.

Astrup, T., and Thorsen, S.: The Physiology of Fibrinolysis. Med. Clin. North Am., 56:153, 1972.

Baker, H., and Blair, C. P.: Cell replacement in the human stratum corneum in old age. Br. J. Dermatol., 80:357, 1968.

Baker, T. J.: Prevention of bleeding following a rhytidectomy. Plast. Reconstr. Surg., 54:651, 1974.

Baker, T. J., and Gordon, H. L.: Complications of rhytidectomy. Plast. Reconstr. Surg., 40:31, 1967.

Baker, T. J., and Gordon, H. L.: Rhytidectomy in males. Plast. Reconstr. Surg., 44:219, 1969.

Beare, R.: Surgical treatment of senile changes in the eyelids: the McIndoe-Beare technique. *In* Converse, J. M., and Smith, B. (Eds.): Proceedings of the 2nd International Symposium on Plastic and Reconstructive Surgery of the Eye and Adnexae. St. Louis, Mo., C. V. Mosby Company, 1967.

Beare, R.: Personal communication, 1975.

Beighton, P., and Bull, J. C.: Plastic surgery in the Ehlers-Danlos syndrome. Plast. Reconstr. Surg., 45:606, 1970.

Berner, R. E., Morain, W. D., and Noe, J. M.: Postoperative hypertension as an etiology factor in hematoma after rhytidectomy. Plast. Reconst. Surg., 57:314, 1976.

Bettman, A. G.: Plastic and cosmetic surgery of the face. Northwest. Med., 19:205, 1920.

Beyer, C. K., Smith, B., and Buerger, G. F.: Ophthalmological aspects of blepharoplasty. Eye, Ear, Nose and Throat Monthly, 49:65, 1970.

Biggs, R., and MacFarlane, R. G.: Observations on fibrinolysis, experimental activity produced by exercise or adrenaline. Lancet, 1:402, 1947.

Black, M. J. M.: Personal communication, 1976.

Borges, A. F.: Elective Incisions and Scar Revision. Boston, Little, Brown and Company, 1973.

Bouissou, H., Pieraggi, M. T., Julian, M., and Blazy, L. D.: Cutaneous aging. *In* Frontiers of Matrix Biology. Vol. 1. Aging of Connective Tissue—Skin. Basel, S. Karger, 1973.

Bourguet, J.: V. Les hernies graisseuses de l'orbite. Notre traitement chirurgical. Bull. Acad. Méd. (Paris), 92:1270, 1924.

Cannon, B., and Pantazelos, H. H.: W-plasty approach to submandibular lipectomy. *In* Transactions of the Fifth International Congress of Plastic and Reconstructive Surgery. Australia, Butterworths, 1971, p. 1113.

Castañares, S.: Blepharoplasty for herniated intraorbital fat: Anatomical basis for a new approach. Plast. Reconstr. Surg., 8:46, 1951.

Castañares, S.: Forehead wrinkles, glabellar frown, and ptosis of the eyebrows. Plast. Reconstr. Surg., 34:406, 1964.

Castañares, S.: Facial nerve paralysis coincident with, or subsequent to, rhytidectomy. Plast. Reconst. Surg., 54:637, 1974.

Castanares, S.: Personal communication, 1975.

Castañares, S.: Personal communication, 1976.

Cauna, N.: The effects of aging on the receptor organs of the human dermis. *In* Montagna, W. (Ed.): Advances in Biology of Skin. Vol. 6. Aging. Oxford, Pergamon Press, 1965.

Cies, W. A., and Baylis, H. I.: Surgical revision of upper eyelid fold. Am. J. Ophthalmol., 80:1019, 1975.

Colick, J. A., and Fisher, L. M.: A review of the basic mechanisms of fibrinogen to fibrin conversion and of fibrinolysis: Intravascular coagulation versus primary fibrinolysis. Virginia Med. Monthly, 97:310, 1970.

Conley, J.: Face-lift Operation. Springfield, Ill., Charles C Thomas, Publisher, 1968.

Conley, J.: Personal communication, 1976.

Converse, J. M.: Clinical note: Treatment of epithelized suture tracts of the eyelid by marsupialization. Plast. Reconstr. Surg., 38:576, 1966.

Converse, J. M.: Personal communication, 1975.

Converse, J. M., and Coburn, R. J.: The twitching scar. Br. J. Plast. Surg., 24:272, 1971.

Converse, J. M., and Rogers, B. O.: Unpublished technique, 1976.

Conway, H.: Factors underlying prolonged pain following rhytidectomy. Transactions of the Fourth International Congress of Plastic and Reconstructive Surgery. Amsterdam, Excerpta Medica Foundation, 1969, p. 1120.

Conway, H.: The surgical face-lift rhytidectomy. Plast. Reconstr. Surg., 45:124, 1970.

Cronin, T. D.: Marginal incision for upper blepharoplasty. Plast. Reconstr. Surg., 48:14, 1972.

Cronin, T. D., and Biggs, T. M.: The T-Z plasty for the male "turkey gobbler" neck. Plast. Reconstr. Surg., 47:534, 1971.

DeMere, M., Wood, T., and Austin, W.: Eye complications with blepharoplasty or other eyelid surgery. Plast. Reconstr. Surg., 53:634, 1974.

Dingman, R. O., Grabb, W. C., and Oneal, R. M.: Cutis laxa congenita—generalized elastosis. Plast. Reconstr. Surg., 44:431, 1969.

Duke-Elder, S.: Systems of Ophthalmology. St. Louis, Mo., C. V. Mosby Company, 1972.

Dupuis, C., and Rees, T. D.: Historical notes on blepharoplasty. Plast. Reconstr. Surg., 47:246, 1971.

Dupuytren, G.: De e'oedème chronique et des tumeurs enkystées des paupières. Leçons Orales de Clinique Chirurgicale. Vol. 3. 2nd Ed. Paris, Germer-Baillère, 1839.

Edgerton, M. T.: Causes and prevention of lower lid ectropion following blepharoplasty. Plast. Reconstr. Surg., 49:367, 1972.

Ellis, R. A., Montagna, W., and Fanger, H.: Histology and cytochemistry of human skin. XIV. The blood supply of the cutaneous glands. J. Invest. Dermatol., 30:137, 1958.

Fitzpatrick, T. B., Szabo, G., and Mitchell, R. E.: Age Changes in the Human Melanocyte System. *In* Montagna, W. (Eds.): Advances in Biology of Skin. Vol. 6. Aging. Oxford, Pergamon Press, 1965.

Fleischmajer, R., and Nedwich, A.: Werner's syndrome. Am. J. Med., 54:111, 1973.

Fleischmajer, R., Perlish, J. S., and Bashey, R. I.: Aging of Human Dermis. *In* Frontiers of Matrix Biology. Vol. 1. Aging of Connective Tissue-Skin. Basel, S. Karger, 1973.

Flowers, R. S.: Anchor blepharoplasty. Personal communication, 1975.

Fox, S. A.: Ophthalmic Plastic Surgery. Grune & Stratton, New York, 1952.

Freeman, R. G.: Effects of aging on the skin. *In* Helwig, E. B., and Mostofi, F. K. (Eds.): The Skin. Baltimore, The Williams & Wilkins Company, 1971.

Frühwald, V.: Über einen Fall von Hängewange behoben durch eine Modifikation der Joseph'schen Operation. Wien. Med. Wochenschr., 32:1336, 1922.

Fuchs, E.: Ueber Blepharochalasis (Erschlaffung der Lidhaut) Wien Kein. Wochenschr., 9:109, 1896.

Furnas, D. W.: Landmarks for the trunk and the temporofacial division of the facial nerve. Br. J. Surg., 52:694, 1965.

Gerstein, W., and Freeman, R. G.: Transplantation of actinically damaged skin. J. Invest. Dermatol., 41:445, 1963.

Gersuny, R.: Ueber eine subcutane Prosthese. Ztscher. f. Heilk., 1:199, 1900.

Gleason, M. C.: Browlifting through a temporal scalp approach. Plast. Reconstr. Surg., *52*:141, 1973.

Goltz, R. W., Hult, A., Goldfarb, M., and Gorlin, R. J.: Cutis laxa—a manifestation of generalized elastolysis. Arch. Dermatol., *92*:373, 1965.

Gonzalez-Ulloa, M., and Flores, E. S.: Senility of the face—Basic study to understand its causes and effects. Plast. Reconstr. Surg., *36*:239, 1965.

Gonzalez-Ulloa M., Simonin, F., and Flores, E.: The anatomy of the ageing face. *In* Transactions of the Fifth International Congress of Plastic and Reconstructive Surgery. Australia, Butterworths, 1971, p. 1059.

Graham, W. P., III, Messner, K. H., and Miller, S. H.: Keratoconjunctivits sicca symptoms appearing after blepharoplasty. Plast. Reconstr. Surg., *57*:57, 1976.

Green, M. F., and Kadri, S. W. M.: Acute closed-angle glaucoma, a complication of blepharoplasty: Report of a case. Br. J. Plast. Surg., *27*:25, 1974.

Guerrero-Santos, J., Espaillat, L., and Morales, F.: Muscular lift in cervical rhytidoplasty. Plast. Reconstr. Surg., *54*:127, 1974.

Hamilton, J. M.: Rhytidectomy in the male. Plast. Reconstr. Surg., *53*:629, 1974.

Hartley, J. H., Lester, J. C., and Schatten, W. E.: Acute retrobulbar hemorrhage during elective blepharoplasty. Plast. Reconstr. Surg., *52*:8, 1973.

Hartman, E., Morax, P. V., and Vergez, A.: Complications visuelles graves de la chirurgie des poches palpébrales. Ann. Oculist. (Paris), *195*:142, 1962.

Holländer, E.: Plastische (kosmetische) Operation: Dritische Darstellung ihres gegenwartigen Standes. *In* Klemperer, G., and Klemper, F. (Eds.): Neue Deutsche Klinik. Berlin, Urban und Schwarzenberg, 1932.

Huber, E.: Evolution of Facial Musculature and Facial Expression. Baltimore, Johns Hopkins University Press, 1931.

Hunt, H. L.: Plastic Surgery of the Head, Face and Neck. Philadelphia, Lea & Febiger, 1926.

Johnson, J. B., and Hadley, R. C.: The Aging Face. *In* Converse, J. M. (Ed.): Reconstructive Plastic Surgery. Philadelphia, W. B. Saunders Company, 1964.

Joseph, J.: Hängewangenplastik (Melomioplastik). Dtsch. Med. Wochenschr., *47*:287, 1921.

Joseph, J.: Verbesserung meiner Hängewangenplastik (Melomioplastik). Dtsch. Med. Wochenschr., *54*:567, 1928.

Katzberg, A.: The influence of age on the rate of desquamation of human epidermis. Anat. Rec., *112*:418, 1952.

Kazanjian, V. H., and Converse, J. M.: The Face. *In* Kazanjian, V. H., and Converse, J. M.: Surgical Treatment of Facial Injuries. 3rd Ed. Baltimore, The Williams & Wilkins Company, 1974.

Kolle, F. S.: Plastic and Cosmetic Surgery. New York, Appleton, 1911.

Kwaan, H. C.: Disorders of fibrinolysis. Med. Clin. North Am., *56*:163, 1972.

LaGarde, M.: Nouvelles techniques pour le traitment des rides de la face et du cou. Paris Chir., *17*:333, 1925.

Lemoine, A. N., Jr.: Discussion of "acute retrobulbar hemorrhage during elective blepharoplasty" by Hartley, H. H., Lester, J. C., and Schatten, W. E.: Plast. Reconstr. Surg., *52*:12, 1973.

Lexer, E.: Die gesamte Wiederherstellungschirurgie. Vol. 2. Leipzig, J. A. Barth, 1931.

McDowell, A. J.: Effective practical steps to avoid complications in face-lifting. Plast. Reconstr. Surg., *50*:563, 1972.

MacFarlane, R. G., and Biggs, R.: Observations on fibrinolysis, spontaneous activity associated with surgical operations, trauma, etc. Lancet, *2*:862, 1946.

McGregor, M. W., and Greenberg, R. L.: Complications of face-lifting. *In* Transactions of the Fifth International Congress of Plastic and Reconstructive Surgery. Australia, Butterworths, 1971, p. 1091.

McIndoe, A. H.: Personal communication, 1960.

Maciera-Coelho, A.: Aging and cell division. *In* Frontiers of Matrix Biology. Vol. 1. Aging of Connective Tissue-Skin. Basel, S. Karger, 1973.

Mihan, R.: Personal communication, 1962.

Millard, D. R., Pigott, R. W., and Hedo, A.: Submandibular lipectomy. Plast. Reconstr. Surg., *41*:513, 1968.

Millard, D. R., Jr., Garst, W. P., Beck, R. L., and Thompson, I. D.: Submental and submandibular lipectomy in conjunction with a face lift, in the male or female. Plast. Reconstr. Surg., *49*:385, 1972.

Miller, C. C.: The excision of bag-like folds of skin from the region about the eyes. Med. Brief, *34*:648, 1906.

Miller, C. C., and Miller, F.: Folds, bags and wrinkles of the skin about the eyes and their eradication by simple surgical methods. Med. Brief, *35*:540, 1907.

Montagna, W.: Morphology of the aging skin: The cutaneous appendages. *In* Montagna, W. (Ed.): Advances in Biology of Skin. Vol. 6. Aging. Oxford, Pergamon Press, 1965.

Montagna, W., and Parakkal, P. K.: The Structure and Function of Skin. London, Academic Press, 1974.

Morel-Fatio, D.: Cosmetic surgery of the face. *In* Gibson, R. (Ed.): Modern Trends in Plastic Surgery. Washington, D.C., Butterworths, 1964.

Morgan, B. L.: The aftercare of rhytidectomies with the "no dressing" technique. Plast. Reconstr. Surg., *51*:576, 1973.

Moser, M. H., DiPirro, E., and McCoy, F. J.: Sudden blindness following blepharoplasty. Plast. Reconstr. Surg., *51*:364, 1973.

Nöel, A.: La Chirurgie Esthétique: Son Rôle Social. Paris, Masson et Cie, 1926.

Oberste-Lehn, H.: Effects of aging on the papillary body of the hair follicles and on the eccrine sweat glands. *In* Montagna, W. (Ed.): Advances in Biology of Skin. Vol. 6. Aging. Oxford, Pergamon Press, 1965.

Panneton, P.: Le blepharochalazis. A propos de 51 cas dans la même famille. Arch. Ophthalmol. (French), *53*:724, 1936.

Passot, R.: La chirurgie esthétique des rides du visage. Presse Med., *27*:258, 1919; Bull. Acad. Med., *82*:112, 1919.

Pearce, R. H., and Grimmer, B. J.: Age and the chemical constitution of normal human dermis. *In* Frontiers of Matrix Biology. Vol. 1. Aging of Connective Tissue-Skin. Basel, S. Karger, 1973.

Peterson, R.: Personal communication, 1976.

Pierce, G. W., Klabunde, E. H., and Bergeron, V. L.: Useful procedures in plastic surgery. Plast. Reconstr. Surg., *2*:358, 1947.

Pinto, J.: The Dermis. *In* Montagna, W., and Parakkal, P. F. (Eds.): The Structure and Function of Skin. New York, Academic Press, 1974.

Pitanguy, I., and Matta, S. R.: Detalhes úteis em blefaroplastias obtidos de 2175 casos consecutivos. Rev. Bras. Chirurg., *65*:1, 1975.

Pitanguy, I., Pinto, A. R., Garcia, L. C., and Lessa, S. F.: Rhytidoplasty in men. Rev. Bras. Cirurg., *63*:109, 1973.

Pochi, P. E., and Strauss, J. S.: The Effect of aging on the activity of the sebaceous gland in man. *In* Montagna, W. (Ed.): Advances in Biology of Skin. Vol. 6. Aging. Oxford, Pergamon Press, 1965.

Prunieras, M.: Aging of the epidermis. *In* Frontiers of Matrix Biology. Vol. 1. Aging of Connective Tissue-Skin. Basel, S. Karger, 1973.

Rasmusson, D. M., Wakim, K. G., and Winkelman, R. K.: Effect of aging on human dermis: Studies of thermal shrinkage and tension. *In* Montagna, W. (Ed.): Advances in Biology of Skin. Vol. 6. Aging. Oxford, Pergamon Press, 1965.

Rees, T. D.: Technical aids in blepharoplasty. Plast. Reconstr. Surg., *41*:497, 1968.

Rees, T. D.: Technical considerations in blepharoplasty. *In* Transactions of the Fourth International Congress of Plastic and Reconstructive Surgery. Australia, Butterworths, 1971, p. 1067.

Rees, T. D.: The "dry eye" complication after blepharoplasty. Plast. Reconstr. Surg., *56*:375, 1975a.

Rees, T. D.: Personal communication, 1975b.

Rees, T. D., and Guy, C. L.: Patient selection and techniques in blepharoplasty. Surg. Clin. North Am., *51*:353, 1971.

Rees, T. D., and Wood-Smith, D.: Cosmetic Facial Surgery. Philadelphia, W. B. Saunders Company, 1973.

Rees, T. D., Wood-Smith, D., and Converse, J. M.: The Ehlers-Danlos syndrome. Plast. Reconstr. Surg., *32*:39, 1963.

Rees, T. D., Lee, Y. C., and Coburn, R. J.: Expanding hematoma after rhytidectomy. Plast. Reconstr. Surg., *51*:149, 1973.

Rogers, B. O.: A chronologic history of cosmetic surgery. Bull. N.Y. Acad. Med., *47*:265, 1971a.

Rogers, B. O.: A brief history of cosmetic surgery. Surg. Clin. North Am., *51*:265, 1971b.

Rosing, D. R., Brakman, P., Redwood, D. R., Gotostein, R. E., Beiser, G. D., Astrup, T., and Epstein, S. E.: Blood fibrinolytis in man. Diurnal variation and the response to varying intensities of exercise. Circ. Res., *27*:171, 1970.

Roth, R. F., Saunders, D. E., Stark, R. B., and DeHaan, C. R.: Operative blood loss in common plastic surgical procedures. Plast. Reconstr. Surg., *31*:399, 1963.

Rybka, E. J., and O'Hara, E. T.: Surgical significance of the Ehlers-Danlos syndrome. Am. J. Surg., *113*:431, 1967.

Sams, W. M., and Smith, J. G.: Alterations in human dermal fibrous connective tissue with age and chronic sun damage. *In* Montagna, W. (Ed.): Advances in Biology of Skin. Vol. 6. Aging. Oxford, Pergamon Press, 1965.

Serson Neto, D.: Rhytidoplasties: Study of 170 consecutive cases. J. Int. Coll. Surg., *42*:208, 1964.

Sheen, J.: Supratarsal fixation in upper blepharoplasty. Plast. Reconstr. Surg., *54*:424, 1974.

Sichel, J.: Aphorismes pratiques sur divers points d'opthalmologie. Ann. Oculist., *12*:187, 1844.

Sichel, J.: A blépharoplastie. Bull. Mém. Soc. Chir. Paris, *1*:445, 1875.

Silver, A. F., Montagna, W., and Karacan, T.: The effect of age on human eccrine sweating. *In* Montagna, W. (Ed.): Advances in Biology of Skin. Vol. 6. Aging. Oxford, Pergamon Press, 1965.

Skoog, T.: Plastic Surgery. New Methods and Refinements. Stockholm, Almqvist & Wiksell International, and Philadelphia, W. B. Saunders Company, 1974.

Smith, J. G.: The dermal elastoses. Arch. Dermatol., *88*:382, 1963.

Snyder, G. B.: Cervico-mentoplasty with rhytidectomy. Plast. Reconstr. Surg., *54*:404, 1974.

Stark, R. B.: Deliberate hypotension for blepharoplasty and rhytidectomy. Plast. Reconstr. Surg., *49*:453, 1972.

Swartz, R. M., Schultz, R. C., and Seaton, J. R.: "Dry eye" following blepharoplasty. Plast. Reconstr. Surg., *54*:644, 1974.

Tipton, J. B.: Should the subcutaneous tissue be plicated in a face lift? Plast. Reconstr. Surg., *54*:1, 1974.

Viñas, J. C., Lyrio, H., Corujo, M., and Parcansky, J.: Surgical treatment of double chin. Plast. Reconstr. Surg., *50*:119, 1972.

Webster, G. V.: The ischemic face-lift. Plast. Reconstr. Surg., *50*:560, 1972.

Weisman, P. A.: Simplified technique in submental lipectomy. Plast. Reconstr. Surg., *48*:443, 1971.

Wilkinson, T. S.: The repair of a submental depression occurring after rhytidectomy. Plast. Reconstr. Surg., *57*:33, 1976.

Williams, W. J., Beatler, E., Erslev, A. J., and Runoles, R. W.: Hematology. New York, McGraw-Hill, 1972.

Wintrobe, M. M., Lee, G. R., Boggs, D. R., Bitheu, T. C., Athens, J. W., and Foerster, J.: Clinical Hematology. 7th Ed. Philadelphia, Lea & Febiger, 1974.

INDEX